THE
MEDICAL
WORD
BOOK

A spelling and vocabulary guide to medical transcription

SHEILA B. SLOANE

President, Medi-Phone, Incorporated

1973

W. B. Saunders Company • Philadelphia • London • Toronto

W. B. Saunders Company: West Washington Square
Philadelphia, PA   19105

12 Dyott Street
London, WC1A   1DB

833 Oxford Street
Toronto 18, Canada

The Medical Word Book   ISBN 0-7216-8364-9

Print No: 9   8   7   6   5   4   3   2   1

Dedicated
to
My Beloved Mother
In Loving and Devoted Memory

PREFACE

There was a time when hospitals and doctors' offices were small enough to handle all of their records and paper work with the aid of one or two reasonably competent clerks or secretaries. Perhaps, the doctor's wife would come into his office once or twice a week to bring his patients' records up to date. The physician, visiting his patient at the hospital, would scribble a few undecipherable notes on his chart and his duty was executed.

Advancement and progress in research, and the careful division of the highly specialized fields of medicine, have brought about the inevitable need for more space in which to care for the ill. Older hospitals have added floors and wings to their overcrowded facilities. Modern new hospitals have sprung up throughout the country. The requirements for accurate record keeping have grown proportionately. No longer are a few scribbled notes acceptable.

Accreditation boards have set up high standards for the hospital medical record department. The physician is required to dictate a series of reports on each of his patients, and the Medical Record Librarian, in the effort to see that these are transcribed accurately and within the time allotted, soon learns that the supply of competent transcribers falls far below the demand. The training of medical transcribers is a slow and tedious process and only through constant exposure to the highly technical terminology of medical science does she become familiar enough with it to produce a neat and accurate report acceptable as a permanent part of the hospital records.

It is the purpose of this book to provide a simple method of locating the sought-after term with ease and speed. No attempt has been made to make this a complete listing of medical terms. Such an undertaking would be overwhelming and cumbersome. The attempt here is to give the reader a listing of commonly used uncommon medical terms to ease the burden of searching many books for what can now be found in a single volume. In this attempt, the special needs of the transcriber have guided both the organization and arrangement of the content. Particular emphasis was given to her need for quick reference and her reliance on the spoken word.

Organization. The book is divided into nineteen sections: four arranged alphabetically by general categories of information and fourteen by specialty or organ system; a final section lists abbreviations and symbols. With the alphabetical arrangement in mind, any section can be readily located by flipping through the pages and noting the section title at the top of each page.

General Sections. The first general section comprises a series of color plates of anatomical structures. The remaining three cover broad fields. For example, in General Surgical Terms are listed specific incisions, sutures, positions, and anesthetics; in Laboratory Terminology are listed specific tests, pathogenic organisms, and a table of normal values.

Specialty Sections. Through the method of keeping each specialty section complete within itself, the time spent in seeking out a word is greatly reduced. The transcriber is also relieved of the responsibility of guessing whether a disease entity, an instrument, or the like, is listed in one particular specialty rather than another. If it applies to several specialties, it will be listed in each of the appropriate sections. In this respect, repetition of a term has not been avoided, rather it has been sought out. For example, "sarcoidosis" appears in the sections on Internal Medicine, Respiratory System, Cardiovascular System, and Orthopedics, thus making it unnecessary to flip pages back and forth between sections to find the proper spelling.

Arrangement of Terms. Within each section terms are listed so that the familiar term will lead to the unfamiliar; that is, unfamiliar terms are given as subentries under familiar main entries. If, for example, the transcriber is doing a report for a urologist and runs across "Brown-Buerger" cystoscope, she need only turn to the section on Urology to find the proper spelling listed under "cystoscope."

Phonetic spellings. Selected entries and combining forms are given in two forms: the correct spelling and, at its own alphabetical place, a phonetic spelling. The latter is given in italicized form, with a cross-reference to the proper spelling. If, for example, while doing a report for an ophthalmologist, the transcriber hears the unfamiliar term "ptosis," she would turn to the Ophthalmology section and look for what sounds to her like "tosis." At that place, she would find the italicized entry *"tosis.* See *ptosis,"* the cross-reference indicating the proper spelling.

Medications. All appropriate drugs are listed in the specialty sections (with the exception of Internal Medicine) under the main entry *Medications.* Nonproprietary names are given in lower-case letters, and proprietary names with the first letter capitalized.

As originator and owner of an extremely busy medical transcription service for the past six years, I have watched the needs of my transcribers become more apparent daily. The years of observing their requirements and concerns are responsible for the conception of *The Medical Word Book.* It is my hope that this book will answer their needs and be a valuable tool for all those concerned with the usage of medical terminology.

Sheila B. Sloane

ACKNOWLEDGMENTS

I am deeply grateful to the following physicians who so kindly advised me in the development of those sections pertinent to their specialty: Dr. Allen E. Henkin, Obstetrician and Gynecologist; Dr. Jay L. Helfgott, Ophthalmologist; Dr. Timothy J. Tehan, Urologist; and Dr. G. Lennard Gold, Internist. My deep appreciation is also extended to the staff of W. B. Saunders and especially to Mr. John P. Friel, whose kindness and guidance will always be remembered. Particular thanks go to the transcribers of Medi-Phone, Incorporated, whose suggestions and support throughout have been invaluable.

CONTENTS

GENERAL ANATOMY

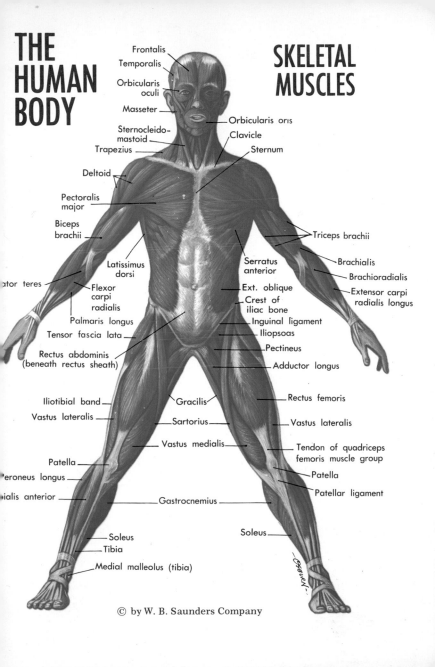

THE HUMAN BODY

SKELETAL MUSCLES

Frontalis
Temporalis
Orbicularis oculi
Masseter
Sternocleidomastoid
Trapezius
Deltoid
Pectoralis major
Biceps brachii
Latissimus dorsi
ator teres
Flexor carpi radialis
Palmaris longus
Tensor fascia lata
Rectus abdominis (beneath rectus sheath)
Iliotibial band
Vastus lateralis
Patella
Peroneus longus
ialis anterior
Soleus
Tibia
Medial malleolus (tibia)

Orbicularis oris
Clavicle
Sternum
Triceps brachii
Brachialis
Brachioradialis
Extensor carpi radialis longus
Serratus anterior
Ext. oblique
Crest of iliac bone
Inguinal ligament
Iliopsoas
Pectineus
Adductor longus
Rectus femoris
Vastus lateralis
Tendon of quadriceps femoris muscle group
Patella
Patellar ligament
Soleus

Gracilis
Sartorius
Vastus medialis
Gastrocnemius

© by W. B. Saunders Company

BONES

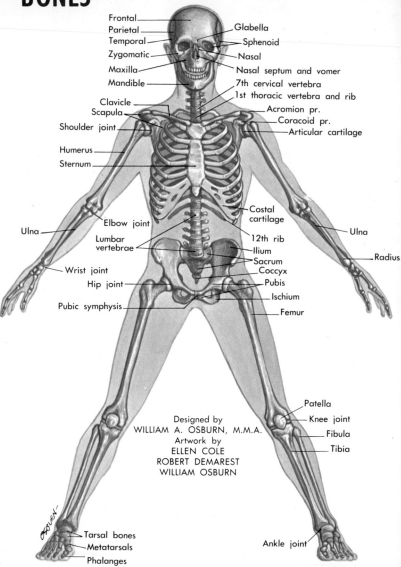

Frontal
Parietal
Temporal
Zygomatic
Maxilla
Mandible
Glabella
Sphenoid
Nasal
Nasal septum and vomer
7th cervical vertebra
1st thoracic vertebra and rib
Clavicle
Scapula
Shoulder joint
Acromion pr.
Coracoid pr.
Articular cartilage
Humerus
Sternum
Costal cartilage
Ulna
Elbow joint
Lumbar vertebrae
Ulna
12th rib
Ilium
Radius
Wrist joint
Hip joint
Pubic symphysis
Sacrum
Coccyx
Pubis
Ischium
Femur
Patella
Knee joint
Fibula
Tibia
Tarsal bones
Metatarsals
Phalanges
Ankle joint

Designed by
WILLIAM A. OSBURN, M.M.A.
Artwork by
ELLEN COLE
ROBERT DEMAREST
WILLIAM OSBURN

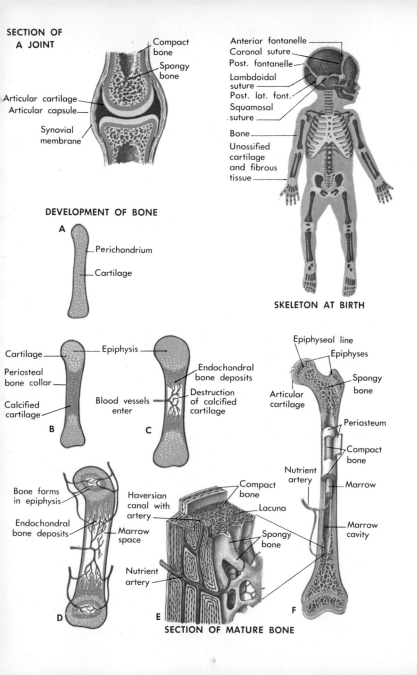

SECTION OF
A JOINT

Compact bone
Spongy bone

Articular cartilage
Articular capsule
Synovial membrane

Anterior fontanelle
Coronal suture
Post. fontanelle
Lambdoidal suture
Post. lat. font.
Squamosal suture
Bone
Unossified cartilage and fibrous tissue

SKELETON AT BIRTH

DEVELOPMENT OF BONE

A

Perichondrium
Cartilage

Cartilage
Periosteal bone collar
Calcified cartilage

Epiphysis

B

Endochondral bone deposits
Blood vessels enter
Destruction of calcified cartilage

C

Epiphyseal line
Epiphyses
Spongy bone
Articular cartilage
Periosteum
Nutrient artery
Compact bone
Marrow
Marrow cavity

F

Bone forms in epiphysis
Endochondral bone deposits
Marrow space
Nutrient artery

D

Haversian canal with artery
Compact bone
Lacuna
Spongy bone
Nutrient artery

E

SECTION OF MATURE BONE

THE ORGANS OF DIGESTION

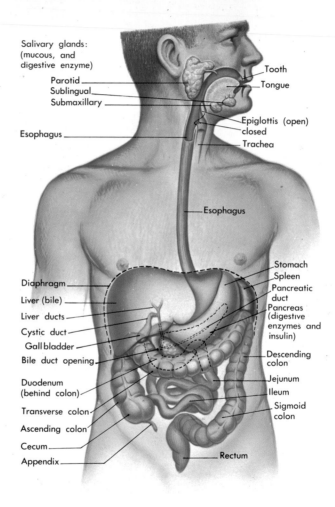

Salivary glands:
(mucous, and
digestive enzyme)

Parotid

Sublingual

Submaxillary

Esophagus

Tooth

Tongue

Epiglottis (open)
closed

Trachea

Esophagus

Diaphragm

Liver (bile)

Liver ducts

Cystic duct

Gall bladder

Bile duct opening

Duodenum
(behind colon)

Transverse colon

Ascending colon

Cecum

Appendix

Stomach

Spleen

Pancreatic
duct

Pancreas
(digestive
enzymes and
insulin)

Descending
colon

Jejunum

Ileum

Sigmoid
colon

Rectum

SECTION OF STOMACH WALL

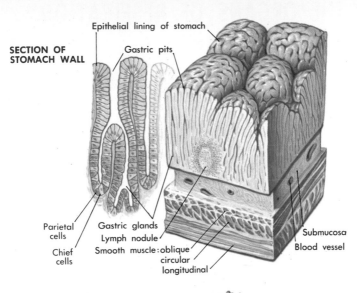

Epithelial lining of stomach

Gastric pits

Parietal cells

Chief cells

Gastric glands

Lymph nodule

Smooth muscle: oblique
circular
longitudinal

Submucosa

Blood vessel

Villi

Epithelium

Mucosal muscle

Blood vessels in submucosa

Smooth muscle
circular
longitudinal

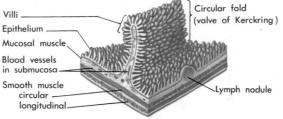

Circular fold (valve of Kerckring)

Lymph nodule

SECTIONS OF SMALL INTESTINE WALL

SECTION OF LARGE INTESTINE (COLON)

Epithelial lining

Openings of glands

Intestinal gland

Submucosal blood vessels

Smooth muscle (circular)

Tenia coli (longitudinal muscle band)

DEMAREST

THE ORGANS OF RESPIRATION AND THE HEART

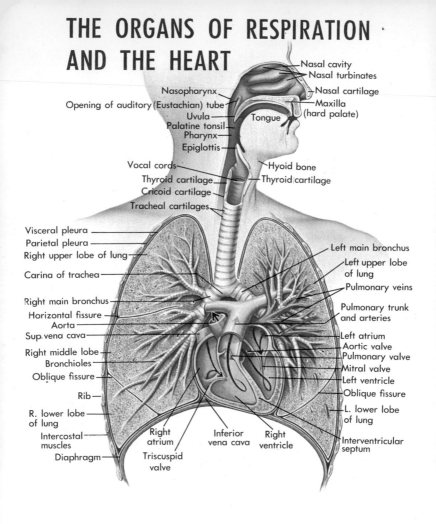

Nasal cavity
Nasal turbinates
Nasopharynx
Nasal cartilage
Opening of auditory (Eustachian) tube
Maxilla (hard palate)
Uvula
Palatine tonsil
Tongue
Pharynx
Epiglottis
Vocal cords
Hyoid bone
Thyroid cartilage
Thyroid cartilage
Cricoid cartilage
Tracheal cartilages
Visceral pleura
Parietal pleura
Left main bronchus
Right upper lobe of lung
Left upper lobe of lung
Carina of trachea
Pulmonary veins
Right main bronchus
Pulmonary trunk and arteries
Horizontal fissure
Aorta
Left atrium
Sup. vena cava
Aortic valve
Pulmonary valve
Right middle lobe
Mitral valve
Bronchioles
Left ventricle
Oblique fissure
Oblique fissure
Rib
L. lower lobe of lung
R. lower lobe of lung
Interventricular septum
Intercostal muscles
Right atrium
Inferior vena cava
Right ventricle
Diaphragm
Triscuspid valve

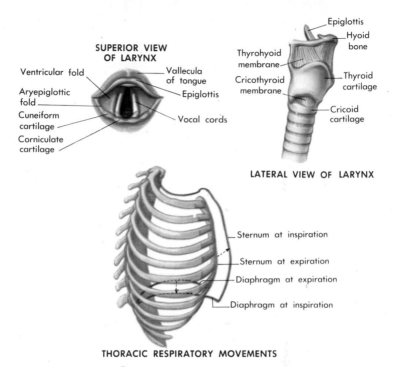

SUPERIOR VIEW OF LARYNX

Ventricular fold

Aryepiglottic fold

Cuneiform cartilage

Corniculate cartilage

Vallecula of tongue

Epiglottis

Vocal cords

Epiglottis

Hyoid bone

Thyrohyoid membrane

Cricothyroid membrane

Thyroid cartilage

Cricoid cartilage

LATERAL VIEW OF LARYNX

Sternum at inspiration

Sternum at expiration

Diaphragm at expiration

Diaphragm at inspiration

THORACIC RESPIRATORY MOVEMENTS

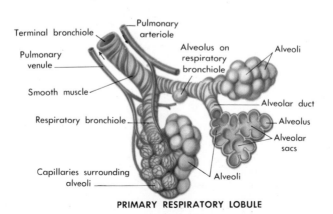

Terminal bronchiole

Pulmonary arteriole

Pulmonary venule

Smooth muscle

Respiratory bronchiole

Capillaries surrounding alveoli

Alveolus on respiratory bronchiole

Alveoli

Alveolar duct

Alveolus

Alveolar sacs

Alveoli

PRIMARY RESPIRATORY LOBULE

THE MAJOR BLOOD VESSELS

VEINS

ARTERIES

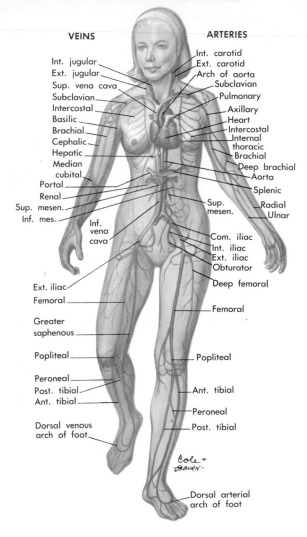

Int. jugular
Ext. jugular
Sup. vena cava
Subclavian
Intercostal
Basilic
Brachial
Cephalic
Hepatic
Median cubital
Portal
Renal
Sup. mesen.
Inf. mes.
Inf. vena cava
Ext. iliac
Femoral
Greater saphenous
Popliteal
Peroneal
Post. tibial
Ant. tibial
Dorsal venous arch of foot

Int. carotid
Ext. carotid
Arch of aorta
Subclavian
Pulmonary
Axillary
Heart
Intercostal
Internal thoracic
Brachial
Deep brachial
Aorta
Splenic
Sup. mesen.
Radial
Ulnar
Com. iliac
Int. iliac
Ext. iliac
Obturator
Deep femoral
Femoral
Popliteal
Ant. tibial
Peroneal
Post. tibial
Dorsal arterial arch of foot

Cole &
OSBURN

DETAILS OF CIRCULATORY STRUCTURES

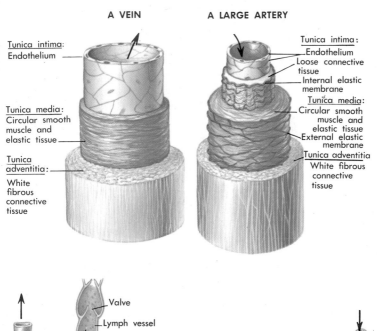

A VEIN

Tunica intima:
Endothelium

Tunica media:
Circular smooth
muscle and
elastic tissue

Tunica
adventitia:
White
fibrous
connective
tissue

A LARGE ARTERY

Tunica intima:
Endothelium
Loose connective
tissue
Internal elastic
membrane
Tunica media:
Circular smooth
muscle and
elastic tissue
External elastic
membrane
Tunica adventitia
White fibrous
connective
tissue

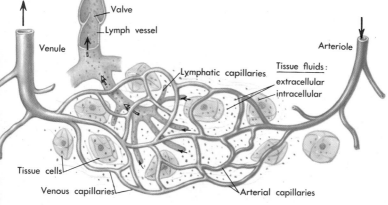

Valve

Lymph vessel

Venule

Lymphatic capillaries

Arteriole

Tissue fluids:
extracellular
intracellular

Tissue cells

Venous capillaries

Arterial capillaries

A CAPILLARY BED

THE BRAIN AND SPINAL NERVES

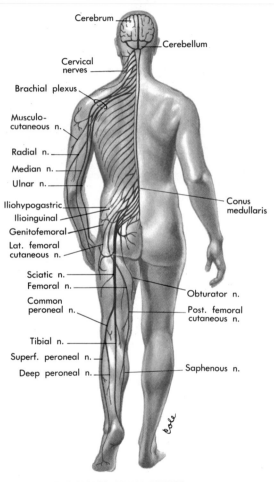

Cerebrum

Cerebellum

Cervical nerves

Brachial plexus

Musculo-cutaneous n.

Radial n.

Median n.

Ulnar n.

Iliohypogastric

Ilioinguinal

Genitofemoral

Lat. femoral cutaneous n.

Sciatic n.

Femoral n.

Common peroneal n.

Tibial n.

Superf. peroneal n.

Deep peroneal n.

Conus medullaris

Obturator n.

Post. femoral cutaneous n.

Saphenous n.

THE MAJOR SPINAL NERVES

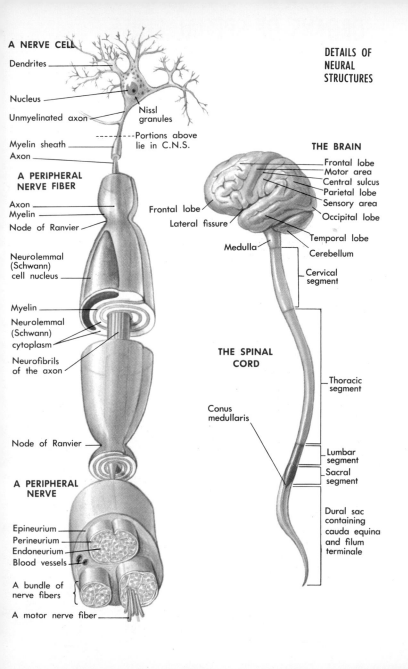

A NERVE CELL

Dendrites

Nucleus

Unmyelinated axon

Nissl granules

Myelin sheath

Axon

- - - Portions above lie in C.N.S.

A PERIPHERAL NERVE FIBER

Axon
Myelin
Node of Ranvier

Neurolemmal (Schwann) cell nucleus

Myelin

Neurolemmal (Schwann) cytoplasm

Neurofibrils of the axon

Node of Ranvier

A PERIPHERAL NERVE

Epineurium
Perineurium
Endoneurium
Blood vessels

A bundle of nerve fibers

A motor nerve fiber

DETAILS OF NEURAL STRUCTURES

THE BRAIN

Frontal lobe
Motor area
Central sulcus
Parietal lobe
Sensory area
Occipital lobe

Frontal lobe

Lateral fissure

Temporal lobe

Medulla

Cerebellum

Cervical segment

THE SPINAL CORD

Conus medullaris

Thoracic segment

Lumbar segment

Sacral segment

Dural sac containing cauda equina and filum terminale

ORGANS OF SPECIAL SENSE THE EAR

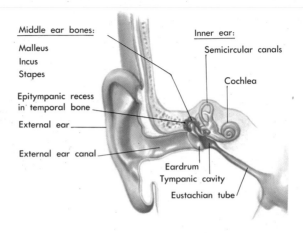

Middle ear bones:

Malleus
Incus
Stapes

Epitympanic recess
in temporal bone

External ear

External ear canal

Inner ear:

Semicircular canals

Cochlea

Eardrum
Tympanic cavity
Eustachian tube

THE ORGAN OF HEARING

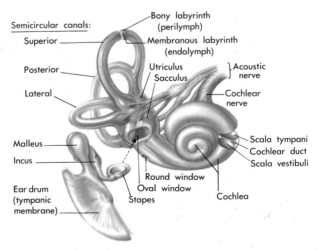

Semicircular canals:

Superior

Posterior

Lateral

Malleus

Incus

Ear drum
(tympanic
membrane)

Bony labyrinth
(perilymph)

Membranous labyrinth
(endolymph)

Utriculus
Sacculus

Acoustic
nerve

Cochlear
nerve

Scala tympani
Cochlear duct
Scala vestibuli

Round window
Oval window
Stapes

Cochlea

THE MIDDLE EAR AND INNER EAR

THE LACRIMAL APPARATUS AND THE EYE

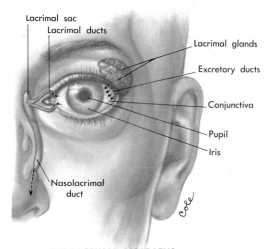

Lacrimal sac
Lacrimal ducts
Lacrimal glands
Excretory ducts
Conjunctiva
Pupil
Iris
Nasolacrimal duct

THE LACRIMAL APPARATUS

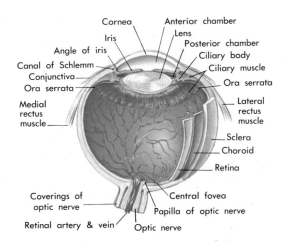

Cornea
Anterior chamber
Iris
Lens
Angle of iris
Posterior chamber
Ciliary body
Canal of Schlemm
Ciliary muscle
Conjunctiva
Ora serrata
Ora serrata
Medial rectus muscle
Lateral rectus muscle
Sclera
Choroid
Retina
Coverings of optic nerve
Central fovea
Papilla of optic nerve
Retinal artery & vein
Optic nerve

HORIZONTAL SECTION OF THE EYE

STRUCTURAL DETAILS

SKELETAL MUSCLE

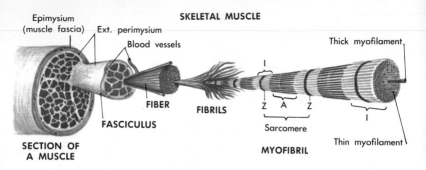

Epimysium (muscle fascia)

Ext. perimysium

Blood vessels

Thick myofilament

FIBER

FIBRILS

I

Z A Z

Sarcomere

I

Thin myofilament

FASCICULUS

SECTION OF A MUSCLE

MYOFIBRIL

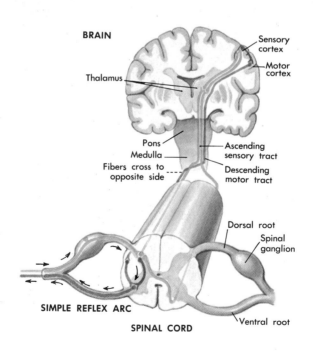

BRAIN

Sensory cortex

Motor cortex

Thalamus

Pons

Medulla

Fibers cross to opposite side

Ascending sensory tract

Descending motor tract

Dorsal root

Spinal ganglion

SIMPLE REFLEX ARC

Ventral root

SPINAL CORD

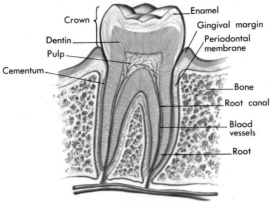

SECTION OF A MOLAR TOOTH

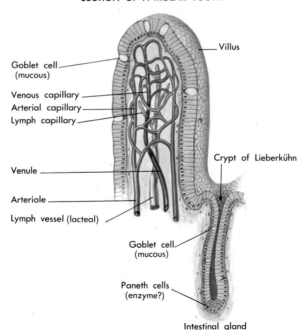

SECTIONS OF SMALL INTESTINE WALL

THE PARANASAL SINUSES

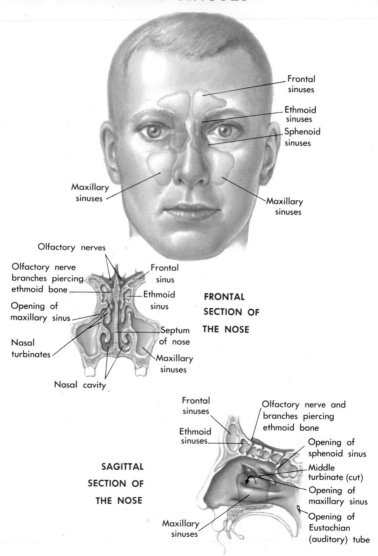

Frontal sinuses

Ethmoid sinuses

Sphenoid sinuses

Maxillary sinuses

Maxillary sinuses

Olfactory nerves

Olfactory nerve branches piercing ethmoid bone

Opening of maxillary sinus

Nasal turbinates

Frontal sinus

Ethmoid sinus

Septum of nose

Maxillary sinuses

Nasal cavity

FRONTAL SECTION OF THE NOSE

SAGITTAL SECTION OF THE NOSE

Frontal sinuses

Ethmoid sinuses

Olfactory nerve and branches piercing ethmoid bone

Opening of sphenoid sinus

Middle turbinate (cut)

Opening of maxillary sinus

Opening of Eustachian (auditory) tube

Maxillary sinuses

GENERAL MEDICAL TERMS

abacterial
abaissement
abate
abatement
abdomen
abducens
abducent
abduct
abduction
aberrant
aberration
abeyance
ablate
ablation
abnormal
abnormality
abradant
abrasion
abrasive
abscess
absorbent
absorption
a capite ad calcem
acatastasia
acathexia
accentuation
accessory
achalasia
ache

acinus
acne
acosmia
acoustic
acquired
acuclosure
acuminate
acute
adduct
adduction
adenitis
adenocarcinoma
adenoma
adenomatous
adenopathy
adhere
adherent
adhesion
adhesive
adhesiveness
adipose
adiposis
aditus
adjunct
adjunctive
adjuvant
ad nauseam
adnerval
adolescence

adolescent
adventitia
adventitious
adynamia
adynamic
aerate
aerophagia
afebrile
afferent
afunction
agenesis
agitated
agonal
ailment
akinesia
akinetic
ala
alae
alar
alba
albinism
algogenesia
alimentary
alimentation
allergic
allergy
alopecia
altricious
alveolus
ambidexterity
ambidextrous
ambient
ambulant
ambulatory
ambustion
amebiasis
amelioration
amnesia

amorphous
ampule
ampulla
ampullae
anacatharsis
analgesia
analgesic
anaphylactic
anasarca
anastomosis
anatomical
anatomy
anemia
anemic
anesthesia
aneurysm
angulus
anhidrosis
annectent
annular
annulus
anomalous
anomaly
anorectic
anorexia
anoxemia
anoxia
ansa
antacid
ante cibum – before meals
anteflexion
antegrade
anterior
anteroexternal
anterograde
anteroinferior
anterointernal
anterolateral

anteromedian
anteroposterior
anterosuperior
anteroventral
anteversion
anteverted
antexed
anthorisma
antibiotic
antibody
anticholinergic
anticoagulant
antidepressant
antidote
antigen
antihistamine
antipyretic
antisepsis
antiseptic
antitoxin
antitussive
antral
antrum
anus
anxiety
apertura
aperture
apex
aphagia
    a. algera
aphasia
aphasic
apical
apices
aplasia
apnea
apogee
aponeurosis

apposition
approximal
approximate
apyretic
apyrexia
apyrexial
apyrogenic
apyrogenetic
aqueduct
aqueductus
aqueous
arcate
archetype
arciform
arctation
arcual
arcuate
arcuation
arcus
areola
areolar
arrhythmia
arrhythmic
arterial
arteriola
arteriole
arteriosclerosis
artery
arthritis
articulate
articulation
articulo
    a. mortis
artifact
artificial
ascending
ascites
asepsis

aseptic

aspect

    dorsal a.

    ventral a.

asphyxia

asphyxiation

aspirate

aspiration

aspirator

asterixis

asteroid

asthenia

asthenic

asthma

asymmetrical

asymmetry

asymptomatic

asynchronism

ataxia

atelectasis

atonic

atonicity

atony

atopic

atopy

atraumatic

atresia

atretic

atrial

atrophy

attenuant

attenuate

attenuation

atypia

atypical

aura

auscultation

autogenesis

autogenous

autopsy

avascular

avulsion

axilla

axillae

axillary

azotemia

bacteria

basal

basilar

belching

benign

bifid

bifurcate

bifurcation

bigeminal

bigeminy

bilateral

bilious

biliousness

bimanual

biochemistry

biochemorphology

biology

biomicroscopy

biophysics

biophysiology

biopsy

bleb

blennogenic

blister

bolus

borborygmus

boss

bosselated

bout

BP — blood pressure

bradycardia
bradykinesia
breadth
brisement
bronchitis
bruise
bruit
bruxism
brwe. See *bruit.*
buccal
bulbar
bulboid
bulbous
bulla
bursa
buttock
cachectic
cachexia
cacoethic
cadaver
caduceus
calcification
calix
calor
calorie
canaliculus
cannula
capillary
capsule
caput
cardiomegaly
cardiovascular
carphology
cartilage
cartilaginous
caruncle
catamnesis
catharsis

catheter
cauda
caudad
caudae
caudal
caudalis
caudalward
causalgia
cauterization
cautery
cavum
CC – chief complaint
        clinical course
cecal
cellula
cellular
cellulitis
cephalad
cephalalgia
cephalic
channel
chemotherapy
chorda
chronic
cicatrix
circinate
circulation
circulus
circumferential
circumflex
circumscribed
claudication
cleft
clinical
clonus
clubbing
clysis
coagulate

coagulation
coalescence
coapt
coarctate
coccyx
coherent
coitus
colic
colicky
collagen
coma
comatose
compatible
compensation
competence
complaint
compress
compression
concavity
concentric
concomitant
concrescence
configuration
confluent
congenital
congested
conical
consanguinity
conscious
consciousness
conservative
constipated
constipation
constitutional
constriction
consultant
consultation
contagious

contamination
contiguity
contiguous
contour
contraction
contraindication
contralateral
contusion
convalescence
convalescent
convexity
convoluted
convolution
convulsion
coroner
corpse
corpus
corpuscle
cortex
coryza
crepitant
crepitation
crepitus
crescent
cribriform
crisis
criterion
critical
croupette
crus
cryoprecipitability
cryoprecipitate
cryotherapy
crypt
cryptogenetic
cul-de-sac
curet
curettage

cutaneous
cyanosis
cyanotic
cyst
debilitate
debility
débouchement
debride
debridement
debris
deceleration
deciduous
decompression
decontamination
decortication
decrement
decrepitate
decrepitation
decrudescence
decrustation
decubation
decubitus
defecation
defervescence
defervescent
deformity
degeneration
deglutition
dehiscence
dehydration
deleterious
delirious
delirium
delitescence
deltoid
demarcation
demise
demulcent

density
denudation
dermatitis
descending
desiccate
deterioration
detumescence
deviation
dextroposition
diagnose
diagnosis
    biological d.
    clinical d.
    cytohistologic d.
    cytologic d.
    differential d.
    d. ex juvantibus
    niveau d.
    pathologic d.
    provocative d.
    roentgen d.
    serum d.
diagnostic
diagnostician
dialysis
dialyzed
diaphoresis
diaphoretic
diaphragm
diarrhea
diastasis
diathermy
diathesis
dichotomy
differentiate
differentiation
diffuse
digestion

digestive
digit
digital
dilatation
dilation
dilator
dilution
diminution
dimpling
diplopia
disciform
discoid
discrete
discus
disease
disesthesia
disinfect
disintegration
disorganization
disorientation
disparate
displacement
disposition
disseminated
distad
distal
distalis
distally
distention
distortion
diuresis
diuretic
diurnal
divergent
diverticulum
divulsion
dizziness
donor

dorsal
dorsum
dressing
droplet
duct
ductulus
dysarthria
dysbarism
dyschezia
dyscrasia
dysentery
dysfunction
dyspepsia
dysphagia
dysphasia
dysplasia
dyspnea
dyspneic
dysponderal
dyspragia
dysrhythmia
dyssymmetry
dystonia
dystonic
dysuria
ebrietas
ebriety
eccentric
ecchymoses
ecchymosis
ecchymotic
eclampsia
écouvillon
écouvillonage
ectad
ectal
ecto-entad
ectopic

eczema
edema
edematous
edentulous
efferent
efflux
effraction
effusion
egophony
elastica
elective
electrocautery
electrotherapy
electrophoresis
electropyrexia
elicited
elongation
emaciated
embedding
embolism
embryo
embryonic
emesis
emetic
emetocathartic
empiric
en bloc
encapsulated
endemic
endocrine
endoscopy
engorged
engorgement
entad
ental
enucleate
enucleation
environment

eparsalgia
epidemic
epigastric
epigastrium
epiphenomenon
epistaxis
epithelium
equilibrium
erosion
erosive
eructation
eruption
erythema
esophagitis
ethanol
etiological
etiology
eucrasia
euphoria
euthanasia
euthyroid
evacuation
evanescent
eversion
evert
evisceration
exacerbation
excavation
excise
excoriation
excrescence
excretion
excretory
exenteration
exhaustion
exogenous
expiration
expire

exsanguinate
exstrophy
extraocular
extravasation
extremity
extrinsic
extrude
extubate
extubation
exudate
facial
facies
facilitation
Fahrenheit Thermometer
fahrma. See words beginning
   pharma-.
falces
falciform
falx
familial
fascia
fascial
fascicle
fasciculation
fasciculus
fatigability
fatigue
FB — foreign body
    fingerbreadth
febrile
fecal
feces
fenomenon. See *phenomenon.*
fenestra
fenestrated
fervescence
fetid
fetor

fever
FH — family history
fiber
fibra
fibrillation
fibroma
fimbria
fimbriated
fingerbreadth
fissure
fistula
flaccid
flank
flatulence
flatus
flexibility
flexion
flexure
florid
fluctuant
fluctuation
fluoroscope
folium
follicle
folliculus
fontanelle
fonticulus
foramen
foramina
forceps
    bayonet f.
    mosquito f.
    mouse-tooth f.
    sequestrum f.
    speculum f.
    tubular f.
    vulsella f.
    vulsellum f.

forme
    f. fruste
    f. tradive
fornix
fossa
fovea
foveola
fragility
fremitus
frenulum
friable
fulgurate
fulguration
fulminant
fulminate
fumigation
function
functional
fundus
funiculus
FUO – fever of undetermined
       origin
      fever of unknown
       origin
furuncle
fusiform
gait
ganglion
gangrene
gangrenous
gaseous
gauze
genetic
genitalia
genu
glomerulus
gonorrhea
gradient

gram
granulation
grumous
guaiac
halitosis
hemangioma
hematemesis
hematochezia
hematoma
hemiparesis
hemiplegia
hemoptysis
hemorrhage
hemostasis
hepatitis
hereditary
heredity
heterogenic
heterotopia
heterotopic
hiatus
hiccup
hidrorrhea
hilus
hirsute
hirsutism
homogeneous
homogenous
homologous
hormone
hospital
H & P – history and physical
HPE – history and physical
    examination
HPI – history of present
    illness
hyaline
hyalinization

hydration
hydrotherapy
hygiene
hygienic
hygroma
hypalgesia
hypasthenia
hyperemia
hyperesthesia
hyperhidrosis
hyperplasia
hyperthermia
hypertonic
hypertonicity
hypertrophy
hyperventilation
hypervolemia
hypochondriac
hypodermic
hypodermoclysis
hypothermal
hypothermia
hypotonia
hypotonic
hypoxia
iatrogenic
icteric
icterus
ictus
idiopathic
idiopathy
idiosyncrasy
illumination
IM – intramuscularly
imbed
imbricated
imbrication
immature

immediate
immobility
immobilization
immune
immunity
immunization
impalpable
impatency
impatent
imperforate
impermeable
implant
implantation
impressio
in articulo mortis
incarcerated
incidence
incipient
incisura
incompatibility
incompetence
incontinence
incubation
incurable
indigenous
indigestion
indisposition
indolent
induced
indurated
induration
inebriation
inebriety
inert
inertia
in extremis
infantile
infarct

infarction
infection
infectious
inferior
inferolateral
inferomedian
inferoposterior
infestation
infiltrate
infiltration
infirm
infirmity
inflammation
inflammatory
inflation
inflexion
infundibulum
infusion
ingestion
ingravescent
inhalation
inherent
initial
injection
injury
innominate
inoculate
inoculation
insalubrious
insenescence
in situ
inspiration
inspissated
instillation
insufficiency
insufflation
integration
integument

integumentary
intensity
intensive
intention
intermittent
interstitial
intestine
in toto
intoxication
intractable
intramuscular
intravenous
intra vitam
intrinsic
introflexion
introversion
intubate
intubation
intumescent
invaginate
inversion
in vivo
involuntary
ipsilateral
irradiation
irreducible
irregular
irregularity
irreversible
irrigation
irritability
irritant
ischemia
isolate
isolateral
isolation
isolette
isotonia

isotonic

isotope

    radioactive i.

isthmus

IV – intravenous

jactitation

jaundice

jugulation

junction

junctura

juvenile

juxtaposition

kahkekseah. See *cachexia.*

kahkektik. See *cachectic.*

kakoethik. See *cacoethic.*

keloid

keratosis

kilogram

kinetic

kyphosis

labile

labium

lacerated

laceration

lacuna

lamina

laminated

laser

lassitude

laterad

lateral

lateralis

latissimus

lavage

lesion

lethal

lethargy

limbus

limen

linear

lipoma

lobe

lobule

lobulus

lobus

longitudinal

lumen

lymph

lymphatic

lyse

lysis

ma – milliampere

maceration

macula

maim

malabsorption

malacia

malady

malaise

malar

malformation

malfunction

malignancy

malignant

malingerer

malleable

malnutrition

malposition

malpractice

malum

mandible

mandibula

maneuver

manipulation

manual

marasmus

marcid
margin
marginal
margo
marital
marsupialization
masculine
maser
massa
massage
mastication
masticatory
matrix
maxillary
maximum
meatus
medial
medialis
median
medianus
medicable
medicate
medication
medicinal
medicochirurgic
mediolateral
medius
medulla
medusa
melanemesis
melanoma
melena
melenemesis
melu. See *milieu.*
membrana
membrane
membranous
membrum

mentoanterior
mentoposterior
mentotransverse
mEq — milliequivalent
meridian
meridianus
meridional
mesad
mesal
mesiad
mesial
mesentery
metabolic
metabolism
metamorphosis
metastases
metastasis
metastasize
metastatic
MFB — metallic foreign body
mg — milligram
mgm — milligram
MH — marital history
        medical history
mication
microbiology
microgram
milliampere
millicurie
milliequivalent
milligram
milliliter
millimeter
millimicrocurie
millimicrogram
millisecond
milliunit
millivolt

milieu
ml — milliliter
mm — millimeter
mmm — micromillimeter
modality
mongolism
mongoloid
monitor
morbid
morbidity
moribund
morphology
mortality
motile
motility
msec — millisecond
mucopurulent
mucosa
mucosanguineous
mucus
mummification
mummying
mural
muscle
mutilation
myalgia
myelitis
myelopathy
myoma
myositis
myxedema
myxoma
nausea
nauseous
nebulization
necropsy
necrosis
neoplasm

neoplastic
nerve
neural
neurasthenia
niche
nocturia
nocturnal
node
nodular
nodule
nodulus
nodus
nonspecific
normoactive
normocephalic
normotensive
normothermia
normotonia
normotopia
normotrophic
noxious
NPO — nothing by mouth
    (nulla per os)
NTP — normal temperature
    and pressure
nucha
nucleus
nutrition
N & V — nausea and vomiting
obese
obesity
    exogenous o.
obfuscation
oblique
obliteration
obsolescence
obsolete
obstipation

obstruction
obtund
obturation
obtuse
occipital
occiput
occlusion
occult
oncology
opacity
opaque
OPD – outpatient department
optimum
orbicular
organic
organism
organomegaly
orifice
orthopnea
orthostatic
orthotopic
os
oscillation
osculum
osteoid
ostium
P & A – percussion and
    auscultation
pain
    lancinating p.
palliate
palliative
pallor
palpable
palpate
palpation
palpitation
panhidrosis

panhyperemia
panniculus
papilla
papule
paracenesthesia
paradoxical
paralyses
paralysis
parenchyma
parenchymal
parenteral
paresis
paresthesia
paries
parietal
pari passu
paroxysm
paroxysmal
patent
pathogen
pathogenesis
pathologic
pathological
pathology
pathosis
PC – after meals (post cibum)
PE – physical examination
peau
    p. d'orange
pectinate
pedal
pedicle
peduncle
peduncular
pedunculated
pendulous
percussion
percutaneous

periosteum
peripheral
periphery
permeability
permeation
pernicious
per os – by mouth
per primam intentionem
per rectum
perspiration
per tubam
pestilence
petechia
petekeah. See *petechia.*
petrous
PH – past history
pharmaceutical
pharmacist
phenomenon
phthisis
physician
physiologic
physiological
physique
pica
pillion
placebo
plantar
plica
plication
PO – period of onset
po dorahnj. See *peau d'orange.*
polydipsia
polyuria
posterior
posteroinferior
posterolateral
posteromedial

postictal
postmortem
postprandial
poudrage
poultice
prandial
premonitory
preponderance
prescription
preventive
primary
procedure
process
prodrome
prodromic
profundus
progeria
prognosis
pronation
prone
prophylactic
prophylaxis
proprioceptive
prosthesis
prosthetics
prostration
protuberance
provisional
provocative
proximal
proximalis
pruritus
psychic
psychogenic
psychosomatic
ptosis
puberty
pulsatile

pulsion
punctate
punctum
purulent
pustular
pustule
putrescence
putrid
pyemesis
pyemia
pyknic
pyogenesis
pyogenic
pyramid
pyramidal
pyretic
pyrexia
pyrosis
quadrant
qualitative
quantitative
quarantine
quiescent
radial
radialis
radiant
radiate
radiathermy
radiatio
radiation
radical
radioactivity
radioisotope
radiology
radiolucent
radix
rakoma. See *rhacoma.*
rale

ramification
ramus
raphe
rarefaction
rebound
recapitulation
recidivation
recrudescence
recrudescent
rectus
recumbent
recuperation
recurrence
reducible
redundant
refractory
regimen
regio
regional
regma. See *rhegma.*
regurgitant
regurgitation
rehabilitation
rehydration
reksis. See *rhexis.*
relapse
remedy
remission
remittent
rentgen. See *roentgen.*
resection
reservoir
residual
resilience
resolution
resorption
respiration
respiratory

restitutio
    r. integrum
restitution
restoration
resuscitation
retching
rete
retention
retrograde
retroversion
reversion
rhacoma
rhegma
rhexis
rhonchal
rhonchial
rhonchus
rictus
rigidity
    nuchal r.
rigor
    r. mortis
rima
roentgen
rong. See words beginning
   rhonc-.
rongeur
rostrum
rotation
rotexion
rubedo
rubefacient
rubella
rubor
ructus
rudiment
rudimentary
ruga

rugae
rugosity
rumination
rupture
sac
saccular
sacculus
saccus
sacroiliac
sagittal
saliva
salivary
salivation
salubrious
salutary
sanguine
sanguineous
sarcoma
scalpel
scanning
    radioisotope s.
scanography
scaphoid
sciatica
scirrhous
scirrhus
sclerosing
sclerosis
sclerotic
scyphoid
scythropasmus
sebaceous
seborrhea
secretion
secretory
sedation
sedative
sedentary

seizure
semicomatose
senescence
senile
senility
sensitivity
sensitization
sensorium
sensory
sepsis
septic
septicemia
septulum
sequela
sequelae
sersinat. See *circinate.*
serial
serially
seropurulent
seropus
serosa
serosanguineous
serous
serpiginous
serrated
serum
sessile
sexual
sexuality
shivering
shock
    anaphylactic s.
SI – seriously ill
sibling
sign
    vital s's.
silastic
sinister

sinistrad
sinus
sithropazmus. See
   scythropasmus.
siphon
skeleton
skeletonized
sluf. See *slough.*
slough
sloughing
soluble
somnolence
spasm
spasmodic
species
specific
specimen
spes
    s. phthisica
spheroid
spontaneous
spurious
stability
stamina
stat – statim (immediately)
status
stellate
stenosis
stenotic
sterile
sterilely
stigma
stigmata
stimulant
stimulation
stimulus
stoma
strangulation

stratum
stria
striae
striated
stricture
stridor
stroma
stupor
stuporous
subacute
subcutaneous
subcuticular
sulcus
superficial
superficialis
supernumerary
supination
suppuration
suppurative
susceptible
symmetrical
symphysis
symptom
symptomatic
symptomatology
syncopal
syncope
syndrome
tabes
tabescent
tabez. See *tabes.*
tachycardia
tachypnea
tactile
takipneah. See *tachypnea.*
tampon
technique
tegmen

tela
telangiectasis
temperature
tenacious
tenaculum
ter in die
terminal
terminus
tertiary
tessellated
tetralogy
texture
therapeutic
therapist
therapy
thermometer
    centigrade t.
    Fahrenheit t.
thoracic
thoracocentesis
thorax
threshold
throbbing
thyroid
thyromegaly
tinnitus
tisis. See *phthisis.*
tissue
tolerance
tomogram
tonicity
topical
topography
torpid
torpidity
torpor
torsion
tortuous

torus
tosis. See *ptosis.*
tourniquet
toxemia
toxic
toxicity
trabecula
trachea
tract
tractus
trajector
tranquilizer
transfusion
transillumination
translucent
transmigration
transmissible
transmission
transplantation
trauma
traumatic
treatment
tremor
tremulous
trigeminy
trigone
trigonum
trocar
troche
trochlea
truncus
tuba
tubal
tubercle
tuberculum
tuberosity
tubule
tubulus

tumefacient
tumefaction
tumescence
tumid
tumor
tunic
tunica
tunnel
turbid
turbidity
turgescence
turgescent
turgid
turgor
tussive
twinge
tympanic
uforeah. See *euphoria.*
ukraseah. See *eucrasia.*
ulcerate
ulceration
ultrasonic
ultraviolet
umbilicus
umbo
unconscious
undernutrition
unicentral
unilateral
uremia
URI — upper respiratory
    infection
urogenital
urticaria
uthahnazeah. See *euthanasia.*
uthiroid. See *euthyroid.*
uvula
vaccinate

vaccine
vacillate
vallecula
valve
variable
variability
vas
vascular
velamen
velamentum
velum
venter
ventral
ventralis
vertex
vertical
vertigo
vesicle
vesicula
vestibule
vestibulum
vestigial
viable
villus
viral
virile
virulent
virus
viscera

viscus
vital
vitality
vitamin
vitium
volar
volvulate
vomit
vomiting
vomitus
    v. cruentus
vortex
vulsella
vulsellum
wakefulness
wart
well-developed
well-nourished
wheal
wheeze
whelk
whorl
wound
xiphoid
zifoid. See *xiphoid.*
zona
zonula
zoster

GENERAL SURGICAL TERMS

Aaron's sign
Abbe's
    operation
    rings
Abbott-Rawson tube
abdomen
abdominal
abdominocentesis
abdominoperineal
abdominoscopy
Abernethy's operation
aberrant
abscess
    amebic a.
    appendiceal a.
    ischiorectal a.
    mammary a.
    perianal a.
    perirectal a.
    pyogenic a.
    subphrenic a.
achalasia
    pelvirectal a.
    sphincteral a.
ACMI
    forceps
    gastroscope
    proctoscope
Acrel's ganglion
ACTH — adrenocorticotropic
    hormone

actinomycosis
acupuncture
Adair's forceps
Adams'
    operation
    position
adenectomy
adenitis
    mesenteric a.
adenocarcinoma
adenofibroma
adenoma
adenomammectomy
adenomatosis
adenopathy
    axillary a.
adhesion
    attic a's.
adhesiotomy
adipectomy
adipocele
adipose
adiposis
adrenalectomize
adrenalectomy
Adson's forceps
agraffe
akahlazea. See *achalasia.*
Akerlund's deformity
alar
Albert's

43

Albert's *(continued)*
    position
    suture
Alexander's incision
alimentary
alimentation
Allarton's operation
Allen's
    clamp
    trocar
Allingham's
    operation
    speculum
    ulcer
Allis' forceps
Allis-Ochsner forceps
Alm's retractor
ampulla
    a. of Vater
amputation
Amussat's operation
anal
anastomosis
    antiperistaltic a.
    Braun's a.
    Clado's a.
    end-to-end a.
    end-to-side a.
    intestinal a.
    isoperistaltic a.
    side-to-end a.
    side-to-side a.
anastomotic
Andrews' operation
anesthesia
    basal a.
    Bier's local a.
    block a.

anesthesia *(continued)*
    caudal a.
    chloroform a.
    closed a.
    colonic a.
    electric a.
    endobronchial a.
    endotracheal a.
    epidural a.
    general a.
    Gwathmey's oil-ether a.
    high pressure a.
    hypnosis a.
    hypotensive a.
    hypothermic a.
    infiltration a.
    inhalation a.
    insufflation a.
    intercostal a.
    intranasal a.
    intraoral a.
    intraspinal a.
    intravenous a.
    Kulenkampff's a.
    local a.
    Meltzer's a.
    mixed a.
    nerve blocking a.
    open a.
    paraneural a.
    parasacral a.
    paravertebral a.
    partial a.
    pentothal a.
    peridural a.
    perineural a.
    periodontal a.
    permeation a.

anesthesia *(continued)*
    plexus a.
    pressure a.
    rectal a.
    refrigeration a.
    regional a.
    sacral a.
    saddle block a.
    semiclosed a.
    semiopen a.
    sodium pentothal a.
    spinal a.
    splanchnic a.
    subarachnoid a.
    surface a.
    surgical a.
    topical a.
    transsacral a.
    twilight a.
anesthesiologist
anesthesiology
anesthetic
anesthetist
anesthetize
aneurysm
aneurysmal
aneurysmectomy
angiitis
angiopancreatitis
ankyloproctia
annular
annulorrhaphy
annulus
anoperineal
anoplasty
anorectal
anorectocolonic
anorectum

anoscope
    Bacon's a.
    Bodenheimer's a.
    Boehm's a.
    Brinkerhoff's a.
    Buie-Hirschman a.
    Fansler's a.
    Goldbacher's a.
    Hirschman's a.
    Ives' a.
    Muer's a.
    Otis' a.
    Pratt's a.
    Pruitt's a.
    Sims' a.
    Welch-Allyn a.
anoscopy
anosigmoidoscopic
anosigmoidoscopy
anospinal
Anson-McVay operation
antecubital
anteversion
antiperistalsis
antiperistaltic
antrum
    pyloric a.
    a. pyloricum
    a. of Willis
anus
apepsia
    achlorhydria a.
aplooshahzh. See *épluchage.*
aponeurosis
aponeurotic
aponeurotomy
appendalgia
appendectomy

appendekthlipsia
appendical
appendiceal
appendicealgia
appendicectasis
appendicectomy
appendices
appendicism
appendicitis
    a. by contiguity
    fulminating a.
    gangrenous a.
    a. granulosa
    helminthic a.
    a. larvata
    myxoglobulosis a.
    necro-purulent a.
    a. obliterans
    perforating a.
    perforative a.
    stercoral a.
    subperitoneal a.
    suppurative a.
    syncongestive a.
    verminous a.
appendiclausis
appendicocecostomy
appendicocele
appendicoenterostomy
appendicolithiasis
appendicolysis
appendicopathia
appendicopathy
appendicosis
appendicostomy
appendicular
appendiculoradiography
appendix

appendix *(continued)*
    auricular a.
    cecal a.
    a. cerebri
    ensiform a.
    vermiform a.
    a. vermiformis
appendolithiasis
appendoroentgenography
appendotome
Appolito's
    operation
    suture
apposition
approximate
areola
areolae
areolar
areolitis
Armsby's operation
artery
    appendicular a.
    brachial a.
    calcareous a.
    epigastric a.
    femoral a.
    hepatic a.
    intramural a.
    sternocleidomastoid a.
    suprascapular a.
    temporal a.
    thoracoacromial a.
ascites
asepsis
aseptic
Ashford's mamilliplasty
aspirate
aspiration

aspirator
    Thorek's a.
asymmetry
atheromatosis
    a. cutis
athyreosis
atony
atresia
atretic
atrophy
Auvray's incision
aw bissahk. See *en bissac.*
axilla
axillae
axillary
Babcock's
    clamp
    forceps
    operation
Backhaus' forceps
Bacon's anoscope
Bainbridge's forceps
Bake's dilator
Baker's cyst
Balfour's
    gastroenterostomy
    retractor
ballooning
ballottement
    abdominal b.
Ball's operation
bandage
    Elastoplast b.
    Esmarch's b.
Bardenheuer's incision
Bard-Parker blades
Barnes'
    dilator

Barnes'
    trocar
Barrett's forceps
Barr's
    hook
    probe
    speculum
Bar's incision
Barth's hernia
Bassini's operation
"basting stitch"
    Parker-Kerr b.s.
bath
    sitz b.
Battle-Jalaguier-Kammerer
    incision
Battle's
    incision
    operation
Baynton's operation
Beardsley's clamp
Beatson's operation
Beaver's blades
Beck-Jianu gastrostomy
Beckman's retractor
Beck's gastrostomy scoop
Béclard's
    hernia
    suture
Beebe's forceps
Bell's suture
Belmas' operation
Benedict's gastroscope
benign
Berbridge's scissors
Berens'
    retractor
    scoop

Bergman-Israel incision
Bergmann's incision
Berna's retractor
Bernstein's gastroscope
Best's
    clamp
    operation
Bevan's
    forceps
    incision
    operation
Beyea's operation
Bier's anesthesia
bifurcation
biliary
Billroth's
    forceps
    gastroenterostomy I and
      II
    operation
biopsy
    aspiration b.
    excisional b.
    fractional b.
    needle b.
    punch b.
    sponge b.
    surface b.
Bircher's operation
Birkett's hernia
bistoury
    b. blade
blade
    Bard-Parker b.'s.
    Beaver's b's.
Blake's forceps
Blanchard's
    cryptotome

Blanchard's
    forceps
Bloodgood's operation
Boari button
Bobb's operation
Bochdalek's foramen
Bodenheimer's anoscope
body
    malpighian b's.
Boehm's
    anoscope
    proctoscope
    sigmoidoscope
Bogue's operation
bolus
Bonta's knife
borborygmus
Bose's operation
bosselated
Bovie unit
bowel
Boyce's position
Boys-Allis forceps
Bozeman's
    position
    suture
Brackin's incision
Bradford's forceps
Braun and Jaboulay
    gastroenterostomy
Braun's anastomosis
Brenner's operation
Brinkerhoff's anoscope
Brinton's disease
Brock's incision
Brooks' scissors
Brophy's forceps
Brown-Adson forceps

Brown's forceps
bruit
    b. de clapotement (brwe
        duh klahpotmaw)
Brunner's
    dissector
    forceps
Brunschwig's operation
brwe. See *bruit.*
Bryant's operation
bubo
Buckstein's insufflator
Buerger's disease
Buie-Hirschman
    anoscope
    clamp
Buie-Smith
    retractor
    speculum
Buie's
    clamp
    forceps
    irrigator
    position
    probe
    procedure
    scissors
    sigmoidoscope
    technique
    tube
bunion
bunionectomy
Burnham's scissors
Butcher's saw
buttock
button
    Boari's b.
    Chlumsky's b.

button *(continued)*
    Jaboulay's b.
    Lardennois's b.
    Murphy's b.
    peritoneal b.
    Villard's b.
Byford's retractor
calculus
Callisen's operation
Calot's triangle
Camper's fascia
canal
    crural c.
    c. of Nuck
canaliculus
canalization
cannula
    Ingals' c.
cannulation
Cantor's tube
capitonnage
capsule
carbuncle
carcinoma
    basal cell c.
    ductal c.
    infiltrating ductal cell c.
    lobular c.
    metastatic c.
    squamous cell c.
Cargile's membrane
Carmalt's forceps
Carman's tube
Carmody's forceps
carrier
    Deschamps' c.
    Lahey's c.
    Mayo's c.

carrier *(continued)*
    Wangensteen's c.
Carter's
    clamp
    splenectomy
caruncle
Casselberry's position
Cassidy-Brophy forceps
catheter
    Foley's c.
    indwelling c.
    Lane's c.
    mushroom c.
    retention c.
    self-retaining c.
    Virden's c.
    Weber's c.
    whistle-tip c.
catheterization
catheterize
Cattell's operation
cauterization
cautery
cavernous
cavity
    peritoneal c.
cecal
cecectomy
cecocele
cecocolic
cecocolon
cecocoloplicopexy
cecocolostomy
cecoileostomy
cecopexy
cecoplication
cecoptosis
cecorectal

cecorrhaphy
cecosigmoidostomy
cecostomy
cecotomy
cecum
    hepatic c.
    c. mobile
celiac
celiectomy
celiocentesis
celioenterotomy
celiogastrotomy
celioparacentesis
celiopyosis
celiorrhaphy
celioscopy
celiotomy
    ventral c.
cellulitis
centesis
cephalic
Chaput's operation
Chelsea-Eaton speculum
chemosurgery
Cherney's incision
Chevalier-Jackson gastroscope
Cheyne's operation
Chiazzi's operation
Chiene's incision
Child's operation
Childs-Phillips needle
Chlumsky's button
cholangiectasis
cholangiocholecystocholedo-
    chectomy
cholangioenterostomy
cholangiogastrostomy
cholangiogram

cholangiography
    operative c.
cholangiojejunostomy
    intrahepatic c.
cholangiostomy
cholangiotomy
cholecyst
cholecystectomy
cholecystelectrocoagulectomy
cholecystendysis
cholecystenteric
cholecystenteroanastomosis
cholecystenterorrhaphy
cholecystenterostomy
cholecystgastrostomy
cholecystic
cholecystis
cholecystitis
cholecystnephrostomy
cholecystocholangiogram
cholecystocolostomy
cholecystocolotomy
cholecystoduodenostomy
cholecystoenterostomy
cholecystogastric
cholecystogastrostomy
cholecystogram
cholecystography
cholecystoileostomy
cholecystojejunostomy
cholecystokinetic
cholecystolithiasis
cholecystolithotripsy
cholecystopexy
cholecystoptosis
cholecystopyelostomy
cholecystorrhaphy
cholecystostomy

cholecystotomy
choledochal
choledochectomy
choledochitis
choledochocholedochor-
    rhaphy
choledochocholedochostomy
choledochoduodenostomy
choledochoenterostomy
choledochogastrostomy
choledochogram
choledochography
choledochohepatostomy
choledochoileostomy
choledochojejunostomy
choledocholith
choledocholithiasis
choledocholithotomy
choledocholithotripsy
choledochoplasty
choledochorrhaphy
choledochosphincterotomy
choledochostomy
choledochotomy
choledochus
cholelithiasis
cholelithotomy
cholelithotrity
chyle
cicatrectomy
cicatricotomy
cicatrix
cicatrization
cirsectomy
cirsenchysis
cirsodesis
cirsotome
cirsotomy

cisterna
    c. chyli
Clado's anastomosis
clamp
    Allen's c.
    Azchary Cope-DeMartel
      c.
    Babcock's c.
    Beardsley's c.
    Best's c.
    Buie's c.
    Buie-Hirschman c.
    Carter's c.
    Crile's c.
    Daniel's c.
    DeMartel-Wolfson c.
    Dennis' c.
    Dixon-Thomas-Smith c.
    Doyen's c.
    Eastman's c.
    Fehland's c.
    Foss' c.
    Friedrich-Petz c.
    Furniss' c.
    Furniss-Clute c.
    Furniss-McClure-Hinton
      c.
    Glassman's c.
    Hayes' c.
    Herff's c.
    Hunt's c.
    Hurwitz's c.
    Jarvis' c.
    Kapp-Beck c.
    Kelly's c.
    Kocher's c.
    Lane's c.
    Lockwood's c.

clamp *(continued)*
    MacDonald's c.
    Mastin's c.
    Moreno's c.
    mosquito c.
    Moynihan's c.
    Nussbaum's c.
    Ochsner's c.
    Parker's c.
    Payr's c.
    Pean's c.
    Pemberton's c.
    Phillips' c.
    Rankin's c.
    Ranzewski's c.
    Roosevelt's c.
    Schoemaker's c.
    Scudder's c.
    Stevenson's c.
    Stone-Holcombe c.
    Stone's c.
    von Petz's c.
    W. Dean McDonald c.
    Wangensteen's c.
    Watts' c.
    Wolfson's c.
claudication
clavicle
clavicular
cloaca
Cloquet's
    fascia
    hernia
closure
    Smead-Jones c.
Clute's incision
coagulate
coapt

coarctation
coarctotomy
cobalt
coccyx
Codman's incision
Coffey's incision
colectomy
Cole's retractor
colic
colicky
colitis
Collin's forceps
collodion
collum
    c. vesicae felleae
colocentesis
coloclysis
colocolostomy
colocutaneous
colofixation
colohepatopexy
coloileal
cololysis
colon
    c. ascendens
    ascending c.
    c. descendens
    descending c.
    irritable c.
    lead-pipe c.
    pelvic c. of Waldeyer
    sigmoid c.
    c. sigmoideum
    thrifty c.
    transverse c.
    c. transversum
colonorrhagia
colonorrhea

colonoscope
colonoscopy
colopexostomy
colopexotomy
colopexy
coloplication
coloproctectomy
coloproctostomy
coloptosis
colorectostomy
colorrhaphy
colosigmoidostomy
colostomy
    ileotransverse c.
    Wangensteen's c.
colotomy
comedocarcinoma
comedomastitis
concretion
condyloma
    c. acuminatum
confluent
Connell's suture
constriction
    duodenopyloric c.
contracture
    Dupuytren's c.
    Volkmann's c.
convolution
Cook's speculum
Cooper's
    disease
    hernia
    ligament
    operation
cord
    spermatic c.
corpora

corpus
cortex
Cotting's operation
Courvoisier's
 gallbladder
 incision
cremaster
cremasteric
cribriform
Crile's
 clamp
 forceps
 retractor
Cripps's
 obturator
 operation
crural
crus
Cruveilhier's ulcer
cryocautery
cryosurgery
cryotherapy
crypt
 c's of Lieberkühn
 Luschka's c's.
cryptitis
cryptotome
 Blanchard's c.
cul-de-sac
curettage
curetted
Curtis' forceps
curvature
 lesser c.
Curvoisier's gastroenterostomy
Cushing's
 forceps
 suture

Cushing's
 ulcer
cutaneous
cuticle
cyst
 Baker's c.
 blue dome c.
 branchial c.
 echinococcus c.
 inclusion c.
 involution c.
 pilonidal c.
 retention c.
 sacrococcygeal c.
 thyroglossal c.
cystauchenotomy
cystduodenostomy
cystectomy
cystic
cysticolithectomy
cysticolithotripsy
cysticorrhaphy
cysticotomy
cystis
 c. fellea
cystjejunostomy
cystocele
cystodiaphanoscopy
cystogastrostomy
cystojejunostomy
 Roux-en-y c.
cystosarcoma
 c. phylloides
Czerny-Lembert suture
Czerny's
 operation
 suture
dabreedmaw. See *débridement.*

Dacron graft
Dallas' operation
Daniel's clamp
David's speculum
Deaver's
    incision
    retractor
    scissors
DeBakey's scissors
Debove's tube
débride
débridement
decompression
decubitus
defecation
deformity
    Akerlund's d.
dehiscence
    wound d.
dehisens. See *dehiscence.*
DeLee's forceps
Delphian node
DeMartel-Wolfson clamp
Denans' operation
Dennis'
    clamp
    forceps
denudation
DePage-Janeway gastrostomy
Depage's position
descensus
    d. ventriculi
Deschamps' carrier
desiccate
desiccation
Desjardin's
    forceps
    probe

diaphragm
diaphragmatic
diastalsis
diastasis
    d. recti abdominis
Dieffenbach's operation
dieresis
Dieulafoy's
    erosion
    ulcer
digital
dilation
    digital d.
dilator
    Bakes' d.
    Barnes' d.
    Ferris' d.
    Kron's d.
    Mantz's d.
    Murphy's d.
    Ottenheimer's d.
    Ramstedt's d.
    Wales' d.
    Young's d.
dimpling
director
    Larry's d.
    Pratt's d.
discrete
disease
    Brinton's d.
    Buerger's d.
    Cooper's d.
    Gaucher's d.
    Hashimoto's d.
    Hirschsprung's d.
    Paget's d.
    Riedel's d.

dissection
>   blunt d.
>   radical neck d.
>   sharp d.
>   supraomohyoid neck d.

dissector
>   Brunner's d.
>   Kocher's d.
>   Wangensteen's d.

disseminated
distention
diverticulectomy
diverticulitis
diverticulogram
diverticulopexy
diverticulosis
diverticulum
>   Meckel's d.

Dixon-Thomas-Smith clamp
Dowell's operation
Doyen's
>   clamp
>   forceps
>   scissors

drain
>   Penrose d.
>   stab wound d.
>   whistle tip d.

dressing
>   gelfoam d.
>   Kerlex d.
>   Lister's d.
>   stent d.

drugs. See *Medications.*
Drummond-Morison operation
duct
>   biliary d.
>   common bile d.

duct *(continued)*
>   common hepatic d.
>   cystic d.
>   lactiferous d's.
>   pancreatic d.
>   d. of Santorini
>   Stenson's d.
>   Wharton's d.
>   d. of Wirsung

Dudley's hook
Dudley-Smith speculum
Duhrssen's incision
Duke's trocar
Duncan's position
Dunhill's hemostat
duodenal
duodenectomy
duodenitis
duodenocholangeitis
duodenocholecystostomy
duodenocholedochotomy
duodenocolic
duodenocystostomy
duodenoduodenostomy
duodenoenterostomy
duodenogram
duodenohepatic
duodenoileostomy
duodenojejunostomy
duodenolysis
duodenorrhaphy
duodenoscopy
duodenostomy
duodenotomy
duodenum
Dupuytren's
>   contracture
>   enterotome

Dupuytren's
   suture
Duvergier's suture
dysfunction
dyskinesia
   biliary d.
dysplasia
Earle's probe
Eastman's clamp
ecchymosis
echinococcosis
echinococcotomy
ectocolostomy
ectokelostomy
ectopic
Edebohls'
   incision
   position
edema
edematous
Eder-Chamberlin gastroscope
Eder-Hufford gastroscope
Eder-Palmer gastroscope
Eder's gastroscope
Edwards' hook
Ekehorn's operation
Elastoplast bandage
electrocautery
electrocholecystectomy
electrocholecystocausis
electrocoagulation
electrodesiccation
electrogastroenterostomy
electrosurgery
Elliot's position
Elliott's forceps
Ellsner's gastroscope
Elsberg's incision

embolectomy
embolism
embolus
Emerson's stripper
Emmet's suture
en bissac
en bloc
encapsulated
endocholedochal
endoscopy
endothyropexy
engorgement
enterauxe
enterectasis
enterectomy
enterelcosis
enteritis
enteroanastomosis
enteroapokleisis
enterocele
enterocentesis
enterochirurgia
enterocholecystostomy
enterocholecystotomy
enterocleisis
enteroclysis
enterocolectomy
enterocolitis
enterocolostomy
enteroenterostomy
enteroepiplocele
enterogastritis
enterohepatopexy
enterolith
enterolithiasis
enteropexy
enteroplasty
enteroplexy

enteroptosis
enterorrhaphy
enterostomy
    Witzel's e.
enterotome
    Dupuytren's e.
enterotomy
enucleation
epauxesiectomy
epidermoid
epigastric
epigastrium
epigastrocele
epigastrorrhaphy
epiglottis
epiplocele
epiploectomy
epiploenterocele
epiploic
epiploitis
epiplomerocele
epiplomphalocele
epiploon
epiplopexy
epiploplasty
epiplorrhaphy
epiplosarcomphalocele
epiploscheocele
epithelialization
epithelialize
epithelium
épluchage
eponychium
erosion
    Dieulafoy's e.
erythema
erythematous
eschar

Esmarch's
    bandage
    scissors
esofa-. See words beginning
    esopha-.
esogastritis
esophagocardiomyotomy
esophagocologastrostomy
esophagoduodenostomy
esophagoenterostomy
esophagofundopexy
esophagogastrectomy
esophagogastroanastomosis
esophagogastroplasty
esophagogastroscopy
esophagogastrostomy
esophagojejunogastrostomosis
esophagojejunostomy
Ethicon suture
Ethilon suture
euthyroid
evagination
eventration
evisceration
excavation
excision
    wound e.
excoriation
exenteration
exenteritis
exploratory
exteriorize
extirpation
extravasation
extrusion
extubate
exudate
falciform

Fansler's
    anoscope
    proctoscope
    speculum
Farris' forceps
fascia
    Camper's f.
    Cloquet's f.
    cremaster f.
    cribriform f.
    external oblique f.
    infundibuloform f.
    f. lata femoris
    pectineal f.
    prepubic f.
    Scarpa's f.
    f. transversalis
    transverse f.
fascial
fasciaplasty
fascioplasty
fasciorrhaphy
fasciotomy
FB — fingerbreadth
    foreign body
fecal
fecalith
fecopurulent
Federoff's splenectomy
Fehland's clamp
Feilchenfeld's forceps
felon
femoral
femorocele
fenestra
Fenger's probe
feokromositoma. See
    pheochromocytoma.

Ferguson-Coley operation
Ferguson-Moon retractor
Ferguson's
    forceps
    operation
    scissors
    scoop
Fergusson's incision
Ferris'
    dilator
    scoop
Ferris-Smith forceps
fiberscope
    Hirschowitz's f.
fibrin
fibrinopurulent
fibroadenoma
fibroadenosis
fibrocystic
fibroma
fibromectomy
fibromyoma
fibromyomectomy
fibromyotomy
fibrosis
fimbria
fimbriated
fingerbreadth
Finney's
    operation
    pyloroplasty
fissure
fistula
fistulectomy
fistulization
fistuloenterostomy
fistulotomy
fistulous

fitobezor. See *phytobezoar.*
flap
    cellulocutaneous f.
    island f.
    musculocutaneous f.
    skin f.
    sliding f.
    surgical f.
flebektomee. See *phlebectomy*
flebitis. See *phlebitis.*
flebo-. See words beginning
    phlebo-.
flegmon. See *phlegmon.*
flexure
    duodenojejunal f.
    hepatic f.
    iliac f.
    sigmoid f.
    splenic f.
fluctuant
fluctuation
Foerster's forceps
Foley's catheter
follicle
    Lieberkühn's f's.
follicular
folliculi
    f. lymphatici aggregati
    f. lymphatici aggregati
      appendicis vermifor-
      mis
    f. lymphatici gastrici
    f. lymphatici lienales
    f. lymphatici recti
    f. lymphatici solitarii
      intestini crassi
    f. lymphatici solitarii
      intestini tenuis

folliculus
foramen
    f. of Bochdalek
    Morgagni's f.
    f. of Winslow
forceps
    ACMI f.
    Adair's f.
    Adson's f.
    Allis' f.
    Allis-Ochsner f.
    Babcock's f.
    Backhaus' f.
    Bainbridge's f.
    Barrett's f.
    Beebe's f.
    Bevan's f.
    Billroth's f.
    Blake's f.
    Blanchard's f.
    Boys-Allis f.
    Bradford's f.
    Brophy's f.
    Brown-Adson f.
    Brown's f.
    Brunner's f.
    Buie's f.
    Carmalt's f.
    Carmody's f.
    Cassidy-Brophy f.
    Collin's f.
    Crile's f.
    Curtis' f.
    Cushing's f.
    DeLee's f.
    Dennis' f.
    Desjardin's f.
    Doyen's f.

forceps *(continued)*

Elliott's f.
Farris' f.
Feilchenfeld's f.
Ferguson's f.
Ferris-Smith f.
Foerster's f.
Foss' f.
Frankfeldt's f.
Fulpit's f.
Glassman-Allis f.
Glassman's f.
Gray's f.
Halsted's f.
Harrington's f.
Healy's f.
Heaney's f.
Hirschman's f.
Hoxworth's f.
Hudson's f.
Jackson's f.
Jones' f.
Judd-Allis f.
Judd-DeMartel f.
Kelly's f.
Kocher's f.
Lahey-Pean f.
Lahey's f.
Lillie's f.
Lockwood's f.
Lovelace's f.
Lower's f.
Maier's f.
Martin's f.
Mayo-Blake f.
Mayo-Ochsner f.
Mayo-Robson f.
Mayo's f.

forceps *(continued)*

McNealy-Glassman-
    Babcock f.
McNealy-Glassman-
    Mixter f.
Mixter's f.
Moynihan's f.
New's f.
Ochsner-Dixon f.
Ochsner's f.
Parker-Kerr f.
Pean's f.
Pennington's f.
Percy's f.
Porter's f.
Potts-Smith f.
Pratt-Smith f.
Providence f.
Rankin's f.
Ratliff-Blake f.
Rochester-Ewald f.
Rochester-Mixter f.
Rochester-Rankin f.
Rochester's f.
Roeder's f.
Russian f.
Schoenberg's f.
Schutz's f.
Scudder's f.
Semken's f.
Shallcross' f.
Singley's f.
Spencer Wells f.
Stille's f.
Stone's f.
Thoms' f.
Thorek-Mixter f.
Virtus' f.

forceps *(continued)*
    Walter's f.
    Walther's f.
    Wangensteen's f.
    Weisenbach's f.
    Welch-Allyn f.
    Williams' f.
    Yeomans' f.
Foss'
  clamp
    forceps
    retractor
fossa
    Hartmann's f.
    Landzert's f.
    Mohrenheim's f.
Fowler's
    incision
    position
Fowler-Weir incision
fragmentation
Frankfeldt's
    forceps
    needle
    sigmoidoscope
    snare
Frank's operation
Franz's retractor
Fredet-Ramstedt
    operation
    pyloromyotomy
fren-. See words beginning
  phren-.
frenulum
frenum
Freund's operation
friable
Friedrich-Petz clamp

FSH — follicle stimulating
  hormone
fulguration
fulminant
fulminate
Fulpit's forceps
fundus
fundusectomy
funiculopexy
funiculus
    f. spermaticus
Furniss'
    clamp
    incision
Furniss-Clute clamp
Furniss-McClure-Hinton clamp
furuncle
furuncular
furunculosis
Gabriel's proctoscope
galactocele
gallbladder
    Courvoisier's g.
Gallie's
    operation
    transplant
gallstone
Gamgee tissue
Gamna nodules
Gandy-Gamna nodules
ganglion
    Acrel's g.
ganglionectomy
ganglionostomy
gangliosympathectomy
gangrene
gangrenous
gasserectomy

gastrectomy
gastritis
    cirrhotic g.
    hypertrophic g.
gastrocele
gastrocolic
gastrocolitis
gastrocolostomy
gastrocolotomy
gastrodiaphany
gastroduodenal
gastroduodenoscopy
gastroduodenostomy
gastroenteritis
gastroenteroanastomosis
gastroenterocolostomy
gastroenteroplasty
gastroenterostomy
    Balfour's g.
    Billroth's g. I and II
    Braun and Jaboulay g.
    Curvoisier's g.
    Heineke-Mikulicz g.
    Hofmeister's g.
    Polya's g.
    Roux's g.
    Schoemaker's g.
    Von Haberer-Finney g.
    Wölfler's g.
gastroenterotomy
gastroepiploic
gastroesophagostomy
gastrogalvanization
gastrogastrostomy
gastrogavage
gastrohepatic
gastroileitis
gastroileostomy

gastrointestinal
gastrojejunocolic
gastrojejunostomy
gastrolysis
gastromegaly
gastromyotomy
gastronesteostomy
gastropexy
gastroplasty
gastroplication
gastroptosis
gastropylorectomy
gastropyloric
gastrorrhaphy
gastrorrhexis
gastroscope
    ACMI g.
    Benedict's g.
    Bernstein's g.
    Chevalier-Jackson g.
    Eder's g.
    Eder-Chamberlin g.
    Eder-Hufford g.
    Eder-Palmer g.
    Ellsner's g.
    Herman-Taylor g.
    Housset-Debray g.
    Janeway's g.
    Kelling's g.
    Schindler's g.
    Wolf-Schindler g.
gastroscopy
gastrosplenic
gastrostomy
    Beck-Jianu g.
    Beck's g.
    DePage-Janeway g.
    Janeway's g.

gastrostomy *(continued)*
> Kader's g.
> Marwedel's g.
> Spivack's g.
> Ssabanajew-Frank g.
> Stamm's g.
> Witzel's g.

gastrotome

gastrotomy

Gatellier's incision

Gaucher's disease

gauze
> Surgicel g.

Gelfilm

Gelfoam

Gély's suture

Gersuny's operation

GI — gastrointestinal

Gibbon's hernia

Gibson-Balfour retractor

Gimbernat's ligament

gland
> adrenal g's.
> Lieberkühn's g's.
> parotid g.
> pineal g.
> pituitary g.
> salivary g.
> sublingual g.
> submaxillary g.
> thyroid g.

Glassman-Allis forceps

Glassman's
> clamp
> forceps

glioma

glossectomy

glossitis

glossoplasty

glossorrhaphy

glossotomy

Goelet's retractor

goiter
> adenomatous g.
> colloid g.
> cystic g.
> exophthalmic g.
> fibrous g.
> nodular g.
> papillomatous g.
> parenchymatous g.
> substernal g.
> toxic g.

Goldbacher's
> anoscope
> needle
> proctoscope
> speculum

Gosset's retractor

Gould's suture

Goyrand's hernia

graft
> cutis g.
> Dacron g.
> fascial g.
> fiber glass g.
> full-thickness skin g.
> Marlex g.
> split thickness skin g.
> tantalum mesh g.
> Teflon g.

Graham-Roscie operation

granulation

granuloma

granulomatous

Gray's forceps

Green's retractor
Greiling's tube
Gridiron's incision
Grieshaber's retractor
Gruber's hernia
Grynfelt's hernia
guarding
Guild-Pratt speculum
Gussenbauer's suture
Gwathmey's oil-ether
    anesthesia
gynecomastia
Hagedorn's needle
Hahn's operation
hallux
        h. malleus
        h. valgus
        h. varus
Halsted's
        forceps
        hemostat
        incision
        operation
        suture
hamartoma
Handley's
        incision
        operation
Harmon's incision
Harrington-Pemberton
        retractor
Harrington's
        forceps
        retractor
Harris's suture
Hartmann's
        fossa
        point

Hartmann's
        pouch
Hashimoto's disease
haustra coli
haustration
haustrum
Hayes' clamp
healing
        h. by first intention
        h. by granulation
        h. by second intention
        h. by third intention
Healy's forceps
Heaney's forceps
Heaton's operation
Heerman's incision
Heineke-Mikulicz
        gastroenterostomy
        operation
        pyloroplasty
Heineke's operation
Heller's operation
hemangioma
hemangiosarcoma
hematemesis
hematoma
hemicolectomy
hemicorporectomy
hemigastrectomy
hemihepatectomy
hemipylorectomy
hemisection
hemithyroidectomy
hemoptysis
hemorrhage
hemorrhagic
hemorrhoid
        combined h.

hemorrhoid *(continued)*
    external h.
    internal h.
    lingual h.
    mixed h.
    mucocutaneous h.
    prolapsed h.
    strangulated h.
    thrombosed h.
hemorrhoidal
hemorrhoidectomy
hemostasis
hemostat
    Dunhill's h.
    Halsted's h.
    Maingot's h.
hemovac
Henke's triangle
Henry's
    incision
    operation
    splenectomy
hepatectomize
hepatectomy
hepatic
hepaticocholangiocholecyst-
    enterostomy
hepaticocholangiojejunostomy
hepaticodochotomy
hepaticoduodenostomy
hepaticoenterostomy
hepaticogastrostomy
hepaticojejunostomy
hepaticolithotomy
hepaticolithotripsy
hepaticostomy
hepaticotomy
hepatitis

hepatobiliary
hepatocele
hepatocholangiocystoduo-
    denostomy
hepatocholangioduodenos-
    tomy
hepatocholangioenterostomy
hepatocholangiogastrostomy
hepatocholangiostomy
hepatocirrhosis
hepatoduodenostomy
hepatoenterostomy
hepatogastric
hepatolithectomy
hepatomegaly
hepatopexy
hepatorrhaphy
hepatosplenomegaly
hepatostomy
hepatotomy
hephestiorrhaphy
Herff's clamp
Herman-Taylor gastroscope
hernia
    abdominal h.
    acquired h.
    h. adiposa
    amniotic h.
    Barth's h.
    Béclard's h.
    Birkett's h.
    cecal h.
    Cloquet's h.
    Cooper's h.
    crural h.
    diaphragmatic h.
    diverticular h.
    duodenojejunal h.

hernia *(continued)*
- encysted h.
- epigastric h.
- extrasaccular h.
- femoral h.
- foraminal h.
- funicular h.
- gastroesophageal h.
- Gibbon's h.
- gluteal h.
- Goyrand's h.
- Gruber's h.
- Grynfelt's h.
- Hesselbach's h.
- Hey's h.
- hiatal h.
- hiatus h.
- Holthouse's h.
- incarcerated h.
- incisional h.
- indirect h.
- infantile h.
- inguinal h.
- inguinocrural h.
- inguinofemoral h.
- inguinoproperitoneal h.
- inguinosuperficial h.
- h. in recto
- intermuscular h.
- interparietal h.
- intersigmoid h.
- interstitial h.
- irreducible h.
- ischiatic h.
- ischiorectal h.
- Krönlein's h.
- Küster's h.
- labial h.

hernia *(continued)*
- Laugier's h.
- levator h.
- linea alba h.
- Littre-Richter h.
- Littre's h.
- lumbar h.
- Maydl's h.
- mesenteric h.
- mesocolic h.
- mucosal h.
- oblique h.
- obturator h.
- omental h.
- ovarian h.
- pantaloon h.
- paraduodenal h.
- paraesophageal h.
- paraperitoneal h.
- parasaccular h.
- h. par glissement
- parietal h.
- parumbilical h.
- pectineal h.
- perineal h.
- Petit's h.
- properitoneal h.
- pudendal h.
- pulsion h.
- rectal h.
- reducible h.
- retrocecal h.
- retrograde h.
- retroperitoneal h.
- Richter's h.
- Riex's h.
- Rokitansky's h.
- sciatic h.

hernia *(continued)*
    scrotal h.
    sliding h.
    spigelian h.
    strangulated h.
    subpubic h.
    synovial h.
    thyroidal h.
    Treitz's h.
    tunicary h.
    umbilical h.
    uterine h.
    vaginal h.
    vaginolabial h.
    Velpeau's h.
    ventral h.
    vesical h.
    voluminous h.
    Von Bergmann's h.
    w h.
hernial
herniary
herniated
herniation
hernioappendectomy
hernioenterotomy
hernioid
herniolaparotomy
hernioplasty
herniopuncture
herniorrhaphy
herniotome
herniotomy
Hesselbach's
    hernia
    ligament
    triangle
heteroautoplasty

Hey-Grooves' operation
Hey's hernia
hiatal
hiatopexy
hiatus
hidradenitis
    h. suppurativa
Higgins' incision
Hill-Ferguson retractor
hilum
hilus
Hinckle-James speculum
Hirschman-Martin proctoscope
Hirschman's
    anoscope
    forceps
    proctoscope
Hirschowitz's fiberscope
Hirschsprung's disease
Hochenegg's operation
Hofmeister's gastroenteros-
    tomy
Hoguet's maneuver
Holthouse's hernia
homograft
homoplastic
homoplasty
Hood and Kirklin incision
hook
    Barr's h.
    Dudley's h.
    Edwards' h.
    Pratt's h.
    Rosser's h.
    Stewart's h.
    Welch-Allyn h.
Hopkins' operation
Horsley's pyloroplasty

Hotchkiss' operation
Houget's operation
Housset-Debray gastroscope
Houston's valve
Hoxworth's forceps
Hudson's forceps
Hunt's
    clamp
    operation
Hurwitz's clamp
hydrocele
hydrocelectomy
hydroperitoneum
hydrops
    h. abdominis
hygroma
hyperemic
hyperinsulinism
hyperparathyroidism
hyperpituitarism
hyperplasia
hyperthyroidism
hypertonic
hypertrophic
hypertrophy
hypochondrium
hypocystotomy
hypodermatomy
hypogastric
hypoparathyroidism
hypophysectomy
hypopituitarism
hypoplasia
hypothermia
hypothyroidism
hypotonic
Hyrtl's sphincter
I^{131} — radioactive iodine

I & D — incision and drainage
ileac
ileal
ileectomy
ileitis
    distal i.
    regional i.
    terminal i.
ileocecal
ileocecostomy
ileocecum
ileocolic
ileocolitis
    i. ulcerosa chronica
ileocolostomy
ileocolotomy
ileocystoplasty
ileoileostomy
ileoproctostomy
ileorectal
ileorectostomy
ileorrhaphy
ileosigmoid
ileosigmoidostomy
ileostomy
ileotomy
ileotransversostomy
ileum
    terminal i.
ileus
iliocolotomy
iliohypogastric
ilioinguinal
iliolumbocostoabdominal
iliopectineal
iliopubic
imbricated
imbrication

impaction
implant
    Silastic i.
incarcerated
incarceration
incised
incision
    abdominal i.
    abdominothoracic i.
    Alexander's i.
    arcuate i.
    areolar i.
    Auvray's i.
    Bardenheuer's i.
    Bar's i.
    Battle-Jalaguier-
      Kammerer i.
    Battle's i.
    Bergman-Israel i.
    Bergmann's i.
    Bevan's i.
    Brackin's i.
    Brock's i.
    buttonhole i.
    celiotomy i.
    Cherney's i.
    Chiene's i.
    circular i.
    circumareolar i.
    circumferential i.
    circumlimbar i.
    circumscribing i.
    Clute's i.
    Codman's i.
    Coffey's i.
    collar i.
    confirmatory i.
    Courvoisier's i.

incision *(continued)*
    crescent i.
    crosshatch i.
    cruciate i.
    curved i.
    curvilinear i.
    Deaver's i.
    Duhrssen's i.
    Edebohls' i.
    elliptical i.
    Elsberg's i.
    endaural i.
    exploratory i.
    Fergusson's i.
    flank i.
    Fowler's i.
    Fowler-Weir i.
    Furniss' i.
    Gatellier's i.
    Gridiron's i.
    Halsted's i.
    Handley's i.
    Harmon's i.
    Heerman's i.
    Henry's i.
    Higgins' i.
    hockey-stick i.
    Hood and Kirklin i.
    infraumbilical i.
    inguinal i.
    Jackson's i.
    J-shaped i.
    Kammerer's i.
    Kehr's i.
    Kocher's i.
    Küstner's i.
    Lamm's i.
    Langenbeck's i.

incision *(continued)*
- lateral flank i.
- lateral rectus i.
- Lempert's i.
- Lilienthal's i.
- linear i.
- longitudinal i.
- Lonquet's i.
- Mackenrodt's i.
- Mason's i.
- Mayo-Robson i.
- McArthur's i.
- McBurney's i.
- McLaughlin's i.
- median i.
- Meyer's hockey stick i.
- midline i.
- Morison's i.
- muscle splitting i.
- oblique i.
- Ollier's i.
- Orr's i.
- paracostal i.
- paramedian i.
- paramuscular i.
- pararectus i.
- parascapular i.
- Parker's i.
- Pean's i.
- periareolar i.
- perilimbal i.
- Perthes' i.
- Pfannenstiel's i.
- Phemister's i.
- pyelotomy i.
- racquet i.
- radial i.
- rectus muscle splitting i.

incision *(continued)*
- recumbent i.
- relaxing i.
- relief i.
- Risdon's extraoral i.
- Rocky-Davis' i.
- Rodman's i.
- Rollet's i.
- Rosen's i.
- Roux-en-y jejunal loop i.
- saber-cut i.
- Sanders' i.
- Schobinger's i.
- Schuchardt's i.
- scratch type i.
- semicircular i.
- semilunar i.
- serpentine i.
- shoulder-strap i.
- Simon's i.
- Singleton's i.
- skinline i.
- Sloan's i.
- Smith-Peterson i.
- stab wound i.
- stellate i.
- Stewart's i.
- subcostal i.
- subumbilical i.
- supracervical i.
- suprapubic i.
- supraumbilical i.
- T-shaped i.
- Thomas-Warren i.
- thoracoabdominal i.
- Timbrall-Fisher i.
- transmeatal i.
- transrectus i.

incision *(continued)*
>   transverse i.
>   T-shaped i.
>   U-shaped i.
>   V-shaped i.
>   vertical i.
>   Vischer's i.
>   Warren's i.
>   Watson-Jones i.
>   Weber-Fergusson i.
>   Whipple's i.
>   Wilde's i.
>   Willie-Meyer i.
>   Y-type i.
>   Z-flap i.
>   Z-plasty i.
>   Z-shaped i.

incisura
>   i. angularis ventriculi
>   i. cardiaca ventriculi

inclusion
incontinence
indurated
induration
infarction
>   intestinal i.

infiltration
inflammation
inframamillary
inframammary
infundibula
infundibuliform
infundibulopelvic
infundibulum
Ingals' cannula
inguinal
inguinoabdominal
inguinocrural

inguinolabial
inguinoscrotal
Inlay's operation
inoperable
in situ
instillation
insufflation
insufflator
>   Buckstein's i.
>   Weber's i.

intercostal
interstitial
intestinal
intestine
intractable
intracystic
intraductal
intubation
intumescence
intussusception
intussusceptum
intussuscipiens
invagination
inversion
inverted
irradiation
irrigator
>   Buie's i.

ischioanal
ischiococcygeal
ischiorectal
ischochymia
island
>   i's of Langerhans

Israel's retractor
isthmectomy
isthmus
Ives' anoscope

Jaboulay's
  button
  operation
  pyloroplasty
Jackson's
  forceps
  incision
  retractor
Janeway's
  gastroscope
  gastrostomy
Jarvis' clamp
jaundice
jejunectomy
jejunitis
jejunocecostomy
jejunocolostomy
jejunoileitis
jejunoileostomy
jejunojejunostomy
jejunorrhaphy
jejunostomy
jejunotomy
jejunum
Jobert's suture
Johnson's tube
Jones'
  forceps
  scissors
Jorgenson's scissors
Judd-Allis forceps
Judd-DeMartel forceps
Judd's pyloroplasty
juncture
  saphenofemoral j.
Jutte tube
Kader's gastrostomy
Kammerer's incision

Kapp-Beck clamp
Keeley's stripper
Keel's operation
Keen's operation
Kehr's incision
Keith's needle
Kelling's gastroscope
Kelly's
  clamp
  forceps
  proctoscope
  retractor
  sigmoidoscope
  tubes
keloid
keloplasty
kelotomy
kemo-. See words beginning
  chemo-.
keratosis
Kerlex dressing
kyl. See *chyle.*
Killian-King retractor
King's retractor
Kirschner's wire
Klemme's retractor
knife
  Bonta's k.
Knowles' scissors
Kocher-Crotti retractor
kocherization
Kocher's
  clamp
  dissector
  forceps
  incision
  operation
  ulcer

koilonychia
kol-. See words beginning
    chol-.
kolangi-. See words beginning
    cholangi-.
kole-. See words beginning
    chole-.
kolo-. See words beginning
    cholo-.
Kraske's
    position
    retractor
Krönlein's hernia
Kron's
    dilator
    probe
Kulenkampff's anesthesia
Kurten's stripper
Küster's hernia
Küstner's incision
laceration
lacuna
    l. musculorum
    l. vasorum
lacunar
Lahey-Pean forceps
Lahey's
    carrier
    forceps
    operation
    retractor
    tenaculum
lamella
lamina
Lamm's incision
Landzert's fossa
Lane's
    catheter

Lane's
    clamp
Langenbeck's incision
Langerhans' islands
laparectomy
laparocholecystotomy
laparocolostomy
laparocolotomy
laparocystectomy
laparocystidotomy
laparoenterostomy
laparoenterotomy
laparogastroscopy
laparogastrostomy
laparogastrotomy
laparohepatotomy
laparoileotomy
laparomyomectomy
laparorrhaphy
laparoscope
laparoscopy
laparosplenectomy
laparosplenotomy
laparotome
laparotomy
laparotyphlotomy
Lardennois' button
La Roque's technique
Larry's
    director
    probe
laser
Laugier's hernia
lavage
Le Dran's suture
leiomyoma
leiomyomata
Lembert's suture

Lempert's incision
Lempka's stripper
lesion
leukonychia
Levin's tube
Lieberkühn's
    crypts
    follicles
    glands
Lieberman's
    proctoscope
    sigmoidoscope
lien
    l. accessorius
    l. mobilis
lienal
lienculus
lienopancreatic
lienorenal
ligament
    arcuate l.
    Cooper's l.
    gastrohepatic l.
    gastrolienal l.
    gastrophrenic l.
    Gimbernat's l.
    hepatogastric l.
    Hesselbach's l.
    inguinal l.
    lacunar l.
    lienorenal l.
    pancreaticosplenic l.
    pectineal l.
    phrenicocolic l.
    phrenicolienal l.
    phrenicosplenic l.
    Poupart's l.
    splenocolic l.

ligament (*continued*)
    splenorenal l.
    l. of Treitz
ligation
    high saphenous vein l.
ligature
    McGraw's elastic l.
Lilienthal's incision
Lillie's forceps
line
    iliopectineal l.
    pectinate l.
    pectineal l.
    Spieghel's l.
linea
    l. alba
    l. semilunaris
linitis
    l. plastica
lipectomy
lipoma
Lister's
    dressing
    scissors
lithotome
lithotomy
lithotony
lithotresis
Littauer's scissors
Little's retractor
Littre-Richter hernia
Littre's
    hernia
    suture
lobe
    Riedel's l.
lobectomy
lobular

lobule
lobulette
lobulus
Lockwood's
    clamp
    forceps
Löffler's suture
Lonquet's incision
Lotheissen-McVay technique
Lotheissen's operation
Lovelace's forceps
Lower's forceps
Luer-Korte scoop
lumen
lunula
Luschka's crypts
lymphadenectomy
lymphadenitis
lymphadenopathy
    giant follicular l.
lymphosarcoma
Lynch's operation
lyse
lysis
MacDonald's clamp
Macewen's operation
Mackenrodt's incision
Mackid's operation
Maier's forceps
Maingot's hemostat
Mair's operation
malacotomy
malignant
malpighian bodies
mamilla
mamma
mammary
mammectomy

mammiform
mammilliplasty
    Ashford's m.
mammogram
mammography
mammoplasia
mammoplasty
    augmentation m.
maneuver
    Hoguet's m.
Mann-Williamson ulcer
Manson's schistosomiasis
Mantz's dilator
Marcy's operation
Marlex
    graft
    mesh
    suture
marsupialization
Martin's
    forceps
    needle
    retractor
    speculum
Marwedel's
    gastrostomy
    operation
Mason's incision
mastadenitis
mastadenoma
mastectomy
masthelcosis
Mastin's clamp
mastitis
mastocarcinoma
mastochondroma
mastodynia
mastogram

mastography
mastoncus
mastopathia
    m. cystica
mastopathy
    cystic m.
mastopexy
mastoplastia
mastoptosis
mastorrhagia
mastoscirrhus
mastosis
mastostomy
mastotomy
Mathew's speculum
matrix
Maunsell suture
maxilla
Maydl's
    hernia
    operation
Mayo-Blake forceps
Mayo-Collins retractor
Mayo-Harrington scissors
Mayo-Lovelace retractor
Mayo-Noble scissors
Mayo-Ochsner forceps
Mayo-Robson
    forceps
    incision
    operation
    position
    scoop
Mayo-Sims scissors
Mayo's
    carrier
    forceps
    needle

Mayo's *(continued)*
    operation
    probe
    retractor
    scissors
    scoop
    stripper
McArthurs'
    incision
    method
    operation
McBurney's
    incision
    operation
    point
W. Dean McDonald clamp
McEvedy's operation
McGraw's elastic ligature
McLaughlin's incision
McNealy-Glassman-Babcock
    forceps
McNealy-Glassman-Mixter
    forceps
McVay's operation
Meckel's diverticulum
mediastinal
mediastinum
Medications
    Amethocaine
    amobarbital
    Amytal
    Anectine
    Anesthesin
    apothesine
    Aristocort
    Atropine
    Benzocaine
    Brevital

Medications *(continued)*

- Butadiene
- Carbocaine
- chloral hydrate
- chloroform
- chloroprocaine
- Cinchocaine
- Citanest
- cocaine
- Corticotropin
- cortisone
- Cyclaine
- Cyclohexane
- cyclomethycaine
- Cyclopentane
- Cyclopropane
- dibucaine
- diethyl ether
- Dyclone
- dyclonine
- Epinephrine
- ether
- ethyl aminobenzoate
- ethyl chloride
- Ethylene
- Ethyl ether
- Fluothane
- Freon
- Germa-Medica
- halothane
- Hexa-Germ
- hexylcaine
- Kenalog
- Largon
- lidocaine
- mepivacaine
- methohexital
- methylatropine nitrate

Medications *(continued)*

- Nesacaine
- nitrous oxide
- Noctec
- Novocain
- Nupercaine
- Penthrane
- Pentothal
- pHisoderm
- pHisoHex
- Piperocaine
- Pontocaine
- prilocaine
- procaine
- propiomazine
- Propitocaine
- Quelicin
- Sarapin
- scopolamine
- Septisol
- Somnos
- succinylcholine
- Sucostrin
- Surfacaine
- Surital
- tetracaine
- Thiamylal
- thiopental
- triamcinolone acetonide
- vinyl ethyl ether
- Xylocaine

medusa
megacolon
megalogastria
Meltzer's anesthesia
membrane
    Cargile m.
membranous

Menghini's needle
Mercurio's position
Mermingas' operation
Mersilene suture
mesenteric
mesenteriopexy
mesenteriorrhaphy
mesenteriplication
mesentery
mesentorrhaphy
mesh
    Marlex m.
    tantalum m.
    Teflon m.
mesoappendicitis
mesoappendix
mesocecum
mesocolon
    ascending m.
    descending m.
    sigmoid m.
    transverse m.
mesocoloplication
mesogastrium
mesorectum
mesosigmoid
mesosigmoidopexy
metastases
metastasis
metastatic
metatarsal
method
    McArthur's m.
    Morison's m.
Metzenbaum's scissors
Meyerding's retractor
Meyer's
    hockey stick incision

Meyer's
    retractor
MFB — metallic foreign body
microgastria
microsurgery
Mikulicz's operation
Miles' operation
milium
    colloid m.
Miller-Abbott tube
Miller's scissors
Mixter's forceps
Mohrenheim's fossa
Montague's
    proctoscope
    sigmoidoscope
Moore's scoop
Moreno's clamp
Morgagni's foramen
Morison's
    incision
    method
    pouch
Morton's toe
Moschcowitz's operation
motility
Moynihan's
    clamp
    forceps
    operation
    probe
    scoop
mucocutaneous
mucopurulent
mucosa
Mueller-Frazier tube
Mueller-Pool tube
Mueller-Pynchon tube

Mueller-Yankauer tube
Muer's anoscope
multilocular
Murphy's
> button
> dilator
> needle
> retractor

muscle
> cremaster m.
> deltoid m.
> external oblique m.
> internal oblique m.
> latissimus dorsi m.
> masseter m.
> pectineus m.
> pectoralis major m.
> pectoralis minor m.
> pyramidalis m.
> rectococcygeal m.
> rectus m.
> scalene m.
> serratus anterior m.
> serratus magnus m.
> sternohyoid m.
> sternothyroid m.
> subscapularis m.
> transversus m.

Myers' stripper
myoma
myomectomy
myotomy
Nabatoff's stripper
Nachlas' tube
Narath's operation
narcosis
> Nussbaum's n.

necrosis

needle
> Childs-Phillips n.
> Frankfeldt's n.
> Goldbacher's n.
> Hagedorn's n.
> Keith's n.
> Martin's n.
> Mayo's n.
> Menghini's n.
> Murphy's n.
> Reverdin's n.
> Rochester's n.
> Silverman's n.

neoplasm
neoplastic
nerve
> hypogastric n.
> iliohypogastric n.
> ilioinguinal n.
> phrenic n.

neurectomy
> gastric n.

nevus
> melanocytic n.
> pigmented n.

Newman's proctoscope
New's
> forceps
> scissors

nipple
> invaginated n.

Noble's position
node
> axillary n's.
> cervical lymph n's.
> Delphian n.

nodular
nodule

nodule *(continued)*
    Gamna n's.
    Gandy-Gamna n's.
Northbent's scissors
Norwood's snare
NPO – nothing by mouth
    (nulla per os)
Nuck's canal
Nussbaum's
    clamp
    narcosis
Nuttall's operation
O'Beirne's
    sphincter
    tube
Oberst's operation
oblique
    external o.
    internal o.
obliteration
obstruction
    intestinal o.
obturator
    Cripps's o.
occlusion
    enteromesenteric o.
occult
Ochsner-Dixon forceps
Ochsner's
    clamp
    forceps
    scissors
    tube
Oddi's sphincter
Ogilvie's operation
Ollier's incision
omentectomy
omentopexy

omentoplasty
omentorrhaphy
omentosplenopexy
omentotomy
omentum
    gastrocolic o.
    gastrohepatic o.
    gastrosplenic o.
omfal-. See words beginning
    omphal-.
omphalectomy
omphalelcosis
omphalic
omphalitis
omphalocele
onychauxis
onychectomy
onychia
onychomycosis
onychorrhexis
onychotomy
operation
    Abbe's o.
    Abernethy's o.
    Adams' o.
    Allarton's o.
    Allingham's o.
    Amussat's o.
    Andrews' o.
    Anson-McVay o.
    Appolito's o.
    Armsby's o.
    Babcock's o.
    Ball's o.
    Bassini's o.
    Battle's o.
    Baynton's o.
    Beatson's o.

operation *(continued)*

Belmas' o.
Best's o.
Bevans' o.
Beyea's o.
Billroth's o.
Bircher's o.
Bloodgood's o.
Bobb's o.
Bogue's o.
Bose's o.
Brenner's o.
Brunschwig's o.
Bryant's o.
Callisen's o.
Cattell's o.
Chaput's o.
Cheyne's o.
Chiazzi's o.
Child's o.
Cooper's o.
Cotting's o.
Cripp's o.
Czerny's o.
Dallas' o.
Denans' o.
Dieffenbach's o.
Dowell's o.
Drummond-Morison o.
Ekehorn's o.
Ferguson-Coley o.
Ferguson's o.
Finney's o.
Frank's o.
Fredet-Ramstedt o.
Freund's o.
Gallie's o.
Gersuny's o.

operation *(continued)*

Graham-Roscie o.
Hahn's o.
Halsted's o.
Handley's o.
Heaton's o.
Heineke-Mikulicz o.
Heineke's o.
Heller's o.
Henry's o.
Hey-Grooves o.
Hochenegg's o.
Hopkins' o.
Hotchkiss' o.
Houget's o.
Hunt's o.
Inlay's o.
Jaboulay's o.
Keel's o.
Keen's o.
Kocher's o.
Lahey's o.
Lotheissen's o.
Lynch's o.
Macewen's o.
Mackid's o.
Mair's o.
Marcy's o.
Marwedel's o.
Maydl's o.
Mayo-Robson o.
Mayo's o.
McArthur's o.
McBurney's o.
McEvedy's o.
McVay's o.
Mermingas' o.
Mikulicz's o.

operation *(continued)*

    Miles' o.
    Moschcowitz's o.
    Moynihan's o.
    Narath's o.
    Nuttall's o.
    Oberst's o.
    Ogilvie's o.
    Pirogoff's o.
    Polya's o.
    Poth's o.
    Ramstedt's o.
    Rehn-Delorme o.
    Scarpa's o.
    Schede's o.
    Schlatter's o.
    Sotteau's o.
    Talma's o.
    Tanner's o.
    Torek's o.
    Travel's o.
    Trendelenburg's o.
    Turner's o.
    van Buren's o.
    Vermale's o.
    Verneuil's o.
    Wangensteen's o.
    Warren's o.
    Watson's o.
    Waugh's o.
    Weir's o.
    Whipple's o.
    Wise's o.
    Witzel's o.
    Wölfler's o.
    Wützer's o.
    Wyeth's o.
    Wyllys-Andrews o.

operation *(continued)*

    Zieman's o.
    Zimmerman's o.
    Z-plasty
operable
OR – operating room
organomegaly
Orr's incision
os
    o. pubis
O'Sullivan-O'Connor retractor
O'Sullivan's retractor
Otis' anoscope
Ottenheimer's dilator
oxyuriasis
Oxyuris
    O. vermicularis
Pagenstecher's linen thread
Paget's disease
Palfyn's suture
palliative
pampiniform
pancolectomy
pancreas
    Willis' p.
    Winslow's p.
pancreatectomy
pancreatic
pancreaticoduodenostomy
pancreaticoenterostomy
pancreaticogastrostomy
pancreaticojejunostomy
pancreatitis
pancreatoduodenectomy
pancreatography
pancreatolithectomy
pancreatolithotomy
pancreatotomy

panniculus
panproctocolectomy
Panzer's scissors
papilla
    p. of Vater
papillae
papillary
papillate
papillectomy
papilloma
papillosphincterotomy
paracentesis
    abdominal p.
    p. abdominis
    p. vesicae
parathyroid
parathyroidectomy
Paré's suture
parenchyma
parietal
Parker-Kerr
    "basting stitch"
    forceps
Parker's
    clamp
    incision
    retractor
paronychia
parotid
parotidectomy
parotitis
pars
    p. pylorica
    p. superior duodeni
paste
    Unna's p.
patency
patent

Paul Mixter tube
Payr's clamp
Péan's
    clamp
    forceps
    incision
    position
peau
    p. d'orange
pectenotomy
pectineal
pectoral
pectoralis
pedicle
peduncle
pedunculated
pelvis
Pemberton's clamp
pendulous
Pennington's
    forceps
    speculum
Penrose drain
peptic
percutaneous
Percy's forceps
perforation
perianal
periappendicitis
perigastric
perineal
perineorrhaphy
perineum
periphery
perirectal
peristalsis
peristaltic
peritoneal

peritonealize
peritoneocentesis
peritoneoplasty
peritoneoscopy
peritoneotomy
peritoneum
    parietal p.
    visceral p.
peritonitis
peritonization
peritonize
perityphlitis
    p. actinomycotica
periumbilical
per primam intentionem
Perthes' incision
Petit's
    hernia
    suture
Pfannenstiel's incision
phalanx
Phemister's incision
pheochromocytoma
Phillips' clamp
phlebectomy
phlebitis
phlebolith
phlebolithiasis
phleboplasty
phlebosclerosis
phlebothrombosis
phlebotomy
phlegmon
phrenemphraxis
phrenic
phrenicectomized
phrenicectomy
phreniclasis

phrenicoexeresis
phreniconeurectomy
phrenicotomy
phrenicotripsy
phytobezoar
pillar
pilonidal
pinealectomy
pinealoma
Pirogoff's operation
pituitectomy
plantar
platysma
pledget
plexus
    brachial p.
    pampiniform p.
plica
    p. duodenalis
    p. duodenojejunalis
    p. duodenomesocolica
    p. epigastrica
    p. gastropancreatica
    p. ileocecalis
    p. paraduodenalis
    p. umbilicalis
plication
plombage
po dorahnj. See *peau d'orange.*
point
    Hartmann's p.
    McBurney's p.
pollicization
Polya's
    gastroenterostomy
    operation
Polydek suture
polyethylene

polyp
polypectomy
polypoid
polyposis
    p. gastrica
    p. intestinalis
    p. ventriculi
polypotome
polyunguia
pons
    p. hepatis
Pool's tube
porta
    p. hepatis
    p. lienis
portacaval
portal
    intestinal p.
Porter's forceps
position
    Adams' p.
    Albert's p.
    anatomical p.
    arm-extension p.
    Boyce's p.
    Bozeman's p.
    Buie's p.
    Casselberry's p.
    chest p.
    coiled p.
    decubitus p.
    Depage's p.
    dorsal p.
    dorsal elevated p.
    dorsal inertia p.
    dorsal lithotomy p.
    dorsal recumbent p.
    dorsal rigid p.

position *(continued)*
    dorsosacral p.
    Duncan's p.
    Edebohls' p.
    Elliot's p.
    emprosthotonos p.
    Fowler's p.
    frog-legged p.
    genucubital p.
    genupectoral p.
    head dependent p.
    hinge p.
    horizontal p.
    hornpipe p.
    jacknife p.
    knee-chest p.
    knee-elbow p.
    kneeling-squatting p.
    Kraske's p.
    lateral prone p.
    lateral recumbent p.
    lithotomy p.
    Mayo-Robson p.
    Mercurio's p.
    neck extension p.
    Noble's p.
    opisthotonos p.
    orthopnea p.
    orthotonos p.
    Péan's p.
    Proetz's p.
    prone p.
    rest p.
    Robson's p.
    Rose's p.
    Scultetus' p.
    semiprone p.
    semireclining p.

position *(continued)*
    shoe-and-stocking p.
    Simon's position
    Sims' p.
    Stern's p.
    supine p.
    Trendelenburg's p.
    Valentine's p.
    Walcher's p.
    Wolfenden's p.
Poth's operation
Potts-Smith forceps
pouch
    Hartmann's p.
    Morison's p.
Poupart's
    ligament
    shelving edge, of P's.
      ligament
Pratt-Smith forceps
Pratt's
    anoscope
    director
    hook
    probe
    scissors
    speculum
prepped and draped
probe
    Barr's p.
    Buie's p.
    Desjardin's p.
    Earle's p.
    Fenger's p.
    Kron's p.
    Larry's p.
    Mayo's p.
    Moynihan's p.

probe *(continued)*
    Pratt's p.
    Welch-Allyn p.
procedure
    Buie's p.
procidentia
proctalgia
    p. fugax
proctectasia
proctectomy
procteurynter
proctitis
proctococcypexy
proctocolectomy
proctocolitis
proctocolpoplasty
proctocystoplasty
proctocystotomy
procto–elytroplasty
proctologic
proctology
proctoperineoplasty
proctopexy
proctoplasty
proctoptosis
proctorrhaphy
proctoscope
    ACMI
    Boehm's p.
    Fansler's p.
    Gabriel's p.
    Goldbacher's p.
    Hirschman-Martin p.
    Hirschman's p.
    Kelly's p.
    Lieberman's p.
    Montague's p.
    Newman's p.

proctoscope *(continued)*
    Pruitt's p.
    Turell's p.
    Tuttle's p.
    Vernon-David p.
    Welch-Allyn p.
    Yeomans' p.
proctoscopy
proctosigmoidectomy
proctosigmoiditis
proctosigmoidoscopy
proctostenosis
proctostomy
proctotome
proctotomy
proctovalvotomy
Proetz's position
prolapse
    rectal p.
prolapsus
    p. ani
    p. recti
proliferation
properitoneal
prosthesis
protrusion
Providence forceps
Pruitt's
    anoscope
    proctoscope
pruritus
    p. ani
pseudocyst
    pancreatic p.
psoas
pubic
pubioplasty
pubiotomy

pubis
pudendal
pudic
pulsatile
punctate
puncture
    epigastric p.
Purcell's retractor
purulent
pylon
pylorectomy
pyloric
pyloristenosis
pylorodilator
pylorodiosis
pyloroduodenitis
pylorogastrectomy
pyloromyotomy
    Fredet-Ramstedt p.
pyloroplasty
    Finney's p.
    Heineke-Mikulicz p.
    Horsley's p.
    Jaboulay's p.
    Judd's p.
    Ramstedt's p.
pyloroptosis
pyloroscopy
pylorospasm
pylorostomy
pylorotomy
pylorus
Pynchon's tube
pyocelia
pyramid
    p. of thyroid
pyramidalis
raclage

radioisotope
rafe. See *raphe.*
Ramdohr's suture
Ramstedt's
    dilator
    operation
    pyloroplasty
ramus
Rankin's
    clamp
    forceps
Ranzewski's clamp
ranula
    pancreatic r.
raphe
Ratliff-Blake forceps
rectal
rectectomy
rectocele
rectorectostomy
rectoromanoscopy
rectoscopy
rectosigmoid
rectosigmoidectomy
rectostomy
rectovaginal
rectovesical
rectum
redundant
Rehn-Delorme operation
reperitonealize
resection
    gastric r.
retinaculum
retractor
    Alm's r.
    Balfour's r.
    Beckman's r.

retractor *(continued)*
    Berens' r.
    Berna's r.
    Buie-Smith r.
    Byford's r.
    Cole's r.
    Crile's r.
    Deaver's r.
    Ferguson-Moon r.
    Foss' retractor
    Franz's r.
    Gibson-Balfour r.
    Goelet's r.
    Gosset's r.
    Green's r.
    Grieshaber's r.
    Harrington-Pemberton r.
    Harrington's r.
    Hill-Ferguson r.
    Israel's r.
    Jackson's r.
    Kelly's r.
    Killian-King r.
    King's r.
    Klemme's r.
    Kocher-Crotti r.
    Krasky's r.
    Lahey's r.
    Little's r.
    Martin's r.
    Mayo-Collins r.
    Mayo-Lovelace r.
    Mayo's r.
    Meyerding's r.
    Meyer's r.
    Murphy's r.
    O'Sullivan's r.
    Parker's r.

retractor *(continued)*
    Purcell's r.
    Richardson-Eastman r.
    Richardson's r.
    Rigby's r.
    Rochester-Ferguson r.
    Roux's r.
    Senn's r.
    Sistrunk's r.
    Sloan's r.
    Smith-Buie r.
    Theis' r.
    Volkmann's r.
    Walker's r.
    Walter-Deaver r.
    Webster's r.
    Weinberg's r.
    Weitlaner's r.
    Wolfson's r.
retrocecal
retroflexion
retrograde
retromammary
retroperitoneal
retroversion
Reverdin's needle
Richardson-Eastman retractor
Richardson's retractor
Richter's
    hernia
    suture
Riedel's
    disease
    lobe
    struma
Riex's hernia
Rigal's suture
Rigby's retractor

rima
ring
    Abbe's r's.
    inguinal r.
Ringer's lactate solution
Risdon's extraoral incision
Ritisch's suture
Rives' splenectomy
Robson's position
Rochester-Ewald forceps
Rochester-Ferguson
    retractor
    scissors
Rochester-Mixter forceps
Rochester-Rankin forceps
Rochester's
    forceps
    needle
Rocky-Davis' incision
Rodman's incision
Roeder's forceps
Rokitansky's hernia
Rollet's incision
Roosevelt's clamp
Rosen's incision
Rose's position
rosette
Rosser's hook
Roux-en-y
    cystojejunostomy
    jejunal loop incision
Roux's
    gastroenterostomy
    retractor
    sign
Rovsing's sign
RR — Recovery Room
ruga

ruga
    r. gastrica
rugae
rupture
Russian forceps
Ryle's tube
sac
    hernial s.
saccular
sacculation
sacculus
Sanders' incision
sanguineous
Santorini's duct
saphenectomy
saphenofemoral
saphenous
sarcoid
sarcoma
saucerization
saw
    Butcher's s.
scalene
scalenectomy
scalenotomy
scalenus
scalpel
Scarpa's
    fascia
    operation
    sheath
    triangle
Schede's operation
Schindler's gastroscope
schistosomiasis
    intestinal s.
    Manson's s.
Schlange's sign

Schlatter's operation
Schobinger's incision
Schoemaker's
    clamp
    gastroenterostomy
Schoenberg's forceps
Schuchardt's incision
Schutz's forceps
scirrhous
scirrhus
scissors
    Berbridge's s.
    Brooks' s.
    Buie's s.
    Burnham's s.
    Deaver's s.
    DeBakey's s.
    Doyen's s.
    Esmarch's s.
    Ferguson's s.
    Jones' s.
    Jorgenson's s.
    Knowles' s.
    Lister's s.
    Littauer's s.
    Mayo-Harrington s.
    Mayo-Noble s.
    Mayo-Sims s.
    Mayo's s.
    Metzenbaum's s.
    Miller's s.
    New's s.
    Northbent's s.
    Ochsner's s.
    Panzer's s.
    Pratt's s.
    Rochester-Ferguson s.
    Shortbent's s.

scissors *(continued)*
>> Sistrunk's s.
>> Thorek-Feldman s.
>> Thorek's s.
>> Vezien's s.

sclerotherapy

sclerosis
> gastric s.

scoop
>> Beck's s.
>> Berens' s.
>> Desjardin's s.
>> Ferguson's s.
>> Ferris' s.
>> Luer-Korte s.
>> Mayo-Robson s.
>> Mayo's s.
>> Moore's s.
>> Moynihan's s.

scrotal

scrotectomy

scrotocele

scrotoplasty

scrotum

Scudder's
> clamp
> forceps

Scultetus' position

scybalous

scybalum

sebaceous

section
> frozen s.

Semken's forceps

Senn's retractor

sentinel pile

sepsis

septic

septum
> crural s.
> s. femorale

serosa

serosanguineous

serositis

serous

sessile

sfinkter-. See words beginning *sphincter-.*

Shallcross's forceps

sheath
>> rectus s.
>> s. of rectus abdominis muscle
>> Scarpa's s.

Shortbent's scissors

shunt
> portacaval s.
> postcaval s.

sibah-. See words beginning *scyba-.*

sigmoid

sigmoidectomy

sigmoiditis

sigmoidopexy

sigmoidoproctostomy

sigmoidorectostomy

sigmoidoscope
>> Boehm's s.
>> Buie's s.
>> Frankfeldt's s.
>> Kelly's s.
>> Lieberman's s.
>> Montague's s.
>> Solow's s.
>> Turell's s.
>> Tuttle's s.

sigmoidoscope *(continued)*
> Vernon-David s.
> Welch-Allyn s.

sigmoidoscopy
sigmoidosigmoidostomy
sigmoidostomy
sigmoidotomy
sigmoidovesical
sign
> Aaron's s.
> Roux's s.
> Rovsing's s.
> Schlange's s.
> Stokes's s.
> Tansini's s.
> Thomayer's s.
> Toma's s.
> Volkovitsch's s.
> Wachenheim-Reder s.
> Wahl's s.
> Wölfler's s.
> Wolkowitsch's s.
> Wreden's s.

Silastic implant
silicone
Silverman's needle
Simon's
> incision
> position
> suture

Sims'
> anoscope
> position
> speculum
> suture

Singleton's incision
Singley's forceps
sinus

sinus
> pilonidal s.
> sacrococcygeal s.
> thyroglossal s.

siphon
Sistrunk's
> retractor
> scissors

situs
> s. inversus viscerum
> s. perversus
> s. solitus
> s. transversus

skeletonize
Sloan's
> incision
> retractor

sloughing
sluffing. See *sloughing.*
Smead-Jones closure
Smith-Buie retractor
Smith-Peterson incision
snare
> Frankfeldt's s.
> Norwood's s.

sois. See *psoas.*
Solow's sigmoidoscope
solution
> Ringer's lactate s.

Sotteau's operation
Southey's trocar
speculum
> Allingham's s.
> Barr's s.
> Buie-Smith s.
> Chelsea-Eaton s.
> Cook's s.
> David's s.

speculum *(continued)*
    Dudley-Smith s.
    Fansler's s.
    Goldbacher's s.
    Guild-Pratt s.
    Hinckle-James s.
    Martin's s.
    Mathew's s.
    Pennington's s.
    Pratt's s.
    Sims' s.
    Vernon-David s.
Spencer Wells forceps
sphincter
    Hyrtl's s.
    O'Beirne's s.
    Oddi's s.
    prepyloric s.
sphincteralgia
sphincterectomy
sphincterismus
sphincteritis
sphincteroplasty
sphincteroscope
sphincteroscopy
sphincterotome
sphincterotomy
    choledochal s.
spicular
spiculated
spicule
spiculum
Spieghel's line
Spivack's gastrostomy
splanchnicectomy
spleen
    accessory s.
splenectomize

splenectomy
    Carter's thoraco-
      abdominal s.
    Federoff's s.
    Henry's s.
    Rives' s.
    subcapsular s.
splenectopia
splenic
splenitis
splenocele
splenocleisis
splenomegaly
splenoncus
splenopexy
splenoportography
splenoptosis
splenorenal
splenorrhagia
splenorrhaphy
splenotomy
splenulus
Ssabanajew-Frank gastrostomy
Stamm's gastrostomy
stasis
steatorrhea
stenosis
    pyloric s.
stenotic
Stenson's duct
stent
stercoraceous
sterile
sterilely
Steri-strip
Stern's position
sternal
sternum

Stevenson's clamp
Stewart's
    hook
    incision
Stille's forceps
Stokes's sign
stoma
stomach
    dumping s.
    leather bottle s.
Stone-Holcombe clamp
Stone's
    clamp
    forceps
strangulation
stratum
stria
stricture
stripper
    Emerson's s.
    intraluminal s.
    Keeley's s.
    Kurten's s.
    Lempka's s.
    Mayo's s.
    Myers' s.
    Nabatoff's s.
    Webb's s.
    Wilson's s.
stroma
struma
    Riedel's s.
strumectomy
stump
    invaginated s.
subareolar
subcutaneous
submammary

subscapular
sudosist. See *pseudocyst.*
sulcus
    s. intermedius
supernumerary
suppuration
suppurative
surgical procedures. See
    operation.
Surgicel gauze
suture
    absorbable s.
    Albert's s.
    Appolito's s.
    apposition s.
    approximation s.
    arcuate s.
    atraumatic s.
    basilar s.
    bastard s.
    Béclard's s.
    Bell's s.
    biparietal s.
    bolster s.
    Bozeman's s.
    bregmatomastoid s.
    buried s.
    button s.
    catgut s.
    chain s.
    chromic catgut s.
    circular s.
    clavate s.
    coaptation s.
    cobblers' s.
    collagen s.
    compound s.
    Connell's s.

suture *(continued)*

continuous s.
coronal s.
Cushing's s.
cutaneous s.
Czerny's s.
Czerny-Lembert s.
dacron s.
dekalon s.
deknatel silk s.
dentate s.
dermalon s.
dexon s.
double-button s.
Dupuytren's s.
Duvergier's s.
Emmet's s.
Ethicon s.
Ethilon s.
everting s.
false s.
figure-of-eight s.
furrier's s.
Gély's s.
glovers' s.
Gould's s.
Gussenbauer's s.
Halsted's s.
Harris's s.
hemostatic s.
interrupted s.
intradermic s.
inverting s.
Jobert's s.
lace s.
Le Dran's s.
Lembert's s.
Littre's s.

suture *(continued)*

living s.
lock-stitch s.
Löffler's s.
Marlex s.
mattress s., horizontal
mattress s., right-angle
mattress s., vertical
Maunsell s.
Mersilene s.
monofilament s.
near-and-far s.
nonabsorbable s.
noose s.
nylon s.
over-and-over s.
overlapping s.
Palfyn's s.
Paré's s.
Petit's s.
pin s.
plicating s.
Polydek s.
polyethylene s.
polypropylene s.
presection s.
primary s.
prolene s.
pursestring s.
quilled s.
quilt s.
Ramdohr's s.
relaxation s.
retention s.
Richter's s.
Rigal's s.
Ritisch's s.
rubber s.

suture *(continued)*
    secondary s.
    seroserous s.
    serrated s.
    shotted s.
    silk s.
    silk braided s.
    silkworm gut s.
    Simon's s.
    Sims's s.
    stainless steel s.
    staple s.
    stay s.
    stick-tie s.
    subcuticular s.
    superficial s.
    Taylor's s.
    tension s.
    Tevdek s.
    through-and-through s.
    tongue-and-groove s.
    transfixing s.
    twisted s.
    uninterrupted s.
    visceroparietal s.
    Wölfler's s.
    Wysler's s.
    Zytor's s.
sympathectomy
syndrome
    Wermer's s.
    Zollinger-Ellison s.
syringectomy
syringotome
syringotomy
Talma's operation
Tanner's operation
Tansini's sign

tantalum mesh
Taylor's suture
technique
    Buie t.
    La Roque's t.
    Lotheissen-McVay t.
    vest-over-pants t.
Teflon
    graft
    mesh
tenaculum
    Lahey's t.
tendon
    conjoined t.
tenectomy
tenesmus
tenomyoplasty
tenotomy
teratoma
testicle
Tevdek suture
Theis' retractor
theleplasty
thelerethism
thelitis
thelorrhagia
thenar eminence
Thomas-Warren incision
Thomayer's sign
Thoms' forceps
thoracotomy
Thorek-Feldman scissors
Thorek-Mixter forceps
Thorek's
    aspirator
    scissors
thread
    Pagenstecher's linen t.

thrombectomy
thrombophlebitis
thymectomize
thymectomy
thymus
thyroglossal
thyrohyal
thyroid
thyroidea
    t. accessoria
    t. ima
thyroidectomize
thyroidectomy
thyroiditis
thyroidotomy
thyromegaly
thyroparathyroidectomy
thyrotomy
thyrotoxicosis
Timbrall-Fisher incision
tissue
    Gamgee t.
toe
    Morton's t.
toilet
Toma's sign
Torek's operation
torsion
tortuous
tourniquet
trabeculae
    t. lienis
    t. of spleen
trabecular
tracheostomy
tract
    alimentary t.
    biliary t.

transduodenal
transection
transfixion
transfusion
transplant
    Gallie t.
transplantation
transposition
transversalis
transversostomy
Travel's operation
Treitz's
    hernia
    ligament of T.
Trendelenburg's
    operation
    position
triangle
    Calot's t.
    Henke's t.
    Hesselbach's t.
    Scarpa's t.
trigone
trigonectomy
trocar
    Allen's t.
    Barnes' t.
    Duke's t.
    Ochsner's t.
    Southey's t.
TSH – thyroid stimulating
    hormone
T-tube
tube
    Abbott-Rawson t.
    Buie's t.
    Cantor t.
    Carman's t.

tube *(continued)*
  Debove's t.
  Greiling's t.
  Johnson's t.
  Jutte's t.
  Kelly's t's.
  Levin's t.
  Miller-Abbott t.
  Mueller-Frazier t.
  Mueller-Pool t.
  Mueller-Pynchon t.
  Mueller-Yankauer t.
  Nachlas' t.
  O'Beirne's t.
  Ochsner's t.
  Paul-Mixter t.
  Pool's t.
  Pynchon's t.
  Ryle's t.
  Wangensteen t.
  Yankauer's t.
tuber
 t. omental
tubercle
 pubic t.
tumor
tunica
 t. abdominalis
 t. adventitia
 t. albuginea
 t. dartos
 t. fibrosa hepatis
 t. fibrosa lienis
 t. mucosa ventriculi
 t. mucosa vesicae felleae
 t. muscularis coli
 t. muscularis intestini
  tenuis

tunica *(continued)*
 t. muscularis recti
 t. muscularis ventriculi
 t. serosa
 t. serosa coli
 t. serosa hepatis
 t. serosa intestini tenuis
 t. serosa lienis
 t. serosa peritonei
 t. serosa ventriculi
 t. serosa vesicae felleae
Turell's
 proctoscope
 sigmoidoscope
Turner's operation
Tuttle's
 proctoscope
 sigmoidoscope
ulcer
 Allingham's u.
 Cruveilhier's u.
 Cushing's u.
 decubitus u.
 Dieulafoy's u.
 duodenal u.
 gastric u.
 gastroduodenal u.
 gastrojejunal u.
 jejunal u.
 Kocher's dilatation u.
 Mann-Williamson u.
 marginal u.
 peptic u.
 perforating u.
 stomal u.
ulceration
umbilectomy
umbilical

umbilicus
unguis
    u. incarnatus
Unna's paste
unit
    Bovie u.
urachus
U-shaped incision
uthiroid. See *euthyroid.*
vagal
vagotomy
vagus
Valentine's position
valve
    Houston's v.
valvula
    v. ileocolica
    v. pylori
van Buren's operation
varicocele
varicose
varicosity
varicotomy
varix
vas
    v. deferens
vasa
    v. brevia
vasectomy
vascular
Vater's
    ampulla
    papilla
vein
    azygos v.
    femoral v.
    portal v.
    saphenous v.

Velpeau's hernia
vena
    v. cava
venesection
venipuncture
venoperitoneostomy
ventral
ventrocystorrhaphy
verge
    anal v.
Vermale's operation
vermicular
vermiculation
vermiculous
vermiform
vermifugal
Verneuil's operation
Vernon-David
    proctoscope
    sigmoidoscope
    speculum
verruca
    v. acuminata
    v. digitata
    v. filiformis
    v. plana
    v. plantaris
    v. vulgaris
vesicointestinal
vessel
    circumflex v.
    external pudic v.
    hypogastric v.
    iliac v.
    pudendal v.
    pudic v.
vest-over-pants technique
Vezien's scissors

Vi-drape
Villard's button
villus
Virden's catheter
Virtus' forceps
viscera
visceral
visceroparietal
visceroperitoneal
visceropleural
Vischer's incision
viscid
viscus
Volkmann's
    contracture
    retractor
Volkovitsch's sign
volvulus
Von Bergmann's hernia
Von Haberer-Finney
   gastroenterostomy
von Petz's clamp
V-shaped incision
Wachenheim-Reder sign
Wahl's sign
Walcher's position
Waldeyer's colon
Wales' dilator
Walker's retractor
Walter-Deaver retractor
Walter's forceps
Walther's forceps
Wangensteen's
    carrier
    clamp
    colostomy
    dissector
    forceps

Wangensteen's *(continued)*
    operation
    tube
Warren's
    incision
    operation
wart
    plantar w.
Watson-Jones incision
Watson's operation
Watts' clamp
Waugh's operation
Webb's stripper
Weber-Fergusson incision
Weber's
    catheter
    insufflator
Webster's retractor
Weinberg's retractor
Weir's operation
Weisenbach's forceps
Weitlaner's retractor
Welch-Allyn
    anoscope
    forceps
    hook
    probe
    proctoscope
    sigmoidoscope
Wermer's syndrome
Wharton's duct
Whipple's
    incision
    operation
whitlow
    melanotic w.
    thecal w.
Wilde's incision

Williams' forceps
Willie-Meyer incision
Willis'
    antrum
    pancreas
Wilson's stripper
Winslow's
    foramen
    pancreas
wire
    Kirschner's w.
Wirsung's duct
Wise's operation
Witzel's
    enterostomy
    gastrostomy
    operation
Wolfenden's position
Wölfler's
    gastroenterostomy
    operation
    sign
    suture
Wolf-Schindler gastroscope
Wolfson's
    clamp
    retractor

Wolkowitsch's sign
Wreden's sign
Wützer's operation
Wyeth's operation
Wyllys-Andrews operation
Wysler's suture
xiphoid
xyster
Yankauer's tube
Yeomans'
    forceps
    protoscope
Young's dilator
Y-type incision
Zachary Cope-DeMartel
   clamp
Zieman's operation
Zimmerman's operation
zister. See *xyster.*
Z-flap incision
Zollinger-Ellison syndrome
Z-plasty
    incision
    operation
Z-shaped incision
Zytor's suture

LABORATORY TERMINOLOGY
STAINS & CULTURES
Normal Laboratory Values

AA — acetic acid
abetalipoproteinemia
ablastin
ABO — blood groups (named
    for agglutinogens)
Abrams' test
Absidia
absorption
    fat a.
    iron a.
Acanthameba
Acanthocheilonema perstans
acanthocyte
acanthocytosis
Acaridae
Acaulium
ACD — acid, citrate, dextrose
Acetest
Acetobacter
    A. aceti
    A. melanogenus
    A. oxydans
    A. rancens
    A. roseus
    A. suboxydans
    A. xylinus
acetone

acetonemia
Achorion
achroacyte
achromia
Achromobacter
Achromobacteraceae
acid
    aceto-acetic a.
    acetylsalicylic a.
    amino a.
    argininosuccinic a.
    ascorbic a.
    diacetic a.
    folic a.
    hippuric a.
    homogentisic a.
    hydrochloric a.
    lactic a.
    phenylpyruvic a.
    uric a.
acid-fast
acidifiable
acidifier
acidify
acidimetry
acidity
acidocyte

acidocytopenia
acidocytosis
acidogenic
acidophil
acidophilic
acidosis
acid phosphatase
Acinetobacter
    A. anitratum
    A. parapertussis
Acladium
Acremonium
Acrotheca pedrosoi
Acrothesium floccosum
ACTH – adrenocorticotropic
   hormone
ACTH test
Actinobacillus
    A. mallei
    A. pseudomallei
actinomyces
Actinomyces
    A. bovis
    A. israelii
Actinomycetaceae
Actinomycetales
actinomycetes
actinomycetic
actinomycin
actinomycosis
Actinoplanaceae
Actinoplanes
Actinopoda
Actonia
Adamkiewicz's test
Addis count
ADH – antidiuretic hormone
adjuvant

adjuvant
   Freund a.
Adler's test
ADP – adenosine diphosphate
Aedes
    A. aegypti
    A. albopictus
    A. cinereus
    A. flavescens
    A. leucocelaenus
    A. scutellaris pseudo-
      scutellaris
    A. sollicitans
    A. spencerii
    A. taeniorhynchus
Aerobacter
    A. aerogenes
    A. cloacae
aerobe
aerobia
aerobian
aerobic
aerobiotic
aerogenic
aerogenous
Aeromonas
    A. hydrophila
    A. liquefaciens
    A. punctata
    A. salmonicida
AFB – acid-fast bacillus
agammaglobulinemia
   Bruton's a.
   Swiss type a.
Agamodistomum
    A. ophthalmobium
Agamonema
Agamonematodum migrans

A/G ratio — albumin-globulin
    ratio
agar
Agarbacterium
agglutination
    bacteriogenic a.
    H a.
    intravascular a.
    macroscopic a.
    mediate a.
    microscopic a.
    O a.
    platelet a.
    salt a.
    T-a.
    Vi a.
agglutinin
    alpha a.
    anti-Rh a.
    beta a.
    chief a.
    cold a.
    febrile a.
    flagellar a.
    group a.
    H a.
    haupt a.
    immune a.
    leukocyte a.
    O a.
    platelet a.
    Rh a.
    somatic a.
    warm a.
agglutinogen
aglobulia
aglobuliosis
aglobulism

aglycemia
aglycogenosis
agranulocyte
agranuloplastic
ahaptoglobinemia
AHF — antihemophilic factor
AHG — antihemophilic
      globulin
      antihuman globulin
AHT — antihyaluronidase
    titer
akaryocyte
akoreon. See *Achorion.*
akro-. See words beginning
    achro-
ALA — aminolevulinic acid
albumin
    a. A
    acetosoluble a.
    acid a.
    alkali a.
    a. of Bence Jones
    caseiniform a.
    coagulated a.
    derived a.
    hematin a.
    iodinated serum a.
    normal human serum a.
    Patein's a.
    radio-iodinated serum a.
    serum a.
    a. tannate
    triphenyl a.
albuminuria
albumosuria
    Bence Jones a.
    Bradshaw's a.
    enterogenic a.

albumosuria
    pyogenic a.
Alcaligenes
    A. bookeri
    A. bronchosepticus
    A. faecalis
    A. marshallii
    A. metalcaligenes
    A. recti
    A. viscolactis
alcohol
aldolase
aldosterone
aldosteronism
aleukocytosis
Alginobacter
Alginomonas
alkalemia
alkalescence
alkali
alkaline
    a. phosphatase
allergen
Allescheria
    A. boydii
Alpha$_1$
Alpha$_2$
alpha
    a. amino acids
    a. amino nitrogen
    a. amylase
    a. antitrypsin
    a. -beta variation
    a. cells
    a. chain
    a. globulin antibodies
    A-1 globulins
    A-2 globulins

alpha *(continued)*
    a-1-4 glucosidase
      deficiency
    a. lipoproteins
    a. methyl dopa
    a. particles
    a. receptors
Alternaria
Amanita
    A. muscaria
    A. pantherina
    A. phalloides
    A. rubescens
    A. verna
ameba
    coprozoic a.
amebiasis
Ames Lab-Tek cryostat
amino
    a. acid
aminoaciduria
aminopeptidase
    leucine a.
Amoeba
    A. buccalis
    A. cachexica
    A. coli
    A. coli mitis
    A. dentalis
    A. dysenteriae
    A. histolytica
    A. limax
    A. meleagridis
    A. urinae granulata
    A. urogenitalis
    A. verrucosa
amylase
    pancreatic a.

amylase *(continued)*
    salivary a.
    serum a.
    urinary a.
amyloclast
amyloid
amyloidosis
ANA – antinuclear antibody
anaerobe
    facultative a's.
    obligate a's.
anaerobia
anaerobian
anaerobiase
anaerobic
anaerogenic
Anaplasma
Anaplasmataceae
Ancylostoma
    A. braziliense
    A. duodenale
anemia
    aplastic a.
    Cooley's a.
    hemolytic a.
    hypochromic a.
    macrocytic a.
    microcytic a.
    normochromic a.
    normocytic a.
    pernicious a.
    sickle cell a.
anisocytosis
anisohypercytosis
anisohypocytosis
anisokaryosis
anisoleukocytosis
Anopheles

Anopheles
    A. maculipennis
Anoplura
anoxemia
anoxemic
Anthomyia
    A. canicularis
    A. incisura
    A. manicata
    A. saltatrix
    A. scalaris
Anthomyiidae
    A. Fannia
    A. Hydrotea
    A. Hylemyia
anthrax
antibiotic
    bactericidal a.
    bacteriostatic a.
    broad spectrum a.
    oral a.
antibody
    Duffy a's., Fy^a, Fy^b
    Lewis a's.; Le^a, Le^b
anticoagulant
anticoagulative
anticoagulin
anticolibacillary
anticollagenase
anticolloidoclastic
anti-DNA
antigen
antigenic
antigenicity
antigenotherapy
antiglobulin
antihemagglutinin
antihemolysin

antihemolytic
antihemophilic
antiheterolysin
antihyaluronidase
    a. titer
antinuclear
antistaphylolysin
antistreptococcic
antistreptococcin
antistreptokinase
antistreptolysin
    a. O
aplasmic
aplastic
appliqué form
Argas
    A. reflexus
arginine
argininosuccinicaciduria
Arizona organism
Armanni-Ebstein cell
Arthrographis
    A. langeroni
Arthropoda
arthrospore
ASA – acetylsalicylic acid
    argininosuccinic acid
ascariasis
ascaricidal
ascaricide
ascarides
Ascaris
    A. lumbricoides
Aschheim-Zondek test
Ascomycetes
ascorbate
ascospore
ascotrophosome

ascus
ASO titer – antistreptolysin
    O titer
Aspergillus
    A. auricularis
    A. barbae
    A. bouffardi
    A. clavatus
    A. concentricus
    A. flavus
    A. fumigatus
    A. giganteus
    A. glaucus
    A. gliocladium
    A. mucoroides
    A. nidulans
    A. niger
    A. ochraceus
    A. pictor
    A. repens
Asterococcus
astrocyte
Atelosaccharomyces
atypia
atypical
Auer's bodies
aurococcus
Australian X disease virus
autoagglutination
autoagglutinin
autoantibody
autoanticomplement
autoantigen
autoantitoxin
autoerythrophagocytosis
AZ test – Aschheim-Zondek
    test
bacilli

bacilli
    acid-fast b.
Bacillus
    B. acidi lactici
    B. aerogenes capsulatus
    B. aertrycke
    B. alvei
    B. anthracis
    B. botulinus
    B. brevis
    B. bronchisepticus
    B. circulans
    B. coli
    B. diphtheriae
    B. dysenteriae
    B. enteritidis
    B. faecalis alcaligenes
    B. influenzae
    B. larvae
    B. leprae
    B. mallei
    B. oedematiens
    B. oedematis maligni
      No. II
    B. pertussis
    B. pestis
    B. pneumoniae
    B. polymyxa
    B. proteus
    B. pseudomallei
    B. pumilus
    B. pyocyaneus
    B. stearothermophilus
    B. subtilis
    B. suipestifer
    B. tetani
    B. tuberculosis
    B. tularense

Bacillus *(continued)*
    B. typhi
    B. typhosus
    B. welchii
    B. whitmori
bacillus
    b. abortivus equinus
    Bang's b.
    Battey bacilli
    Boas-Oppler b.
    Bordet-Gengou b.
    Calmette-Guerin b.
    Döderlein's b.
    Ducrey's b.
    Escherich's b.
    Fick's b.
    Flexner-Strong b.
    Flexner's b.
    Friedländer's b.
    Gärtner's b.
    Ghon-Sachs b.
    glanders b.
    Hansen's b.
    Hofmann's b.
    Johne's b.
    Klebs-Löffler b.
    Klein's b.
    Koch-Weeks b.
    Morax-Axenfeld b.
    Morgan's b.
    Newcastle-Manchester b.
    Nocard's b.
    paracolon b.
    Pfeiffer's b.
    Preisz-Nocard b.
    rhinoscleroma b.
    Schmitz's b.
    Schmorl's b.

bacillus *(continued)*
> Shiga's b.
> smegma b.
> Sonne-Duval b.
> Strong's b.
> swine rotlauf b.
> Timothy b.
> tubercle b.
> typhoid b.
> vole b.
> Whitmore's b.

bacteremia
bacterioagglutinin
bacteriophage
Bacterium
> B. aerogenes
> B. aeruginosum
> B. cholerae suis
> B. cloacae
> B. coli
> B. dysenteriae
> B. pestis bubonicae
> B. sonnei
> B. tularense
> B. typhosum

bacteriuria
Balantidium
> B. coli

bands
Bang's bacillus
Bargen's streptococcus
Barr body
Bartonella
> B. bacilliformis

Bartonellaceae
BASO – basophil
basophil
basophilia

basophilic
basophilism
> Cushing's b.
> pituitary b.

Battey bacilli
BEI – butanol extractable iodine
Bence Jones
> albumin
> albumosuria
> protein test
> proteinuria
> reaction

Benedict's test
Bessey-Lowry unit
Beta 1, 2, 3, 2A, 2M
Bethesda-Ballerup Citrobacter
BFP – biologically false positivity
BFT – bentonite flocculation test
bile
bilirubin
bilirubinemia
Blastomyces
> B. brasiliensis
> B. coccidioides
> B. dermatitidis

blastomycin
blastomycosis
bleeding time
> Duke's method b.t.
> Ivy's method b.t.

blood
> cord b.

blood serum
> Löffler's b.s.

blood urea nitrogen

Bloor's test
Bloxam's test
BMR – basal metabolic rate
Boas' test
Boas-Oppler
    bacillus
    lactobacillus
Bodansky unit
Bodo
    B. caudatus
    B. saltans
    B. urinaria
Bodonidae
body
    Auer's b's.
    Barr b.
    Cabot's ring b's.
    Donovan's b's.
    Heinz b's.
    Heinz-Ehrlich b's.
    Howell-Jolly b's.
    Howell's b's.
    inclusion b's.
    Jolly's b's.
    Leishman-Donovan b's.
    Maragiliano b.
    Negri b's.
    Todd's b.
Bonanno's test
bone marrow
Bordet-Gengou bacillus
Bordetella
    B. bronchiseptica
    B. parapertussis
    B. pertussis
Borrelia
    B. anserina
    B. berbera

Borrelia *(continued)*
    B. buccalis
    B. carteri
    B. caucasica
    B. duttonii
    B. hermsii
    B. hispanica
    B. kochii
    B. parkeri
    B. persica
    B. recurrentis
    B. refringens
    B. turicatae
    B. venezuelensis
    B. vincentii
Bowie's stain
Bradshaw's albumosuria
British anti-lewisite
Brucella
    B. abortus
    B. bronchiseptica
    B. melitensis
    B. suis
Brucellaceae
brucellosis
Brunhilde virus
Bruton's agammaglobulinemia
BSP – bromsulphalein
BUN – blood urea nitrogen
Bunyamwera virus
Busse's Saccharomyces
Butyribacterium
Bwamba fever virus
C – centigrade
C_{alb} – albumin clearance
C_{am} – amylase clearance
C_{cr} – creatinine clearance
C_{in} – insulin clearance

C_{pah} — para-aminohippurate clearance

C_u — urea clearance

Cabot's ring bodies

Cache valley virus

calcium

California virus

Calliphora
    C. vomitoria

Calmette-Guerin bacillus

Candida
    C. albicans
    C. guilliermondi
    C. krusei
    C. parakrusei
    C. pseudotropicalis
    C. stellatoidea
    C. tropicalis

candidiasis

carbon
    c. dioxide
    c. monoxide

carboxyhemoglobin

carboxypeptidase

cardiolipin

Carpoglyphus
    C. passularum

Casoni's intradermal test

cast
    granular c.
    hyaline c.
    waxy c.

Castellanella
    C. castellani

Castellani's test

Catalpa

cataphylaxis

catecholamine

Catenabacterium

CA virus — croup associated virus

CBC — complete blood count

Celebes' vibrio

cell
    alpha c's.
    Armanni-Ebstein c.
    band c's.
    beta c's.
    buffy coated c's.
    delta c's.
    epithelial c's.
    erythroid c's.
    Ferrata's c's.
    gamma c's.
    Gaucher's c.
    HeLa c's.
    islet c's.
    Leydig's c's.
    mast c's.
    packed c's.
    plasma c's.
    reticulum c's.
    sickle c.
    target c.

cellular

Cellvibrio
    C. flavescens
    C. fulvus
    C. ochraceus
    C. vulgaris

cephalin

Cephalosporium
    C. granulomatis

CEPH FLOC — cephalin flocculation

cercaria

ceruloplasmin
cestode
cestodiasis
CF – complement fixation
Chagas' disease
Charcot-Leyden crystals
Cheyletiella
    C. parasitovorax
Chikungunya virus
Chilomastix
    C. mesnili
Chlamydia
    C. oculogenitalis
    C. trachomatis
Chlamydiaceae
Chlamydobacteriaceae
Chlamydobacteriales
Chlamydophrys
chlamydospore
Chlamydozoaceae
Chlamydozoon
chloride
chloroleukemia
cholesterol
cholinesterase
chorionic gonadotropin
chromatin
chromoblastomycosis
chromosome
    Philadelphia c.
    X, Y c.
chymotrypsin
CI – colloidal iron
    crystalline insulin
Citrobacter
    Bethesda-Ballerup C.
Cladosporium
    C. werneckii

clasmatocyte
Clathrochloris
Clathrocystis
clearance
    blood urea c.
    creatinine c.
    urea c.
Clinitest
clonorchiasis
Clonorchis
    C. endemicus
    C. sinensis
clostridia
Clostridium
    C. acetobutylicum
    C. aerofoetidum
    C. agni
    C. bifermentans
    C. botulinum
    C. butylicum
    C. chauvoei
    C. cochlearium
    C. fallax
    C. feseri
    C. haemolyticum
    C. histolyticum
    C. kluyveri
    C. multifermentans
    C. nigrificans
    C. novyi
    C. oedematiens
    C. ovitoxicus
    C. paludis
    C. parabotulinum
    C. parabotulinum equi
    C. pasteurianum
    C. pastorianum
    C. perfringens

Clostridium *(continued)*
    C. septicum
    C. sordellii
    C. sporogenes
    C. sticklandii
    C. tertium
    C. tetani
    C. tetanomorphum
    C. thermosaccharolyti-
        cum
    C. tyrosinogenes
    C. welchii
clumping
CO_2 – carbon dioxide
coagulase
coagulate
coagulation
coagulin
coagulogram
Coccidioides
    C. immitis
coccidioidin
coccidioidomycosis
Coccidium
coccus
Coe virus
colibacillary
coliform
collagenase
colloid
colloidal gold
colony
Colorado tick fever virus
complex
    Ghon c.
condenser
conglutination
Congo Red

Congo Red *(continued)*
    stain
    test
contagium
    c. animatum
    c. vivum
contaminant
conversion
    Mantoux c.
Cooley's anemia
Coombs' test
    direct
    indirect
coprohematology
Copromastix
    C. prowazeki
Copromonas
    C. subtilis
coproporphyria
coproporphyrin
coproporphyrinogen
Cordylobia
    C. anthropophaga
corpuscle
Corynebacteriaceae
Corynebacterium
    C. acnes
    C. diphtheriae
    C. enzymicum
    C. equi
    C. hemolyticum
    C. hofmannii
    C. minutissimum
    C. murisepticum
    C. mycetoides
    C. ovis
    C. pseudodiphtheriticum
    C. pseudotuberculosis

Corynebacterium *(continued)*
  C. pyogenes
  C. renale
  C. ulcerans
  C. xerosis
count
  Addis c.
  reticulocyte c.
  Schilling blood c.
Coxiella
  C. burnetii
Coxsackie virus
CPK – creatine phospho-
  kinase
C-reactive protein test
creatinase
creatine
creatininase
creatinine
crenation
crossmatching
CRP – C-reactive protein
cryocrit
cryofibrinogen
cryogammaglobulin
cryoglobulin
cryostat
  Ames Lab-Tek c.
cryptococcosis
Cryptococcus
  C. capsulatus
  C. epidermidis
  C. gilchristi
  C. histolyticus
  C. hominis
  C. meningitidis
  C. neoformans
cryptozoite

crystal
  Charcot-Leyden c's.
C & S – culture and
  sensitivity
CSF – cerebrospinal fluid
Ctenocephalides
culture
  attenuated c.
  blood c.
  chorioallantoic c.
  direct c.
  flask c.
  hanging-block c.
  hanging-drop c.
  needle c.
  plate c.
  sensitized c.
  shake c.
  slant c.
  smear c.
  stab c.
  stock c.
  streak c.
  stroke c.
  thrust c.
  tissue c.
  tube c.
  type c.
Cushing's basophilism
C virus – Coxsackie virus
cylindroid
cysticerci
Cysticercus
  C. acanthrotrias
  C. bovis
  C. cellulosae
  C. fasciolaris
  C. ovis

Cysticercus
  C. tenuicollis
cysticercus
cytology
cytolysate
  blood c.
cytomegalovirus
cytoplasm
Dale-Laidlaw's clotting time
  method
dehydrogenase
  isocitric d.
  lactic d.
dehydropeptidase
Dematium
Demodex
  D. folliculorum
dengue
Dermacentor
  D. andersoni
  D. occidentalis
  D. variabilis
Dermacentroxenus
Dermanyssus
  D. avium et gallinae
Dermatobia
  D. hominis
Dermatophilus
  D. penetrans
diacetate
Diagnex Blue test
Dialister
  D. pneumosintes
diastase
Dick test
Dicrocoelium
  D. dendriticum
Dientamoeba

Dientamoeba
  D. fragilis
differential
difilo-. See words beginning
  diphyllo-.
Dimastigamoeba
diphyllobothriasis
Diphyllobothrium
  D. latum
  D. parvum
  D. taenioides
diplobacillus
diplobacterium
Diplococcus
  D. pneumoniae
diplococcus
  d. of Morax-Axenfeld
  d. of Neisser
  Weichselbaum's d.
Diplogonoporus
  D. brauni
  D. grandis
Dipylidium
  D. caninum
dis-. See also words beginning
  dys-.
disease
  Chagas' d.
  Gaisböck's d.
  Gaucher's d.
  Osler's d.
  Schottmüller's d.
  Vaquez-Osler d.
  Vaquez's d.
dish
  Petri's d.
Distoma
distomiasis
DNA – deoxyribonucleic acid

Döderlein's bacillus
Donath-Landsteiner test
Donovan's bodies
Dracunculus
    D. medinensis
drepanocyte
drepanocytemia
drepanocytic
Drepanospira
drumstick
Ducrey's bacillus
Duffy antibodies, Fy^a, Fy^b
Duke's method bleeding time
dyscrasia
    blood d.
    lymphatic d.
dysdiemorrhysis
dysemia
dysentery
    amebic d.
    bacillary d.
    balantidial d.
    bilharzial d.
    catarrhal d.
    ciliary d.
    ciliate d.
    flagellate d.
    Flexner's d.
    fulminant d.
    malarial d.
    protozoal d.
    scorbutic d.
    Sonne d.
    spirillar d.
    sporadic d.
    viral d.
dysgammaglobulinemia
Eberthella

ECBO virus – enteric cyto-
    pathogenic bovine orphan
    virus
ECDO virus – enteric cyto-
    pathogenic dog orphan
    virus
ECG – electrocardiogram
echinococcosis
Echinococcus
    E. granulosus
    E. multilocularis
Echinorhynchus
echinosis
Echinostoma
ECHO virus – enteric cyto-
    pathogenic human orphan
    virus
ECMO virus – enteric cyto-
    pathogenic monkey
    orphan virus
E. coli – Escherichia coli
ECSO virus – enteric cyto-
    pathogenic swine orphan
    virus
ectoplasm
EEE virus – Eastern equine
    encephalomyelitis virus
EEG – electroencephalogram
eelworm
Ehrlich's
    reaction
    test
EKG – electrocardiogram
ekino-. See words beginning
    echino-.
elastase
electrocardiogram
electrocardiograph

electroencephalogram
electrolyte
    amphoteric e.
    colloidal e.
    protein e.
    serum e.
Ellsworth-Howard test
El Tor's vibrios
EMC virus — encephalomyo-
    carditis
Endamoeba
    E. blattae
Endolimax
    E. nana
Endomyces
    E. albicans
    E. capsulatus
    E. epidermatidis
    E. epidermidis
endomycosis
endotheliocyte
Entamoeba
    E. buccalis
    E. buetschlii
    E. coli
    E. gingivalis
    E. histolytica
    E. kartulisi
    E. nana
    E. nipponica
    E. tetragena
    E. tropicalis
    E. undulans
Enterobacter
    E. aerogenes
    E. alvei
    E. cloacae
Enterobacteriaceae

enterobiasis
Enterobius
    E. vermicularis
enterococcus
Enteromonas
    E. hominis
enzyme
EOS — eosinophils
eosinophil
    polymorphonuclear e.
eosinophilia
Epidermophyton
    E. floccosum
    E. inguinale
    E. rubrum
epithelium
eratirus. See *Eratyrus.*
Eratyrus
erisip-. See words beginning
    erysip-.
erithremea. See *erythremia.*
erithro-. See words beginning
    erythro-.
Erysipelothrix
    E. insidiosa
    E. rhusiopathiae
erythremia
Erythrobacillus
erythroblast
erythroblastoma
erythroblastosis
    e. fetalis
    e. neonatorum
erythrocyte
erythrocythemia
erythrocytosis
    leukemic e.
    e. megalosplenica

erythrokinetics
erythron
erythroneocytosis
erythropenia
erythropoiesis
Escherichia
    E. aerogenes
    E. alkalescens
    E. aurescens
    E. coli
    E. dispar
    E. dispar var. ceylonensis
    E. dispar var. madam-
        pensis
    E. freundii
    E. intermedia
Escherichieae
Escherich's bacillus
esherikea. See *Escherichia.*
esherikiee. See *Escherichieae.*
ESR – erythrocyte sedimentation rate
ester
esterase
estrogen
estrus. See *Oestrus.*
Eubacteriales
Eubacterium
Euglena
    E. gracilis
euglobulin
eugonic
Euproctis
    E. chrysorrhoea
Eurotium
    E. malignum
Eusimulium
Eutriatoma

Eutrombicula
    E. alfreddugesi
exfoliative
extracellular
extracorpuscular
exudate
F – Fahrenheit
factor
   coagulation f's, I, II, III,
      IV, V, VII, VIII,
      IX, X, XI, XII
fago-. See words beginning
   phago-.
FANA – flourescent anti-
   nuclear antibody
faneroplazm. See *phaneroplasm.*
Fannia
    F. canicularis
Fasciola
    F. gigantica
    F. hepatica
Fasciolopsis
    F. buski
FBS – fasting blood sugar
Fehleisen's streptococcus
Fehling's test
fenilketonurea. See
   phenylketonuria.
fenistiks. See *Phenistix.*
feno-. See words beginning
   pheno-.
feo-. See words beginning
   pheo-.
fermentation
   mannitol f.
Ferrata's cells
Ferribacterium

Feulgen test
fibrin
fibrinogen
fibrinogenase
fibrinolysin
    seminal f.
Fick's bacillus
fiferz. See *Pfeiffer's.*
Filaria
    F. bancrofti
    F. conjunctivae
    F. hominis oris
    F. juncea
    F. labialis
    F. lentis
    F. lymphatica
    F. palpebralis
    F. philippinensis
filariasis
Filarioidea
fisaloptera. See *Physaloptera.*
Fishberg's concentration test
fixative
    Heidenhain's Susa f.
    Zenker's f.
Flagellata
flagellate
flagellum
Flavobacterium
    F. meningosepticum
flebotomus. See *Phlebotomus.*
Flexner-Strong bacillus
Flexner's
    bacillus
    dysentery
flocculation
    cephalin f.
    Ramon f.

floccule
    toxoid-antitoxin f.
flocculoreaction
flora
fluke
Fonsecaea pedrosoi
fos-. See words beginning
    phos-.
fragility
    erythrocyte f.
    osmotic f.
    red cell f.
Frei test
Freund adjuvant
Friedländer's
    bacillus
    pneumobacillus
Friedman's test
FSH — follicle stimulating
    hormone
FTA — fluorescent
    treponemal antibody
FTI — free thyroxine index
Fungi Imperfecti
fungus
Fusiformis
Fusobacterium
    F. fusiforme
    F. plautivincenti
fusocellular
fusospirillary
fusospirillosis
fusospirochetal
fusospirochetosis
fusotreptococciosis
Gaffkya
    G. tetragena
Gaisböck's disease

galactose
Gamma A, D, E, G, M
gamma globulin
Gärtner's bacillus
gastrin
Gaucher's
    cell
    disease
GC – gonococcus
    gonorrhea
    granular casts
Geotrichum
Gerhardt's test
GFR – glomerular filtration
  rate
GG – gamma globulin
Ghon complex
Ghon-Sachs bacillus
Giardia
    G. lamblia
Giemsa's stain
globulin
    alpha g's.
    beta g's.
    gamma g's.
    immune serum g.
    g. X
glucose
glucosuria
glutaminase
glutamine
Glyciphagus
    G. buski
    G. domesticus
glycosuria
gonadotropin
    chorionic g.
Gongylonema

Gongylonema
    G. pulchrum
gongylonemiasis
gonococcus
gonorrhea
G6PD – glucose-6-phosphate
    dehydrogenase
GPT – glutamic pyruvic
    transaminase
gram-negative
gram-positive
Gram stain
granulocyte
Gravindex test
gravity
    specific g.
Gruber-Widal reaction
GTT – glucose tolerance test
guaiac
Guaroa virus
Guthrie test
Gutman unit
Haemonchus
    H. contortus
Haemophilus
    H. aegyptius
    H. aprophilus
    H. ducreyi
    H. duplex
    H. hemoglobinophilus
    H. hemolyticus
    H. influenzae
    H. parahemolyticus
    H. parainfluenzae
    H. pertussis
    H. suis
    H. vaginalis
Haemosporidia

Hageman factor
Ham's test
Hanger's test
Hansen's bacillus
haptoglobin, Hp^1 and Hp^2
Harrison's test
Hartmanella
     H. hyalina
Haverhillia multiformis
HB — hemoglobin
HBD — hydroxybutyrate
   dehydrogenase
HCG — human chorionic
   gonadotropin
HCT — hematocrit
H & E — hematoxylin and
   eosin stain
Heidenhain's Susa fixative
Heinz bodies
Heinz-Ehrlich bodies
HeLa cells
helminth
Helophilus
hemagglutinin
Hemastix
Hematest
hematocrit
hematocrystallin
hematogen
hematogenesis
hematogenous
hematohyaloid
hematologist
hematology
hematopoiesis
    extramedullary h.
heme
Hemispora stellata

hemocytoblast
hemofilus. See *Haemophilus.*
hemoglobin
hemoglobinemia
hemoglobinuria
hemogram
hemohistioblast
hemolysin
hemolysis
hemolytic
hemolyze
hemonkus. See *Haemonchus.*
hemophil
hemophilia
Hemophilus
    H. aegypti
    H. bovis
    H. bronchisepticus
    H. ducreyi
    H. duplex
    H. influenzae
    H. parapertussis
    H. pertussis
hemophilus
    h. of Koch-Weeks
    h. of Morax-Axenfeld
hemosiderin
hemosiderinuria
hemosporidea. See
    Haemosporidia.
hemostasis
Hemostix
heparin
hepatocellular
hepatogram
Hermetia illucens
heterophil
Heterophyes

Heterophyes *(continued)*
  H. heterophyes
  H. katsuradai
heterophyiasis
HF — Hageman factor
HGF — hyperglycemic-
  glycogenolytic factor
HIAA — hydroxyindoleacetic
  acid
Hicks-Pitney thromboplastin
  generation test
histamine
histiocyte
histiocytosis
histology
Histoplasma
  H. capsulatum
  H. duboisii
histoplasmin
histoplasmosis
Hofmann's bacillus
Hogben test
Homalomyia
hookworm
Hormodendron
  H. carrionii
  H. compactum
  H. pedrosoi
Howard test
Howell-Jolly bodies
Howell's bodies
HPF — high power field
Huebener-Thomsen-
  Friedenreich phenomenon
hyaline
hyalinization
Hydatigera
  H. infantis

17-hydroxycorticosteroid
5-hydroxyindoleacetic acid
17-hydroxysteroid
5-hydroxytryptamine
hymenolepiasis
Hymenolepis
  H. diminuta
  H. murina
  H. nana
hyperbetalipoproteinemia
hyperbilirubinemia
hypercalcemia
hypercholesterolemia
hyperchromasia
hyperchromatism
hyperchromemia
hyperchromia
hypergammaglobulinemia
hyperglycemia
hyperimmunoglobulinemia
hyperkalemia
hypochromasia
hypochromemia
  idiopathic h.
hypochromia
hypochrosis
Hypoderma
  H. bovis
hypogammaglobulinemia
hypoglycemia
hypokalemia
hyponatremia
hypovolemic
IBC — iron-binding capacity
ICD — isocitric dehydrogenase
icteric index
I^{131} uptake test (radioactive
  iodine)

Ig — immunoglobulin
IgA — gamma A
    immunoglobulin
IgD — gamma D
    immunoglobulin
IgE — gamma E
    immunoglobulin
IgG — gamma G
    immunoglobulin
IgM — gamma M
    immunoglobulin
iksodez. See *Ixodes.*
iksodiasis. See *ixodiasis.*
Ilheus virus
immunoelectrophoresis
immunofluorescent
immunoglobulin
    gamma A i. (IgA)
    gamma D i. (IgD)
    gamma E i. (IgE)
    gamma G i. (IgG)
    gamma M i. (IgM)
index
    acidophilic i.
    hematopneic i.
    hemolytic i.
    icteric i.
    Krebs' leukocyte i.
    maturation i.
    phagocytic i.
    pyknotic i.
    sedimentation i.
indican
Indigo-carmine test
indole
Infusoria
INH — isonicotinic acid
    hydrazide

insulin
intracellular
iodameba. See *Iodamoeba.*
Iodamoeba
    I. büetschlii
    I. williamsi
iodine
iontophoresis
isoenzyme
isohemagglutination
isohemagglutinin
isoimmunization
isolation
Isoparoichis
    I. trisimilitubis
Isospora
    I. belli
    I. hominis
isotope
Ivy's method bleeding time
Ixodes
    I. bicornis
    I. calvepalpus
    I. frequens
ixodiasis
Japanese B encephalitis virus
jaundice
Jenner-Giemsa stain
JH virus
Johne's bacillus
Jolly's bodies
Jones-Cantarow test
Junin virus
K — potassium
Kahn test
karyocyte
KAU — King-Armstrong units
ketogenic

ketone
ketonuria
ketosis
17-ketosteroid
Ketostix
kilomastiks. See *Chilomastix.*
kimotripsin. See *chymotryp-sin.*
kinetocyte
kinetoplast
King-Armstrong unit
klahmidea. See *Chlamydia.*
klahmideasee. See *Chlamy-diaceae.*
klahmido-. See words beginning *Chlamydo-.*
Klebs-Löffler bacillus
Klebsiella
    K. friedländeri
    K. ozaenae
    K. pneumoniae
    K. rhinoscleromatis
Klein's bacillus
klorid. See *chloride.*
kloro-. See words beginning *chloro-.*
Koch-Weeks
    bacillus
    hemophilus
koksakee. See *Coxsackie.*
kokseela. See *Coxiella.*
koksidi-. See words beginning *coccidi-.*
kol-. See words beginning *chol-.*
Kolmer's test
koreonik. See *chorionic.*
korinee-. See words beginning *Coryne-.*

Krebs' leukocyte index
kromatin. See *chromatin.*
kromo-. See words beginning *chromo-.*
Kumba virus
Kunkel's test
Kyasanur Forest disease virus
Lactobacillaceae
Lactobacilleae
Lactobacillus
    L. acidophilus
    L. arabinosus
    L. bifidus
    L. bulgaricus
    L. casei
    L. fermentans
    L. fermenti
    L. leichmannii
    L. plantarum
lactobacillus
    l. of Boas-Oppler
Lactobacteriaceae
lactose
Ladendorff's test
Laelaps
Lansing virus
larva
LDH – lactic dehydrogenase
LE – lupus erythematosus
lecithin
lecithinase
Lee-White clotting time method
Leishman-Donovan bodies
Leishmania
    L. braziliensis
    L. donovani

Leishmania *(continued)*
    L. infantum
    L. tropica
leishmaniasis
    cutaneous l.
    mucocutaneous l.
    naso-oral l.
    nasopharyngeal l.
    visceral l.
Leishman's stain
lelaps. See *Laelaps.*
Leon virus
leptocyte
leptocytosis
Leptomitus
    L. epidermidis
    L. urophilus
    L. vaginae
Leptospira
    L. australis
    L. autumnalis
    L. canicola
    L. grippotyphosa
    L. hebdomadis
    L. hyos
    L. icterohaemorrhagiae
    L. pomona
leptospirosis
    l. icterohemorrhagica
Leptothrix
Leptotrichia
    L. buccalis
    L. placoides
lesithin. See *lecithin.*
lesithinas. See *lecithinase.*
leucine
leukemia
    lymphoblastic l.

leukemia *(continued)*
    lymphocytic l.
    monocytic l.
    myeloblastic l.
    myelocytic l.
    myelogenous l.
    reticuloendothelial cell l.
leukocyte
leukocytosis
    eosinophilic l.
    lymphocytic l.
leukopenia
level
    barbiturate l.
    ethanol l.
    lead l.
Levinson test
Lewis antibodies; Le^a, Le^b
Leydig's cells
Lichtheimia corymbifera
likthimea korimbifera. See
    Lichtheimia corymbifera.
Limnatis
    L. granulosa
    L. mysomelas
    L. nilotica
lipase
lipid
lipidase
lipocyte
lipoid
liponisus. See *Lyponyssus.*
lipoprotein
Lissoflagellata
Listeria
    L. monocytogenes
Loa
    L. loa

Löffler's blood serum
LPF – low power field
lukemea. See *leukemia.*
luko-. See words beginning
   leuko-.
Lunyo virus
lupus
    l. erythematosus
lusin. See *leucine.*
lymphoblast
lymphoblastomid
lymphoblastosis
lymphocyte
    atypical l.
    plasmacytoid l.
lymphocytosis
    neutrophilic l.
LYMPHS – lymphocytes
Lyponyssus
macroblast
macrocyte
macrocythemia
    hyperchromatic m.
macroglobulin
macroglobulinemia
    Waldenström's m.
Macromonas
    M. bipunctata
    M. mobilis
macromonocyte
macromyeloblast
macronormoblast
macrophage
macropolycyte
Macrostoma mesnili
Madurella
magnesium
malabsorption

malaria
malasezeah. See *Malassezia.*
Malassezia
    M. furfur
    M. macfadyani
    M. tropica
mallein
Malleomyces
    M. mallei
    M. pseudomallei
    M. whitmori
Malmejde's test
Mansonella ozzardi
Mantoux
    conversion
    skin test
Maragiliano body
marrow
    bone m.
Mastigophora
materia
Mayaro virus
May-Grunwald-Giemsa stain
MCD – mean cell diameter
    mean corpuscular
      diameter
MCH – mean corpuscular
    hemoglobin
MCHC – mean corpuscular
    hemoglobin concentration
MCV – mean corpuscular
    volume
mean corpuscular hemoglobin
mean corpuscular hemoglobin
    concentration
mean corpuscular volume
megakaryoblast
megakaryocyte

megaloblast
meiosis
melanin
Melanolestes
    M. picipes
Mengo virus
meningococci
meningococcin
meningococcus
meningocyte
meniscocyte
Merulius
    M. lacrimans
mesobacterium
metagglutinin
metaglobulin
metagonimiasis
Metagonimus
    M. ovatus
    M. yokogawai
metamyelocyte
Methanobacterium
Methanococcus
methemalbumin
methemalbuminemia
methemoglobin
methemoglobinemia
methemoglobinuria
method
    Dale-Laidlaw's clotting
      time m.
    Lee-White clotting
      time m.
methyl
    m. methacrylate
Metopirone test
Microbacterium
microbiology

microchemistry
Micrococcaceae
Micrococcus
    M. pyogenes var. aureus
microcyte
Microfilaria
    M. bancrofti
    M. streptocerca
microne
microscope
microscopic
microscopy
    electron m.
microspherocyte
Microsporon furfur
Microsporum
    M. audouini
    M. canis
    M. felineum
    M. fulvum
    M. furfur
    M. gypseum
    M. lanosum
miksopod. See *myxopod.*
miksosporidea. See
    Myxosporidia.
miosis. See *meiosis.*
mitochondria
mitosis
Miyagawanella
    M. illinii
    M. louisianae
    M. lymphogranulomato-
      sus
    M. ornithosis
    M. pneumoniae
    M. psittaci
Monadina

Monas
Monilia
monilial
Moniliformis
monoblast
monocyte
mononuclear
MONOS – monocytes
monosomy G, X
Monosporium
    M. apiospermum
Monotricha
Morax-Axenfeld
    bacillus
    diplococcus
    hemophilus
Moraxella
    M. lacunata
    M. liquefaciens
Morgan's bacillus
morococcus
morphology
Mosenthal's test
motile
motility
mouse unit
MU – mouse unit
mucoprotein
Mucor
    M. corymbifer
    M. mucedo
    M. pusillus
    M. racemosus
    M. ramosus
    M. rhizopodiformis
mucormycosis
mucus
Murphy-Pattee test

Murray Valley encephalitis
    virus
murtofilum. See
    Myrtophyllum.
mycoagglutinin
Mycobacteriaceae
mycobacteriosis
Mycobacterium
    M. avium
    M. berolinenis
    M. bovis
    M. butyricum
    M. fortuitum
    M. intracellularis
    M. kansasii
    M. leprae
    M. leprae murium
    M. luciflavum
    M. marinum
    M. microti
    M. paratuberculosis
    M. phlei
    M. scrofulaceum
    M. smegmatis
    M. tuberculosis
    M. tuberculosis var.
        avium
    M. tuberculosis var.
        bovis
    M. tuberculosis var.
        hominis
    M. ulcerans
Mycocandida
Mycococcus
Mycoderma
    M. aceti
    M. dermatitis
    M. immite

mycology
Myconostoc
    M. gregarium
Mycoplana
    M. bullata
    M. dimorpha
Mycoplasma
    M. pneumoniae
Mycoplasmataceae
Mycoplasmatales
mycosis
    m. fungoides
myeloblast
myeloclast
myelocyte
myoglobin
Myriapoda
Myrtophyllum
    M. hepatis
myxopod
Myxosporidia
NANA — N-acetylneur-
    aminic acid
Necator
    N. americanus
Negri bodies
Neisseria
    N. catarrhalis
    N. flava
    N. gonorrhoeae
    N. intracellularis
    N. meningitidis
    N. sicca
Neisseriaceae
Neisser's diplococcus
Nematoda
nematode
neocyte

neocytosis
neutropenia
neutrophil
    band n.
neutrophile
    juvenile n.
    mature n.
    polymorphonuclear n.
    segmented n.
neutrophilia
Newcastle disease virus
Newcastle-Manchester bacillus
Nitrobacter
Nitrobacteraceae
Nitrocystis
Nocardia
    N. asteroides
    N. brasiliensis
    N. madurae
Nocard's bacillus
normoblast
    andacidophilic n.
    basophilic n.
    intermediate n.
    orthochromatophilic n.
    polychromatophilic n.
normoblastosis
normocyte
normocytic
normocytosis
normo-orthocytosis
NPN — nonprotein nitrogen
NSQ — not sufficient quantity
nucleus
numo-. See words beginning
    pneumo-.
Obermayer's test
Obermeier's spirillum

Obermüller's test
occult blood
Ochromyia
    O. anthropophaga
OCT – ornithine carbamyl
    transferase
Octomitus
    O. hominis
Octomyces
    O. etiennei
Oestrus
    O. hominis
    O. ovis
OHCS – hydroxycortico-
    steroid
Oidiomycetes
oidiomycosis
oligemia
oligocythemia
Onchocerca
    O. caecutiens
    O. volvulus
onchocerciasis
O'nyong-nyong virus
Oospora
opisthorchiasis
Opisthorchis
    O. felineus
    O. noverca
    O. viverrini
organic
organism
    Arizona o.
    Rickett's o.
    Vincent's o's.
Oropouche virus
Osler's disease
osmosis

Ostertag
    Streptococcus of O.
Otomyces
    O. hageni
    O. purpureus
otomycosis
    o. aspergillina
ova
ovum
oxalate
oxygen
oxyhemoglobin
oxyhemogram
oxyhemograph
oxysteroid
Oxyuris
    O. incognita
    O. vermicularis
PAH – para-aminohippurate
pancytopenia
Pandy's test
panhematopoietic
panhemocytophthisis
Papanicolaou's
    smear
    stain
    test
Pappenheim's stain
Parachordodes
Paracoccidioides brasiliensis
paracoccidioidomycosis
Paracolobactrum
    P. aerogenoides
    P. arizonae
    P. coliforme
    P. intermedium
Paragonimus
    P. westermani

Paragordius
    P. cintus
    P. tricuspidatus
    P. varius
Parasaccharomyces
    P. ashfordi
parasite
Paratyphi S.C.
paratyphoid A and B
Parvobacteriaceae
PAS – para-aminosalicylic
    acid
Pasteurella
    P. multocida
    P. pestis
    P. pseudotuberculosis
    P. tularensis
Patein's albumin
pathogen
Paul-Bunnell-Barrett test
Paul-Bunnell test
PBG – porphobilinogen
PBI – protein bound iodine
pCO_2 – carbon dioxide
    pressure
PCV – packed cell volume
Pediculoides
    P. ventricosus
Pediculus
    P. humanus var. capitis
    P. humanus var. corporis
    P. inguinalis
    P. pubis
pellicle
Penicillium
    P. barbae
    P. bouffardi
    P. minimum

Penicillium *(continued)*
    P. montoyai
    P. notatum
    P. patulum
    P. spinulosum
Pentastoma
    P. constrictum
    P. denticulatum
    P. taenioides
pentastomiasis
Pentatrichomonas
    P. ardin delteili
pentatrichomoniasis
pentolysis
pentosan
pentosazon
pentose
pepsin
peptidase
    leucine amino p.
Peptostreptococcus
pericyte
peroxidase
Petri's
    dish
    test
Pfeiffer's bacillus
pH – hydrogen ion concen-
    tration
phagocyte
phagocytosis
phaneroplasm
Phenistix
phenol
    p. liquefactum
    p. red
    p. salicylate
phenolphthalein

phenolsulfonphthalein
phenomenon
    Heubener-Thomsen-
      Friedenreich p.
phenotype
phenylketonuria
pheochromocyte
pheochromocytoma
Phialophora
    P. verrucosa
Philadelphia chromosome
Phlebotomus
    P. argentipes
    P. chinensis
    P. intermedius
    P. macedonicum
    P. noguchi
    P. papatasii
    P. sergenti
    P. verrucarum
    P. vexator
phosphatase
    acid p.
    alkaline p.
    serum p.
phosphate
phospholipase
phospholipid
phosphorus
phosphorylase
Physaloptera
    P. caucasica
    P. mordens
Piazza's test
picogram
Piedrai
    P. hortai
Piedraia
pigment

pinworm
Pityrosporon
    P. orbiculare
    P. ovale
PKU – phenylketonuria
plasma
plasmablast
plasmacyte
plasmocyte
Plasmodium
    P. falciparum
    P. malariae
    P. ovale
    P. pleurodyniae
    P. vivax
    P. vivax minuta
plasmodium
    exoerythrocytic p.
platelet
pleokaryocyte
pleomorphic
pneumobacillus
    Friedländer's p.
pneumococcal
pneumococcus
pO_2 – partial pressure of
    oxygen
poikiloblast
poikilocyte
poikilocytosis
POLY – polymorphonuclear
    leukocyte
polychromasia
polychromatophilia
polychromatosis
polychromemia
polycyte
polycythemia
    p. hypertonica

polycythemia *(continued)*
    myelopathic p.
    p. rubra
    splenomegalic p.
    p. vera
polycytosis
polyemia
    p. aquosa
    p. hyperalbuminosa
    p. polycythaemica
    p. serosa
polymorphocyte
polymorphonuclear
    p. basophil
    p. eosinophil
    p. leukocyte
    p. neutrophil
polynuclear
polysaccharide
polysomaty
polysomy X
Porges-Meier test
Porges-Salomon test
Porocephalus
    P. armillatus
    P. clavatus
    P. constrictus
    P. denticulatus
porphobilinogen
porphyria
porphyrin
postprandial
potassium
Powassan virus
PP – postprandial
PPD – purified protein
    derivative
pregnanediol

pregnanetriol
Preisz-Nocard bacillus
premyeloblast
premyelocyte
proerythroblast
proerythrocyte
profile
    liver p.
Proflagellata
proliferate
proliferation
prolymphocyte
promegaloblast
promonocyte
promyelocyte
pronormoblast
Propeomyces
proplasmacyte
Proteeae
proteidin
    pyocyanase p.
protein
    Bence Jones p.
    C-reactive p.
proteinemia
proteinosis
proteinuria
    Bence Jones p.
proteoclastic
proteolipid
proteose
proteosuria
Proteus
    P. inconstans
    P. mirabilis
    P. morganii
    P. rettgeri
    P. vulgaris

prothrombin
prothrombinase
prothrombinogen
prothrombinokinase
prothrombinopenia
protoanemonin
Protobacterieae
protocoproporphyria
protoporphyrin
Protozoa
protozoan
protozoon
protozoophage
Prowazekia
Pseudamphistomum
    truncatum
Pseudomonadaceae
Pseudomonadales
Pseudomonadineae
Pseudomonas
    P. aeruginosa
    P. eisenbergii
    P. fluorescens
    P. fragi
    P. non-liquefaciens
    P. pseudomallei
    P. pyocyanea
    P. syncyanea
    P. viscosa
Pseudomonilia
PSP – phenolsulfonphthalein
PTA – plasma thromboplastin
    antecedent
PTC – plasma thromboplastin
    component
PTT – partial thromboplastin
    time
Pulex

Pulex
    P. irritans
Pulicidae
Pullularia
purpura
    thrombocytopenic p.
pyocyanase
pyogenic
pyroglobulin
QNS – quantity not sufficient
qualitative
quantitative
Quick's test
RA – rheumatoid arthritis
rabdo-. See words beginning
    rhabdo-.
RAI – radioactive iodine
Ramon flocculation
rate
    sedimentation r.
ratio
    myeloid-erythroid r.
RBC – red blood cell
    red blood count
RBC/hpf – red blood cells
    per high power field
RBE – relative biological
    effectiveness
reaction
    Bence Jones r.
    Ehrlich's r.
    Gruber-Widal r.
    Wasserman r.
    Weil-Felix r.
    Widal r.
renin
renogram
reticulin

reticulocyte
reticuloendothelial
Rh — Rhesus (factor)
rhabdocyte
Rhabdomonas
Rhinocladium
Rhizobiaceae
Rhizobium
Rhizoglyphus
    R. parasiticus
Rhizopoda
Rhizopus
    R. equinus
    R. niger
    R. nigricans
RhoGAM vaccine
riboflavin
Rickett's organism
Rickettsia
    R. akamushi
    R. akari
    R. australis
    R. conorii
    R. diaporica
    R. mooseri
    R. muricola
    R. nipponica
    R. orientalis
    R. pediculi
    R. prowazekii
    R. quintana
    R. rickettsii
    R. tsutsugamushi
    R. typhi
    R. wolhynica
Rickettsiaceae
rickettsial
Rift Valley fever virus

Ringer's solution
rinokladeum. See
    Rhinocladium.
RISA — radioiodinated serum
    albumin
rizo-. See words beginning
    Rhizo-.
RNA — ribonucleic acid
rod-shaped
roolo. See *rouleau* and
    rouleaux.
Rose's test
Rose-Waaler test
Rothera's test
rouleau
rouleaux
roundworm
Rourke-Ernstein sedimenta-
    tion rate
Rowntree and Geraghty's test
RPF — renal plasma flow
RS virus
rubella
rubrum
Russell unit
Russian spring-summer
    encephalitis v.
Saccharomyces
    S. albicans
    S. anginae
    S. apiculatus
    Busse's s.
    S. cantliei
    S. capillitii
    S. carlsbergensis
    S. cerevisiae
    S. coprogenus
    S. epidermica

Saccharomyces *(continued)*
- S. galacticolus
- S. glutinis
- S. lemonnieri
- S. mellis
- S. mycoderma
- S. neoformans

Salmonella
- S. choleraesuis
- S. derby
- S. durazzo
- S. enteritidis
- S. gallinarum
- S. montevideo
- S. muenchen
- S. paratyphi A, B, C
- S. pullorum
- S. schottmülleri
- S. sendai
- S. typhi
- S. typhimurium
- S. typhisuis
- S. typhosa

Sappinia diploidea
Saprospira
Sarcina
Sarcocystis
sarcocyte
Sarcodina
Sarcophaga
- S. carnaria
- S. dux
- S. fuscicauda
- S. haemorrhoidalis
- S. nificornis

Sarcoptes
- S. scabiei

scan

scan
- brain s.
- kidney s.
- liver s.
- RAI s.
- risa s.
- spleen s.

SCG — serum chemistry graph
Schick test
Schilling
- blood count
- test

schistocyte
Schistosoma
- S. haematobium
- S. intercalatum
- S. japonicum
- S. mansoni

schistosome
schistosomiasis
Schizoblastosporion
schizogony
Schmitz's bacillus
Schmorl's bacillus
Schottmüller's disease
schwannoma
Schwann's white substance
scolecoid
scolex
Scopulariopsis
- S. americana
- S. aureus
- S. blochi
- S. brevicaulis
- S. cinereus
- S. koningi
- S. minimus

scopulariopsosis
sediment

sedimentation
    erythrocyte s.
sedimentation rate
    Rourke-Ernstein s.r.
    Westergren's s.r.
    Wintrobe's s.r.
sefalin. See *cephalin.*
sefalosporeum. See
    Cephalosporium.
SEGS — segmented cells
Semliki Forest virus
Sendai virus
sensitivity
septicemia
serkarea. See *cercaria.*
serology
serotonin
serotype
serous
Serratia
    S. indica
    S. kiliensis
    S. marcescens
    S. piscatorum
    S. plymuthica
Serratieae
serum creatinine
sfero-. See words beginning
    with *sphero-.*
SGOT — serum glutamic
    oxaloacetic transaminase
SGPT — serum glutamic
    pyruvic transaminase
SH - serum hepatitis
shaletela. See *Cheyletiella.*
Shiga's bacillus
Shigella
    S. alkalescens

Shigella *(continued)*
    S. ambigua
    S. arabinotarda Type A,
        B
    S. boydii
    S. ceylonensis
    S. dispar
    S. dysenteriae
    S. etousae
    S. flexneri
    S. madampensis
    S. newcastle
    S. paradysenteriae
    S. parashigae
    S. schmitzii
    S. shigae
    S. sonnei
    S. wakefield
Shinowara-Jones-Reinhard
    unit
sickle cell
sickling
Siderobacter
Siderocapsa
Siderocapsaceae
Siderococcus
siderocyte
sifasea. See *Syphacia.*
Simbu virus
Sims-Huhner test
Sindbis virus
skisto-. See words beginning
    schisto-.
skizo-. See words beginning
    schizo-.
SMA-12 profile test
smear
    fungi s.

smear *(continued)*
    Papanicolaou's s.
    TB s.
sodium
solution
    Ringer's s.
Somogyi unit
Sonne-Duval bacillus
Sonne dysentery
SPCA — serum prothrombin-
   conversion accelarator
SPF — specific pathogen free
sp. gr. — specific gravity
spherocyte
spherocytosis
Spirillaceae
Spirillum
    S. minus
Spirochaeta
    S. daxensis
    S. eurystrepta
    S. marina
    S. pallida
    S. plicatilis
    S. stenostrepta
    S. vincenti
Spirochete
Sporotrichum
    S. schenckii
Sporozoa
sporozoite
sporozoon
sputum
SSKI — saturated solution of
   potassium iodide
STAB — stabnuclear neutrophil
steroid
St. Louis encephalitis virus

staf-. See words beginning
   staph-.
stain
    alcian blue s.
    Bowie's s.
    Congo red s.
    Giemsa's s.
    Gram's s.
    Jenner-Giemsa s.
    Leishman's s.
    May-Grunwald-Giemsa s.
    Papanicolaou's s.
    Pappenheim's s.
    van Gieson's s.
    Wade-Fite-Faraco s.
    Weigert's s.
    Wright's s.
    Ziehl-Neelsen's s.
staphylocoagulase
staphylococcal
staphylococcemia
staphylococci
Staphylococcus
    S. albus
    S. aureus
    S. citreus
    S. epidermidis
staphylolysin
    α s., alpha s.
    β s., beta s.
    δ s., delta s.
    ϵ s., epsilon s.
    γ s., gamma s.
stippling
    basophilic s.
Stormer viscosimeter
Streptobacillus
    S. moniliformis

Streptococceae
streptococci
Streptococcus
    S. agalactiae
    S. anginosus
    S. bovis
    S. cremoris
    S. durans
    S. equi
    S. equisimilis
    S. faecalis
    S. faecium
    S. fecalis
    S. hemolyticus
    S. lactis
    S. liquefaciens
    S. MG
    S. mitis
    S. pyogenes
    S. salivarius
    S. uberis
    S. viridans
    S. zooepidemicus
    S. zymogenes
streptococcus
   alpha s.
   anhemolytic s.
   Bargen's s.
   beta s.
   Fehleisen's s.
   gamma s.
   hemolytic s.
   nonhemolytic s.
   s. of Ostertag
streptolysin O, S
Streptomyces
    S. madurae
    S. pelletieri

Streptomyces
    S. somaliensis
Streptothrix
Strong's bacillus
Strongyloides
    S. stercoralis
strongyloidiasis
STS – serologic test for
     syphilis
    standard test for
     syphilis
STU – skin test unit
study
    erythrokinetic s's.
    fat absorption s's.
substance
    white s. of Schwann
    zymoplastic s.
suda-. See words beginning
    pseuda-.
Sudan black
Sudan
    S. I
    S. II
    S. G. S. III
    S. IV
    S. yellow G
sudo-. See words beginning
    pseudo-.
sulfhemoglobin
sulfmethemoglobin
sulfobromophthalein
Sulkowitch's test
survival
    red blood cell s.
Swiss type agammaglobulin-
    emia
Syphacia

Syphacia
    S. obvelata
Taenia
    T. africana
    T. brunerri
    T. confusa
    T. echinococcus
    T. philippina
    T. saginata
    T. solium
Takata-Ara test
tapeworm
target cell
TAT – toxin-antitoxin
TB – tubercle bacillus
    tuberculosis
TBC – tuberculosis
TBG – thyroxine-binding
    globulin
TBI – thyroxine binding index
tenea. See *Taenia.*
tenosefalidez. See
    Ctenocephalides.
T_3 – triiodothyronine
T_4 – thyroxine, levothyroxine,
    tetralodothyronine
Teschen virus
test
    Abrams' t.
    acetic acid t.
    acetic acid and potassium
      ferrocyanide t.
    aceto-acetic acid t.
    acetone t.
    acidosis t.
    acid phosphatase t.
    ACTH t.
    Adamkiewicz's t.

test *(continued)*
    Adler's t.
    adrenalin t.
    adrenocortical
      inhibition t.
    A/G ratio t.
    agglutination t.
    albumin t.
    aldolase t.
    aldosterone t.
    alizarin t.
    alkali t.
    alkali denaturation t.
    alkali tolerance t.
    alkaline phosphatase t.
    alkaloid t.
    alpha amino nitrogen t.
    amylase t.
    arginine t.
    Aschheim-Zondek t.
    ascorbic acid t.
    Bence Jones protein t.
    Benedict's t.
    bile acid t.
    bile pigment t.
    bile solubility t.
    bilirubin t., direct,
      indirect
    blood urea nitrogen t.
    Bloor's t.
    Bloxam's t.
    Boas' t.
    Bonanno's t.
    bromsulfalein t.
    butanol extractable
      iodine t.
    calcium t.
    capillary fragility t.

test *(continued)*

carbon dioxide combing
power t.
Casoni's intradermal t.
Castellani's t.
catecholamine t.
cephalin-cholesterol
flocculation t.
cephalin flocculation t.
cholesterol t.
cholinesterase t.
coagulation t.
colloidal gold t.
Congo Red t.
Coombs' t., direct,
indirect
coproporphyrin t.
cortisone-glucose
tolerance t.
C-reactive protein t.
creatine t.
creatinine t.
dextrose t.
Diagnex Blue t.
Dick t.
Donath-Landsteiner t.
Ehrlich's t.
Ellsworth-Howard t.
Fehling's t.
Feulgen t.
fibrinogen t.
Fishberg's concentration
t.
flocculation t.
fluorescent treponemal
antibody t.
formol-gel t.
fragility t.

test *(continued)*

Frei t.
Friedman's t.
frog t.
galactose tolerance t.
Gerhardt's t.
glucagon t.
glucose tolerance t.
glycogen storage t.
Gravindex t.
Guthrie t.
Ham's t.
Hanger's t.
Harrison's t.
heterophile antibody t.
Hicks-Pitney thrombo-
plastin generation t.
hippuric acid t.
Hogben t.
homogentisic acid t.
Howard t.
17-hydroxycortico-
steroid t.
5-hydroxyindoleacetic
acid t.
I^{131} uptake t.
(radioactive iodine)
icterus index t.
indican t.
indigo-carmine t.
insulin clearance t.
insulin tolerance t.
iron binding capacity t.
isoiodeikon t.
Jones-Cantarow t.
Kahn t.
17-ketosteroid t.
Kolmer's t.

test *(continued)*

- Kunkel's t.
- lactic acid t.
- lactic dehydrogenase t.
- lactose tolerance t.
- Ladendorff's t.
- latex fixation t.
- latex slide agglutination t.
- LE t.
- leucine aminopeptidase t.
- Levinson t.
- levulose tolerance t.
- lipase t.
- lipid t.
- lymphocyte transfer t.
- magnesium t.
- malaria film t.
- mallein t.
- Malmejde's t.
- Mantoux skin t.
- mastic t.
- melanin t.
- methylene blue t.
- Metopirone t.
- Mosenthal's t.
- mucoprotein t.
- Murphy-Pattee t.
- nonprotein nitrogen t.
- Obermayer's t.
- Obermüller's t.
- occult blood t.
- osazone t.
- Pandy's t.
- Papanicolaou's t.
- partial thromboplastin time t.

test *(continued)*

- Paul-Bunnell t.
- Paul-Bunnell-Barrett t.
- Petri's t.
- phenolphthalein t.
- phenolsulfonphthalein t.
- phenylketonuria t.
- phosphatase t.
- phospholipid t.
- phosphoric acid t.
- Piazza's t.
- Porges-Meier t.
- Porges-Salomon t.
- porphobilinogen t.
- porphyrin t.
- potassium t.
- precipitin t.
- protein t.
- protein bound iodine t.
- prothrombin t.
- purine bodies t.
- Quick's t.
- RA latex fixation t.
- radioactive iodine t.
- rose bengal t.
- Rose's t.
- Rose-Waaler t.
- Rothera's t.
- Rowntree and Geraghty's t.
- Schick t.
- Schilling t.
- sedimentation t.
- serology t.
- sickle cell t.
- sickling t.
- Sims-Huhner t.

test *(continued)*
    SMA-12 profile t.
    sodium t.
    Sulkowitch's t.
    T-3 uptake t.
    Takata-Ara t.
    Thorn t.
    thromboplastin
      generation t.
    thymol turbidity t.
    thyroxine binding
      index t.
    Tine t.
    tolbutamide tolerance t.
    transaminase t. (SGOT -
      SGPT)
    trypsin t.
    tyrosine t.
    Uffelmann's t.
    urea clearance t.
    urea nitrogen t.
    uric acid t.
    urobilinogen t.
    van den Bergh t.
    vanilmandelic acid t.
    Van Slyke t.
    VDRL t.
    Voges-Proskauer t.
    Volhard's t.
    Wassermann t.
    wire loop t.
    xylose concentration t.
    d-xylose tolerance t.
    zinc flocculation t.
    zinc turbidity t.
tetraploidy
TGT – thromboplastin
    generation test

TGT – thromboplastin
    generation time
thalassemia
THAM – trihydroxymethyl-
    aminomethane
Theiler's virus
thermogram
thiocyanate
Thorn test
thread
    mucous t's.
thrombasthenia
thrombin
thrombocyte
thrombocytopenia
thrombocytopoiesis
thrombocytosis
thrombometer
thromboplastic
thromboplastin
thromboplastinogen
thrombostasis
thrombosthenin
thrombotest
thymol turbidity
TIBC – total iron-binding
    capacity
Tine test
titer
    agglutination t.
    antihyaluronidase t.
titration
TNTC – too numerous to
    count
Todd's bodies
Todd units
Torula
    T. capsulatus

Torula
    T. histolytica
toxin
Toxocara
    T. canis
    T. cati
toxocariasis
toxoid
toxoid-antitoxoid
Toxoplasma
    T. gondii
    T. pyrogenes
toxoplasmosis
TPI — Treponema pallidium
    immobilization
TPTZ — tripyridyltriazine
Trachybdella bistriata
Trematoda
    T. Clonorchis
    T. Dicrocoelium
    T. Echinostoma
    T. Fasciola
    T. Fasciolopsis
    T. Gastrodiscoides
    T. Heterophyes
    T. Metagonimus
    T. Opisthorchis
    T. Paragonimus
    T. Schistosoma
trematode
Treponema
    T. calligyrum
    T. carateum
    T. genitalis
    T. macrodentium
    T. microdentium
    T. mucosum
    T. pallidum

Treponema *(continued)*
    T. pertenue
    T. pintae
Tricercomonas
Trichinella
    T. spiralis
trichinosis
trichomonad
Trichomonas
    T. buccalis
    T. hominis
    T. intestinalis
    T. pulmonalis
    T. vaginalis
trichomoniasis
Trichophyton
    T. concentricum
    T. epilans
    T. ferrugineum
    T. mentagrophytes
    T. rosaceum
    T. rubrum
    T. sabouraudi
    T. schoenleini
    T. sulfureum
    T. tonsurans
    T. verrucosum
    T. violaceum
trichophytosis
Trichoptera
Trichosporon
    T. beigelii
    T. cutaneum
    T. pedrosianum
Trichostrongylus
    T. instabilis
    T. orientalis
    T. vitrinus

Trichothecium
  T. roseum
Trichuris
  T. trichiura
triglyceride
Triodontophorus
  T. diminutus
Triphleps insidiosus
triploidy
trisomies
trisomy C, mosaic
trisomy D
trisomy E
trisomy G
trisomy X
trisomy 18
Trombicula
  T. autumnalis
  T. irritans
  T. tsalsahuati
  T. vandersandi
Trombiculidae
trophoplasm
trophozoite
TRP — tubular reabsorption
  of phosphate
Trypanosoma
  T. cruzi
  T. escomeli
  T. gambiense
  T. rhodesiense
trypanosomiasis
trypsin
tryptase
TSH — thyroid stimulating
  hormone
tularemia
Tunga

Tunga
  T. penetrans
typhoid
typhus
Tyroglyphus
  T. siro
tyrosine
tyrosinosis
ubakterealez. See
  Eubacteriales.
ubaktereum. See
  Eubacterium.
Uffelmann's test
Uganda S virus
uglena. See *Euglena.*
uglobulin. See *euglobulin.*
ugonik. See *eugonic.*
unit
  Bessey-Lowry u.
  Bodansky u.
  Gutman u.
  King-Armstrong u.
  mouse u.
  rat u.
  Russell u.
  Shinowara-Jones-
    Reinhard u.
  Somogyi u.
  Todd u's.
  Wohlgemuth u.
uproktis. See *Euproctis.*
uptake
  RAI u.
  resin u.
urea
uric
urinalysis
urobilin

urobilinogen
Uronema caudatum
uropepsin
uroporphyrin
uroreaction
urosheum. See *Eurotium.*
Uruma virus
usimuleum. See *Eusimulium.*
utriatoma. See *Eutriatoma.*
utrombikula. See
  Eutrombicula.
vaccine
Vahlkampfia
van den Bergh test
van Gieson's stain
Van Slyke test
Vaquez-Osler disease
Vaquez's disease
VDRL – Venereal Disease
  Research Laboratories
VEE virus – Venezuelan
  equine encephalomyelitis
Veillonella
    V. alcalescens
    V. discoides
    V. orbiculus
    V. parvula
    V. reniformis
    V. vulvovaginitidis
venipuncture
Verticillium
    V. graphii
Vibrio
    V. alginolyticus
    V. bulbulus
    V. cholerae
    V. cholerae-asiaticae
    V. coli

Vibrio *(continued)*
    V. comma
    V. danubicus
    V. fecalis
    V. fetus
    V. finkleri
    V. ghinda
    V. jejuni
    V. massauah
    V. metchnikovii
    V. niger
    V. parahemolyticus
    V. phosphorescens
    V. proteus
    V. septicus
    V. tyrogenus
vibrio
    Celebes' v.
    cholera v.
    El Tor's v's.
    non-agglutinating v's.
    paracholera v's.
vibrion
    v. septique
Vincent's organisms
viral
virus
    animal v's.
    v. animatum
    arbor v's.
    attenuated v.
    Australian X disease v.
    bacterial v.
    Brunhilde v.
    Bunyamwera v.
    Bwamba fever v.
    C v.
    CA v.

virus *(continued)*

- Cache valley v.
- California v.
- Chikungunya v.
- Coe v.
- Colorado tick fever v.
- coryza v.
- Coxsackie v.
- croup associated v.
- cytomegalic inclusion disease v.
- dengue v.
- ECBO v.
- ECDO v.
- ECHO v.
- ECHO 28 v.
- ECMO v.
- ECSO v.
- EEE v.
- EMC v.
- encephalomyocarditis v.
- enteric orphan v's.
- epidemic keratoconjunctivitis v.
- equine encephalomyelitis v.
- filterable v.
- fixed v.
- Guaroa v.
- hemadsorption v. types 1 and 2
- hepatitis v.
- herpangina v.
- herpes v.
- Ilheus v.
- inclusion conjunctivitis v.
- Japanese B encephalitis v.

virus *(continued)*

- JH v.
- Junin v.
- Kumba v.
- Kyasanur Forest disease v.
- Lansing v.
- latent v.
- Leon v.
- louping ill v.
- Lunyo v.
- lymphogranuloma venereum v.
- masked v.
- Mayaro v.
- Mengo v.
- Murray Valley encephalitis v.
- Newcastle disease v.
- O'nyong-nyong v.
- ornithosis v.
- Oropouche v.
- orphan v's.
- pappataci fever v.
- parainfluenza v.
- parrot v.
- pharyngoconjunctival fever v.
- pneumonitis v.
- poliomyelitis v.
- polyoma v.
- Powassan v.
- poxvirus v.
- psittacosis v.
- rabies v.
- respiratory syncytial v.
- Rift Valley fever v.
- RS v.

virus *(continued)*
    Russian spring-summer
      encephalitis v.
    salivary gland v.
    Semliki Forest v.
    Sendai v.
    Simbu v.
    simian v's.
    Sindbis v.
    St. Louis encephalitis v.
    street v.
    Teschen v.
    Theiler's v.
    tick-borne v's.
    trachoma v.
    2060 v.
    Uganda S v.
    unorganized v.
    Uruma v.
    vaccine v.
    VEE v.
    WEE v.
    Wesselsbron v.
    West Nile v.
viscosimeter
    Stormer v.
viscosity
viscous
VMA – vanillylmandelic acid
Voges-Proskauer test
Volhard's test
volumetric
Wade-Fite-Faraco stain
Waldenström's macroglobulin-
    emia
washing
    bronchial w.
Wasserman

Wasserman *(continued)*
    reaction
    test
WBC – white blood cell
    white blood count
WBC/hpf – white blood cells
    per high power field
WEE virus – Western equine
    encephalomyelitis virus
Weichselbaum's diplococcus
Weigert's stain
Weil-Felix reaction
Wesselsbron virus
Westergren's sedimentation
    rate
West Nile virus
whipworm
Whitmore's bacillus
Widal reaction
Wintrobe's sedimentation
    rate
Wohlgemuth unit
Wright's stain
Wuchereria
    W. bancrofti
    W. malayi
wuchereriasis
xanthochromatic
xanthocyte
xanthomatous
Xanthomonas
Xenopsylla
    X. cheopis
zantho-. See words beginning
    xantho-.
Zenker's fixative
Ziehl-Neelsen's stain
Zoogloea

Zuberella   zymogen
Zymobacterium

NORMAL LABORATORY VALUES*

NORMAL HEMATOLOGIC VALUES

Acid hemolysis test (Ham)			No hemolysis
Alkaline phosphatase, leukocyte			Total score 14–100
Bleeding time			
Ivy			Less than 5 min.
Duke			1–5 min.
Carboxyhemoglobin			Up to 5% of total

Cell counts

Erythrocytes:	Males		4.6–6.2 million/cu. mm.
	Females		4.2–5.4 million/cu. mm.
	Children (varies with age)		4.5–5.1 million/cu. mm.

Leukocytes

Total			5000–10,000/cu. mm.

Differential	*Percentage*	*Absolute*
Myelocytes	0	0/cu. mm.
Juvenile neutrophils	3– 5	150– 400/cu. mm.
Segmented neutrophils	54–62	3000–5800/cu. mm.
Lymphocytes	25–33	1500–3000/cu. mm.
Monocytes	3– 7	285– 500/cu. mm.
Eosinophils	1– 3	50– 250/cu. mm.
Basophils	0– 0.75	15– 50/cu. mm.

(Infants and children have greater relative numbers of lymphocytes and monocytes)

Platelets	150,000–350,000/cu. mm.
Reticulocytes	25,000– 75,000/cu. mm.
	0.5–1.5% of erythrocytes
Clot retraction, qualitative	Begins in 30–60 min.
	Complete in 24 hrs.
Coagulation time (Lee-White)	5–15 min. (glass tubes)
	19–60 min. (siliconized tubes)
Cold hemolysin test (Donath-Landsteiner)	No hemolysis

Corpuscular values of erythrocytes
(Values are for adults; in children, values vary with age)

M.C.H. (mean corpuscular hemoglobin)	27–31 picogm.
M.C.V. (mean corpuscular volume)	82–92 cu. micra
M.C.H.C. (mean corpuscular hemoglobin concentration)	32–36%
Fibrinogen	200–400 mg./100 ml.
Fibrinolysins	0

Hematocrit

Males	40–54 ml./100 ml.
Females	37–47 ml./100 ml.
Newborn	49–54 ml./100 ml.
Children (varies with age)	35–49 ml./100 ml.

*Prepared by REX B. CONN, M.D.,
The Johns Hopkins School of Medicine, Baltimore

Hemoglobin
  Males   14.0–18.0 grams/100 ml.
  Females   12.0–16.0 grams/100 ml.
  Newborn   16.5–19.5 grams/100 ml.
  Children (varies with age)   11.2–16.5 grams/100 ml.
Hemoglobin, fetal   Less than 1% of total
Hemoglobin A_2 1.5–3.0% of total
Hemoglobin, plasma   0–5.0 mg./100 ml.
Methemoglobin   0.03–0.13 grams/100 ml.
Osmotic fragility of erythrocytes   Begins in 0.45–0.39% NaCl
                                      Complete in 0.33–0.30% NaCl

Partial thromboplastin time   60–70 sec.
  Kaolin activated   35–45 sec.
Prothrombin consumption   Over 80% consumed in 1 hr.
Prothrombin content   100% (calculated from
                                      prothrombin time)
Prothrombin time (one stage)   12.0–14.0 sec.
Sedimentation rate
  Wintrobe: Males   0–5 mm. in 1 hr.
             Females   0–15 mm. in 1 hr.
  Westergren: Males   0–15 mm. in 1 hr.
             Females   0–20 mm. in 1 hr.
  (May be slightly higher in children and
  during pregnancy)
Thromboplastin generation test   Compared to normal control
Tourniquet test   Ten or fewer petechiae in a
                                    2.5 cm. circle after 5 min.
                                    with cuff at 100 mm. Hg

Bone marrow, differential cell count	*Range*	*Average*
Myeloblasts	0.3– 5.0%	2.0%
Promyelocytes	1.0– 8.0%	5.0%
Myelocytes: Neutrophilic	5.0–19.0%	12.0%
Eosinophilic	0.5– 3.0%	1.5%
Basophilic	0.0– 0.5%	0.3%
Metamyelocytes ("juvenile" forms)	13.0–32.0%	22.0%
Polymorphonuclear neutrophils	7.0–30.0%	20.0%
Polymorphonuclear eosinophils	0.5– 4.0%	2.0%
Polymorphonuclear basophils	0.0– 0.7%	0.2%
Lymphocytes	3.0–17.0%	10.0%
Plasma cells	0.0– 2.0%	0.4%
Monocytes	0.5– 5.0%	2.0%
Reticulum cells	0.1– 2.0%	0.2%
Megakaryocytes	0.03– 3.0%	0.4%
Pronormoblasts	1.0– 8.0%	4.0%
Normoblasts	7.0–32.0%	18.0%

NORMAL BLOOD, PLASMA, AND SERUM VALUES

For some procedures the normal values may vary depending upon the methods used.

Acetone, serum	
Qualitative	Negative
Quantitative	0.3–2.0 mg./100 ml.
Aldolase, serum	0.8–3.0 ml.U./ml. (30°)
	(Sibley-Lehninger)
Alpha amino nitrogen, serum	4–6 mg./100 ml.
Ammonia nitrogen, blood	75–196 mcg./100 ml.
plasma	56-122 mcg./100 ml.
Amylase, serum	80–160 Somogyi units/100 ml.
Ascorbic acid	See Vitamin C
Base, total, serum	145–160 mEq./liter
Bilirubin, serum	
Direct	0.1–0.4 mg./100 ml.
Indirect	0.2–0.7 mg./100 ml.
	(Total minus direct)
Total	0.3–1.1 mg./100 ml.
Calcium, serum	4.5–5.5 mEq./liter
	(9.0–11.0 mg./100 ml.)
	(Slightly higher in children)
	(Varies with protein concentration)
Calcium, serum, ionized	2.1–2.6 mEq./liter
	(4.25–5.25 mg./100 ml.)
Carbon dioxide content, serum	24–30 mEq./liter
	Infants: 20–28 mEq./liter
Carbon dioxide tension (Pco_2), blood	35–45 mm. Hg
Carotene, serum	50–300 mcg./100 ml.
Ceruloplasmin, serum	23–44 mg./100 ml.
Chloride, serum	96–106 mEq./liter
Cholesterol, serum	
Total	150–250 mg./100 ml.
Esters	68–76% of total cholesterol
Cholinesterase, serum	0.5–1.3 pH units
RBC	0.5–1.0 pH units
Copper, serum	
Male	70–140 mcg./100 ml.
Female	85–155 mcg./100 ml.
Cortisol, plasma	6–16 mcg./100 ml.
Creatine, serum	0.2–0.8 mg./100 ml.

Creatine phosphokinase, serum
   Male   0–50 mI.U./ml. (30°)
                                         (Oliver-Rosalki)
   Female   0–30 mI.U./ml. (30°)
                                         (Oliver-Rosalki)

Creatine phosphokinase, serum	
Male	0–50 mI.U./ml. (30°) (Oliver-Rosalki)
Female	0–30 mI.U./ml. (30°) (Oliver-Rosalki)
Creatinine, serum	0.7–1.5 mg./100 ml.
Cryoglobulins, serum	0
Fatty acids, total, serum	190–420 mg./100 ml.
Fibrinogen, plasma	200–400 mg./100 ml.
Folic acid, serum	7–16 nanogm./ml.
Glucose (fasting)	
blood, true	60–100 mg./100 ml.
Folin	80–120 mg./100 ml.
plasma or serum, true	70–115 mg./100 ml.
Haptoglobin, serum	40–170 mg./100 ml.
Hydroxybutyric dehydrogenase, serum	0–180 mI.U./ml. (30°) (Rosalki-Wilkinson) 114–290 units/ml. (Wroblewski)
17-Hydroxycorticosteroids, plasma	8–18 mcg./100 ml.
Icterus index, serum	4–7
Immunoglobulins, serum	
IgG	800–1500 mg./100 ml.
IgA	50–200 mg./100 ml.
IgM	40–120 mg./100 ml.
Iodine, butanol extractable, serum	3.2–6.4 mcg./100 ml.
Iodine, protein bound, serum	3.5–8.0 mcg./100 ml. (May be slightly higher in infants)
Iron, serum	75–175 mcg./100 ml.
Iron binding capacity, total, serum	250–410 mcg./100 ml.
% saturation	20–55%
17-Ketosteroids, plasma	25–125 mcg./100 ml.
Lactic acid, blood	6–16 mg./100 ml.
Lactic dehydrogenase, serum	0–300 mI.U./ml. (30°) (Wroblewski modified) 150–450 units/ml. (Wroblewski) 80–120 units/ml. (Wacker)
Lipase, serum	0–1.5 units (Cherry-Crandall)
Lipids, total, serum	450–850 mg./100 ml.

Magnesium, serum		1.5–2.5 mEq./liter
		(1.8–3.0 mg./100 ml.)
Nitrogen, nonprotein, serum		15–35 mg./100 ml.
Osmolality, serum		285–295 mOsm./liter
Oxygen, blood		
Capacity		16–24 vol. % (varies with Hb)
Content	Arterial	15–23 vol. %
	Venous	10–16 vol. %
Saturation	Arterial	94–100% of capacity
	Venous	60–85% of capacity
Tension, Po$_2$ Arterial		75–100 mm. Hg
pH, arterial, blood		7.35–7.45
Phenylalanine, serum		Less than 3 mg./100 ml.
Phosphatase, acid, serum		1.0–5.0 units (King-Armstrong)
		0.5–2.0 units (Bodansky)
		0.5–2.0 units (Gutman)
		0.0–1.1 units (Shinowara)
		0.1–0.63 unit (Bessey-Lowry)
Phosphatase, alkaline, serum		5.0–13.0 units (King-Armstrong)
		2.0–4.5 units (Bodansky)
		3.0–10.0 units (Gutman)
		2.2–8.6 units (Shinowara)
		0.8–2.3 units (Bassey-Lowry)
		30–85 milliunits/ml. (I.U.)
		(Values are higher in children)
Phosphate, inorganic, serum		3.0–4.5 mg./100 ml.
		(Children: 4.0–7.0 mg./100 ml.)
Phospholipids, serum		6–12 mg./100 ml. as lipid phosphorus
Potassium, serum		3.5–5.0 mEq./liter
Proteins, serum		
Total		6.0–8.0 grams/100 ml.
Albumin		3.5–5.5 grams/100 ml.
Globulin		2.5–3.5 grams/100 ml.
Electrophoresis		
Albumin		3.5–5.5 grams/100 ml.
		52–68% of total
Globulin		
Alpha$_1$		0.2–0.4 gram/100 ml.
		2–5% of total

Alpha$_2$	0.5–0.9 gram/100 ml.
	7–14% of total
Beta	0.6–1.1 grams/100 ml.
	9–15% of total
Gamma	0.7–1.7 grams/100 ml.
	11–21% of total
Pyruvic acid, plasma	1.0–2.0 mg./100 ml.
Serotonin, platelet suspension	0.1–0.3 mcg./ml. blood
serum	0.10–0.32 mcg./ml.
Sodium, serum	136–145 mEq./liter
Sulfates, inorganic, serum	0.8–1.2 mg./100 ml. (as S)
Thyroxine, free, serum	1.0–2.1 nanogm./100 ml.
Thyroxine binding globulin	
(TBG), serum	10–26 mcg./100 ml.
Thyroxine iodine (T$_4$), serum	2.9–6.4 mcg./100 ml.
Transaminase, serum: SGOT	0.19 mI.U./ml. (30°)
	(Karmen modified)
	15–40 units/ml. (Karmen)
	18–40 units/ml.
	(Reitman-Frankel)
SGPT	0.17 mI.U./ml. (30°)
	(Karmen modified)
	6–35 units/ml. (Karmen)
	5–35 units/ml.
	(Reitman-Frankel)
Triglycerides, serum	0–150 mg./100 ml.
Urea, blood	21–43 mg./100 ml.
plasma or serum	24–49 mg./100 ml.
Urea nitrogen, blood (BUN)	10–20 mg./100 ml.
plasma or serum	11–23 mg./100 ml.
Uric acid, serum	
Male	2.5–8.0 mg./100 ml.
Female	1.5–6.0 mg./100 ml.
Vitamin A, serum	20–80 mcg./100 ml.
Vitamin B$_{12}$, serum	200–800 picogm./ml.
Vitamin C, blood	0.4–1.5 mg./100 ml.

NORMAL URINE VALUES

Acetone and acetoacetate	0
Addis count	
Erythrocytes	0–130,000/24 hrs.
Leukocytes	0–650,000/24 hrs.
Casts (hyaline)	0–2000/24 hrs.
Alcapton bodies	Negative
Aldosterone	3–20 mcg./24 hrs.
Alpha amino nitrogen	50–200 mg./24 hrs.
	(Not over 1.5% of total nitrogen)
Ammonia nitrogen	20–70 mEq./24 hrs.
Amylase	35–260 Somogyi units/hr.
Bence Jones protein	Negative
Bilirubin (bile)	Negative
Calcium	
Low Ca diet (Bauer-Aub)	Less than 150 mg./24 hrs.
Usual diet	Less than 250 mg./24 hrs.
Catecholamines	
Epinephrine	Less than 10 mcg./24 hrs.
Norepinephrine	Less than 100 mcg./24 hrs.
Chloride	110–250 mEq./24 hrs.
	(Varies with intake)
Chorionic gonadotrophin	0
Copper	0–30 mcg./24 hrs.
Creatine	
Male	0–40 mg./24 hrs.
Female	0–100 mg./24 hrs.
	(Higher in children and during pregnancy)
Creatinine	15–25 mg./kg. of body weight/24 hrs.
Cystine or cysteine, qualitative	Negative
Delta aminolevulinic acid	1.3–7.0 mg./24 hrs.

Estrogens	Male	Female
Estrone	3–8	4–31
Estradiol	0–6	0–14
Estriol	1–11	0–72
Total	4–25	5–100

(Units above are mcg./24 hours.)
(Markedly increased during pregnancy)

Glucose (reducing substances)	Less than 250 mg./24 hrs.
Gonadotrophins, pituitary	5–10 rat units/24 hrs.
	10–50 mouse units/24 hrs.
	(Increased after menopause)
Hemoglobin and myoglobin	Negative
Homogentisic acid, qualitative	Negative

17-Hydroxycorticosteroids
    Male — 3–9 mg./24 hrs.
    Female — 2–8 mg./24 hrs.
    (Varies with method used)

5-Hydroxyindole-acetic acid (5-HIAA)
    Qualitative — Negative
    Quantitative — Less than 16 mg./24 hrs.

17-Ketosteroids
    Male — 6–18 mg./24 hrs.
    Female — 4–13 mg./24 hrs.

Osmolality — 38–1400 mOsm./kg. water

pH — 4.6–8.0, average 6.0
    (Depends on diet)

Phenylpyruvic acid, qualitative — Negative

Phosphorus — 0.9–1.3 gm./24 hrs.
    (Varies with intake)

Porphobilinogen
    Qualitative — Negative
    Quantitative — 0–0.2 mg./100 ml.
    Less than 2.0 mg./24 hrs.

Porphyrins
    Coproporphyrin — 50–250 mcg./24 hrs.
    Uroporphyrin — 10–30 mcg./24 hrs.

Potassium — 25–100 mEq./24 hrs.
    (Varies with intake)

Pregnanetriol — Less than 2.5 mg./24 hrs. in adults

Protein
    Qualitative — 0
    Quantitative — 10–150 mg./24 hrs.

Sodium — 130–260 mEq./24 hrs.
    (Varies with intake)

Solids, total — 30–70 grams/liter, average
    50 grams/liter
    (To estimate total solids per liter, multiply last two figures of specific gravity by 2.66, Long's coefficient)

Specific gravity — 1.003–1.030

Sugar — 0

Titratable acidity — 20–40 mEq./24 hrs.

Urobilinogen — Up to 1.0 Ehrlich unit/2 hrs. (1–3 P.M.)
    0–4.0 mg./24 hrs.

Vanillylmandelic acid (VMA) — 1–8 mg./24 hrs.

NORMAL VALUES FOR GASTRIC ANALYSIS

Basal gastric secretion (one hour)

	Concentration Mean ± 1 S.D.	Output Mean ± 1 S.D.
Male	25.8 ± 1.8 mEq./liter	2.57 ± 0.16 mEq./hr.
Female	20.3 ± 3.0 mEq./liter	1.61 ± 0.18 mEq./hr.

After histamine stimulation
  Normal   Mean output = 11.8 mEq./hr.
  Duodenal ulcer Mean output = 15.2 mEq./hr.
After maximal histamine stimulation
  Normal   Mean output   22.6 mEq./hr.
  Duodenal ulcer Mean output   44.6 mEq./hr.

Diagnex blue (Squibb):	Anacidity	0–0.3 mg. in 2 hrs.
	Doubtful	0.3–0.6 mg. in 2 hrs.
	Normal	Greater than 0.6 mg. in 2 hrs.

Volume, fasting stomach content	50–100 ml.
Emptying time	3–6 hrs.
Color	Opalescent or colorless
Specific gravity	1.006–1.009
pH (adults)	0.9–1.5

NORMAL VALUES FOR CEREBROSPINAL FLUID

Cells	Fewer than 5 cu. mm., all mononuclear
Chloride	120–130 mEq./liter
	(20 mEq./liter higher than serum)
Colloidal gold test	Not more than 1 in any tube
Glucose	50–75 mg./100 ml.
	(20 mg./100 ml. less than blood)
Pressure	70–180 mm. water
Protein, total	15–45 mg./100 ml.
Albumin	52%
Alpha₁ globulin	5%
Alpha₂ globulin	14%
Beta globulin	10%
Gamma globulin	19%

NORMAL VALUES FOR SEMEN

Volume	2–5 ml., usually 3–4 ml.
Liquefaction	Complete in 15 min.
pH	7.2–8.0; average 7.8
Leukocytes	Occasional or absent
Count	60–150 million/ml.
	Below 60 million/ml. is abnormal
Motility	80% or more motile
Morphology	80–90% normal forms

NORMAL VALUES FOR FECES

Bulk	100–200 grams/24 hrs.
Dry matter	23–32 grams/24 hrs.
Fat, total	Less than 6.0 grams/24 hrs.
Nitrogen, total	Less than 2.0 grams/24 hrs.
Urobilinogen	40–280 mg./24 hrs.
Water	Approximately 65%

NORMAL VALUES FOR SEROLOGIC PROCEDURES

Anti-hyaluronidase	Less than 1:200. Significant if rising titer can be demonstrated at weekly intervals.
Anti-streptolysin O titer	Normal up to 1:128. Single test usually has little significance. Rise in titer or persistently elevated titer is significant.
Bacterial agglutinins	Significant only if rise in titer is demonstrated or if antibodies are absent.
Complement fixation tests	Titers of 1:8 or less are usually not significant. Paired sera showing rise in titer of more than two tubes are usually considered significant.
C reactive protein (CRP)	Negative

Heterophile titer

	Unabsorbed	Absorbed With G.P.	Absorbed With Beef
Normal	1:160	1:10	1:160
Inf. mono.	1:160	1:320	1:10
Serum sickness	1:160	1:5	1:10

Proteus OX-19 agglutinins

1:80	Negative
1:160	Doubtful
1:320	Positive

R. A. test (latex)

1:40	Negative
1:80 –1:160	Doubtful
1:320	Positive

Rose test

1:10	Negative
1:20 –1:40	Doubtful
1:80	Positive

Tularemia agglutinins

1:80	Negative
1:160	Doubtful
1:320	Positive

TOXICOLOGY

Arsenic, blood	3.5–7.2 mcg./100 ml.
Arsenic, urine	Less than 100 mcg./24 hrs.
Barbiturates, serum	0
	Coma level: Phenobarbital approximately 11 mg./100 ml.; most other barbiturates 1.5 mg./100 ml.
Bromides, serum	0
	Toxic levels above 17 mEq./liter
Carbon monoxide, blood	Up to 5% saturation
	Symptoms occur with 20% saturation
Dilantin, blood or serum	Therapeutic levels 1–11 mcg./ml.
Ethanol, blood	Less than 0.005%
Marked intoxication	0.3–0.4%
Alcoholic stupor	0.4–0.5%
Coma	Above 0.5%
Lead, blood	0–40 mcg./100 ml.
Lead, urine	Less than 100 mcg./24 hrs.
Lithium, serum	0
	Therapeutic levels 0.5–1.5 mEq./liter
	Toxic levels above 2 mEq./liter
Mercury, urine	Less than 10 mcg./24 hrs.
Salicylate, plasma	0
Therapeutic range	20–25 mg./100 ml.
Toxic range	Over 30 mg./100 ml.
Death	45–75 mg./100 ml.

LIVER FUNCTION TESTS

Bromsulphalein (B.S.P.)	Less than 5% remaining in serum 45 minutes after injection of 5 mg./kg. of body weight
Cephalin cholesterol flocculation	0–1 in 24 hours.
Galactose tolerance	Excretion of not more than 3.0 grams galactose in the urine 5 hours after ingestion of 40 grams of galactose.
Glycogen storage	Increase of blood glucose 45 mg./100 ml. over fasting level 45 minutes after subcutaneous injection of 0.01 mg./kg. body weight of epinephrine.
Hippuric acid	Excretion of 3.0–3.5 grams hippuric acid in urine within 4 hours after ingestion of 6.0 grams sodium benzoate.

or

Excretion of 0.7 gram hippuric acid in urine within 1 hour after intravenous injection of 1.77 grams sodium benzoate.

Thymol turbidity	0–5 units.
Zinc turbidity	2–12 units.

PANCREATIC (ISLET) FUNCTION TESTS

Glucose tolerance tests Patient should be on a diet containing 300 grams of carbohydrate per day for 3 days prior to test.

Oral After ingestion of 100 grams of glucose or 1.75 grams glucose/kg. body weight, blood glucose is not more than 160 mg./100 ml. after 60 minutes, 140 mg./100 ml. after 90 minutes, and 120 mg./100 ml. after 120 minutes. Values are for blood; serum measurements are approximately 15% higher.

Intravenous Blood glucose does not exceed 200 mg./100 ml. after infusion of 0.5 gram of glucose/kg. body weight over 30 minutes. Glucose concentration falls below initial level at 2 hours and returns to preinfusion levels in 3 hours or 1 hour. Values are for blood; serum measurements are approximately 15% higher.

Cortisone-glucose tolerance test The patient should be on a diet containing 300 grams of carbohydrate per day for 3 days prior to test. At 8½ and again 2 hours prior to glucose load patient is given cortisone acetate by mouth (50 mg. if patient's ideal weight is less than 160 lb., 62.5 mg. if ideal weight is greater than 160 lb.). An oral dose of glucose 1.75 grams/kg. body weight, is given and blood samples are taken at 0, 30, 60, 90, and 120 minutes. Test is considered positive if true blood glucose exceeds 160 mg./100 ml. at 60 minutes, 140 mg./100 ml. at 90 minutes, and 120 mg./100 ml. at 120 minutes. Values are for blood; serum measurements are approximately 15% higher.

RENAL FUNCTION TESTS

Clearance tests (corrected to 1.73 sq. meters body surface area)

Glomerular filtration rate (G.F.R.)

Inulin clearance,
Mannitol clearance, or
Endogenous creatinine clearance

| Males | 110–150 ml./min. |
| Females | 105–132 ml./min. |

Renal plasma flow (R.P.F.)

p-Aminohippurate (P.A.H.), or
Diodrast

| Males | 560–830 ml./min. |
| Females | 490–700 ml./min. |

Filtration fraction (F.F.)

$$FF = \frac{G.F.R.}{R.P.F.}$$

| Males | 17–21% |
| Females | 17–23% |

Urea clearance (C_u)

Standard 40–65 ml./min.
Maximal 60–100 ml./min.

Concentration and dilution

Specific gravity · 1.025 on dry day
Specific gravity · 1.003 on water day

Maximal Diodrast excretory capacity T_{M_D}

Males 43–59 mg./min.
Females 33–51 mg./min.

Maximal glucose reabsorptive capacity T_{M_G}

Males 300–450 mg./min.
Females 250–350 mg./min.

Maximal PAH excretory capacity $T_{M_{PAH}}$

80–90 mg./min.

Phenolsulfonphthalein excretion (P.S.P.)

25% or more in 15 min.
40% or more in 30 min.
55% or more in 2 hrs.
After injection of 1 ml. P.S.P. intravenously.

THYROID FUNCTION TESTS

Protein bound iodine, serum (P.B.I.)	3.5–8.0 mcg./100 ml.
Butanol extractable iodine, serum (B.E.I.)	3.2–6.4 mcg./100 ml.
Thyroxine iodine, serum (T_4)	2.9–6.4 mcg./100 ml.
Free thyroxine, serum	1.4–2.5 nanogram/100 ml.
T_3 (index of unsaturated T.B.G.)	10.0–14.6%
Thyroxine-binding globulin, serum (T.B.G.)	10–26 mcg. T_4/100 ml.
Thyroid-stimulating hormone, serum (T.S.H.)	0 up to 0.2 milliunits/ml.
Radioactive iodine (I^{131}) uptake (R.A.I.)	20–50% of administered dose in 24 hrs.
Radioactive iodine (I^{131}) excretion	30–70% of administered dose in 24 hrs.
Radioactive iodine (I^{131}), protein bound	Less than 0.3% of administered dose per liter of plasma at 72 hrs.
Basal metabolic rate	Minus 10% to plus 10% of mean standard

GASTROINTESTINAL ABSORPTION TESTS

d-Xylose absorption test	After an 8 hour fast 10 ml./kg. body weight of a 5% solution of d-xylose is given by mouth. Nothing further by mouth is given until the test has been completed. All urine voided during the following 5 hours is pooled, and blood samples are taken at 0, 60, and 120 minutes. Normally 26% (range 16–33%) of ingested xylose is excreted within 5 hours, and the serum xylose reaches a level between 25 and 40 mg./100 ml. after 1 hour and is maintained at this level for another 60 minutes.
Vitamin A absorption test	A fasting blood specimen is obtained and 200,000 units of vitamin A in oil is given by mouth. Serum vitamin A level should rise to twice fasting level in 3 to 5 hours.

CARDIOVASCULAR SYSTEM

AA — ascending aorta
A₂ — aortic second sound
ABE — acute bacterial
  endocarditis
Abée's support
aberrant
AC — anŏdal closure
  aortic closure
ACC — anodal closing
  contraction
accelerans
accretio
    a. cordis
    a. pericardii
ACD — absolute cardiac
  dullness
achalasia
acromioclavicular
Adams' disease
Adams-Stokes
    disease
    syncope
    syndrome
Addison's disease
adipositas
    a. cordis
Adson's
    forceps
    hook
    needle
    retractor

adventitious
aerendocardia
AF — aortic flow
    atrial fibrillation
    atrial flutter
AG — atrial gallop
AHD — atherosclerotic heart
  disease
AI — aortic incompetence
    aortic insufficiency
    apical impulse
Alexander-Farabeuf
    periosteotome
Alfred M. Large's clamp
ALG — antilymphocyte
    globulin
Allen's test
Allison's retractor
allorhythmia
allorhythmic
all or none law
Allport-Babcock searcher
alternans
    a. of the heart
AMI — acute myocardial
    infarction
amyloid
anastomosis
aneurysm
    abdominal a.
    aortic arch a.

aneurysm *(continued)*
    arteriovenous a.
    axial a.
    Bérard's a.
    cylindroid a.
    cystogenic a.
    ectatic a.
    embolic a.
    embolomycotic a.
    endogenous a.
    erosive a.
    exogenous a.
    fusiform a.
    Park's a.
    popliteal a.
    Pott's a.
    Richet's a.
    Rodrigues's a.
    thoracic a.
aneurysmal
aneurysmectomy
aneurysmogram
aneurysmoplasty
aneurysmorrhaphy
aneurysmotomy
angialgia
angiasthenia
angiectasis
angiectatic
angiectid
angiectomy
angiectopia
angiemphraxis
angiitis
angileucitis
angina
    a. ducubitis

angina *(continued)*
    a. dyspeptica
    a. pectoris
    a. pectoris vasomotoria
anginal
anginiform
anginoid
anginose
anginosis
angioataxia
angioblast
angioblastic
angioblastoma
angiocardiography
angiocardiokinetic
angiocardiopathy
angiocarditis
angioclast
angiodiascopy
angiodiathermy
angiogenesis
angiogenic
angiogram
angiograph
angiography
angiohypertonia
angiohypotonia
angioinvasive
angiokinesis
angiokinetic
angiolipoma
angiolith
angiolithic
angiologia
angiology
angioma
angiomatosis

angiometer
angiomyocardiac
angioneoplasm
angioneumography
angioneurosis
angioneurotomy
angionoma
angioparalysis
angioparesis
angiopathology
angiopathy
angioplasty
angiopressure
angiorrhaphy
angiosclerosis
angiosclerotic
angiospasm
angiostomy
angiotelectasis
angiotribe
angloid
anomaly
 Ebstein's a.
anoxemia
anoxia
 stagnant a.
anteroposterior
anticoagulant
AO – anodal opening
 aorta
 aortic opening
 opening of the atrio-
  ventricular valves
aorta
 abdominal a.
 a. abdominalis
 a. angusta
 a. ascendens

aorta *(continued)*
 ascending a.
 a. chlorotica
 a. descendens
 descending a.
 dynamic a.
 palpable a.
 primitive a.
 a. sacrococcygea
 a. thoracalis
 thoracic a.
 a. thoracica
 throbbing a.
 ventral a.
aortae
aortal
aortalgia
aortarctia
aortectasia
aortectasis
aortectomy
aortic
aorticorenal
aortism
aortismus
 a. abdominalis
aortitis
 Dohle-Heller a.
 nummular a.
 syphilitic a.
 a. syphilitica
 a. syphilitica obliterans
aortoclasia
aortogram
 transbrachial arch a.
 translumbar a.
aortography
 retrograde a.

aortolith
aortomalacia
aortopathy
aortoptosia
aortorrhaphy
aortosclerosis
aortostenosis
aortotomy
AP – angina pectoris
    anteroposterior
    arterial pressure
APB – atrial premature beat
    auricular premature
      beat
APC – atrial premature
      contraction
apex
    a. cordis
apical
apices
apnea
apneic
appendage
    atrial a.
    auricular a.
AR – aortic regurgitation
    artificial respiration
arcus
    a. aortae
Argyle's catheter
arrest
    cardiac a.
    sinus a.
arrhythmia
    inotropic a.
    nodal a.
    respiratory a.

arrhythmia *(continued)*
    sinus a.
    vagus a.
arrhythmic
arterial
arterialization
arteriarctia
arteriasis
arteriectasis
arteriectomy
arterioatony
arteriocapillary
arteriochalasis
arteriodilating
arteriofibrosia
arteriogram
    femoral a.
    subclavian a.
arteriograph
arteriography
arteriolae
arteriolar
arteriole
arteriolith
arteriolonecrosis
arteriolosclerosis
arteriolosclerotic
arteriomalacia
arteriometer
arteriomotor
arteriomyomatosis
arterionecrosis
arteriopalmus
arteriopathy
    hypertensive a.
arteriophlebotomy
arterioplania
arterioplasty

arteriorenal
arteriorrhagia
arteriorrhaphy
arteriorrhexis
arteriosclerosis
    cerebral a.
    coronary a.
    decrescent a.
    diffuse a.
    infantile a.
    intimal a.
    Mönckeberg's a.
    nodose a.
    nodular a.
    a. obliterans
    peripheral a.
    senile a.
arteriosclerotic
arteriospasm
arteriostenosis
arteriosteogenesis
arteriostosis
arteriostrepsis
arteriosus
    patent ductus a.
arteriosympathectomy
arteriotome
arteriotomy
arteriotony
arteriovenous
arterioversion
arteritis
    a. deformans
    a. hyperplastica
    necrosing a.
    a. nodosa
    a. obliterans
    temporal a.

arteritis *(continued)*
    a. umbilicalis
    a. verrucosa
artery
    brachial a.
    carotid a.
    coronary a.
    innominate a.
    interventricular a.
    peroneal a.
    pulmonary a.
    subclavian a.
    tibial a.
artifact
AS − aortic stenosis
    arteriosclerosis
Aschoff's
    bodies
    node
Aschoff-Tawara node
ascites
ASCVD − arteriosclerotic
        cardiovascular
        disease
        atherosclerotic
        cardiovascular
        disease
ASD − atrial septal defect
asequence
ASHD − arteriosclerotic
        heart disease
ASMI − anteroseptal
        myocardial infarct
ASO − arteriosclerosis
        obliterans
asphygmia
asthenia
    neurocirculatory a.

asynchronism
asystole
atelocardia
atheroma
atheromatous
atheronecrosis
atherosclerosis
atresia
    aortic a.
    tricuspid a.
atrial
atriocommissuropexy
atriomegaly
atrionector
atrioseptopexy
atriotome
atriotomy
atrioventricular
atrium
    a. cordis
    a. dextrum
    a. pulmonale
    pulmonary a.
    a. sinistrum
auricle
auricula
    a. atrii
    a. atrii dextri
    a. atrii sinistri
    a. cordis
    a. dextra cordis
    a. sinistra cordis
auricular
auriculoventricular
auscultation
auscultatory
Austin Flint murmur
AV – arteriovenous

AV – atrioventricular
A-V dissociation
avascular
AVR – aortic valve
        replacement
AVRP – atrioventricular
            refractory period
A wave
awbooshma. See
    embouchment.
AWI – anterior wall infarction
awl
        Rochester's a.
        Wangensteen's a.
AWMI – anterior wall myo-
            cardial infarction
axis
Ayerza's syndrome
azotemia
azygography
azygos
Babinski's syndrome
Bachmann's bundle
Bahnson's clamp
Bailey-Gibbon rib contractor
Bailey-Glover-O'Neil knife
Bailey-Morse knife
Bailey's
        clamp
        rib contractor
ballistocardiogram
ballistocardiograph
ballistocardiography
Bamberger's bulbar pulse
Barraya's forceps
Baylor's sump
BE – bacterial endocarditis
Beardsley's dilator

beat
    ectopic b's.
    nodal b's.
    premature auricular b's.
Beau's
    disease
    syndrome
Beck's
    clamp
    rasp
Bengolea's forceps
Bérard's aneurysm
Bernheim's syndrome
Bethune's rib shears
bifurcation
bigeminal
bigeminy
    nodal b.
bipolar
Bishop's sphygmoscope
blade
    Cooley-Pontius b.
    DeBakey's b.
Blalock-Taussig operation
block
    atrioventricular b.
    A-V b.
    bundle-branch b.
    sino-auricular b.
blow
    diastolic b.
body
    Aschoff's b's.
Boettcher's forceps
Bosher's knife
Botallo's duct
Bouillaud's tinkle
Bradshaw-O'Neill clamp

bradycardia
    Branham's b.
    cardiomuscular b.
    clinostatic b.
    nodal b.
    postinfective b.
    sinus b.
    vagal b.
bradycardiac
bradycrotic
bradydiastole
bradydiastolia
Branham's bradycardia
Brauer's operation
Bright's murmur
Broadbent's sign
Brock's
    knife
    operation
    punch
bruit
    aneurysmal b.
    b. de canon (brwe duh
        kahnaw)
    b. de choc (brwe duh
        shawk)
    b. de craquement (brwe
        duh krak maw)
    b. de cuir neuf (brwe
        duh kwer nuf)
    b. de diable (brwe duh
        de ahbl)
    b. de frolement (brwe
        duh frolmaw)
    b. de lime (brwe duh
        lem)
    b. de moulin (brwe duh
        moola)

bruit *(continued)*
  b. de parchemin (brwe duh parshmaw)
  b. de piaulement (brwe duh pyolmaw)
  b. de rape (brwe duh rahp)
  b. de rappel (brwe duh rahpel)
  b. de Roger (brwe duh rozha)
  b. de scie (brwe duh se)
  Roger's b.
  systolic b.
brwe. See *bruit.*
Buerger's disease
bulbus
  b. aortae
  b. arteriosus
  b. caroticus
  b. cordis
  b. venae jugularis
bundle
  atrioventricular b.
  a-v. b.
  Bachmann's b.
  b. branch block
  b. of His
  Keith's b.
  Kent-His b.
  Kent's b.
  sino-atrial b.
  b. of Stanley-Kent
  Thorel's b.
Burford's rib spreader
Burger's triangle
by-pass
  aortoiliac b.

by-pass *(continued)*
  cardiopulmonary b.
  coronary artery b.
  femoropopliteal b.
CA – cardiac arrest
  coronary artery
cachexia
Cameron-Haight elevator
canalization
Cannon's endarterectomy loop
cannula
  Rockey's c.
  Silastic coronary artery c.
  Soresi's c.
cannulate
cannulation
capillary
  Meig's c's.
cardiac
cardialgia
cardianastrophe
cardiasthenia
cardiasthma
cardiectasis
cardiectomy
cardioaccelerator
cardioaortic
cardioarterial
cardiocairograph
cardiocele
cardiocentesis
cardiocirrhosis
cardioclasis
cardiodiaphragmatic
cardiodilator
cardiodiosis

cardiogram
    echo c.
cardiograph
cardiography
cardio-green
cardiohepatic
cardiohepatomegaly
cardioinhibitory
cardiokinetic
cardiolith
cardiologist
cardiology
cardiolysis
cardiomalacia
cardiomegalia
    c. glycogenica
      circumscripta
cardiomegaly
cardiomelanosis
cardiometer
cardiometry
cardiomotility
cardiomyoliposis
cardiomyopathy
cardiomyopexy
cardiomyotomy
cardionecrosis
cardionector
cardionephric
cardioneural
cardioneurosis
cardio-omentopexy
cardiopalmus
cardiopaludism
cardiopathy
cardiopericardiopexy
cardiopericarditis
cardiophone

cardioplegia
cardiopneumograph
cardiopneumonopexy
cardioptosis
cardiopulmonary
cardiorrhaphy
cardiorrhexis
cardioschisis
cardiosclerosis
cardioscope
cardiospasm
cardiosphygmogram
cardiosphygmograph
cardiosplenopexy
cardiosymphysis
cardiotachometer
cardiotomy
cardiotoxic
cardiovalvular
cardiovalvulitis
cardiovalvulotomy
cardiovascular
cardioversion
carditis
    rheumatic c.
    Sterges' c.
carotid
Carter's retractor
Cartwright's prosthesis
catheter
    Argyle's c.
    Edwards' c.
    Fogarty's c.
    Lehman's c.
    NIH c.
    Teflon c.
catheterization
    cardiac c.

catheterization
    hepatic vein c.
CC – cardiac cycle
CD – cardiac disease
    cardiac dullness
    cardiovascular disease
CE – cardiac enlargement
cerebrocardiac
CF – cardiac failure
change
    QRS c's.
    QRS-T c's.
    ST segment c's.
    T wave c's.
CHB – complete heart block
CHD – congenital heart
       disease
    coronary heart disease
Cheyne-Stokes respiration
CHF – congestive heart
       failure
choc
    c. en dome
cholesterol
chorda
    c. tendineae cordis
CI – cardiac index
    cardiac insufficiency
    coronary insufficiency
CICU – cardiology intensive
       care unit
    coronary intensive
      care unit
cineangiocardiography
cineangiography
cineradiography
circle
    c. of Willis

circulation
circulatory
circulus
    c. arteriosus
    c. arteriosus cerebri
    c. articuli vasculosus
clamp
    Alfred M. Large's c.
    Bahnson's c.
    Bailey's c.
    Beck's c.
    Bradshaw-O'Neill c.
    Cooley's c.
    Crafoord's c.
    Crutchfield's c.
    Davis' c.
    DeBakey's c.
    Derra's c.
    Diethrich's shunt c.
    Glover's c.
    Gross' c.
    Herbert-Adams c.
    Hopkins' c.
    Hufnagel's c.
    Hume's c.
    Humphries' c.
    Jacobson's c.
    Javid's by-pass c.
    Johns Hopkins c.
    Juevenell's c.
    Kantrowicz's c.
    Kapp-Beck c.
    McDonald's c.
    Nichols' c.
    Poppen-Blalock c.
    Poppen's c.
    Potts' c.
    Potts-Niedner c.

clamp *(continued)*
    Potts-Smith c.
    Reich-Nechtow c.
    Rienhoff's c.
    Rumel's c.
    Salibi's c.
    Satinsky's c.
    Selverstone's c.
    Shoemaker's c.
    Trandelenburg-
      Crafoord c.
claudication
    intermittent c.
    venous c.
clip
    Scoville-Lewis c.
    Smith's c.
    Sugar's c.
clubbing
coarctation
    c. of the aorta
coeur
    c. en sabot
collateral
columnae
    c. carneae cordis
commissure
commissurorrhaphy
commissurotomy
compensation
complex
    Eisenmenger's c.
    Lutembacher's c.
    QRS c.
    QS c.
    ventricular c.
      (Q,R,S,T waves)
concretio

concretio
    c. cordis
conduction
    ventricular c.
congenital
congestion
congestive
contraction
    atrial premature c.
    nodal premature c.
    supraventricular
      premature c.
conus
    c. arteriosus
conversion
Cooley-Pontius blade
Cooley's
    clamp
    dilator
    forceps
    retractor
    scissors
cor
    c. adiposum
    c. arteriosum
    c. biloculare
    c. bovinum
    c. dextrum
    c. hirsutum
    c. juvenum
    c. mobile
    c. pendulum
    c. pseudotriloculare
      biatriatum
    c. pulmonale
    c. sinistrum
    c. taurinum
    c. tomentosum

cor *(continued)*
    c. triatriatum
    c. triloculare biatriatum
    c. triloculare
        biventriculare
    c. venosum
    c. villosum
Cordis' pacemaker
Cordis-Ectocor pacemaker
coronarism
coronaritis
coronary
Corrigan's
    disease
    pulse
    respiration
    sign
Corvisart's
    disease
    facies
Coryllos'
    raspatory
    retractor
costotome
    Tudor-Edwards c.
CPB – cardiopulmonary
        bypass
Crafoord's
    clamp
    forceps
Crawford-Cooley tunneler
Crawford's retractor
crista
    c. supraventricularis
    c. terminalis atrii dextri
crus
    c. fasciculi atrioventri-
      cularis dextrum

crus
    c. fasciculi atrioventri-
      cularis sinistrum
Crutchfield's clamp
crux
    c. of heart
cryocardioplegia
CT – cardiothoracic (ratio)
    carotid tracing
CTR – cardiothoracic ratio
Curry's needle
curve
    Traube's c's.
Cushing's
    forceps
    needle
cusp
cuspis
    c. anterior valvae
      atrioventricularis
      dextrae
    c. anterior valvae
      atrioventricularis
      sinistrae
    c. anterior valvulae
      bicuspidalis
    c. anterior valvulae
      tricuspidalis
    c. medialis valvulae
      tricuspidalis
    c. posterior valvae
      atrioventricularis
      dextrae
    c. posterior valvae
      atrioventicularis
      sinistrae
    c. posterior valvulae
      bicuspidalis

cuspis *(continued)*
    c. posterior valvulae
       tricuspidalis
    c. septalis valvae
       atrioventricularis
       dextrae
CVA − cardiovascular accident
    cerebrovascular
       accident
CVS − cardiovascular surgery
    cardiovascular system
cyanosis
    shunt c.
    tardive c.
cyanotic
Dacron prosthesis
DAH − disordered action of
       the heart
Davidson's retractor
Davis' clamp
DeBakey-Bahnson forceps
DeBakey-Bainbridge forceps
DeBakey-Balfour retractor
DeBakey-Cooley
    dilator
    forceps
    retractor
DeBakey-Metzenbaum scissors
DeBakey's
    blade
    clamp
    forceps
    graft
    prosthesis
    scissors
    tunneler
decompensation
decortication

decortication
    arterial d.
defect
    atrial septal d.
    ventricular septal d.
defibrillation
defibrillator
deflection
    Q-S d's.
degeneration
    Mönckeberg's d.
    Quain's d.
Dehio's test
Delorme's operation
de Musset's sign
depolarization
depressant
    cardiac d.
depression
    ST d
Derra's
    clamp
    dilator
    knife
Desault's ligation
devasation
devascularization
deviation
    right axis d.
    ST-T d's.
dextrocardia
    mirror-image d.
dextrocardiogram
dextroversion
DG − diastolic gallop
diaphoresis
diastasis
    d. cordis

diastole
diastolic
DIC — diffuse intravascular
    coagulation
    disseminated intra-
    vascular coagulation
Dick's dilator
dicliditis
diclidostosis
diet
    Karell's d.
    Kempner's d.
Diethrich's shunt clamp
Dieuaide's sign
digitalism
digitalization
dilator
    Beardsley's d.
    Cooley's d.
    DeBakey-Cooley d.
    Derra's d.
    Dick's d.
    Gohrbrand's d.
    Jackson-Mosher d.
    Tubbs' d.
    Tucker's d.
diplocardia
disease
    Adams' d.
    Adams-Stokes d.
    Addison's d.
    Beau's d.
    Buerger's d.
    Corrigan's d.
    Corvisart's d.
    Eisenmenger's d.
    Hamman's d.
    Libman-Sacks d.

disease *(continued)*
    Lutembacher's d.
    Pick's d.
    Raynaud's d.
    Roger's d.
    Rummo's d.
    thyrotoxic heart d.
    von Willebrand's d.
    Wenckebach's d.
dissociation
    A-V d.
    auriculoventricular d.
Dittrich's stenosis
diuresis
diuretic
DM — diastolic murmur
DOE — dyspnea on exercise
    dyspnea on exertion
Dohle-Heller aortitis
Doyen's elevator
drugs. See *Medications.*
Drummond's sign
duct
    d. of Botallo
ductus
    d. arteriosus
Duroziez's
    murmur
    sign
dysphagia
dyspnea
    cardiac d.
    exertional d.
    orthostatic d.
    paroxysmal d.
dyspneic
dyspneoneurosis
dyssystole

Ebstein's anomaly
ECG – electrocardiogram
echo
    metallic e.
Eck's fistula
ectopia
    e. cordis
    e. cordis abdominalis
    e. cordis pectoral
edema
    pulmonary e.
Edward's
    catheter
    patch
effusion
    pericardial e.
Einthoven's
    law
    triangle
Eisenmenger's
    complex
    disease
    syndrome
EKG – electrocardiogram
electrocardiogram
electrocardiograph
electrocardiography
    precordial e.
electrocardiophonogram
electrocardiophonograph
electrocardioscopy
electrocardioversion
electrode
Electrodyne pacemaker
electrofluoroscopy
electrokymography
electrophysiology
    cardiac e.

electrostethograph
elevator
    Cameron-Haight e.
    Doyen's e.
    Hedblom's e.
    Matson's e.
    Overholt's e.
    Phemister's e.
    Sedillot's e.
EM – ejection murmur
embolectomy
emboli
embolism
    air e.
    pulmonary e.
embolus
embouchment
empyema
    e. of pericardium
    pulsating e.
endaortic
endaortitis
endarterectomize
endarterectomy
endarterial
endarteritis
    e. deformans
    Heubner's specific e.
    e. obliterans
    e. proliferans
endarterium
endarteropathy
endartery
endoaneurysmorrhaphy
endocardial
endocarditis
    acute bacterial e.
    benigna

endocarditis *(continued)*
    e. chordalis
    e. lenta
    Löffler's e.
    mural e.
    mycotic e.
    nonbacterial thrombotic
      e.
    plastic e.
    polypous e.
    pulmonic e.
    pustulous e.
    rheumatic e.
    septic e.
    subacute bacterial e.
    ulcerative e.
    valvular e.
    vegetative e.
    verrucous e.
    viridans e.
endocardium
endophlebitis
    e. hepatica obliterans
    proliferative e.
endosthethoscope
endothelium
endovasculitis
engorgement
eparterial
epicardia
epicardiectomy
epicardiolysis
epicardium
Erb's point
Erlanger's sphygmomanometer
erythromelalgia
ESM — ejection systolic
    murmur

ethmocarditis
Eustace Smith's murmur
Evans' forceps
Ewart's sign
excitation
    anomalous atrioventri-
      cular e.
extrasystole
    auricular e.
    auriculoventricular e.
    infranodal e.
    interpolated e.
    nodal e.
    retrograde e.
    ventricular e.
facies
    Corvisart's f.
Fallot
    pentalogy of F.
    tetralogy of F.
Faught's sphygmomanometer
fenestration
    aortopulmonary f.
feokromositoma. See
    pheochromocytoma.
fever
    rheumatic f.
fiber
    Purkinje's f's.
fibrillation
    auricular f.
    ventricular f.
fibroelastosis
    endocardial f.
fibrosis
    arteriocapillary f.
Fiedler's myocarditis
Finochietto's rib spreader

Fisher's murmur
fissure
    Henle's f's.
fistula
    arteriovenous f.
    Eck's f.
Fitzgerald's forceps
Flack's node
fleb-. See words beginning
    phleb-.
Flint's murmur
flucticulus
flutter
    atrial f.
    auricular f.
    impure f.
Flynt's needle
Fogarty's catheter
foramen
    f. ovale cordis
forceps
    Adson's f.
    Barraya's f.
    Bengolea's f.
    Boettcher's f.
    Cooley's f.
    Crafoord's f.
    Cushing's f.
    DeBakey-Bahnson f.
    DeBakey-Bainbridge f.
    DeBakey-Cooley f.
    DeBakey's f.
    Evans' f.
    Fitzgerald's f.
    Foss' f.
    Glover's f.
    Harken's f.
    Harrington's f.

forceps *(continued)*
    Hendren's f.
    Horsley's f.
    Jacobson's f.
    Johns Hopkins f.
    Julian's f.
    Lebsche's f.
    Leland-Jones f.
    Leriche's f.
    Liston-Stille f.
    Love-Gruenwald f.
    McNealy-Glassman-
      Mixter f.
    Mixter's f.
    Mount-Mayfield f.
    O'Shaughnessy's f.
    Potts-Smith f.
    Rienhoff's f.
    Rumel's f.
    Ruskin's f.
    Satinsky's f.
    Sauerbruch's f.
    Selman's f.
    Semb's f.
    Stille-Luer f.
    Stille's f.
    Vanderbilt's f.
Foss' forceps
fossa
    f. ovalis cordis
F & R — force and rhythm
Fraentzel's murmur
fragmentation
    f. of myocardium
Fränkel's treatment
fremitus
    pericardial f.

fren-. See words beginning
   phren-.
frolement
furrow
   atrioventricular f.
gasendarterectomy
George Lewis technique
Gibson's
   murmur
   vestibule
Giertz-Shoemaker rib shears
glomera
   g. aortica
glomus
   g. carotideum
Glover's
   clamp
   forceps
Gluck's rib shears
glycosuria
Gohrbrand's dilator
Goldberg-MPC mediastino-
   scope
gradient
   ventricular g.
graft
   autogenous vein g.
   dacron g.
   DeBakey's g.
   Weavenit's patch g.
Graham Steell murmur
Gross'
   clamp
   retractor
Gross-Pomeranz-Watkins
   retractor
Hamman's disease
Harken's

Harken's *(continued)*
   forceps
   rib spreader
Harrington-Pemberton
   retractor
Harrington's
   forceps
   operation
   retractor
HB – heart block
HCVD – hypertensive
   cardiovascular disease
HD – heart disease
HDH – heart disease history
heart
   chaotic h.
   flask-shaped h.
   hypoplastic h.
   irritable h.
   luxus h.
   Quain's fatty h.
   tabby cat h.
   Traube's h.
heart-block
   arborization h.
   atrioventricular h.
   auriculoventricular h.
   bundle-branch h.
   interventricular h.
   sino-auricular h.
heart-failure
   congestive h.
Hedblom's
   elevator
   retractor
hemartoma
hemithorax
hemodynamic

hemopericardium
hemopneumopericardium
hemoptysis
    cardiac h.
hemorrhage
Hendren's forceps
Henle's
    fissures
    membrane
heparinize
Herbert-Adams clamp
Heubner's specific endarteritis
HHD – hypertensive heart
  disease
hiatus
    aortic h.
Hibbs' retractor
His
    bundle of H.
His-Tawara node
holodiastolic
holosystolic
hook
    Adson's h.
Hopkins' clamp
Horsley's forceps
Hufnagel's
    clamp
    knife
    operation
    prosthesis
Hume's clamp
Humphries' clamp
HVD – hypertensive vascular
  disease
hydropericarditis
hydropericardium
hydropneumopericardium

hypercalcemia
hypercholesterolemia
hyperemia
hyperkalemia
hypertension
    essential h.
    portal h.
    pulmonary h.
    vascular h.
hypertrophy
    ventricular h.
hyperventilation
hypocalcemia
hypokalemia
hypokinemia
hyponatremia
hypoproteinemia
hypoprothrombinemia
hypotension
    orthostatic h.
hypothermia
hypovolemia
hypoxia
hysterosystole
IA – intra-aortic
    intra-arterial
IABP – intra-aortic balloon
  pumping
IASD – interatrial septal
  defect
ICC – intensive coronary care
ICCU – intensive coronary
  care unit
ictometer
ictus
    i. cordis
ICU – intensive care unit
idioventricular

IHD — ischemic heart disease
imbalance
    electrolyte i.
IMH — idiopathic myocardial
   hypertrophy
implantation
impressio
    i. cardiaca pulmonis
impulse
    apex i.
    apical i.
    episternal i.
incisura
    i. apicis cordis
incompetence
infarct
infarction
    anterolateral i.
    anteroposterior i.
    anteroseptal i.
    cardiac i.
    diaphragmatic i.
    myocardial i.
    Roesler-Dressler i.
    septal i.
    subendocardial i.
    transmural i.
infundibular
infundibulum
    i. of heart
insufficiency
    aortic i.
    cardiac i.
    coronary i.
    mitral i.
    myocardial i.
    myovascular i.
    pseudoaortic i.

insufficiency *(continued)*
    tricuspid i.
    valvular i.
    venous i.
interatrial
intercostal
interval
    a.-c. i.
    atriocarotid i.
    atrioventricular i.
    auriculocarotid i.
    auriculoventricular i.
    a.-v. i.
    c.-a. i.
    cardioarterial i.
    P-Q i.
    P-R i.
    Q-M i.
    QRST i.
    Q-T. i.
    QU i.
    T-P i.
interventricular
intimal
intima-pia
intimectomy
intimitis
intra-arterial
intra-atrial
intra-auricular
intracardiac
intramyocardial
intraventricular
irregularity
    i. of pulse
ischemia
    i. cordis intermittens
ischemic

IVC – inferior vena cava
IVSD – interventricular septal defect
IWMI – inferior wall myocardial infarction
Jackson-Mosher dilator
Jacobson's
    clamp
    forceps
    scissors
    spatula
Janeway's sphygmomanometer
Javid's by-pass clamp
Johns Hopkins
    clamp
    forceps
Jorgenson's scissors
Juevenell's clamp
Julian's forceps
JV – jugular vein
    jugular venous
JVP – jugular venous pulse
Kantrowicz's clamp
Kapp-Beck clamp
Karell's
    diet
    treatment
Katz-Wachtel phenomenon
Keith's bundle
Kempner's diet
Kent-His bundle
Kent's bundle
ker-on-sabo. See *coeur en sabot.*
knife
    Bailey-Glover-O'Neil k.
    Bailey-Morse k.
    Bosher's k.

knife *(continued)*
    Brock's k.
    Derra's k.
    Hufnagel's k.
    Lebsche's k.
    Niedner's k.
    Nunez-Nunez k.
    Rochester's k.
    Sellor's k.
Korotkoff's
    method
    sounds
    test
Krasky's retractor
Kronecker's
    needle
    puncture
Krönig's steps
Kussmaul's pulse
LAE – left atrial enlargement
LAH – left atrial hypertrophy
LAP – left atrial pressure
law
    all or none l.
    Einthoven's l.
LBBB – left bundle branch block
lead
    precordial l's.
    sternal l.
    V l's., 1 through 6
    Wilson l's.
Lebsche's
    forceps
    knife
    shears
Lehman's catheter
Leksell's rongeur

Leland-Jones forceps
Lemmon's rib spreader
Leriche's
        forceps
        operation
        syndrome
Libman-Sacks disease
ligamentum
        l. arteriosum
ligation
        Desault's l.
        proximal l.
ligature
        Woodbridge's l.
Lilienthal-Sauerbruch rib
    spreader
limbus
        l. fossae ovalis
line
        midclavicular l.
Liston-Stille forceps
Litwak's scissors
Livierato's test
Löffler's endocarditis
loop
        Cannon's endarterec-
            tomy l.
        P l.
Love-Gruenwald forceps
LSM – late systolic murmur
LSV – left subclavian vein
lubb
lubb-dupp
Lukens' retractor
lumen
Lutembacher's
        complex
        disease

Lutembacher's *(continued)*
        syndrome
luxus
Lyon-Horgan operation
MABP – mean arterial blood
    pressure
machine
        heart-lung m.
M_2 – mitral second sound
Makins' murmur
manometric
Marfan's syndrome
Master "2-step" exercise test
Master's two-step test
Matson's elevator
McDonald's clamp
McGinn-White sign
MCI – mean cardiac index
McNealy-Glassman-Mixter
        forceps
MCL – midclavicular line
mediastinal
mediastinitis
mediastinopericarditis
mediastinoscope
        Goldberg-MPC m.
mediastinum
Medications
        Acenocoumarin
        acenocoumarol
        acetylcholine
        acetyldigitoxin
        Acylanid
        adrenalin
        Aldactone
        Aldomet
        alkavervir
        alseroxylon

Medications *(continued)*
- aluminum nicotinate
- Amicar
- aminocaproic acid
- aminophylline
- amyl nitrite
- Angio-Conray (contrast material)
- anisindione
- Ansolysen bitartrate
- Apresoline
- Aramine
- Arfonad
- Arlidin
- Atabrine
- Athrombin
- Atromid-S
- Atropine
- azapetine phosphate
- Benemid
- betahistine
- Bio-Heprin
- bishydroxycoumarin
- Capla
- Cardilate
- Cedilanid
- Cedilanid-D
- Chlorphenisate
- Choloxin
- clofibrate
- Conray (contrast material)
- Coumadin
- cryptenamine
- Crystodigin
- cyclandelate
- Cyclospasmol
- Cytellin

Medications *(continued)*
- Danilone
- Davoxin
- deserpidine
- deslanoside
- dextrothyroxine
- Diamox
- Dicumarol
- Digitaline Nativelle
- digitalis
- digitoxin
- digoxin
- dioxyline
- dipyridamole
- Diuretin
- Diuril
- D-Thyroxine sodium
- ephedrine
- epinephrine
- erythrityl tetranitrate
- erythrol tetranitrate
- Etamon
- Eutonyl
- Frusemide
- furosemide
- Gitaligin
- gitalin
- glyceryl trinitrate
- G-Strophanthin
- guanethidine sulfate
- Harmonyl
- Hedulin
- heparin
- Hepathrom
- Histamine acid phosphate
- Histamine diphosphate
- histamine phosphate

Medications *(continued)*

hydralazine
Hypaque (contrast
   material)
Ilidar
Inderal
Indon
Innovar
Inversine
Ismelin sulfate
Isoamyl nitrite
Isordil
isosorbide dinitrate
isoxsuprine
Isuprel
Kaon
Kay Ciel
KCI
khellin
lanatoside
Lanoxin
Lasix
levarterenol bitartrate
Levophed
lidocaine
Lignocaine
Lipo-Hepin
Liquaemin sodium
Liquamar
magnesium sulfate
mannitol hexanitrate
mebutamate
mecamylamine
Mecholyl
mephentermine
mercaptomerin
Metamine
metaraminol bitartrate

Medications *(continued)*

methoxamine
methyldopa
Miradon
Moderil
morphine
Myodigin
neostigmine
Neosynephrine
nicotinyl alcohol
Nitranitol
Nitretamin
Nitroglycerin
Norepinephrine
nylidrin
ouabain
Panheprin
Panwarfin
papaverine
Paredrine
pargyline
Paveril
penicillin
pentaerythritol
Pentapyrrolidinium
   bitartrate
pentolinium tartrate
Pentritol
Peritrate
Persantin
PETN
phenindione
phenprocoumon
phentolamine
phenylephrine
   hydrochloride
P.I.D.
potassium

Medications *(continued)*
  Pressonex
  Priscoline
  probenecid
  procainamide
  procainamide
    hydrochloride
  Pronestyl
  propranolol
  propylthiouracil
  Prostigmin
  Protalba
  protamine sulfate
  protoveratrine A
  Provell
  Purodigin
  quinidine
  Raudixin
  Rau-Sed
  Rautensin
  Rautina
  Rautotal
  Rauwiloid
  Rauwoldin
  rauwolfia serpentina
  Regitine
  rescinnamine
  reserpine
  Reserpoid
  Roniacol
  Sandril
  Saroxin
  scopolamine
  Ser-Ap-Es
  Serc
  Serfin
  Serpasil
  Singoserp

Medications *(continued)*
  Sintrom
  sitosterols
  spironolactone
  syrosingopine
  tetraethylammonium
    chloride
  theobrominal
  theobromine
  Theocalcin
  Theominal
  theophylline
  Thiomerin
  Thiouracil
  tolazoline
  transaminase
  trimethaphan camsylate
  trolnitrate
  Unitensen
  Vasodilan
  Vasoxyl
  Veralba
  Veriloid
  warfarin
  Wyamine
  Xylocaine
Medtronic demand pacemaker
Meigs's capillaries
membrane
    Henle's m.
mesaortitis
mesarteritis
mesoaortitis
    m. syphilitica
mesocardia
mesocardium
method
    Korotkoff's m.

method *(continued)*
    Orsi-Grocco m.
Meyerding's retractor
MI – mitral incompetence
    mitral insufficiency
    myocardial infarction
mitral
mitrale
    P m.
mitralization
mitroarterial
Mixter's forceps
Mönckeberg's
    arteriosclerosis
    degeneration
monitor
Monneret's pulse
Morgagni's sinus
Morse's scissors
Mount-Mayfield forceps
Moure-Coryllos rib shears
MR – mitral reflux
    mitral regurgitation
MRF – mitral regurgitant
    flow
MS – mitral stenosis
MSL – midsternal line
multifocal
mural
murmur
    amphoric m.
    aneurysmal m.
    aortic m.
    apex m.
    arterial m.
    attrition m.
    Austin Flint m.
    bellows m.

murmur *(continued)*
    blowing m.
    Bright's m.
    cardiac m.
    cardiopulmonary m.
    cardiorespiratory m.
    crescendo m.
    decrescendo m.
    deglutition m.
    diastolic m.
    Duroziez's m.
    dynamic m.
    ejection m.
    endocardial m.
    Eustace Smith's m.
    exocardial m.
    expiratory m.
    Fisher's m.
    Flint's m.
    Fraentzel's m.
    friction m.
    functional m.
    Gibson's m.
    grade 1, 2, 3, 4, 5, or 6 m.
    Graham Steell m.
    harsh m.
    hemic m.
    holosystolic m.
    hour-glass m.
    humming-top m.
    inorganic m.
    inspiratory m.
    lapping m.
    machinery m.
    Makins' m.
    mitral m.
    musical m.
    nun's m.

murmur *(continued)*
    obstructive m.
    organic m.
    pansystolic m.
    Parrot's m.
    pericardial m.
    pleuropericardial m.
    prediastolic m.
    presystolic m.
    pulmonic m.
    reduplication m.
    regurgitant m.
    respiratory m.
    Roger's m.
    sea-gull m.
    seesaw m.
    Steell's m.
    stenosal m.
    subclavicular m.
    systolic m.
    to-and-fro m.
    Traube's m.
    tricuspid m.
    vascular m.
    venous m.
    vesicular m.
    water-wheel m.
muscle
    papillary m.
    pectinate m.
MV – mitral valve
myocardial
myocardiogram
myocardiograph
myocardiorrhaphy
myocarditis
    acute bacterial m.
    Fiedler's m.

myocarditis *(continued)*
    fragmentation m.
    indurative m.
    interstitial m.
    parenchymatous m.
    m. scarlatinosa
myocardium
myocardosis
    Riesman's m.
myofibrosis
    m. cordis
myomalacia
    m. cordis
myopathia
    m. cordis
myxedema
myxoma
needle
    Adson's n.
    Curry's n.
    Cushing's n.
    Flynt's n.
    Kronecker's n.
    Parhad-Poppen n.
    Retter's n.
    Rochester's n.
    Sanders-Brown-Shaw n.
    Sheldon-Spatz n.
    Smiley-Williams n.
    Tuohy's n.
    Wood's n.
nephrectomy
nephritis
nerve
    vagal n.
network
    Purkinje's n.
Nichols' clamp

Niedner's knife
NIH catheter
nodal
node
 Aschoff's n.
 n. of Aschoff and
  Tawara
 atrioventricular n.
 Flack's n.
 His-Tawara n.
 Osler's n's.
 sinoatrial n.
notch
 Sibson's n.
NPB – nodal premature beat
NSR – normal sinus rhythm
Nunez-Nunez knife
occlusion
 coronary o.
occlusive
Oertel's treatment
Öhnell
 X wave of O.
omentopexy
OMI – old myocardial
 infarction
operation
 Blalock-Taussig o.
 Brauer's o.
 Brock's o.
 Delorme's o.
 Harrington's o.
 Hufnagel's o.
 Leriche's o.
 Lyon-Horgan o.
 Potts' o.
 Potts-Smith-Gibson o.
 Vineberg's o.

Orsi-Grocco method
orthopnea
orthopneic
orthostatic
oscillation
oscillograph
oscillometer
oscillometric
oscillometry
oscilloscope
O'Shaughnessy's forceps
Osler's
 nodes
 sign
ostia
 o. atrioventricularia
  dextrum
 o. atrioventricularis
  sinistrum
 o. venarum pulmonalium
ostium
 o. aortae
 o. arteriosum cordis
 o. cardiacum
 o. primum
 o. secundum
 sinusoidal o.
 o. trunci pulmonalis
 o. venosum cordis
Overholt's elevator
oximetry
oxygen
oxygenate
oxygenator
P_2 – pulmonic second sound
PAC – premature auricular
 contraction
pacemaker

pacemaker *(continued)*
    Cordis' p.
    Cordis-Ectocor p.
    Electrodyne p.
    Medtronic demand p.
    transvenous p.
    wandering p.
    Zoll's p.
PAH – pulmonary artery
   hypertension
palpitation
panangiitis
    diffuse necrotizing p.
panarteritis
pansphygmograph
paracentesis
    p. cordis
    p. pericardii
paradoxical
parasternal
parasystole
Parhad-Poppen needle
paries
    p. caroticus cavi
      tympani
Park's aneurysm
paroxysmal
Parrot's murmur
PAT – paroxysmal atrial
   tachycardia
patch
    Edwards' p.
    Teflon p.
patent ductus arteriosus
paulocardia
PDA – patent ductus
   arteriosus
pectoral

pectoralis
pentalogy
    p. of Fallot
perfusion
periaortitis
periarteritis
    p. nodosa
periatrial
periauricular
pericardial
pericardicentesis
pericardiectomy
pericardiolysis
pericardiomediastinitis
pericardiophrenic
pericardiopleural
pericardiorrhaphy
pericardiostomy
pericardiosymphysis
pericardiotomy
pericarditis
    acute fibrinous p.
    adhesive p.
    bacterial p.
    p. calculosa
    p. callosa
    carcinomatous p.
    constrictive p.
    p. epistenocardiaca
    p. externa et interna
    fibrous p.
    obliterating p.
    purulent p.
    rheumatic p.
    serofibrinous p.
    p. sicca
    suppurative p.
    p. villosa

pericardium
  adherent p.
  bread-and-butter p.
  calcified p.
  fibrous p.
  parietal p.
  serous p.
  shaggy p.
  visceral p.
pericardosis
period
  Wenckebach's p.
periosteotome
  Alexander-Farabeuf p.
peripericarditis
peripheral
periphlebitis
petechia
Phemister's elevator
phenomenon
  Katz-Wachtel p.
  Raynaud's p.
pheochromocytoma
phlebangioma
phlebarteriectasia
phlebarteriodialysis
phlebasthenia
phlebectasia
phlebectomy
phlebectopia
phlebemphraxis
phlebexairesis
phlebismus
phlebitis
phlebocarcinoma
phlebocholosis
phlebogram
phlebography

phlebolith
phlebolithiasis
phlebomanometer
phlebomyomatosis
phlebophlebostomy
phlebopiezometry
phleboplasty
phleborrhagia
phleborrhaphy
phleborrhexis
phlebosclerosis
phlebosis
phlebostasis
phlebostenosis
phlebostrepsis
phlebothrombosis
phlebotome
phlebotomy
phonocardiogram
phonocardiograph
phonocardiographic
phonocardiography
  intracardiac p.
phonoelectrocardioscope
phonogram
phrenocardia
phrenopericarditis
Pick's
  disease
  syndrome
plethora
plethysmometer
plethysmometry
pleuropericardial
pleuropericarditis
plexus
  cardiac p.
  p. cardiacus profundus

plexus *(continued)*
- p. cardiacus superficialis
- p. caroticus communis
- p. caroticus externus
- p. caroticus internus
- coronarius cordis
- vascular p.
- p. venosus caroticus internus
- venous p.

P loop

PMI – point of maximal impulse

P mitrale

PND – paroxysmal nocturnal dyspnea

pneumocardial

pneumohemia

pneumohemopericardium

pneumohydropericardium

pneumopericardium

pneumoprecordium

pneumopyopericardium

point
- Erb's p.

polyarteritis

poodrazh. See *poudrage.*

Poppen-Blalock clamp

Poppen's clamp

potassium

Potts'
- aneurysm
- clamp
- operation
- rib shears
- scissors

Potts-Niedner clamp

Potts-Smith

Potts-Smith *(continued)*
- clamp
- forceps
- scissors

Potts-Smith-Gibson operation

poudrage

P-pulmonale

P-Q interval

P-Q segment

P-R interval

P-R segment

precardiac

precordial

precordium

preponderance
- ventricular p.

presbycardia

presystolic

preventriculosis

preventriculus

prosthesis
- Cartwright's p.
- Dacron p.
- DeBakey's p.
- discoid aortic p.
- Hufnagel's p.
- tri-leaflet aortic p.
- Wada's p.
- Weavenit's p.

protodiastolic

pseudoanemia
- p. angiospastica

pseudoangina

pseudoangioma

pulmonale
- P. p.

pulmonary

pulsate

pulsatile
pulsation
    expansile p.
    suprasternal p.
pulse
    allorhythmic p.
    anacrotic p.
    anadicrotic p.
    anatricrotic p.
    arachnoid p.
    auriculovenous p.
    Bamberger's bulbar p.
    bigeminal p.
    bisferious p.
    cannon ball p.
    catacrotic p.
    catadicrotic p.
    catatricrotic p.
    centripetal venous p.
    collapsing p.
    cordy p.
    Corrigan's p.
    coupled p.
    decurtate p.
    dicrotic p.
    digitalate p.
    elastic p.
    entoptic p.
    filiform p.
    formicant p.
    gaseous p.
    guttural p.
    high-tension p.
    hyperdicrotic p.
    jugular p.
    Kussmaul's p.
    Monneret's p.
    monocrotic p.

pulse *(continued)*
    mouse tail p.
    paradoxical p.
    pistol-shot p.
    plateau p.
    polycrotic p.
    pulmonary p.
    quadrigeminal p.
    Quincke's p.
    Riegel's p.
    thready p.
    tremulous p.
    tricrotic p.
    trigeminal p.
    undulating p.
    vagus p.
    ventricular venous p.
    vermicular p.
    vibrating p.
    water-hammer p.
pulsus
    p. alternans
    p. bigeminus
    p. bisferiens
    p. celer
    p. contractus
    p. cordis
    p. debilis
    p. deficiens
    p. deletus
    p. differens
    p. duplex
    p. durus
    p. filiformis
    p. formicans
    p. frequens
    p. heterochronicus
    p. intercurrens

pulsus *(continued)*
    p. irregularis perpetuus
    p. magnus et celer
    p. mollis
    p. monocrotus
    p. oppressus
    p. paradoxus
    p. parvus et tardus
    p. plenus
    p. pseudo-intermittens
    p. rarus
    p. tardus
    p. trigeminus
    p. undulosus
    p. vacuus
    p. venosus
    p. vibrans
punch
    Brock's p.
puncture
    Kronecker's p.
Purkinje's
    fibers
    network
PVC – premature ventricular
   contraction
PVS – premature ventricular
   systole
PVT – paroxysmal ventricular
   tachycardia
P wave
pyelophlebitis
pyemia
    arterial p.
    portal p.
pyopneumopericardium
Q wave
Q-M interval

QRS changes
QRS complex
QRS-T changes
QRST interval
QS complex
Q-S deflections
QT interval
QU interval
Quain's
    degeneration
    fatty heart
Quincke's pulse
R wave
ramus
rankenangioma
raphe
rasp
      Beck's r.
raspatory
      Coryllos' r.
ratio
      R/S r.
Raynaud's
    disease
    phenomenon
RBBB – right bundle branch
   block
RCD – relative cardiac
   dullness
regurgitant
regurgitation
    aortic r.
    mitral r.
    pulmonic r.
Reich-Nechtow clamp
respiration
      Cheyne-Stokes' r.
      Corrigan's r.

resuscitation

rete
  r. arteriosum
  r. mirabile
  r. vasculosum
  r. venosum

retractor
  Adson's r.
  Allison's r.
  Carter's r.
  Cooley's r.
  Coryllos' r.
  Crawford's r.
  Davidson's r.
  DeBakey-Balfour r.
  DeBakey-Cooley r.
  Gross' r.
  Gross-Pomeranz-
    Watkins r.
  Harrington-Pemberton r.
  Harrington's r.
  Hedblom's r.
  Hibbs' r.
  Krasky's r.
  Lukens' r.
  Meyerding's r.
  Richardson's r.
  Ross' r.
  Sauerbruch's r.
  Semb's r.
  Walter-Deaver r.
Retter's needle
RF — rheumatic fever
RHD — rheumatic heart
  disease
rheumapyra
rheumatic
rhythm

rhythm *(continued)*
  atrial r.
  auriculoventricular r.
  cantering r.
  coupled r.
  gallop r.
  idioventricular r.
  nodal r.
  pendulum r.
  reversed r.
  sinus r.
  triple r.
  ventricular r.
rhythmophone
rib contractor
  Bailey-Gibbon r.c.
  Bailey's r.c.
  Sellors' r.c.
rib shears
  Bethune's r.s.
  Giertz-Shoemaker r.s.
  Gluck's r.s.
  Moure-Coryllos r.s.
  Potts' r.s.
  Sauerbruch's r.s.
  Shoemaker's r.s.
rib spreader
  Burford's r.s.
  Finochietto's r.s.
  Harken's r.s.
  Lemmon's r.s.
  Lilienthal-Sauerbruch r.s.
  Reinhoff-Finochietto r.s.
  Tuffier's r.s.
  Wilson's r.s.
Richardson's retractor
Richet's aneurysm
Riegel's pulse

Rienhoff-Finochietto rib
   spreader
Rienhoff's
   clamp
   forceps
Riesman's myocardosis
Riva-Rocci sphygmomano-
   meter
Rochester's
   awl
   knife
   needle
Rockey's cannula
Rodrigues's aneurysm
roentgenocardiogram
roentgenography
Roesler-Dressler infarction
Roger's
   bruit
   disease
   murmur
   sphygmomanometer
rongeur
   Leksell's r.
rooma-. See words beginning
   rheuma-.
Rose's tamponade
Ross' retractor
RSR — regular sinus rhythm
R/S ratio
RS-T segment
rumble
   diastolic r.
Rumel's
   clamp
   forceps
   tourniquet
Rummo's disease

Ruskin's forceps
RVE — right ventricular
   enlargement
RVH — right ventricular
   hypertrophy
Salibi's clamp
Sanders-Brown-Shaw needle
sanguis
saphenofemoral
saphenous
sarcoid
sarcoidosis
   s. cordis
Satinsky's
   clamp
   forceps
   scissors
Sauerbruch's
   forceps
   retractor
   rib shears
SBE — subacute bacterial
   endocarditis
scissors
   Cooley's s.
   DeBakey-Metzenbaum s.
   DeBakey's s.
   Jacobson's s.
   Jorgenson's s.
   Litwak's s.
   Morse's s.
   Potts' s.
   Potts-Smith s.
   Satinsky's s.
   Thorek-Feldman s.
   Thorek's s.
   Toennis' s.
scleroderma

sclerosis
    arterial s.
sclerotic
Scoville-Lewis clip
searcher
    Allport-Babcock s.
Sedillot's elevator
segment
    P-Q s.
    P-R s.
    RS-T s.
    S-T s.
    T-P s.
Sellor's
    knife
    rib contractor
selman's forceps
Selverstone's clamp
Semb's
    forceps
    retractor
semilunar
septal
septum
    s. atriorum cordis
    s. atrioventriculare
        cordis
    s. interatriale cordis
    interauricular s.
    interventricular s.
    s. interventriculare
        cordis
    s. membranaceum
        ventriculorum cordis
    s. musculare
        ventriculorum cordis
    s. primum
    s. secundum

septum *(continued)*
    s. ventriculorum cordis
serrefine
sfigmo-. See words beginning
    sphygmo-.
Shaw's stripper
shears
    Lebsche's s.
Sheldon-Spatz needle
Shoemaker's clamp
Shoemaker's rib shears
shunt
    portacaval s.
    postcaval s.
Sibson's
    notch
    vestibule
sign
    Broadbent's s.
    Corrigan's s.
    de Musset's s.
    Dieuaide's s.
    Drummond's s.
    Duroziez's s.
    Ewart's s.
    McGinn-White s.
    Osler's s.
    Wenckebach's s.
Silastic coronary artery
    cannula
silhouette
    cardiovascular s.
sinoatrial
sinoauricular
sinospiral
sinoventricular
sinus
    carotid s.

sinus *(continued)*
  s. caroticus
  coronary s.
  s. of Morgagni
  s. transversus pericardii
  s. of Valsalva
sinusoid
  myocardial s.'s.
Smiley-Williams needle
Smith's clip
Soresi's cannula
souffle
  cardiac s.
sound
  bellows s.
  flapping s.
  heart s.'s., first s.;
    second s.
  Korotkoff's s.'s.
  pistol-shot s.
  tick-tack s.'s.
Southey-Leech tubes
spatula
  Jacobson's s.
sphygmobologram
sphygmobolometer
sphygmocardiogram
sphygmocardiograph
sphygmocardioscope
sphygmodynamometer
sphygmogram
sphygmography
sphygmomanometer
  Erlanger's s.
  Faught's s.
  Janeway's s.
  Riva-Rocci s.
  Rogers' s.

sphygmomanometer
  (continued)
  Staunton's s.
  Tycos' s.
sphygmomanometroscope
sphygmometer
sphygmometrograph
sphygmometroscope
sphygmo-oscillometer
sphygmopalpation
sphygmophone
sphygmoplethysmograph
sphygmoscope
  Bishop's s.
sphygmosignal
sphygmosystole
sphygmotonogram
sphygmotonograph
sphygmotonometer
sphygmoviscosimetry
splenosis
  pericardial s.
ST depression
S-T segment
ST segment changes
standstill
  atrial s.
  auricular s.
  cardiac s.
  respiratory s.
  ventricular s.
Stanley-Kent bundle
stasis
  venous s.
Staunton's
  sphygmomanometer
Steell's murmur
stellectomy

stenocardia
stenosis
    aortic s.
    Dittrich's s.
    mitral s.
    preventricular s.
    pulmonary s.
    tricuspid s.
steotic
step
    Krönig's s's.
Sterges' carditis
sternopericardial
sternotomy
sternum
stethoscope
Stille-Luer forceps
Stille's forceps
stimulation
    vagus s.
striation
    tabby cat s.
    tigroid s.
stripper
    Shaw's s.
    Wylie's s.
ST-T deviations
stylet
subclavian
subclavicular
suffusion
Sugar's clip
sulcus
    s. aorticus
    atrioventricular s.
    s. coronarius cordis
    interventricular s. of
      heart

sulcus *(continued)*
    longitudinal s. of heart
    s. of subclavian artery
    transverse s. of heart
sump
    Baylor's s.
support
    Abée's s.
supraclavicular
surgical procedures. See
    operation.
suture
    Tevdek s.
    Tycron s.
SVC – superior vena cava
S wave
sympathectomy
symphysis
    cardiac s.
synanastomosis
synchronous
syncopal
syncope
    Adams-Stokes s.
    s. anginosa
    carotid s.
    vasovagal s.
syndrome
    Adams-Stokes s.
    Ayerza's s.
    Babinski's s.
    Beau's s.
    Bernheim's s.
    Eisenmenger's s.
    Leriche's s.
    Lutembacher's s.
    Marfan's s.
    Pick's s.

syndrome *(continued)*
>   Takayasu's s.
>   Taussig-Bing s.
>   Wolff-Parkinson-White s.

systole
>   aborted s.
>   arterial s.
>   atrial s.
>   auricular s.
>   catalectic s.
>   extra s.
>   hemic s.
>   ventricular s.

systolic
systolometer
T wave
T wave changes
tachycardia
>   atrial t.
>   alternating bidirectional
>   t.
>   auricular t.
>   nodal t.
>   orthostatic t.
>   paroxysmal ventricular t.
>   sinus t.
>   supraventricular t.
>   ventricular t.

tachycardiac
tachypnea
tachysystole
>   atrial t.
>   auricular t.

taeni
>   t. terminalis

Takayasu's syndrome
takipnea. See *tachypnea.*
tamponade

tamponade *(continued)*
>   cardiac t.
>   Rose's t.

Taussig-Bing syndrome
technique
>   George Lewis t.

Teflon
>   catheter
>   patch

telangiectasis
telecardiogram
telecardiography
test
>   Allen's t.
>   Dehio's t.
>   Korotkoff's t.
>   Livierato's t.
>   Master "2-step"
>   exercise t.
>   Master's two-step t.
>   regitine t.
>   Trendelenburg's t.

tetralogy
>   t. of Fallot

Tevdek suture
thebesian
theca
>   t. cordis

thoracentesis
Thorek-Feldman scissors
Thorek's scissors
Thorel's bundle
thrill
>   aneurysmal t.
>   aortic t.
>   diastolic t.
>   presystolic t.
>   systolic t.

thrombectomy
thromboangiitis
    t. obliterans
thromboarteritis
    t. purulenta
thromboclasis
thromboembolism
thromboendarterectomy
thromboendarteritis
thromboendocarditis
thrombokinesis
thrombolymphangitis
thrombophlebitis
    iliofemoral t.
    t. migrans
    t. purulenta
    t. saltans
thrombopoiesis
thrombosis
    coronary t.
thrombus
TI – tricuspid incompetence
    tricuspid insufficiency
tinkle
    Bouillaud's t.
Toennis' scissors
tourniquet
    Rumel's t.
T-P interval
T-P segment
trabeculae
    t. carneae cordis
trabecular
transplant
transposition
transseptal
transventricular
Traube-Hering waves

Traube's
    curves
    heart
    murmur
treatment
    Fränkel's t.
    Karell's t.
    Oertel's t.
Trendelenburg-Crafoord
  clamp
Trendelenburg's test
triangle
    Burger's t.
    Einthoven's t.
tricuspid
trigeminy
triglyceride
trigona
    t. fibrosa cordis
trilogy
    t. of Fallot
truncus
    t. arteriosus
    t. brachiocephalicus
    t. fasciculi atrioventri-
      cularis
trunk
    brachiocephalic t.
Tubbs' dilator
tube
    Southey-Leech t's.
Tucker's dilator
Tudor-Edwards costotome
Tuffier's rib spreader
tunica
    t. adventitia vasorum
    t. externa vasorum
    t. intima vasorum

tunica *(continued)*
    t. media vasorum
    t. vasculosa
tunneler
    Crawford-Cooley t.
    DeBakey's t.
Tuohy's needle
turgescent
turgid
turgor
    t. vitalis
Tycos' sphygmomanometer
Tycron suture
unipolar
U wave
Valsalva's sinus
valve
    aortic v.
    atrioventricular v.
    auriculoventricular v.
    bicuspid v.
    cardiac v's.
    caval v.
    v. of coronary sinus
    eustachian v.
    mitral v.
    pulmonary v.
    semilunar v's.
    thebesian v.
    tricuspid v.
valvotomy
    mitral v.
valvula
    v. bicuspidalis
    v. semilunaris dextra
      aortae
    v. semilunaris posterior
      aortae

valvula *(continued)*
    v. semilunaris sinistra
      aortae
    v. sinus coronarii
    v. tricuspidalis
    v. venae cavae inferioris
    v. venosa
    v. vestibuli
valvulae semilunares aortae
valvular
valvulitis
    rheumatic v.
valvuloplasty
valvulotome
Vanderbilt's forceps
varicose
varicosity
varix
    aneurysmal v.
    arterial v.
vascular
vascularity
vascularization
vasculitis
vasoconstriction
vasoconstrictor
vasodepression
vasodilation
vasodilator
vasoinhibitor
vasomotor
vector
vectorcardiogram
vectorcardiography
    spatial v.
vein
vena
    v. cava

venipuncture
venoauricular
venofibrosis
venogram
venography
veno-occlusive
venosinal
venostasis
venous
ventricle
ventricular
ventriculomyotomy
ventriculonector
ventriculotomy
ventriculus
    v. cordis
    v. sinister cordis
vessel
vestibule
    Gibson's v.
    Sibson's v.
Vineberg's operation
vitium
    v. cordis
von Willebrand's disease
VPC — ventricular premature
    contraction
VSD — ventricular septal
    defect
Wada's prosthesis
Walter-Deaver retractor
Wangensteen's awl
wave
    A w.
    arterial w.
    delta w.
    dicrotic w.
    F w's.

wave *(continued)*
    fibrillary w's.
    oscillation w.
    overflow w.
    P w.
    percussion w.
    peridicrotic w.
    predicrotic w.
    pre-excitation w.
    Q w.
    R w.
    recoil w.
    respiratory w.
    S w.
    T. w.
    tidal w.
    transverse w.
    Traube-Hering w's.
    tricrotic w.
    U w.
    vasomotor w.
    ventricular w.
    X w. of Öhnell
Weavenit's
    patch graft
    prosthesis
Wenckebach's
    disease
    period
    sign
Willis' circle
Wilson leads
Wilson's rib spreader
Wolff-Parkinson-White
    syndrome
Wood's needle
Woodbridge's ligature

WPW — Wolff-Parkinson-
    White (syndrome)

Wylie's stripper
Zoll's pacemaker

DENTISTRY

AB — axiobuccal
ABC — axiobuccocervical
ABG — axiobuccogingival
ABL — axiobuccolingual
abocclusion
abrasio
 a. dentium
abscess
 apical a.
 dento-alveolar a.
 periodontal a.
abstraction
abutment
AC — axiocervical
acrylic
AD — axiodistal
adamantine
adamantinocarcinoma
adamas
 a. dentis
Adams' clasp
ADC — axiodistocervical
ADG — axiodistogingival
adhesive
 denture a.
ADI — axiodistoincisal
ADO — axiodisto-occlusal
AG — axiogingival
AI — axioincisal
Ainsworth's punch

AL — axiolingual
A.La. — axiolabial
A.LaG — axiolabiogingival
A.LaL — axiolabiolingual
ALC — axiolinguocervical
ALG — axiolinguogingival
alignment
Allen's root pliers
alloy
ALO — axiolinguo-occlusal
alveolalgia
alveolar
alveolectomy
alveolitis
alveoloclasia
alveolocondylean
alveolodental
alveololabial
alveololabialis
alveololingual
alveolomerotomy
alveolonasal
alveolopalatal
alveoloplasty
alveolotomy
alveolus
alveolysis
AM — axiomesial
amalgam
AMC — axiomesiocervical

211

AMD — axiomesiodistal
amelodentinal
amelogenesis
    a. imperfecta
AMG — axiomesiogingival
AMI — axiomesioincisal
AMO — axiomesio-occlusal
anchorage
anesthesia
    nasotracheal intubation
      a.
angina
    Ludwig's a.
ankylosis
anodontia
anteroclusion
antrum
    a. of Highmore
AO — axio-occlusal
AP — axiopulpal
apex
    a. radicis dentis
apical
apices
apicitis
apicoectomy
apicolocator
apicostome
apicostomy
apoxemena
apoxesis
appliance
    Crozat's a.
    Hawley's a.
apposition
arch
    zygomatic a.
arch bar

arch bar *(continued)*
    Erich's a. b.
    Jelanko's a. b.
arcus
    a. dentalis
    a. zygomaticus
articulator
atresia
attachment
    Gottlieb's epithelial a.
attrition
Austin's
    knife
    retractor
avulsion
axiodistal
axiodistogingival
axiodisto-occlusal
axiogingival
axioincisal
axiolabiogingival
axiolingual
axiolinguogingival
axiomesial
axiomesiogingival
axiomesio-occlusal
axio-occlusal
axiopulpal
BA — buccoaxial
BAC — buccoaxiocervical
BAG — buccoaxiogingival
bandage
    Barton's b.
bar
    Erich's arch b.
    Jelanko's arch b.
Barton's bandage
BC — buccocervical

BD – buccodistal
bell-crowned
BG – buccogingival
bicuspid
bicuspoid
bimaxillary
bitegage
bitelock
biteplate
bite-rim
bite-wing
BL – buccolingual
block
    infraorbital b.
BM – buccomesial
BO – bucco-occlusal
BP – buccopulpal
broach
    root-canal b.
Brophy's operation
bruxism
buccal
buccoaxial
buccoaxiocervical
buccoaxiogingival
buccocervical
buccoclination
buccoclusion
buccodistal
buccogingival
buccolingual
buccomesial
bucco-occlusal
buccoplacement
buccopulpal
buccoversion
bunodont
bunolophodont
bunoselenodont

bur
    round b.
CA – cervicoaxial
cacodontia
calcification
calculus
Caldwell-Luc operation
canal
    root c.
canine
carcinoma
caries
carious
Carmichael's crown
cartilage
    gingival c.
carver
catheter
    nasotracheal c.
cavitas
    c. dentis
Cavitron
cellulitis
cementation
cementoperiostitis
cementosis
cementum
ceramics
    dental c.
ceramodontics
cervicoaxial
check-bite
cingulum
clasp
    Adams' c.
    ball c.
cleoid
coagulate

coagulation
collum
    c. dentis
Commando operation
comminution
condylar
condyle
    c. of mandible
contrusion
corona
    c. dentis
coronal
coronoid
crepitation
crepitus
crevice
    gingival c.
crevicular
crista
    c. buccinatoria
Crombie's ulcer
crossbite
crown
    Carmichael's c.
    Davis' c.
    dowel c.
Crozat's appliance
crusta
    c. petrosa dentis
Cryer's elevator
crypt
curet
    Goldman's c.
    Gracey's c.
    Moult c.
curettage
    subgingival c.
cuspid

cyst
    radicular c.
cytology
dam
    rubber d.
Davis' crown
DB — distobuccal
DBO — distobucco-occlusal
DBP — distobuccopulpal
DC — distocervical
debridement
debris
deciduous
dedentition
def
dens
    d. acutus
    d. axis
    d. epistrophei
    d. in dente
    d. sapientia
    d. serotinus
dentata
dentate
dentes
    d. acustici
    d. canini
    d. decidui
    d. incisivi
    d. molares
    d. permanentes
    d. premolares
dentia
dentibuccal
denticle
dentifrice
dentigerous
dentilabial

dentilingual
dentimeter
dentin
dentinogenesis
    d. imperfecta
dentinosteoid
dentition
dentulous
denture
detrition
DG – distogingival
diastema
diazone
dilaceration
diphyodont
discoid
disease
    Fauchard's d.
    periodontal d.
    Spira's d.
disocclude
displacement
dissection
    blunt d.
    sharp d.
distal
distobuccal
distobucco-occlusal
distobuccopulpal
distocervical
distoclination
distoclusion
distogingival
distolabial
distolabioincisal
distolingual
distolinguoincisal
distolinguo-occlusal

distolinguopulpal
distomolar
disto-occlusal
distoplacement
distopulpal
distopulpolabial
distopulpolingual
distoversion
distraction
DLA – distolabial
DLAI – distolabioincisal
DLI – distolinguoincisal
DLO – distolinguo-occlusal
DLP – distolinguopulpal
DO – disto-occlusal
DP – distopulpal
DPL – distopulpolingual
drill
    Hall's surgical d.
    Lentulo spiral d.
    Spirec d.
drip
    succinylcholine d.
drugs. See *Medications.*
duct
    submandibular d.
    Wharton's d.
dysodontiasis
eburnation
eburnitis
edentulous
ekselsimosis. See *exelcymosis.*
eksognatheon. See
    exognathion.
eksolever. See *exolever.*
electrocautery
elevator
    Cryer's e.

embrasure
enamel
enameloma
enamelum
endodontics
endodontium
enucleation
enula
epulis
epulofibroma
equilibration
    occlusal e.
Erich's arch bar
erosion
eruption
erythrodontia
ethmoid
evulsed
excavation
excavator
excementosis
excursion
    protrusive e.
    retrusive e.
exelcymosis
exodontics
exodontology
exognathion
exolever
extirpation
extraction
extrude
extrudoclusion
extrusion
exudation
exuviation
farinks. See *pharynx.*

fatno-. See words beginning
    phatno-.
Fauchard's disease
fetor
    f. exore
    f. oris
fibromatosis
    f. gingivae
fibrosarcoma
    odontogenic f.
fistula
fistulous
flange
    buccal f.
    labial f.
    lingual f.
Fleischmann's hygroma
fluoridation
fluoride
fluoridization
fluorosis
follicular
foramen
    mandibular f.
    mental f.
    Scarpa's f.
Fournier teeth
frena
frenectomy
frenum
    labial f.
    lingual f.
furca
furcae
Fusobacterium
    F. plauti-vincenti
fusospirillary
fusospirillosis

G – gingival
GA – gingivoaxial
GBA – gingivobuccoaxial
Gilmer's splint
gingiva
    alveolar g.
    areolar g.
    buccal g.
    cemented g.
    labial g.
    lingual g.
    marginal g.
    septal g.
gingival
gingivectomy
    Ochsenbein's g.
gingivitis
    necrotizing ulcerative g.
gingivoaxial
gingivobuccoaxial
gingivoglossitis
gingivolabial
gingivolinguoaxial
gingivoplasty
gingivosis
gingivostomatitis
GLA – gingivolinguoaxial
gland
    parotid g.
    submandibular salivary g.
glaze
Goldman's curet
gomphiasis
gomphosis
Goslee tooth
Gottlieb's epithelial
   attachment
Gracey's curet

granuloma
gubernaculum
    g. dentis
gutta-percha
Hall's surgical drill
Hawley's appliance
headgear
    Kloehn's h.
hemisection
hemorrhage
herpes
    h. labialis
Highmore's antrum
Horner's teeth
Huschke's auditory teeth
Hutchinson's teeth
hydrotherapy
hygienist
    dental h.
hygroma
    Fleischmann's h.
hypercementosis
hyperdontia
hyperkeratosis
hyperplasia
hypoconid
hypoconule
hypoconulid
hypoplasia
I & D – incision and drainage
imbrication
immobilization
impacted
impaction
incisive
incisolabial
incisolingual
incisoproximal

incisor
infection
    Vincent's i.
infrabulge
injection
    nasopalatine i.
inlay
interdigitation
intermaxillary
interocclusal
interosseous
interspace
intraoral
Ivy wire
jackscrew
Jelanko's arch bar
Kirkland's knife
Kirschner's wire
Kloehn's headgear
knife
    Austin's k.
    Kirkland's k.
LA – linguoaxial
labiogingival
labioincisal
LAG – labiogingival
LAI – labioincisal
LD – linguodistal
ledging
Lentulo spiral drill
leptodontous
leukoplakia
LI – linguoincisal
line
    Salter's incremental l's.
lingual
linguoaxial
linguocervical

linguoclination
linguoclusion
linguodental
linguodistal
linguogingival
linguoincisal
linguomesial
linguo-occlusal
linguopapillitis
linguoplacement
linguoplate
    palatal l.
linguopulpal
linguotrite
linguoversion
LM – linguomesial
LO – linguo-occlusal
LP – linguopulpal
Ludwig's angina
macrodontia
malalignment
malar
maleruption
malformation
malocclusion
malposition
malturned
malunion
mamelon
mandible
mandibular
marsupialization
mass
    Stent's m.
masseteric
matrix
maxilla
maxillary

maxillodental
maxillomandibular
MB – mesiobuccal
MBO – mesiobucco-occlusal
MBP – mesiobuccopulpal
Medications
    Benadryl
    butacaine
    butethamine
    Butyn
    camphorated
      parachlorophenol
    Carbocaine
    Chloramine-T
    codeine
    Cresatin
    Darvon
    Demerol
    dextro-propoxyphene
    diphenhydramine
    Duocaine
    Dynacaine
    Equanil
    Erythrocin
    erythromycin
    eugenol
    formocresol
    Ilotycin
    isobucaine
    Kincaine
    lidocaine
    mepivacaine
    meprobamate
    meprylcaine
    metabutethamine
    metabutoxycaine
    metacresyl acetate
    Metycaine

Medications *(continued)*
    Miltown
    Monocaine
    Nesacaine
    Novocain
    Oracaine
    penicillin G
    penicillin V-K
    pentobarbital
    Phenergan
    piperocaine
    Pontocaine
    Primacaine
    procaine
    promethazine
    propoxycaine
    pyrrocaine
    Ravocaine
    secobarbital
    Seconal
    sodium pentobarbital
    tetracaine
    tetracycline
    Unacaine
    Xylocaine
membrane
    Nasmyth's m.
    peridental m.
mesial
mesiobuccal
mesiobucco-occlusal
mesiobuccopulpal
mesiocervical
mesioclination
mesioclusion
mesiodens
mesiodistal
mesiogingival

mesioincisodistal
mesiolabial
mesiolabioincisal
mesiolingual
mesiolinguoincisal
mesiolinguo-occlusal
mesiolinguopulpal
mesio-occlusal
mesio-occlusodistal
mesiopalatal
mesiopulpal
mesiopulpolabial
mesiopulpolingual
mesioversion
metacone
metaconid
metaconule
metaplasia
      m. of pulp
metodontiasis
MG – mesiogingival
microdontia
micrognathia
MID – mesioincisodistal
ML – mesiolingual
MLa – mesiolabial
MLaI – mesiolabioincisal
MLI – mesiolinguoincisal
MLO – mesiolinguo-occlusal
MLP – mesiolinguopulpal
MO – mesio-occlusal
MOD – mesio-occlusodistal
Moon's teeth
Moorehead's retractor
Moult curet
mouth prop
MP – mesiopulpal
MPL – mesiopulpolingual

MPLa – mesiopulpolabial
mucobuccal
mucocele
mucoid
mucoperiosteal
mucoperiosteum
mucosa
      buccal m.
      retromolar m.
      retrotuberosity m.
Mummery's pink tooth
muscle
      masseter m.
      masticatory m.
      platysma m.
      sternocleidomastoid m.
mylohyoid
Nasmyth's membrane
neck
      surgical n. of tooth
necrosis
neoplasm
nonocclusion
nonunion
NUG – necrotizing ulcerative
      gingivitis
numatizashun. See
      pneumatization.
OC – occlusocervical
occlude
occlusal
occlusion
      afunctional o.
      buccal o.
      centric o.
      eccentric o.
      edge-to-edge o.
      functional o.

occlusion *(continued)*
    lingual o.
    mesial o.
    traumatogenic o.
occlusocervical
Ochsenbein's gingivectomy
odontagra
odontalgia
    phantom o.
odontatrophia
odontectomy
odontexesis
odontiasis
odontoblast
odontoblastoma
odontobothrion
odontobothritis
odontocele
odontoceramic
odontocia
odontoclasis
odontoclast
odontogen
odontogenesis
    o. imperfecta
odontogenous
odontoglyph
odontography
odontohyperesthesia
odontolith
odontolithiasis
odontoloxia
odontoma
odontonecrosis
odontoneuralgia
odontoparallaxis
odontoplasty
odontoplerosis

odontoptosis
odontoradiograph
odontorrhagia
odontoschism
odontoscope
odontoscopy
odontoseisis
odontosis
odontosteophyte
odontotheca
odontotomy
odontotripsis
odontotrypy
oligodontia
oolo-. See words beginning
    ulo-.
operation
    Brophy's o.
    Caldwell-Luc o.
    Commando o.
operculum
    dental o.
oral
orale
orolingual
oromandibular
oromaxillary
oropharyngeal
oropharynx
orthodontic
orthodontics
orthodontist
osteoma
    o. dentale
osteoperiostitis
    alveolodental o.
osteotome
osteotomy

overbite
PA — pulpoaxial
pack
    oropharyngeal p.
packing
    vaginal p.
palatal
palate
    cleft p.
palatine
papillomatosis
paracone
paraconid
paradental
parallelometer
pararhizoclasia
parodontal
parodontid
PBA — pulpobuccoaxial
PD — pulpodistal
pedodontics
pemphigus
perforation
    root p.
periapical
pericementitis
    apical p.
pericementoclasia
pericementum
pericoronitis
peridens
periodontal
periodontics
periodontitis
periodontium
periodontoclasia
periodontosis
periosteal

periosteum
    p. alveolare
pharynx
phatnoma
phatnorrhagia
pick
    Rhein's p's.
pioreah. See *pyorrhea.*
PL — pulpolingual
PLA — pulpolinguoaxial
PLa — pulpolabial
plaque
pliers
    Allen's root p.
    crown-crimping p's.
PM — pulpomesial
pneumatization
poikilodentosis
polyodontia
pontic
porcelain
pouch
    Rathke's p.
process
    mastoid p.
profile
    prognathic p.
    retrognathic p.
prognathism
prognathous
prophylactodontics
prophylaxis
prosthesis
prosthetic
prosthion
prosthodontics
protrusion
proximobuccal

proximolabial
proximolingual
pulp
    coronal p.
    mummified p.
    necrotic p.
    radicular p.
pulpa
    p. dentis
pulpalgia
pulpectomy
pulpitis
pulpoaxial
pulpobuccoaxial
pulpodistal
pulpolabial
pulpolingual
pulpolinguoaxial
pulpomesial
pulpotomy
punch
    Ainsworth's p.
purchase point
putrescence
pyorrhea
    p. alveolaris
    paradental p.
    Schmutz p.
quadricuspid
radectomy
radicular
radiectomy
radiolucency
radiopacity
radix
    r. dentis
ramus
ranula

Rathke's pouch
reattachment
reciprocation
replantation
    intentional r.
reposition
restoration
    crown r.
retractor
    Austin's r.
    Moorehead's r.
retromolar
retrusion
Retzius' parallel striae
Rhein's picks
rhizodontropy
rhizoid
Risdon's wire
rongeur
root canal
salivary
salivation
Salter's incremental lines
saprodontia
scaler
scaling
Scarpa's foramen
Schmutz pyorrhea
Schreger's striae
separator
septa
    s. interalveolaria
        maxillae
septum
    s. interradiculare
sequestrectomy
sequestrum
sialolithiasis

singulum. See *cingulum.*
socket
    dry s.
spicule
Spira's disease
Spirec drill
splint
    acrylic s.
    canine-to-canine lingual s.
    Gilmer's s.
stenocompressor
Stent's mass
Stim-U-Dents
stomatitis
    aphthous s.
    herpetic s.
    necrotizing ulcerative s.
    s. venenata
    Vincent's s.
    vulcanite s.
stomatorrhagia
    s. gingivarum
stratum
    s. adamantinum
    s. eboris
striae
    Retzius' parallel s.
    Schreger's s.
stylomyloid
sublingual
submandibular
submaxillary
substantia
    s. adamantina dentis
    s. dentalis propria
    s. eburnea dentis
    s. intertubularis dentis

substantia *(continued)*
    s. propria dentis
    s. vitrea dentis
sulcus
    alveolabial s.
    alveolingual s.
    buccal s.
    gingival s.
    labiodental s.
    lingual s.
supernumerary
suppuration
    alveodental s.
supraclusion
surgical procedures. See *operation.*
symphysis
teeth
    accessional t.
    acrylic resin t.
    anatomic t.
    auditory t. of Huschke
    azzle t.
    barred t.
    bicuspid t.
    buccal t.
    canine t.
    cheoplastic t.
    chiaie t.
    connate t.
    cuspid t.
    cuspless t.
    deciduous t.
    diatoric t.
    Fournier t.
    fused t.
    geminate t.
    hag t.

teeth *(continued)*
- hair t.
- Horner's t.
- Hutchinson's t.
- incisor t.
- labial t.
- malacotic t.
- mandibular t.
- maxillary t.
- molar t.
- Moon's t.
- morsal t.
- mottled t.
- premolar t.
- rake t.
- sclerotic t.
- screw-driver t.
- straight-pin t.
- succedaneous t.
- successional t.
- supernumerary t.
- wang t.
- zero degree t.

template
temporomandibular
temporomaxillary
thecodont
tic
- t. douloureux (doo-loo-roo)

tooth
- t. of epistropheus
- Goslee t.
- malposed t.
- mulberry t.
- pink t. of Mummery
- pulpless t.
- snaggle t.

tooth *(continued)*
- stomach t.
- submerged t.
- Turner t.

tooth-borne
tophus
- dental t.

tork-. See words beginning *torq-.*
torque
torquing
torsion
torsiversion
torus
- t. mandibularis
- t. palatinus

tracheostomy
transversion
trigonid
triple-angle
trismus
tube
- endotracheal t.
- nasogastric t.
- tuberosity

Turner tooth
ulcer
- Crombie's u.

ulectomy
ulemorrhagia
ulitis
ulocace
ulocarcinoma
uloglossitis
ulokahse. See *ulocace.*
uloncus
ulorrhagia
ulorrhea

ulotomy
ultrasonic
uvula
vermilion
vestibular
vestibuloplasty
Vincent's
    infection
    stomatitis
vomer
vulcanite
Wharton's duct

wire
    continuous loop w.
    interdental w.
    intraoral w.
    Ivy w.
    Kirschner's w.
    Risdon's w.
xanthodontus
zanthodontus. See
    xanthodontus.
zygoma
zygomatic

DERMATOLOGY AND ALLERGY

Abernethy's sarcoma
abscess
    Monro's a.
    Paget's a.
Absidia
Abt-Letterer-Siwe syndrome
acanthokeratodermia
acantholysis
    a. bullosa
acanthoma
    a. adenoides cysticum
    a. inguinale
    a. tropicum
    a. verrucosa seborrhoeica
acanthosis
    a. nigricans
    a. papulosa nigra
    a. seborrhoeica
    a. verrucosa
acanthotic
acariasis
    chorioptic a.
    demodectic a.
    psoroptic a.
    sarcoptic a.
acarodermatitis
    a. urticarioides
Acarus
    A. folliculorum
    A. gallinae

Acarus *(continued)*
    A. hordei
    A. rhyzoglypticus
      hyacinthi
    A. scabiei
    A. tritici
acetonasthma
achor
achromatosis
achromia
    congenital a.
    a. parasitica
achromoderma
achromotrichia
acladiosis
acne
    adenoid a.
    a. aggregata seu
      conglobata
    a. agminata
    a. albida
    a. artificialis
    a. atrophica
    bromine a.
    a. cachecticorum
    a. cheloidique
    a. ciliaris
    common a.
    a. conglobata
    cystic a.

227

acne *(continued)*
- a. decalvans
- a. disseminata
- a. dorsalis
- epileptic a.
- a. erythematosa
- a. excoriee des jeunes filles
- a. frontalis
- a. generalis
- halogen a.
- halowax a.
- a. hordeolaris
- a. hypertrophica
- a. indurata
- iodine a.
- a. keloid
- lupoid a.
- a. mentagra
- a. necrotica miliaris
- a. necroticans et exulcerans serpiginosa nasi
- a. neonatorum
- pancreatic a.
- a. papulosa
- petroleum a.
- a. picealis
- a. punctata
- a. pustulosa
- a. rodens
- a. rosacea
- a. scorbutica
- a. scrofulosorum
- a. seborrheica
- a. simplex
- a. syphilitica
- tar a.

acne *(continued)*
- a. tarsi
- a. varioliformis
- a. vulgaris
acnegenic
acneiform
acrochordon
acrocyanosis
acrodermatitis
- a. chronica atrophicans
- a. continua
- a. enteropathica
- Hallopeau's a.
- a. hiemalis
- a. perstans
- a. vesiculosa tropica
acrodermatoses
acrodermatosis
acrodynia
acrokeratosis
- a. verruciformis
acroscleroderma
acrosclerosis
actinocutitis
actinodermatitis
actinomycosis
adamantinoma
Addison-Gull disease
Addison's
- disease
- keloid
adenoma
- a. sebaceum
adermia
adermogenesis
adiponecrosis
adjuvant
- Freund a.

aftha. See *aphtha.*
agammaglobulinemia
agglutination
agglutinin
agglutinogen
agranulocytosis
agria
agrius
albinism
albinismus
    a. conscriptus
    a. totalis
    a. universalis
albino
Albright's syndrome
Alibert-Bazin syndrome
Alibert's
    disease
    mentagra
allergen
allergenic
allergic
allergy
alopecia
    androgenetic a.
    a. areata
    a. capitis totalis
    cicatricial a.
    a. cicatrisata
    a. circumscripta
    congenital a.
    a. congenitalis
    a. disseminata
    drug a.
    female pattern a.
    follicular a.
    a. follicularis
    a. hereditaria

alopecia *(continued)*
    hereditary a.
    a. liminaris
    male pattern a.
    marginal a.
    a. marginalis
    a. medicamentosa
    a. mucinosa
    a. orbicularis
    a. perinevica
    physiologic a.
    postpartum a.
    a. prematura
    a. presenilis
    pressure a.
    roentgen a.
    a. seborrheica
    senile a.
    a. senilis
    symptomatic a.
    a. symptomatica
    syphilitic a.
    a. syphilitica
    a. totalis
    toxic a.
    a. toxica
    traction a.
    traumatic a.
    a. traumatica
    a. triangularis
        congenitalis
    a. universalis
    x-ray a.
alopecic
alphodermia
alphos
altauna
amboceptor

amelanotic
ameloblastoma
Amico's
    drill
    extractor
    skin lifter
    nail nipper
amyloid
amyloidosis
    cutaneous a.
    a. cutis
anaphylactic
anaphylactoid
anaphylaxis
Andrews' disease
anergy
anetoderma
angiocavernous
angiodermatitis
angiofibroma
angiokeratoma
angiolupoid
angioma
    a. pigmentosum
    plexiform a.
    a. serpiginosum
anhidrosis
anonychia
anthema
anthracia
anthracoid
anthrax
antibody
    antinuclear a's.
antifungal
antifungoid
antigen
antiserum

antiserum
    Reenstierna a.
antitoxigen
antitoxin
antitoxinogen
aphtha
aphthoid
aphthous
apiotherapy
apisination
appendage
areatus
areola
    Chaussier's a.
    vaccinal a.
arevareva
argyria
ariboflavinosis
Arndt-Gottron disease
Arthus's phenomenon
Asboe-Hansen's disease
aspergillosis
asteatosis
    a. cutis
asthma
    Millar's a.
asthmatic
Asturian leprosy
atheroma
    a. cutis
atheromasia
atheromatosis
    a. cutis
atheromatous
atopen
atopic
atopy
atrichia

atrichosis
atrophodermatosis
aurantiasis
aurid
Auspitz's dermatosis
autoantibody
autoantigen
autodermic
autodesensitization
autoeczematization
autoimmunization
autoinoculation
bacillus
    Ducrey's b.
    Hansen's b.
bacterid
    pustular b.
Baerensprung's erythrasma
Barber's dermatosis
Bard-Parker dermatome
Barker Vacu-tome dermatome
Bazin's disease
Beau's line
Becker's nevus
bejel
Besnier-Boeck disease
Besnier's prurigo
biotripsis
blastomycosis
    cutaneous b.
    systemic b.
bleb
blef-. See words beginning
    bleph-.
blennorrhagia
blennorrhea
blepharitis
blepharochalasis

blister
Bloch's reaction
blotch
    palpebral b.
Bockhart's impetigo
body
    Leishman-Donovan b's.
    Lipschütz's b's.
Boeck's
    disease
    itch
    sarcoid
    scabies
boil
Bowen's
    precancerous dermatosis
    disease
bromhidrosis
Brooke's disease
Brown's dermatome
Bruck's test
bubo
    Frei's b.
bubon
    b. d'emblēe
Buerger's disease
bulla
bullous
Buschke-Ollendorff syndrome
Buschke's scleredema
calcinosis
    c. circumscripta
    c. cutis
callosity
callous
callus
calor
    c. mordax

calor
    c. mordicans
calva
calvities
calvitium
canceroderm
cancroid
cancrum
Candida
    C. albicans
candidiasis
canities
canker
Cantlie's foot tetter
carbuncle
carbuncular
carbunculosis
carcinelcosis
carcinomelcosis
carotenemia
carotenodermia
Carrión's disease
caruncle
caruncula
Casal's necklace
caseation
Castellani's paint
cativi
Cazenave's
    disease
    lupus
    vitiligo
cell
    basal c.
    Langhans' c's.
    Lipschütz's c.
    malpighian c's.
    Paget's c.

cell *(continued)*
    prickle c.
    Touton giant c's.
    Tzank c.
cellulitis
    streptococcus c.
cellulocutaneous
Celsus'
    kerion
    papules
    vitiligo
centrocyte
chalazia
chalazion
chancre
    fungating c.
    indurated c.
    Ricord's c.
    Rollet's c.
    sporotrichotic c.
    sulcus c.
chancriform
chancroid
chapped
Chaussier's areola
cheilitis
    actinic c.
    c. actinica
    apostematous c.
    commissural c.
    exfoliativa c.
    glandularis apostematosa
      c.
    impetiginous c.
    migrating c.
    c. venenata
cheiropompholyx
chigger

chigoe
chilblain
    necrotized c.
chloasma
    c. hepaticum
    c. periorale virginium
    c. phthisicorum
    c. traumaticum
chloracne
chlorosis
cholesterosis
    c. cutis
chondrodermatitis
    c. nodularis chronica
      helicis
chromatophore
chromatosis
chromhidrosis
chromoblastomycosis
chromomycosis
chromophytosis
chrotoplast
Ciarrocchi's disease
cicatrix
cimicosis
circinate
Civatte's poikiloderma
clavus
    c. syphiliticus
Coccidioides
    C. immitis
coccidioidomycosis
collagenosis
Collins' dynamometer
comedo
complex
    EAHF c.
condyloma

condyloma (continued)
    c. acuminatum
    c. latum
    c. subcutaneum
congelation
conjunctivitis
corium
    c. phlogisticum
Corlett's pyosis
cornification
cornified
cornu
    c. cutaneum
corona
    c. seborrheica
    c. veneris
coxsackie virus
croup
crustosus
cryocautery
cryotherapy
cryptococcosis
cuniculus
curet
    Fox's c.
    Piffard's c.
    Walsh's c.
cutaneous
cuticularization
cutireaction
cutis
    c. anserina
    c. elastica
    c. hyperelastica
    c. laxa
    c. marmorata
    c. pendula
    c. pensilis

cutis *(continued)*
    c. rhomboidalis nuchae
    c. testacea
    c. unctuosa
    c. vera
    c. verticis gyrata
cutisector
cutitis
cutization
cyasma
cylindroma
cyst
    dermoid c.
dactylitis
    d. strumosa
    d. syphilitica
    d. tuberculosa
dander
dandruff
Danielssen's disease
Danlos' syndrome
Darier-Roussy sarcoid
Darier's disease
dartre
dartrous
deallergization
debride
debridement
    enzymatic d.
    surgical d.
decalvant
decongestant
decongestive
decubital
decubitus
deficiency
    riboflavin d.
deflorescence

defluxio
    d. capillorum
    d. ciliorum
defurfuration
Degos-Delort-Tricot
    syndrome
Demodex
    D. folliculorum
depigmentation
depilate
depilation
depilatory
derma
dermabrader
    Iverson's d.
    sand paper d.
dermabrasion
dermadrome
dermagen
dermal
dermalaxia
dermametropathism
dermamyiasis
    d. linearis migrans
      oestrosa
dermanaplasty
dermapostasis
dermatalgia
dermataneuria
dermatauxe
dermatergosis
dermathemia
dermatic
dermatitides
dermatitis
    actinic d.
    d. aestivalis
    allergic d.

dermatitis *(continued)*
- d. ambustionis
- ancylostome d.
- arsphenamine d.
- d. artefacta
- atopic d.
- d. atrophicans
- berloque d.
- bhiwanol d.
- blastomycetic d.
- brucella d.
- d. bullosa
- d. calorica
- d. combustionis
- d. congelationis
- contact d.
- d. contusiformis
- cosmetic d.
- dhobie mark d.
- d. dysmenorrhoeica
- d. epidemica
- d. erythematosa
- d. escharotica
- d. excoriativa infantum
- d. exfoliativa
- d. exfoliativa epidemica
- d. exfoliativa infantum
- exudative discoid and lichenoid d.
- d. factitia
- d. gangrenosa
- d. gangrenosa infantum
- d. hemostatica
- d. herpetiformis
- d. hiemalis
- d. hypostatica
- d. infectiosa eczematoides

dermatitis *(continued)*
- Jacquet's d.
- Leiner's d.
- livedoid d.
- d. medicamentosa
- d. multiformis
- mycotic d.
- d. nodosa
- d. nodularis necrotica
- d. papillaris capillitii
- d. pediculoides ventricosus
- pigmented purpuric lichenoid d.
- poison ivy d.
- poison oak d.
- poison sumac d.
- precancerous d.
- d. psoriasiformis nodularis
- purpuric pigmented lichenoid d.
- d. repens
- roentgen-ray d.
- schistosome d.
- seborrheic d.
- d. seborrheica
- d. simplex
- d. skiagraphica
- d. solaris
- stasis d.
- d. traumatica
- uncinarial d.
- d. vegetans
- d. venenata
- d. verrucosa
- weeping d.

dermatoautoplasty

dermatocele
dermatocellulitis
dermatochalasis
dermatoconiosis
dermatoconjunctivitis
dermatocyst
dermatodysplasia
    d. verruciformis
dermatofibroma
    d. protuberans
dermatofibrosarcoma
    d. protuberans
dermatofibrosis
    d. lenticularis
       disseminata
dermatogen
dermatogenous
dermatograph
dermatoheteroplasty
dermatokelidosis
dermatologist
dermatology
dermatolysis
    d. palpebrarum
dermatoma
dermatome
    Bard-Parker d.
    Barker Vacu-tome d.
    Brown's d.
    Hall's d.
    Hood's d.
    Meek-Wall d.
    Padgett's d.
    Reese's d.
    Stryker's d.
dermatomegaly
dermatomucosomyositis
dermatomycosis

dermatomycosis *(continued)*
    blastomycetic d.
    d. furfuracea
    d. microsporina
    d. trichophytina
dermatomyoma
dermatomyositis
dermatoneurology
dermato-ophthalmitis
dermatopathy
dermatophiliasis
Dermatophilus
    D. penetrans
dermatophylaxis
dermatophyte
dermatophytid
dermatophytosis
    d. furfuracea
dermatoplastic
dermatoplasty
dermatopolyneuritis
dermatorrhagia
dermatorrhea
dermatorrhexis
dermatoscopy
dermatosis
    acarine d.
    angioneurotic d.
    Auspitz's d.
    Barber's d.
    Bowen's precancerous d.
    lichenoid d.
    d. papulosa nigra
    precancerous d.
    progressive pigmentary d.
    Schamberg's d.
    stasis d.
    subcorneal pustular d.

dermatosis
    Unna's d.
dermatostomatitis
dermatotome
dermatozoonosus
dermatrophia
dermepenthesis
dermis
dermitis
dermoanergy
dermoblast
dermograph
dermographia
dermohemia
dermoid
dermoidectomy
dermolipoma
dermolysis
dermomycosis
dermopathy
dermophlebitis
dermostenosis
dermostosis
dermosynovitis
dermosyphilography
dermosyphilopathy
dermotactile
dermotropic
dermovaccine
dermovascular
desensitize
desiccation
    electric d.
desquamation
    furfuraceous d.
    membranous d.
    siliquose d.
Devergie's disease

diamonds
diascope
diascopy
Dick test
disease
    Addison-Gull d.
    Addison's d.
    Alibert's d.
    Andrews' d.
    Arndt-Gottron d.
    Asboe-Hansen's d.
    Bazin's d.
    Besnier-Boeck d.
    Boeck's d.
    Bowen's d.
    Brooke's d.
    Buerger's d.
    Carrión's d.
    Cazenave's d.
    Ciarrocchi's d.
    Danielssen's d.
    Darier's d.
    Devergie's d.
    Duhring's d.
    Fordyce's d.
    Fox-Fordyce d.
    Frei's d.
    Gaucher's d.
    Gibert's d.
    Gilchrist's d.
    Hailey and Hailey d.
    Hallopeau's d.
    Hand-Schüller-Christian
      d.
    Hansen's d.
    Hartnup's d.
    Hebra's d.
    Hodgkin's d.

disease *(continued)*
- Hutchinson's d.
- Hyde's d.
- Jadassohn's d.
- Kaposi's d.
- Köbner's d.
- Landouzy's d.
- Leiner's d.
- Leloir's d.
- Letterer-Siwe d.
- Lipschütz's d.
- Lortat-Jacob's d.
- Lutz-Miescher d.
- Majocchi's d.
- Mibelli's d.
- Neumann's d.
- Nicolas-Favre d.
- Niemann-Pick d.
- Osler's d.
- Osler-Vaquez d.
- Pollitzer's d.
- Puente's d.
- Quincke's d.
- Quinquaud's d.
- Rayer's d.
- Raynaud's d.
- Recklinghausen's d.
- Reiter's d.
- Robinson's d.
- Schamberg's d.
- Senear-Usher d.
- Sticker's d.
- Sutton's d.
- Taenzer's d.
- Urbach-Oppenheim d.
- Weber-Christian d.
- Weber's d.
- White's d.

disseminated
distichia
dopaoxidase
dracunculiasis
drill
- Amico's d.
- Ralks' d.

drugs. See *Medications.*
D & S – dermatology and syphilology
Ducrey's bacillus
Duhring's
- disease
- pruritus

dynamometer
- Collins' d.

dyschromia
dyshidrosis
- trichophytic d.

dyskeratosis
- d. congenita
- d. follicularis

dyspigmentation
dystrophy
- median canaliform d. of the nail

EAHF – eczema, asthma, hay fever
ecchymosis
ecthyma
- e. contagiosum
- e. gangrenosum
- e. syphiliticum

ectoderm
ectodermosis
- e. erosiva pluriorificialis

ectothrix
Ectotrichophyton

ectylotic
eczema
    allergic e.
    e. articulorum
    atopic e.
    e. barbae
    e. capitis
    e. craquelé
    e. crustosum
    e. diabeticorum
    e. epilans
    e. epizootica
    e. erythematosum
    flexural e.
    e. herpeticum
    e. hypertrophicum
    infantile e.
    e. intertrigo
    lichenoid e.
    linear e.
    e. madidans
    e. marginatum
    e. neuriticum
    e. nummulare
    e. papulosum
    e. parasiticum
    e. pustulosum
    e. rubrum
    e. scrofuloderma
    e. seborrhoeicum
    e. siccum
    solar e.
    e. solare
    e. squamosum
    stasis e.
    e. tyloticum
    e. vaccinatum
    e. verrucosum

eczema *(continued)*
    e. vesiculosum
    weeping e.
eczematid
eczematization
eczematoid
eczematosis
eczematous
edema
    angioneurotic e.
efelis. See *ephelis.*
efidrosis. See *ephidrosis.*
Ehlers-Danlos syndrome
eksan-. See words beginning
    exan-.
ekzema. See *eczema.*
elastosis
    e. senilis
electrodermogram
electrodermography
electrodesiccation
elephantiasis
    e. arabicum
    e. asturiensis
    e. filariensis
    e. graecorum
    e. leishmaniana
    lymphangiectatic e.
    e. telangiectodes
elevator
    Ralks' e.
emaculation
emollient
emphlysis
emphractic
emulsion
    Pusey's e.
endothelioma

endothelioma *(continued)*
    e. capitis
    e. cutis
endothrix
endotoxin
enzyme
eosinophilia
ephelis
ephidrosis
    e. cruenta
epidermal
epidermatoplasty
epidermidosis
epidermis
epidermitis
epidermization
epidermodysplasia
    e. verruciformis
epidermoid
epidermolysis
    e. acquisita
    e. bullosa
epidermoma
epidermomycosis
epidermophytid
Epidermophyton
    E. floccosum
epidermophytosis
    e. cruris
    e. interdigitale
epidermosis
epilation
epilatory
epiparonychia
epithelial
epithelization
epithelioid
epithelioma

epithelioma *(continued)*
    e. adenoides cysticum
    e. capitis
    e. molluscum
epitheliomatosis
epitheliomatous
epithelium
eponychia
eponychium
ergodermatosis
erisipelas. See *erysipelas.*
erosion
erubescence
eruption
    bullous e.
    creeping e.
    crustaceous e.
    erythematous e.
    Kaposi's varicelliform e.
    macular e.
    papular e.
    petechial e.
    pustular e.
    squamous e.
    serum e.
    tubercular e.
eruptive
erysipelas
    ambulant e.
    gangrenous e.
    e. grave internum
    idiopathic e.
    migrant e.
    e. perstans
    phlegmonous e.
    e. pustulosum
    e. verrucosum
    e. vesiculosum

erysipelas
    zoonotic e.
erysipelatous
erysipeloid
erythema
    e. abigne
    acrodynic e.
    e. annulare
    e. annulare centrifugum
    e. annulare rheumaticum
    e. bullosum
    e. caloricum
    e. circinatum
    e. elevatum diutinum
    e. exudativum
    e. figuratum
    e. fugax
    e. gyratum
    e. induratum
    e. infectiosum
    e. intertrigo
    e. iris
    Jacquet's e.
    e. marginatum
    Milian's e.
    e. multiforme
    e. neonatorum
    e. neonatorum toxicum
    e. nodosum
    e. nodosum syphiliticum
    palmar e.
    e. paratrimma
    e. pernio
    e. perstans
    e. pudicitiae
    e. punctatum
    e. scarlatiniforme
    e. simplex

erythema *(continued)*
    e. solare
    e. streptogenes
    e. toxicum
    e. traumaticum
    e. venenatum
erythematous
erythra
erythralgia
erythrasma
    Baerensprung's e.
erythredema polyneuropathy
erythrocyanosis
    e. crurum puellaris
    e. frigida crurum
        puellarum
    e. supramalleolaris
erythroderma
    atopic e.
    congenital ichthyosi-
        form e.
    e. desquamativum
    exfoliative e.
    e. ichthyosiforme
        congenitum
    lymphomatous e.
    e. psoriaticum
    Sézary e.
    e. squamosum
erythrodermatitis
erythromelia
erythroplasia
    e. of Queyrat
eschar
eskar. See *eschar.*
esthiomene
evanescent
exanthem

exanthem
    vesicular e.
exanthema
    e. subitum
exanthematous
excoriation
excrescence
exfoliation
exfoliative
exocrine
extractor
    Amico's e.
    comedo e.
    Saalfeld's e.
    Schamberg's e.
    Unna's e.
    Walton's e.
exudate
exudation
exulceratio
    e. simplex
exuviae
fajedenah. See *phagedena.*
FANA — fluorescent anti-
    nuclear antibody
favid
favus
    f. circinatus
    f. herpeticus
    f. herpetiformis
    f. pilaris
felon
fester
fever
    scarlet f.
fiber
    Herxheimer's f's.
fibroma

fibroma *(continued)*
    f. cutis
    f. lipomatodes
    f. pendulum
    telangiectatic f.
    f. xanthoma
fibrosis
fitofotodermatitis. See
    phytophotodermatitis.
flare
flumen
flumina pilorum
fluorescence
follicle
    sebaceous f.
follicular
folliculitis
    f. abscedens et
      suffodiens
    agminate f.
    f. barbae
    f. cheloidalis
    f. decalvans
    f. decalvans et lichen
      spinulosus
    f. gonorrhoeica
    f. keloidalis
    f. nares perforans
    f. ulerythematosa
      reticulata
    f. varioliformis
Fordyce's
    disease
    spots
formication
formiciasis
Foshay's test
Fox-Fordyce disease

Fox's
- curet
- impetigo

fragilitas
- f. crinium
- f. unguium

frambesia

frambesioma

freckle

Frei's
- bubo
- disease
- test

frenulum

frenum

Freund adjuvant

fulguration

fulgurize

fungal

fungate

fungous

fungus

furfur

furfuraceous

furuncle

furuncular

furunculoid

furunculosis

furunculus
- f. vulgaris

ganglion

gangrene
- cutaneous g.
- disseminated cutaneous g.
- gaseous g.
- Raynaud's d.

gangrenous

Gaucher's disease

Gennerich's treatment

genodermatology

genodermatosis

Gibert's
- disease
- pityriasis

Gilchrist's disease

gingivitis

glabrous

globulin
- antidiphtheritic g.
- antitoxic g.
- gamma g's.
- immune serum g.

glomus
- cutaneous g.
- digital g.
- neuromyoarterial g.

glossitis
- g. areata exfoliativa
- g. dissecans
- Hunter's g.
- Moeller's g.
- g. parasitica
- parenchymatous g.
- rhomboid g.
- g. rhomboidea mediana

goatpox

gonitis
- fungous g.

gonococcus

gonorrhea

gonorrheal

Gougerot's syndrome

granular

granulation

granuloma

granuloma *(continued)*
    g. annulare
    g. endemicum
    eosinophilic g.
    g. fungoides
    g. gangraenescens
    Hodgkin's g.
    g. inguinale
    lipoid g.
    lycopodium g.
    Majocchi's g.
    g. malignum
    g. pyogenicum
    g. sarcomatodes
    g. telangiectaticum
    g. trichophyticum
    g. venereum
granulomatosis
    Miescher-Leder g.
gumma
gutta
    g. rosacea
guttate
Hailey and Hailey disease
Hallopeau's
    acrodermatitis
    disease
Hall's dermatome
hamartoma
hamartomatosis
hamartomatous
Hand-Schüller-Christian
    disease
Hansen's
    bacillus
    disease
haplodermatitis
Hartnup's disease

Hebra's
    disease
    ointment
    pityriasis
hemangioma
    capillary h.
    cavernous h.
    h. congenitale
    h. hypertrophicum cutis
    h. simplex
hemangiomatosis
hematid
hematidrosis
hemochromatosis
herpangina
herpes
    h. catarrhalis
    h. digitalis
    h. facialis
    h. farinosus
    h. febrilis
    h. generalisatus
    h. iris
    h. labialis
    h. oticus
    h. phlyctaenodes
    h. praeputialis
    h. progenitalis
    h. recurrens
    h. simplex
    h. tonsurans
    h. tonsurans maculosus
    h. vegetans
    h. zoster
    h. zoster oticus
    h. zoster varicellosus
herpetic
herpetiform

Herxheimer's
    fibers
    reaction
    spirals
heterochromia
heterodermic
heterophil
heterophilic
heterotrichosis
    h. supercilliorum
hidradenitis
    h. suppurativa
hidrocystoma
hidrorrhea
hidrosadenitis
    h. axillaris
    h. destruens suppurativa
hidroschesis
hidrosis
hirsuties
hirsutism
histaminase
histamine
histaminia
histiocytoma
    lipoid h.
histiocytomatosis
histiocytosis
histoplasmosis
Hodgkin's
    disease
    granuloma
hodi-potsy
holocrine
homme
    h. rouge
homograft
homologous

Hood'dermatome
hornification
horny
horripilation
Hunter's glossitis
Hutchinson's
    disease
    mask
    triad
hyalin
hyaline
hydatid
Hyde's disease
hydration
hydroa
    h. aestivale
    h. febrile
    h. gestationis
    h. gravidarum
    h. puerorum
    h. vacciniforme
    h. vesiculosum
hydrocystoma
hydrotherapy
hygroma
    cystic h.
    h. cysticum
hyperergia
hyperergy
hypergammaglobulinemia
hyperhidrosis
hyperkeratosis
    h. congenitalis palmaris
        et plantaris
    h. excentrica
    h. figurata centrifuga
        atrophica
    h. linguae

hyperkeratosis *(continued)*
    h. penetrans
    h. subungualis
    h. universalis congenita
hyperpigmentation
hypersarcosis
hypersensibility
hypersensitiveness
hypersensitivity
hypersensitization
hypertrichiasis
hypertrichophrydia
hypertrichosis
hypha
hyphomycetic
hyphomycosis
hypochromotrichia
hypodermis
hypodermolithiasis
hypoergia
hypogammaglobulin
hypogammaglobulinemia
hyponychium
hyponychon
hyposensitive
hyposensitization
ichthyismus
    i. exanthematicus
ichthyosis
    i. congenita
    i. cornea
    follicular i.
    i. follicularis
    i. hystrix
    i. intrauterina
    linear i.
    i. linguae
    nacreous i.

ichthyosis *(continued)*
    i. palmaris
    i. palmaris et plantaris
    i. plantaris
    i. sauroderma
    i. scutulata
    i. sebacea cornea
    i. serpentina
    i. simplex
    i. spinosa
    i. thysanotrichica
    i. uteri
icterus
I & D – incision and drainage
idiosyncrasy
iksodiahsis. See *ixodiasis.*
ikthe-. See words beginning
    ichthy-.
immunity
immunization
immunochemical
immunodiagnosis
immunoelectrophoresis
immunofluorescent
immunoglobulin
immunohistochemical
immunology
immunoreaction
immunotherapy
impetiginization
impetiginous
impetigo
    Bockhart's i.
    i. bullosa
    bullous i.
    i. contagiosa
    i. eczematodes
    follicular i.

impetigo *(continued)*
    Fox's i.
    furfuraceous i.
    i. herpetiformis
    i. neonatorum
    i. simplex
    i. staphylogenes
    i. syphilitica
    i. variolosa
incontinentia
    i. pigmenti
induration
infestation
integument
integumentary
integumentum
    i. commune
intertriginous
intertrigo
    i. labialis
    i. saccharomycetica
intimitis
    proliferative i.
intracutaneous
intradermal
intradermoreaction
itch
    Boeck's i.
    dhobie i.
    grain i.
    Moeller's i.
    seven-year i.
    swimmers' i.
itching
Ito-Reenstierna test
Iverson's dermabrader
ixodiasis
Jacquet's

Jacquet's *(continued)*
    dermatitis
    erythema
Jadassohn-Bloch test
Jadassohn-Lewandosky law
Jadassohn's
    disease
    nevus
Jarisch-Herxheimer reaction
Jarisch's ointment
jaundice
jigger
Jones-Mote reaction
kalazea. See *chalazia.*
kalazeon. See *chalazion.*
Kaposi's
    disease
    sarcoma
    varicelliform eruption
    xeroderma
Keller's ultraviolet test
keloid
    Addison's k.
keloidosis
keratiasis
keratin
keratinocyte
keratinous
keratoacanthoma
keratoderma
    k. blennorrhagica
    k. palmaris et plantaris
keratodermatitis
keratohyalin
keratohyaline
keratolysis
    k. exfoliativa
    k. neonatorum

keratoma
  k. diffusum
  k. hereditaria mutilans
  k. malignum congenitale
  k. palmare et plantare
  k. plantare sulcatum
  k. senile
keratomycosis
  k. linguae
keratonosis
keratoprotein
keratosis
  actinic k.
  k. blennorrhagica
  k. diffusa fetalis
  k. follicularis
  k. follicularis contagiosa
  gonorrheal k.
  k. labialis
  k. linguae
  nevoid k.
  k. nigricans
  k. obturans
  k. palmaris et plantaris
  k. pilaris
  k. punctata
  seborrheic k.
  k. seborrheica
  senile k.
  k. senilis
  k. suprafollicularis
  k. vegetans
keratotic
kerion
  k. celsi
  Celsus' k.
Keyes' dermal punch
kilitis. See *cheilitis.*

kiropomfoliks. See
  cheiropompholyx.
kloazma. See *chloasma.*
klor-. See words beginning
  chlor-.
Köbner's disease
Koebner's phenomenon
koilonychia
Kolmer's test
kondro-. See words beginning
  chondro-.
kraurosis
  k. penis
  k. vulvae
Kveim test
lacuna
Landouzy's
    disease
    purpura
Langhans'
    cells
    layer
lanugo
larva
    l. migrans
Lassar's paste
law
    Jadassohn-Lewandosky l.
layer
    Langhans' l.
    malpighian l.
LE — lupus erythematosus
Leiner's
    dermatitis
    disease
leiodermia
leiomyoma
    l. cutis

Leishman-Donovan body
leishmaniasis
Leloir's disease
lenticula
lentigo
lentigomelanosis
lepidosis
lepothrix
lepra
    l. alba
    l. alphoides
    l. alphos
    l. anaesthetica
    l. arabum
    l. conjunctivae
    l. graecorum
    l. maculosa
    l. mutilans
    l. nervorum
    l. nervosa
    l. tuberculoides
    Willan's l.
leprid
leproma
lepromatous
leprosy
    Asturian l.
    cutaneous l.
    lazarine l.
    lepromatous l.
    Lombardy l.
    macular l.
    maculoanesthetic l.
    neural l.
    nodular l.
    trophoneurotic l.
    tuberculoid l.
leprotic

leprous
leptochroa
lesion
    disseminated l.
    initial syphilitic l.
Letterer-Siwe disease
leukoderma
    l. acquisitum
      centrifugum
leukodermatous
leukonychia
leukoplakia
Libman-Sacks syndrome
lichen
    l. albus
    l. amyloidosus
    l. annularis
    l. chronicus simplex
    l. fibromucinoidosus
    l. frambesianus
    l. leprosus
    l. myxedematosus
    l. nitidus
    l. pilaris
    l. planopilaris
    l. planus
    l. planus et acuminatus
      atrophicans
    l. ruber acuminatus
    l. ruber moniliformis
    l. ruber planus
    l. sclerosus et atrophicus
    l. scrofulosorum
    l. simplex chronicus
    l. spinulosus
    l. striatus
    l. urticatus
licheniasis

lichenification
lichenization
lichenoid
lifter
    Amico's skin l.
line
    Beau's l's.
lipoidosis
lipoidproteinosis
lipoma
lipomatosis
liposarcoma
Lipschütz's
    bodies
    cell
    disease
    ulcer
livedo
    l. annularis
    l. racemosa
    l. reticularis
    l. reticularis idiopathica
    l. reticularis
      symptomatica
    l. telangiectatica
livedoid
livid
Lombardy leprosy
Lortat-Jacob's disease
louse
lues
    l. nervosa
    l. tarda
    l. venerea
lunula
    l. of nail
    l. unguis
lupoid

lupus
    Cazenave's l.
    l. erythematodes
    l. erythematosus
    l. erythematosus
      discoides
    l. erythematosus
      disseminatus
    l. livido
    l. pernio
    l. tuberculosus
    l. tumidus
    l. verrucosus
    l. vorax
    l. vulgaris
Lutz-Miescher disease
Lutz-Splendore-de Almeida
    syndrome
Lyell's syndrome
lymphadenitis
lymphangioma
    l. cavernosum
    l. circumscriptum
    l. cysticum
    l. tuberosum multiplex
    l. xanthelasmoideum
lymphangitis
    l. carcinomatosa
lymphedema
lymphocytoma
lymphodermia
lymphogranuloma
    l. benignum
    l. inguinale
    l. venereum
lymphogranulomatosis
    l. cutis
    l. inguinalis

lymphogranulomatosis
   l. maligna
lymphoma
lymphosarcoma
lymphosarcomatosis
maceration
macroglobulinemia
macula
   m. solaris
maculae
   m. atrophicae
   m. caeruleae
macular
maculate
maculation
maculopapular
maculopapule
maduromycosis
Majocchi's
   disease
   granuloma
   purpura
Malpighi rete
malpighian
   cells
   layer
mange
   demodectic m.
   follicular m.
Mantoux test
mask
   Hutchinson's m.
matrix
   nail m.
   m. unguis
matrixitis
Mauriac's syndrome
measles

Medications
   acetic acid solution
   Achromycin
   Actidil
   acrisorcin
   Adrenalin hydrochloride
   Aerosporin
   Akrinol
   Albamycin
   Alerin
   aluminum acetate
      solution
   Ammonium ichthosul-
      fonate
   amphotericin B
   Anesthesin
   anthralin
   Aristocort
   Aristoderm
   Aureomycin
   Bacitracin
   Barachlor
   Benadryl
   benzalkonium
   benzene hexachloride
   Benzocaine
   benzoic acid
   benzyl benzoate
   Boracic acid
   boric acid
   brompheniramine
      maleate
   Burow's solution
   Cade oil
   calamine
   Candeptin
   candicidin
   carbinoxamine

Medications *(continued)*

carbol-fuchsin solution
carboneol
Carfusin
Cathomycin
Chestamine
Chlo-Amine
Chloramate
chloramphenicol
chlordantoin
chlorhydroxyquinolin
Chloromycetin
chlorpheniramine
chlorquinaldol
chlortetracycline
Chlor-Trimeton
chrysarobin
Chymar
chymotrypsin
Clistin
copper oleate
Copper sulfate
Cordran
Cort-Dome
Cortef
Cortifan
Cortisol
Cortril
crotamiton
Crystal violet
cupric sulfate
cyclomethycaine
cyproheptadine
Decadron
Delta-Cortef
Deltasone
Dendrid
dermatomycin

Medications *(continued)*

Desenex
dexamethasone
dextro pantothenyl
  alcohol
Diafen
diamthazole
dibucaine
diiodohydroxyquin
Diiodohydroxyquinoline
Dimetane
dimethindene
dimethisoquin
Dimethpyrindene
diphenhydramine
  hydrochloride
diphenylpyraline
Drize
Dyclone
dyclonine
Dynazone
Efudex
Elase
Eldezol
ephedrine
epinephrine
Equanil
Erythrocin
erythromycin
ethyl aminobenzoate
Eurax
Euresol
fibrinolysin and
  desoxyribonuclease
fluocinolone acetonide
  N.F.
Fluonid
Fluoroplex

Medications *(continued)*

- fluorouracil
- 5-Fluorouracil
- flurandrenolide
- Forhistal
- 5-FU
- Fulvicin
- Fungizone
- Furacin
- Gamastan
- Gamimune
- Gammagee
- Gamma Globulin
- Gamulin
- Garamycin
- gentamicin
- Gentian violet
- Germa-Medica
- Gexane
- Grifulvin
- griseofulvin
- haloprogin
- Halotex
- Herplex
- hexachlorophene
- Hexadrol
- Hexagerm
- Hispril
- Histachlor
- Histadur
- Histaspan
- Histitrin
- Histrey
- Hydeltrasol
- hydrocortisone
- Hydrocortone
- hydroxyzine pamoate
- ichthammol

Medications *(continued)*

- ichthyol
- idoxuridine
- Ilotycin
- Immu-G
- Immuglobin
- immune serum globulin
- iodochlorhydroxyquin
- juniper tar
- Kenacort
- Kenalog
- Kwell
- lauryl sulfoacetate
- Lidex
- lime solution
- Lindane
- Lowila
- mafenide
- Medrol
- mercury, ammoniated
- methdilazine
- methylprednisolone
- methylrosaniline
- Methyl violet
- Meticortelone
- Meticorten
- Miltown
- Mycifradin
- Mycostatin
- neomycin
- nitrofurazone
- novobiocin
- Nupercaine
- nystatin
- Orthoboric acid
- oxytetracycline
- Panmycin
- Panthenol

Medications *(continued)*

Pantothenylol
parachlormetaxylenol
Periactin
peruvian balsam
Phenergan
Phenetron
pheniramine
phenobarbital
phenol
pHisoHex
Pix Juniperi
Podophyllin
podophyllum resin
Polaramine
Polycycline
polymyxin B
potassium permanganate
  solution
pramoxine
prednisolone
prednisone
promethazine
  hydrochloride
Pyribenzamine
Pyronil
pyrrobutamine
Quotane
Resorcin
resorcinol
rotoxamine
salicylic acid
scarlet red
selenium
Selsun
Septisol
silver nitrate
Sodium Hyposulfite

Medications *(continued)*

sodium sulfathiazole
sodium thiosulfate
Solu-Cortef
Solu-Medrol
Sporostacin
Stanzamine
Steclin
Stoxil
Sudan IV
Sulfamylon
Surfacaine
Synalar
Tacaryl
Teldrin
Temaril
Terramycin
tetracycline
Tetracyn
Tinactin
tolnaftate
triamcinolone
Triburon
triclobisonium
trimeprazine
Trimeton
tripelennamine
  hydrochloride
triprolidine
Tronothane
Twiston
Tylahist
vancomycin
Vanocin
Vioform
Vistaril
Vleminckx' solution
White precipitate

Medications *(continued)*
    Zephiran
    zinchlorundesal
    zincundecate
Meek-Wall dermatome
melanin
melanism
melanocyte
melanoderma
    m. cachecticorum
    senile m.
melanodermatitis
melanoleukoderma
    m. colli
melanoma
    malignant m.
    subungual m.
melanonychia
melanopathy
melanosis
    m. lenticularis
        progressiva
    Riehl's m.
melanotrichia
melasma
    m. universale
melitagra
Melkersson-Rosenthal
    syndrome
membrane
mentagra
    Alibert's m.
Mibelli's disease
microsporosis
    m. capitis
Microsporum
    M. audouini
    M. canis

Microsporum *(continued)*
    M. furfur
    M. lanosum
Miescher-Leder granulomatosis
Milian's
    erythema
    sign
    syndrome
miliaria
    m. pustulosa
    m. rubra
milium
    colloid m.
Millar's asthma
Milton's urticaria
Moeller's
    glossitis
    itch
mole
molluscum
    cholesterinic m.
    m. contagiosum
    m. epitheliale
    m. fibrosum
    m. lipomatodes
    m. pendulum
    m. sebaceum
    m. simplex
    m. varioliformis
    m. verrucosum
monilethrix
moniliasis
Monro's abscess
morphea
    acroteric m.
    m. alba
    m. atrophica
    m. flammea

morphea *(continued)*
    m. guttata
    herpetiform m.
    m. linearis
    m. nigra
mucinosis
    follicular m.
    papular m.
mucocutaneous
mucodermal
mycetoma
mycid
Mycobacterium
    M. leprae
mycoderma
mycodermatitis
mycology
mycosis
    cutaneous m.
    m. cutis chronica
    m. favosa
    m. framboesioides
    m. fungoides
    m. interdigitalis
myiasis
myoepithelium
myringodermatitis
myxodermia
myxoma
nail
    double-edge n's.
    eggshell n.
    hang n.
    ingrown n.
    parrot beak n.
    reedy n.
    spoon n.
    turtle-back n.

necklace
    Casal's n.
necrobiosis
    n. lipoidica
      diabeticorum
necrosis
necrotic
Neumann's disease
neurodermatitis
    n. disseminata
neurodermatosis
neurodermite
nevi
    epithelial n.
nevocarcinoma
nevose
nevoxanthoendothelioma
nevus
    n. anemicus
    n. angiectodes
    n. angiomatodes
    n. arachnoideus
    n. araneosus
    n. araneus
    n. avasculosus
    Becker's n.
    blue n.
    n. cavernosus
    n. cerebelliformis
    compound n.
    connective-tissue n.
    n. depigmentosus
    dermoepidermal n.
    n. fibrosus
    n. flammeus
    n. follicularis
    n. fusco-caeruleus
      ophthalmo-maxillaris

nevus *(continued)*
    halo n.
    Jadassohn's n.
    linear n.
    n. lipomatosus
    n. lymphaticus
    n. maternus
    melanocytic n.
    n. mollusciformis
    n. morus
    multiplex n.
    n. nervosus
    Ota's n.
    n. papillaris
    n. papillomatosus
    n. pigmentosus
    n. pilosus
    polyploid n.
    n. sanguineus
    sebaceous n. of
      Jadassohn
    n. spilus
    n. spongiosus albus
      mucosae
    strawberry n.
    n. syringocystadenosus
      papilliferus
    n. unius lateralis
    Unna's n.
    n. vasculosus
    n. venosus
    n. verrucosus
    n. vinosus
Nicolas-Favre disease
Niemann-Pick disease
Nikolsky's sign
nipper
    Amico's nail n.

Nocardia
    N. madurae
nocardiosis
nodose
nodosity
nodular
nodulus
noli-me-tangere
nonallergic
nummular
oidiomycosis
ointment
    Hebra's o.
    Jarisch's o.
    Whitfield's o.
onchocerciasis
onikalja. See *onychalgia.*
onikatrofea. See
    onychatrophia.
onikawksis. See *onychauxis.*
onikea. See *onychia.*
onikeksalaksis. See
    onychexallaxis.
onikektome. See
    onychectomy.
onikitis. See *onychitis.*
oniko-. See words beginning
    onycho-.
onychalgia
onychatrophia
onychauxis
onychectomy
onychexallaxis
onychia
    o. lateralis
    o. maligna
    o. parasitica
    o. periungualis

onychia
    o. sicca
onychitis
onychoclasis
onychocryptosis
onychodynia
onychogenic
onychograph
onychogryposis
onychohelcosis
onycholysis
onychoma
onychomadesis
onychomalacia
onychomycosis
onychonosus
onychopathic
onychopathology
onychopathy
onychophagist
onychophyma
onychophysis
onychoptosis
onychorrhexis
onychoschizia
onychosis
onychotillomania
onychotomy
ophryitis
Osler's disease
Osler-Vaquez disease
Ota's nevus
Otomyces
    O. hageni
    O. purpureus
otomycosis
otopathy
oxyuriasis

pachyderma
    p. lymphangiectatica
pachydermatocele
pachydermatosis
pachydermatous
pachydermic
pachydermoperiostosis
    p. plicata
pachyhymenic
pachylosis
pachymenia
pachymenic
pachyonychia
Padgett's dermatome
Paget's
    abscess
    cell
paint
    Castellani's p.
panniculitis
    nodular nonsuppurative
    p.
panniculus
    p. adiposus
papilla
papillary
papillocarcinoma
papilloma
    p. diffusum
    intracanalicular p.
    p. lineare
papular
papule
    Celsus' p's.
papuliferous
papuloerythematous
papulopustular
papulopustule

papulosquamous
papulovesicular
paracanthosis
paracoccidioidomycosis
paraeponychia
parakeratosis
    p. ostracea
    p. psoriasiformis
    p. scutularis
    p. variegata
parapsoriasis
    p. atrophicans
    p. varioliformis
parasite
paronychia
    p. tendinosa
paronychial
paronychosis
paste
    Lassar's p.
    Veiel's p.
peau
    p. d'orange
pediculation
Pediculoides
    P. ventricosus
pediculosis
    p. capillitii
    p. capitis
    p. corporis
    p. inguinalis
    p. palpebrarum
    p. pubis
    p. vestimenti
    p. vestimentorum
Pediculus
    P. humanus capitis
    P. humanus corporis

Pediculus *(continued)*
    P. inguinalis
    P. pubis
pellagra
pemphigoid
    bullous p.
pemphigus
    p. acutus
    p. erythematosus
    p. foliaceus
    p. gangrenosus
    p. hemorrhagicus
    p. malignus
    p. neonatorum
    p. syphiliticus
    p. vegetans
    p. vulgaris
periadenitis
    p. mucosa necrotica
      recurrens
periarteritis
    p. gummosa
    p. nodosa
periderm
~~perifollicular~~
perifolliculitis
    p. capitis abscedens et
      suffodiens
    superficial pustular p.
perionychia
perionychium
perionyx
perionyxis
perlèche
perlesh. See *perlèche.*
perna
pernio
petechia

petechial
petechiasis
peteke-. See words beginning
    petechi-.
phacoanaphylaxis
phagedena
    sloughing p.
    tropical p.
phenomenon
    p. of Arthus
    Koebner's p.
    Raynaud's p.
Phialophora
    P. verrucosa
photodermatitis
photosensitive
photosensitization
phthiriasis
    p. inguinalis
    pubic p.
Phthirus
    P. pubis
phthisic
phytophotodermatitis
piedra
Piffard's curet
pigment
pigmentation
pili
    p. multigemini
pilus
    p. annulatus
    p. cuniculatus
    p. incarnatus recurvus
    p. tortus
pimple
pinta
pintado

pintid
pityriasic
pityriasis
    p. alba
    p. amiantacea
    p. capitis
    p. circinata
    p. circinata et marginata
    p. furfuracea
    Gibert's p.
    Hebra's p.
    p. lichenoides
    p. lichenoides et
        varioliformis acuta
    p. linguae
    p. pilaris
    p. rosea
    p. rubra
    p. rubra pilaris
    p. sicca
    p. simplex
    p. steatoides
    p. versicolor
pityroid
Pityrosporon
    P. orbiculare
    P. ovale
plaque
po dorahnj. See *peau d'orange.*
poikiloderma
    p. atrophicans vasculare
    Civatte's p.
    p. congenitale
poikilodermatomyositis
poliosis
    p. eccentrica
pollen
pollinosis

Pollitzer's disease
polyonychia
pomphoid
pompholyx
pomphus
porokeratosis
porphyria
    p. cutanea tarda
      hereditaria
PPD – purified protein
  derivative
pressure ring
    Walsh's p. r.
prophylaxis
prurigo
    Besnier's p.
    p. estivalis
    p. ferox
    p. mitis
    p. nodularis
    p. simplex
    p. universalis
pruritic
pruritus
    p. ani
    Duhring's p.
    p. hiemalis
    p. senilis
    p. vulvae
pseudoxanthoma
    p. elasticum
psora
psorelcosis
psoriasis
    p. annularis
    p. arthropathica
    p. buccalis
    p. circinata

psoriasis *(continued)*
    p. diffusa
    p. discoides
    p. figurata
    p. follicularis
    p. guttata
    p. gyrata
    p. inveterata
    p. linguae
    p. nummularis
    p. ostracea
    p. palmaris et plantaris
    p. punctata
    pustular p.
    p. rupioides
    p. universalis
psoriatic
psoric
psorospermosis
    p. follicularis
psorous
psydracium
pterygium
    p. unguis
Puente's disease
Pulex
    P. irritans
pulicosis
punch
    Keyes' dermal p.
purpura
    allergic p.
    anaphylactoid p.
    p. angioneurotica
    p. annularis telangiec-
      todes
    p. bullosa
    p. cachectica

purpura *(continued)*
    p. fulminans
    p. hemorrhagica
    p. hyperglobulinemica
    p. iodica
    Landouzy's p.
    p. maculosa
    Majocchi's p.
    orthostatic p.
    p. pulicosa
    p. rheumatica
    Schönlein-Henoch p.
    Schönlein's p.
    p. senilis
    p. simplex
    p. symptomatica
    thrombocytopenic p.
    p. urticans
    p. variolosa
purpuric
purulent
purupuru
pus
Pusey's emulsion
pustula
    p. maligna
pustular
pustulation
pustule
pustulocrustaceous
pustulosis
    p. palmaris
    p. vacciniformis acuta
pyemia
pyoderma
    p. chancriforme faciei
    p. faciale
    p. gangrenosum

pyoderma *(continued)*
    p. ulcerosum tropicalum
    p. vegetans
    p. verrucosum
pyodermatitis
    p. vegetans
pyodermatosis
pyodermitis
    p. vegetans
pyogenic
pyonychia
pyosis
    Corlett's p.
Queyrat's erythroplasia
Quincke's disease
Quinquaud's disease
racemose
radioepidermitis
ragadez. See *rhagades.*
rakoma. See *rhacoma.*
Ralks'
    drill
    elevator
rash
Rayer's disease
Raynaud's
    disease
    gangrene
    phenomenon
reaction
    Bloch's r.
    dopa r.
    Herxheimer's r.
    Jarisch-Herxheimer r.
    Jones-Mote r.
    Sanarelli-Shwartzman r.
    Schultz-Charlton r.
    Schultz-Dale r.

Recklinghausen's disease
Reenstierna antiserum
Reese's dermatome
Reiter's disease
rete
    dermal r.
    r. Malpighi
rhacoma
rhagades
rhinophyma
rhinoscleroma
Rhus
    R. diversiloba
    R. toxicodendron
    R. venenata
Ricord's chancre
Riehl's melanosis
ringworm
rino-. See words beginning
    rhino-.
Robinson's disease
Rollet's chancre
rosacea
roseola
rosette
rubella
rubeola
rupia
    r. escharotica
Saalfeld's extractor
Saccharomycetes
saccharomycosis
Sanarelli-Shwartzman reaction
sarcoid
    Boeck's s.
    Darier-Roussy s.
    Spiegler-Fendt s.
sarcoidosis

sarcoma
    Abernethy's s.
    adipose s.
    Kaposi's s.
sarcomatosis
    s. cutis
satellite
sauriasis
sauriderma
sauriosis
scabies
    Boeck's s.
scabrities
    s. unguium
scarification
scarlatiniform
Schamberg's
    dermatosis
    disease
    extractor
Schick test
schistosomiasis
Schönlein-Henoch purpura
Schönlein's purpura
Schultz-Charlton reaction
Schultz-Dale reaction
scleredema
    Buschke's s.
    s. neonatorum
sclerema
    s. neonatorum
sclerodactylia
    s. annularis ainhumoides
sclerodactyly
scleroderma
sclerodermatitis
scleromyxedema
scleronychia

scrofuloderma
  s. gummosa
  papular s.
  pustular s.
  tuberculous s.
  ulcerative s.
  verrucous s.
scrofulophyma
scurf
scutulum
sebaceous
seborrhea
  s. adiposa
  s. capitis
  s. congestiva
  s. corporis
  eczematoid s.
  s. faciei
  s. furfuracea
  s. generalis
  s. nigricans
  s. oleosa
  s. sicca
  s. squamo neonatorum
seborrheic
sebum
Senear-Usher disease
sensibilisinogen
sensitinogen
sensitization
serpiginous
Sézary's
    erythroderma
    syndrome
shanker. See *chancre.*
shankreform. See *chancriform.*
shankroid. See *chancroid.*
shingles

shock
  anaphylactic s.
siazma. See *cyasma.*
sidraseum. See *psydracium.*
sign
    Milian's s.
    Nikolsky's s.
    Silex's s.
Silex's sign
Sjögren's syndrome
SLE – systemic lupus
    erythematosus
slough
sluf. See *slough.*
solenonychia
solum
    s. unguis
sora. See *psora.*
soreatik. See *psoriatic.*
sorelkosis. See *psorelcosis.*
soriasis. See *psoriasis.*
sorik. See *psoric.*
sorospermosis. See
    psorospermosis.
sorus. See *psorous.*
Spiegler-Fendt sarcoid
spiloplania
spiloplaxia
spiradenoma
spiral
    Herxheimer's s's.
sporotrichosis
Sporotrichum
    S. schenckii
spot
    Fordyce's s's.
squarrose
Staphylococcus

Staphylococcus
    S. epidermidis
staphyloderma
staphylodermatitis
steatoma
steatomatosis
Stevens-Johnson syndrome
Sticker's disease
stigmatosis
stomatitis
stratum
    s. basale epidermidis
    s. corneum epidermidis
    s. corneum unguis
    s. filamentosum
    s. germinativum
        epidermidis
    s. germinativum unguis
    s. granulosum
        epidermidis
    s. malpighii
Streptothrix
streptotrichosis
stria
striae
    Wickham's s.
Stryker-Halbeisen syndrome
Stryker's dermatome
subungual
sudamen
sudoriferous
sudorrhea
sudozanthoma. See
    pseudoxanthoma.
sumac
    swamp s.
Sutton's disease
Sweet's syndrome

sycoma
sycosis
    bacillogenic s.
    s. barbae
    coccogenic s.
    s. contagiosa
    s. framboesia
    s. framboesiaeformis
    hyphomycotic c.
    lupoid s.
    nonparasitic s.
    s. nuchae necrotisans
    parasitic s.
    s. staphylogenes
    s. vulgaris
synanthema
syndrome
    Abt-Letterer-Siwe s.
    Albright's s.
    Alibert-Bazin s.
    antibody deficiency s.
    Buschke-Ollendorff s.
    Danlos' s.
    Degos-Delort-Tricot s.
    Ehlers-Danlos s.
    Gougerot's s.
    Libman-Sacks s.
    Lutz-Splendore-de
        Almeida s.
    Lyell's s.
    Mauriac's s.
    Melkersson-Rosenthal s.
    Milian's s.
    Sézary's s.
    Sjögren's s.
    Stevens-Johnson s.
    Stryker-Halbeisen s.
    Sweet's s.

syndrome *(continued)*

> Waterhouse-Friderichsen s.
>
> Weber-Christian s.

syphilid

syphilis

syphilitic

syphiloderm

syphilophyma

syringadenoma

syringocystadenoma

syringocystoma

syringoma

tache

> t. bleuâtre

tachetic

Taenzer's disease

tegument

telangiectasis

telangiectatic

teratoma

terijeum. See *pterygium.*

test

> agglutination t.
>
> basophil degranulation t.
>
> Bruck's t.
>
> coccidioidin skin t.
>
> complement fixation t.
>
> Dick t.
>
> fluorescent antinuclear antibody t.
>
> Foshay's t.
>
> Frei's t.
>
> in vitro t.
>
> Ito-Reenstierna t.
>
> Jadassohn-Bloch t.
>
> Keller's ultraviolet t.
>
> Kolmer's t.

test *(continued)*

> Kveim t.
>
> lepromin t.
>
> Mantoux t.
>
> mast cell degranulation t.
>
> patch t.
>
> PPD t. – purified protein derivative
>
> Schick t.
>
> Tine t.
>
> tuberculin t.
>
> Tzank t.
>
> Vollmer's t.
>
> Wassermann-fast t.
>
> Wassermann reaction t.

tetter

> brawny t.
>
> Cantilie's foot t.
>
> honeycomb t.

thiriasis. See *phthiriasis.*

thrush

Tine test

tinea

> t. amiantacea
>
> t. axillaris
>
> t. barbae
>
> t. capitis
>
> t. ciliorum
>
> t. circinata
>
> t. corporis
>
> t. cruris
>
> t. decalvans
>
> t. favosa
>
> t. furfuracea
>
> t. glabrosa
>
> t. imbricata
>
> t. inguinalis
>
> t. kerion

tinea *(continued)*
 t. nigra
 t. nodosa
 t. pedis
 t. profunda
 t. sycosis
 t. tarsi
 t. tonsurans
 t. unguium
 t. versicolor
tizik. See *phthisic.*
tophus
 t. syphiliticus
Torula
toruli
 t. tactiles
toruloma
torulosis
torulus
Touton giant cells
toxicoderma
toxicodermatitis
treatment
 Gennerich's t.
Treponema
triad
 Hutchinson's t.
trichiasis
trichitis
trichoepithelioma
 t. papillosum multiplex
trichofibroacanthoma
trichofibroepithelioma
trichomatosis
Trichomonas
trichomycosis
 t. axillaris
 t. chromatica

trichomycosis *(continued)*
 t. favosa
 t. nigra
 t. nodosa
 t. palmellina
 t. pustulosa
 t. rubra
trichonocardiasis
trichonodosis
trichonosis
 t. furfuracea
trichophytid
Trichophyton
trichophytosis
 t. barbae
 t. capitis
 t. corporis
 t. cruris
 t. unguium
trichorrhexis
 t. nodosa
trichoschisis
trichostasis spinulosa
Trichothecium
 T. roseum
Triphleps insidiosus
Trombicula
tubercle
tubercular
tuberculid
 papulonecrotic t.
 rosacea-like t.
tuberculoderm
tuberculosis
 t. papulonecrotica
tularemia
Tunga
 T. penetrans

tungiasis
turgor
tylosis
    t. ciliaris
    t. palmaris et plantaris
Tzank
    cell
    test
ulcer
    decubitus u.
    Lipschütz's u.
ulceration
ulcus
    u. ambustiforme
    u. cruris
    u. durum
    u. molle cutis
    u. scorbuticum
    u. syphiliticum
ulerythema
    u. acneiforma
    u. centrifugum
    u. ophryogenes
    u. sycosiforme
ulodermatitis
uloid
ungual
unguinal
unguis
    u. incarnatus
Unna's
    dermatosis
    extractor
    nevus
Urbach-Oppenheim disease
urethritis
    gonorrheal u.
urhidrosis

urtica
urticaria
    u. bullosa
    endemic u.
    u. endemica
    u. epidemica
    u. factitia
    u. gigantea
    u. hemorrhagica
    u. medicamentosa
    Milton's u.
    papular u.
    u. papulosa
    u. perstans
    u. photogenica
    u. pigmentosa
    solar u.
    u. solaris
    u. subcutanea
    subcutaneous u.
urticarial
urticate
vaccination
vaccinia
varicella
    v. gangrenosa
    pustular v.
    v. pustulosa
varicelliform
variola
    v. crystallina
    v. inserta
    v. miliaris
    v. mitigata
    v. pemphigosa
    v. siliquosa
    v. vera
    v. verrucosa

vasculitis
    nodular v.
Veiel's paste
vellus
verruca
    v. acuminata
    v. digitata
    v. filiformis
    v. glabra
    v. necrogenica
    v. peruana
    v. peruviana
    v. plana
    v. plana juvenilis
    v. plantaris
    v. seborrheica
    v. senilis
    v. simplex
    v. tuberculosa
    v. vulgaris
verrucae
verruciform
verrucose
verrucosis
verruga
    v. peruana
vesication
vesicle
vesicular
vesiculation
vesiculobullous
vesiculopapular
vesiculopustular
vespajus
virus
    ECHO v. – enteric
    cytopathogenic
    human orphan v.

virus
    Coxsackie v.
vitiligo
    v. capitis
    Cazenave's v.
    Celsus' v.
    circumnervic v.
    perinevic v.
Vollmer's test
Walsh's
    curet
    pressure ring
Walton's extractor
wart
    anatomical w.
    filiform w.
    mosaic w.
    necrogenic w.
    plantar w.
    seborrheic w.
    telangiectatic w.
    tuberculous w.
    venereal w.
Wassermann-fast test
Wassermann reaction test
Waterhouse-Friderichsen
    syndrome
Weber-Christian
    disease
    syndrome
Weber's disease
wen
wheal
White's disease
Whitfield's ointment
Wickham's striae
Willan's lepra
xanthelasma

xanthoderma
xanthoma
    x. diabeticorum
    x. disseminatum
    x. multiplex
    x. planum
    x. tuberosum
    x. tuberosum multiplex
xanthomatosis
xanthomatous
xanthosis
    x. cutis
XDP – xeroderma
    pigmentosum
xeroderma
    follicular x.
    Kaposi's x.

xeroderma
    x. pigmentosum
xerodermatic
xerodermosteosis
xerosis
    x. cutis
XP – xeroderma pigmentosum
yaws
zan-. See words beginning
    Xan-.
zero-. See words beginning
    xero-.
zoacanthosis
zona
    z. dermatica
    z. epithelioserosa
    z. facialis

GASTROENTEROLOGY

a-beta-lipoproteinemia
abscess
    subphrenic a.
achalasia
achlorhydria
    a. apepsia
acholia
acholic
achylia
    a. gastrica
        haemorrhagica
    a. pancreatica
achylous
acid
    hydrochloric a.
acidity
acidosis
adenasthenia
    a. gastrica
adenia
    angibromic a.
adenitis
    mesenteric a.
adenocarcinoma
adenohypersthenia
    a. gastrica
adenoma
    papillary a.
    villous a.
adenomyoma

adhesion
aerenterectasia
aerocoly
aerogastria
aerogastrocolia
aeroperitoneum
aerophagia
aerophagy
agastroneuria
aglutition
akahlazea. See *achalasia.*
akilea. See *achylia.*
akilus. See *achylous.*
aklorhidreah. See
    achlorhydria.
akoleah. See *acholia.*
akolic. See *acholic.*
alimentation
alkaline
alkalosis
Althausen's test
amebiasis
    intestinal a.
ampulla
    a. hepatopancreatica
    a. of Vater
amyloidosis
anacidity
analysis
    gastric a.

anapepsia
anastomosis
    Billroth I a.
    Billroth II a.
Andresen's diet
angina
    abdominal a.
    a. abdominalis
    a. dyspeptica
    intestinal a.
angiocholecystitis
angiocholitis
    a. proliferans
angulation
angulus
annular
anorexia
antacid
anticholagogic
anticholinergic
antidiarrheal
antimesenteric
antiperistalsis
antispasmodic
    biliary a.
antral
antrectomy
antrum
anus
    imperforate a.
apepsia
    achlorhydria a.
apepsinia
aperistalsis
appendicitis
appendix
    vermiform a.
arachnogastria

arch
    Treitz's a.
argentaffinoma
ascariasis
ascites
aspiration
atony
atresia
atrophy
    gastric mucosal a.
awbarra. See *embarras.*
bacteriocholia
Banti's syndrome
barium
Barrett's syndrome
belching
bezoar
bile
biliary
bilidigestive
bilihumin
bilious
biliousness
biliprasin
bilirubin
bilirubinemia
Billroth
    I anastomosis
    II anastomosis
Billroth's hypertrophy
blood
    occult b.
Boas' test meal
bolus
    alimentary b.
borborygmi
borborygmus
bougie

bowel
  greedy b.
Boyden's test meal
bradypepsia
bradystalsis
brash
Brinton's disease
bronchoscope
bruit
brwe. See *bruit.*
bulb
  duodenal b.
calculi
canaliculus
Cantor's tube
capotement
carcinoid
carcinoma
carcinomatosis
  c. peritonei
cardia
  c. of stomach
cardialgia
cardiospasm
carminative
Carnot's test
carreau
catabolism
cecum
celiac
cholangiectasis
cholangiogram
  percutaneous
    transhepatic c.
cholangiography
cholangiohepatoma
cholangiole
cholangiolitis

cholangioma
cholangitis
  catarrhal c.
  c. lenta
cholecyst
cholecystectomy
cholecystendysis
cholecystenteric
cholecystic
cholecystis
cholecystitis
cholecystocholangiogram
cholecystogastric
cholecystogram
cholecystography
cholecystojejunostomy
cholecystokinetic
cholecystokinin
cholecystolithiasis
cholecystoptosis
choledochal
choledochitis
choledochogram
choledochography
choledocholith
choledocholithiasis
choledochotomy
choledochus
cholelithiasis
cholera
  bilious c.
  c. morbus
  c. nostras
cholerrhagia
cholestasis
cholesterol
choloscopy
chromoscopy

chromoscopy
    gastric c.
chyle
chymase
chyme
chymification
chymorrhea
cicatricial
cirrhosis
    biliary c.
    calculus c.
    cardiac c.
    Maixner's c.
claudication
    intestinal c.
clysma
clyster
colectomy
colic
    biliary c.
    bilious c.
    crapulent c.
    gallstone c.
    hepatic c.
    mucous c.
    pancreatic c.
    pseudomembranous c.
    saburral c.
    stercoral c.
    vermicular c.
    verminous c.
colicky
colicolitis
colitis
    adaptive c.
    amebic c.
    balantidial c.
    fulminating c.

colitis *(continued)*
    granulomatous c.
    c. gravis
    mucous c.
    myxomembranous c.
    c. polyposa
    ulcerative c.
colloid
coloclyster
colocutaneous
colodyspepsia
coloenteritis
colon
    ascending c.
    descending c.
    distal c.
    irritable c.
    lead-pipe c.
    proximal c.
    sigmoid c.
    spastic c.
    transverse c.
    unstable c.
colonorrhea
coloproctitis
colorectitis
colorrhea
colostomy
    end-to-side
        ileotransverse c.
Congo red test
coniasis
constipation
    gastrojejunal c.
copremia
coprolith
coprostasis
Corner's tampon

Courvoisier-Terrier syndrome
craigiasis
crater
crepitus
Crohn's disease
crura
Cruveilhier's disease
curvature
    greater c.
    lesser c.
defecation
deglutition
Degos' disease
dehydration
dehydrocholaneresis
dehydrogenase
    lactic d.
demucosatio
    d. intestini
Diagnex blue test
diaphragm
diarrhea
diastalsis
diastase
    pancreatic d.
diet
    Andresen's d.
    gluten free d.
    Jarotsky's d.
    Meulengracht's d.
    Sippy's d.
Dieulafoy's erosion
digestion
digestive
dilatation
dis-. See also words begin-
    ning dys-.
disease
    Brinton's d.

disease (continued)
    celiac d.
    Crohn's d.
    Cruveilhier's d.
    Degos' d.
    Hanot's d.
    hepatobiliary tract d.
    Hirschsprung's d.
    Menetrier's d.
    Myà's d.
    Patella's d.
    Payr's d.
    Reichmann's d.
    Whipple's d.
distention
distomiasis
    intestinal d.
diverticula
    jejunal d.
diverticulitis
diverticulosis
    jejunal d.
diverticulum
    epiphrenic d.
    hepatic d.
    hypopharyngeal d.
    Meckel's d.
    midesophageal d.
    Zenker's d.
Dock's test meal
drip
    intragastric d.
drugs. See Medications.
Dubin-Johnson syndrome
duct
    common bile d.
    extrahepatic bile d.
duodenal

duodenin
duodenitis
duodenocholangeitis
duodenohepatic
duodenum
d-Xylose absorption test
dyschezia
dysentery
    amebic d.
dyskinesia
    biliary d.
dyspepsia
dysperistalsis
dysphagia
    sideropenic d.
dyspragia
    d. intermittens angio-
      schlerotica intestinalis
d-zylose. See *d-Xylose.*
ecterograph
ectocolon
ectoperitonitis
edema
    alimentary e.
edematous
Ehrmann's alcohol test
    meal
electrogastrogram
electrogastrography
embarras
    e. gastrique
empyema
endocolitis
endoenteritis
endogastric
endogastritis
endometriosis
    e. of colon
endoscopy

enema
    barium e.
enteraden
enteradenitis
enteral
enteralgia
enterauxe
enterectasis
enterelcosis
enteric
enteritides
enteritis
    choleriform e.
    cicatrizing e.
    granulomatous e.
    e. gravis
    myxomembranous e.
    e. nodularis
    pellicular e.
    phlegmonous e.
    e. polyposa
    pseudomembranous e.
    regional e.
    staphylococcal e.
enteroanastomosis
enterobiliary
enterobrosis
enterocolic
enterocolitis
    pseudomembranous e.
enterocystoma
enterodynia
enteroenteric
enteroenterostomy
enterogastritis
enterogastrone
enterogram
enterography

enterohepatitis
enteroidea
enterolith
enterolithiasis
enterology
enteromegaly
enterometer
epigastralgia
epigastric
epigastrium
epigastrocele
epiploon
epithalaxia
erepsin
erosion
    Dieulafoy's e.
eructation
    nervous e.
esofa-. See words beginning
   esopha-.
esogastritis
esophagalgia
esophageal
esophagectasia
esophagism
esophagitis
    peptic e.
    reflux e.
    regurgitant e.
esophagodynia
esophagoscope
esophagoscopy
esophagospasm
esophagus
euchlorhydria
eucholia
euchylia
eupepsia

evacuation
Ewald's test meal
excrement
excreta
excretion
fecalith
feces
fiberscope
    Hirschowitz's f.
fibroblast
Fischer's test meal
fistula
    enterocolic f.
    enteroenteric f.
    gastrojejunocolic f.
    jejunocolic f.
fitobezor. See *phytobezoar.*
flatulence
flatulent
flatus
flexure
    splenic f.
flora
    intestinal f.
fluke
    intestinal f's.
flux
    bilious f.
    celiac f.
fossa
    Treitz's f.
freezing
    gastric f.
fundus
GA – gastric analysis
Galeati's glands
gall
gallbladder

gallstone
gastradenitis
gastralgia
    appendicular g.
gastralgokenosis
gastraneuria
gastrasthenia
gastratrophia
gastrectasia
gastrectomy
gastric
gastricism
gastricsin
gastrin
gastritic
gastritis
    antral g.
    atrophic g.
    catarrhal g.
    cirrhotic g.
    erosive g.
    exfoliative g.
    follicular g.
    giant hypertrophic g.
    g. granulomatosa
      fibroplastica
    hyperpeptic g.
    hypertrophic g.
    interstitial g.
    mycotic g.
    phlegmonous g.
    polypous g.
    pseudomembranous g.
    purulent g.
    suppurating g.
gastroalbumorrhea
gastroatonia
gastroblennorrhea

gastrobrosis
gastrocamera
gastrocardiac
gastrocele
gastrochronorrhea
gastrocolic
gastrocolitis
gastrocoloptosis
gastrocolostomy
gastrocolotomy
gastrocutaneous
gastrodialysis
gastrodiaphane
gastrodiaphany
gastroduodenal
gastroduodenitis
gastroduodenoscopy
gastroduodenostomy
gastrodynia
gastroenteralgia
gastroenteric
gastroenteritis
gastroenteroanastomosis
gastroenterocolic
gastroenterocolitis
gastroenterocolostomy
gastroenterologist
gastroenterology
gastroenteropathy
gastroenteroplasty
gastroenteroptosis
gastroenterostomy
gastroenterotomy
gastroepiploic
gastroesophageal
gastroesophagitis
gastroesophagostomy
gastrogalvanization

gastrogastrostomy
gastrogavage
gastrogenic
gastrograph
gastrohelcoma
gastrohelcosis
gastrohepatic
gastrohepatitis
gastrohydrorrhea
gastrohyperneuria
gastrohypertonic
gastrohyponeuria
gastroileitis
gastroileostomy
gastrointestinal
gastrojejunocolic
gastrojejunostomy
gastrokinesograph
gastrolienal
gastrolith
gastrolithiasis
gastrologist
gastrology
gastrolysis
gastromalacia
gastromegaly
gastromycosis
gastromyxorrhea
gastrone
gastronesteostomy
gastropancreatitis
gastroparalysis
gastroperiodynia
gastroperitonitis
gastropexy
gastrophotography
gastrophthisis
gastroplasty

gastroplication
gastroptosis
gastroptyxis
gastropylorectomy
gastropyloric
gastroradiculitis
gastrorrhagia
gastrorrhaphy
gastrorrhea
   g. continua chronica
gastrorrhexis
gastroschisis
gastroscope
gastroscopic
gastroscopy
gastrosia
   g. fungosa
gastrospasm
gastrosplenic
gastrostaxis
gastrostenosis
gastrostogavage
gastrostolavage
gastrostoma
gastrostomy
gastrosuccorrhea
   digestive g.
   g. mucosa
gastrotomy
gastrotonometer
gastrotoxin
gastroxynsis
   g. fungosa
gavage
geotrichosis
GET – gastric emptying time
GET½ – gastric emptying
   half-time

GI – gastrointestinal
Giardia
    G. lamblia
giardiasis
gland
    Galeati's g's.
    Theile's g's.
Glénard's syndrome
globus
    g. hystericus
GM – gastric mucosa
Gmelin's test
Goldstein's hematemesis
granulation
granulomatosis
    lipophagic intestinal g.
GU – gastric ulcer
gutter
    paracolic g.
Hanot-Rössle syndrome
Hanot's disease
heartburn
helminthemesis
hematemesis
    Goldstein's h.
    h. puellaris
hematobilia
hematochezia
hemidiaphragm
hemocholecystitis
hemolysis
hemoperitoneum
hemorrhage
    petechial h.
Henoch's purpura
hepatitis
    anicteric h.
    serum h.

hepatitis
    viral h.
hepatobiliary
hepatocholangeitis
hepatocolic
hepatocystic
hepatoenteric
hepatogastric
hepatolithiasis
hepatomegaly
hepatorrhea
hepatosplenomegaly
hernia
    diaphragmatic h.
    hiatal h.
    Treitz's h.
heterochylia
hiatus
    esophageal h.
hiccup
Hirschowitz's fiberscope
Hirschsprung's disease
hologastroschisis
Hueter's maneuver
hydraeroperitoneum
hydragogue
hydrepigastrium
hydrocholecystis
hydrocholeresis
hydrolysis
hydroperitoneum
hydrops
    h. abdominis
hyperchlorhydria
hypercholia
hyperemesis
    h. hiemis
hyperemic

hyperpepsia
hyperpepsinia
hyperperistalsis
hypersecretion
    gastric h.
hypertrophy
    Billroth's h.
hypochloremia
hypochlorhydria
hypochondrium
hypochylia
hypogammaglobulinemia
hypogastric
hypogastrium
hypogastroschisis
hypoglycemia
hypokalemia
hypomagnesemia
hyponatremia
hypoxia
hypopepsia
hypopepsinia
hypoperistalsis
hypophrenium
hyposteatolysis
hypothermia
IC – irritable colon
ichthyismus
    i. exanthematicus
icterus
ileitis
    regional i.
    terminal i.
ileocecal
ileocecum
ileocolitis
    i. ulcerosa chronica
ileocolostomy

ileojejunitis
    granulomatous i.
    nongranulomatous i.
ileoproctostomy
ileorectal
ileosigmoid
ileostomy
ileum
    terminal i.
ileus
    adynamic i.
    paralytic i.
    spastic i.
impaction
    fecal i.
incontinence
    fecal i.
indigestion
inertia
    colonic i.
infarction
ingestion
inructation
insufficiency
    pancreatic i.
intestinal
intestine
intestinum
intubated
intubation
intussusception
ischemia
    mesenteric i.
    midgut i.
ischochymia
ischocholia
isko-. See words beginning
    ischo-.

Jarotsky's diet
jaundice
    obstructive j.
jejunal
jejunitis
jejunoileitis
jejunum
junction
    esophagogastric j.
juxtapyloric
kapotmaw. See *capotement.*
karro. See *carreau.*
kil. See *chyle.*
kim. See *chyme.*
kimas. See *chymase.*
kimifikashun. See
    chymification.
kimorea. See *chymorrhea.*
kolange-. See words beginning
    cholangi-.
kole-. See words beginning
    chole-.
kolera. See *cholera.*
lamp
    Wood's l.
laparotomy
lavage
    gastric l.
leiomyoma
leiomyosarcoma
Leube's test meal
leukocytosis
ligament
    gastrohepatic l.
    Treitz's l.
linitis
    l. plastica
liomioma. See *leiomyoma.*

liomiosarkoma. See
    leiomyosarcoma.
lipase
lipodystrophia
    l. intestinalis
lipodystrophy
    intestinal l.
lipophagia
    l. granulomatosis
liver
    biliary cirrhotic l.
loop
    afferent l.
    efferent l.
    jejunal l.
    terminal ileal l.
lumen
lymphangiectasia
lymphenteritis
lymphoma
lysozyme
macrogastria
Maixner's cirrhosis
malabsorption
Mallory-Weiss syndrome
maneuver
    Hueter's m.
McArthur's method
meal
    barium m.
Meckel's diverticulum
Medications
    Acidulin
    Agoral
    Alkets
    Aludrox
    aluminum hydroxide
    aluminum phosphate

Medications *(continued)*
- Alzinox
- ampicillin
- Antifoam
- Antrenyl
- atropine sulfate
- attapulgite
- Banthine
- belladonna
- Bentyl
- bisacodyl
- bismuth subcarbonate
- Bonine
- calcium carbonate
- Cantil
- cascara sagrada
- castor oil
- Cellothyl
- charcoal
- chloramphenicol
- Chrysazin
- citrate of magnesia
- Claysorb
- Colace
- Combid
- Compazine
- Cotazym
- Dactil
- danthron
- Daricon
- Decholin
- dehydrocholic acid
- dicyclomine
- dihydroxyaluminum aminoacetate
- dimenhydrinate
- dioctyl calcium sulfosuccinate

Medications *(continued)*
- dioctyl sodium sulfosuccinate
- diphemanil methylsulfate
- diphenidol
- diphenoxylate
- Donnalate
- Dorbane
- Doxinate
- Dramamine
- Dulcolax
- Elorine
- florantyrone
- Gallogen
- Gelusil
- glutamic acid hydrochloride
- glycopyrrolate
- hexocyclium methylsulfate
- Histalog
- histamine hydrochloride acid
- Hydrolose
- Kalpec
- Kao-con
- kaolin
- Kaopectate
- Kondremul
- Konsyl
- Lactobacillus acidophilus
- Librax
- Librium
- Lipancreatin
- Lomotil
- Maalox

Medications *(continued)*

magaldrate
magnesia magma
magnesium carbonate
magnesium citrate
magnesium oxide
magnesium trisilicate
Malcogel
meclizine hydrochloride
mepenzolate bromide
meprobamate
Mesopin
Metamucil
methacholine
methaminodiazepoxide
methantheline bromide
methixene
methscopolamine
  bromide
methylcellulose
Milk of Magnesia
mineral oil
Monodral
morphine
Mucilose
Mylanta
Mylicon
Nacton
nitroglycerin
Novatrin
Oxaine
ox bile extract
oxethazaine
oxyphencyclimine
  hydrochloride
oxyphenonium bromide
Pamine
pancreatin

Medications *(continued)*

pancrelipase
Panteric
paregoric
Pathilon
pectin
penicillin
pentapiperide
  methylsulfate
penthienate bromide
Petrogalar
Pharmasorb
phenobarbital
phenolphthalein
pipenzolate bromide
piperidolate
  hydrochloride
Piptal
poldine methylsulfate
Prantal
prednisolone
prednisone
Pro-Banthine
prochlorperazine
Procholon
propantheline
psyllium hydrophilic
  mucilloid
psyllium seed
Quilene
Ringer's solution
Riopan
Robalate
Robanul
Setrol
Silain
simethicone
sodium bicarbonate

Medications *(continued)*
    Spasticol
    streptomycin
    Surfak
    Syncuma
    Syntrogel
    taka-diastase
    tetracycline
    thiethylperazine
    thiphenamil
      hydrochloride
    Tigan
    tincture of opium
    Titralac
    tocamphyl
    Torecan
    Tral
    Trest
    Trevidal
    Tricoloid
    tricyclamol chloride
    tridihexethyl chloride
    trimethobenzamide
      hydrochloride
    Trocinate
    Vio-Thene
    Vontrol
    Zanchol
megacolon
megadolichocolon
megaduodenum
megaesophagus
megalobulbus
melena
melenemesis
Menetrier's disease
mesenteric adenitis
mesenteriolum
mesenteritis
mesenterium
mesentery
mesoappendicitis
mesoappendix
mesocecum
mesocolon
metaduodenum
metadysentery
meteorism
method
    McArthur's m.
    Nimeh's m.
Meulengracht's diet
micelle
mikso-. See words beginning
    myxo-.
Miller-Abbott tube
motility
Moynihan's test
mucopolysaccharide
mucoprotein
mucosa
    antral m.
    duodenal m.
    gastric m.
    gastroduodenal m.
    jejunal m.
mucus
Murphy's
    sign
    treatment
muscle
    Treitz's m.
Myà's disease
myasthenia
    m. gastrica
mycogastritis

mycosis
    m. intestinalis
myenteron
myocelialgia
myocelitis
myoneurosis
    colic m.
    intestinal m.
myxoneurosis
    intestinal m.
myxorrhea
    m. intestinalis
nerve
    splanchnic n.
    vagus n.
neurectomy
    gastric n.
neurogastric
neurogenic
NG — nasogastric
Nimeh's method
node
    Troisier's n.
    Virchow's n.
numo-. See words beginning
    pneumo-.
obstipation
obstruction
    biliary tract o.
    intestinal o.
occlusion
occult blood
Ochsner's
    ring
    treatment
Oddi's sphincter
odditis
oil breakfast

oligocholia
oligochylia
oligochymia
oligopepsia
omentum
Osler's syndrome
pancreas
pancreatectomy
pancreaticoduodenal
pancreatitis
pancreatolith
papilla
    duodenal p.
paracholia
paracolitis
parenteral
parepigastric
parietography
    gastric p.
pars
    p. superior duodeni
Patella's disease
Paterson-Brown-Kelly
    syndrome
Payr's disease
pellagra
pepsin
pepsinogen
peptic
perforation
    pyloroduodenal p.
pericecal
pericecitis
pericholangitis
pericholecystitis
    gaseous p.
pericolic
pericolitis

perigastric
perigastritis
peristalsis
peristaltic
peristole
peristolic
peritoneal
peritoneoscope
peritoneoscopy
peritoneum
    visceral p.
peritonitis
    chylous p.
perityphlitis
    p. actinomycotica
periumbilical
petechial
Peutz-Jeghers syndrome
phytobezoar
pleurocholecystitis
plexus
    enteric p.
    myenteric p.
Plummer-Vinson syndrome
pneumatosis
    p. cystoides intestinalis
    p. cystoides intestinorum
    p. intestinales
pneumocholecystitis
pneumocolon
pneumoenteritis
pneumogastric
pneumogastrography
pneumogastroscopy
pneumoperitoneum
pneumoperitonitis
polycholia
polygastria

polyp
    adenomatous p.
polypoid
polyposis
    p. coli
    p. gastrica
    p. intestinalis
    p. ventriculi
postprandial
protoduodenitis
protoduodenum
pseudodiverticula
pseudoleukemia
    p. gastrointestinalis
pseudomegacolon
pseudomyxoma
    p. peritonei
pseudopolyp
psorenteria
psychogenic
PU – peptic ulcer
purpura
    p. abdominalis
    Henoch's p.
    Schönlein-Henoch p.
pylephlebitis
pyloralgia
pyloric
pyloristenosis
pyloritis
pyloroduodenitis
pyloroplasty
pyloroptosis
pylorospasm
pylorotomy
pylorus
pyochezia
pyrosis

reflex
    epigastric r.
    gastroileac r.
    ileogastric r.
    myenteric r.
reflux
regurgitation
Reichmann's disease
renninogen
rentgenograhfe. See
    roentgenography.
resection
    antral r.
    gastric r.
retrocecal
Riegel's test meal
rigidity
ring
    Ochsner's r.
    Schatzki's r.
roentgenography
ruga
    r. gastrica
rugae
rugitus
Sahli's test
Salomon's test
Salzer's test meals
sarcoma
Schatzki's ring
Schilling test
Schönlein-Henoch purpura
scirrhous
scleroderma
sclerosis
    gastric s.
scoretemia
Sengstaken's tube

sepsis
    s. intestinalis
serosal
serosanguineous
serotonin
sialoaerophagy
sialorrhea
    s. pancreatica
sigmoid
sigmoidoscope
sigmoidoscopic
sign
    Murphy's s.
    Trousseau's s.
    Zugsmith's s.
sikwa. See *siqua.*
singultus
    s. gastricus nervosus
Sippy's diet
siqua
sirrosis. See *cirrhosis.*
skirus. See *scirrhous.*
sorenterea. See *psorenteria.*
sphincter
    esophagogastric s.
    Oddi's s.
    pyloric s.
splanchnolith
splanchnologia
splanchnomegaly
splanchnomicria
splanchnopleure
splanchnoptosis
splanchnosclerosis
splanchnostaxis
splank-. See words beginning
    splanch-.
splenomegaly

sprue
    tropical s.
stasis
    ileal s.
    venous s.
status
    s. gastricus
steatorrhea
stenosis
    pyloric s.
stoma
stomach
    leather bottle s.
strangulation
stratum
    s. longitudinale tunicae
      muscularis coli
    s. longitudinale tunicae
      muscularis intestini
      tenuis
stricture
submucosa
succussion
    s. splash
sudo-. See words beginning
    pseudo-
sulcus
    s. intermedius
suppository
    glycerin s.
swallow
    barium s.
syndrome
    Banti's s.
    Barrett's s.
    blind loop s.
    Courvoisier-Terrier s.
    Dubin-Johnson s.

syndrome *(continued)*
    dumping s.
    Glénard's s.
    Hanot-Rössle s.
    malabsorption s.
    Mallory-Weiss s.
    Osler's s.
    Paterson-Brown-Kelly s.
    Peutz-Jeghers s.
    Plummer-Vinson s.
    Wermer's s.
    Zollinger-Ellison s.
Szabo's test
tabes
    t. mesenterica
tampon
    Corner's t.
tamponade
    esophageal t.
telangiectasia
    hemorrhagic t.
telephium
tenesmus
tenia
    t. mesocolica
    t. omentalis
test
    Althausen's t.
    Carnot's t.
    Congo red t.
    Diagnex blue t.
    d-Xylose absorption t.
    fecal fat t.
    glucose absorption t.
    Gmelin's t.
    histamine t.
    Moynihan's t.
    Sahli's t.

test *(continued)*
 Salomon's t.
 Schilling t.
 secretin t.
 secretin-pancreozymin t.
 string t.
 Szabo's t.
 Topfer's t.
 Udránszky's t.
 Vitamin A absorption t.
test meal
 Boas' t. m.
 Boyden's t. m.
 Dock's t. m.
 Ehrmann's alcohol t. m.
 Ewald's t. m.
 Fischer's t. m.
 Leube's t. m.
 motor t. m.
 Riegel's t. m.
 Salzer's t. m's.
Theile's glands
tif-. See words beginning
 typh-.
Topfer's test
torsion
tract
 alimentary t.
 biliary t.
treatment
 Murphy's t.
 Ochsner's t.
Treitz's
 arch
 fossa
 hernia
 ligament
 muscle

trichobezoar
Trichuris
 T. trichiura
Troisier's node
Trousseau's sign
trunci
 t. intestinales
truncus
 t. celiacus
tube
 Cantor's t.
 Miller-Abbott t.
 nasogastric t.
 Sengstaken's t.
 Wangensteen's t.
tuberculosis
 intestinal t.
tumor
 islet cell t.
tunica
 t. fibrosa hepatis
 t. fibrosa lienis
 t. mucosa ventriculi
 t. mucosa vesicae felleae
 t. muscularis coli
 t. muscularis intestini
  tenuis
 t. muscularis recti
 t. muscularis ventriculi
 t. serosa
 t. serosa coli
 t. serosa hepatis
 t. serosa intestini tenuis
 t. serosa lienis
 t. serosa peritonei
 t. serosa ventriculi
 t. serosa vesicae felleae
typhlenteritis

typhlitis
typhlocholecystitis
typhlocolitis
Udránszky's test
ukilea. See *euchylia.*
uklorhidrea. See
    euchlorhydria
ukolea. See *eucholia.*
ulcer
    duodenal u.
    esophageal u.
    gastric u.
    jejunal u.
    peptic u.
    postbulbar u.
    stomal u.
umbilicus
unrest
    peristaltic u.
upepsea. See *eupepsia.*
urease
vagal
vagotomy
vagus
varices
    esophageal v.

vasospasm
Vater's ampulla
villi
    jejunal v.
Virchow's node
Vitamin A absorption test
volvulus
vomit
vomitus
    v. cruentus
    v. matutinus
Wangensteen's tube
Wermer's syndrome
Whipple's disease
Wood's lamp
xiphoid
Zenker's diverticulum
zifoid. See *xiphoid.*
Zollinger-Ellison
    syndrome
Zugsmith's sign
zymogen
    lab z.
zymosis
    z. gastrica

INTERNAL MEDICINE

Abderhalden-Fanconi
  syndrome
abdomen
abdominal
abdominalgia
Abrami's disease
Abrikossoff's tumor
abscess
    caseocavernous a.
    epidural a.
    Pautrier's a.
acalcerosis
acanthocheilonema perstans
acanthocheilonemiasis
acanthocytosis
acantholysis
acanthosis
    a. nigricans
acapnia
acariasis
acatalasia
acaulinosis
achalasia
Achard-Thiers syndrome
achondroplasia
achroacytosis
achylanemia
acidosis
    diabetic a.
    hypercapnic a.

acidosis *(continued)*
    hyperchloremic a.
    metabolic a.
    nonrespiratory a.
    renal tubular a.
    respiratory a.
    starvation a.
aciduria
acinus
acne
    a. pustulosa
    a. vulgaris
Acosta's disease
acremoniosis
acrocyanosis
acrodynia
acromegaly
acropachyderma
actinomycosis
adamantinoma
    pituitary a.
    a. polycysticum
Adams-Stokes
    disease
    syndrome
addisonian
Addison's disease
adenalgia
adenia
    leukemic a.

adenitis
  acute epidemic
    infectious a.
  acute salivary a.
  cervical a.
  phlegmonous a.
adenoacanthoma
adenoangiosarcoma
adenocarcinoma
adenocystoma
  papillary a.
    lymphomatosum
adenofibroma
adenohypophysis
adenoma
adenomata
  colloid a.
  follicular a.
adenomatosis
adenomeloblastoma
adenomyofibroma
adenomyomatosis
adenopathy
adenosarcoma
adenosarcorhabdomyoma
adenosclerosis
adenosis
adenotyphus
adenovirus
adiposis
  a. dolorosa
  a. hepatica
  a. tuberosa simplex
  a. universalis
adrenal
  Marchand's a's.
adrenalectomize
adrenalism

adrenalitis
adrenalopathy
adrenalotropic
adrenarche
adrenergic
adrenic
adrenin
adreninemia
adrenitis
adrenocortical
adrenocorticomimetic
adrenocorticotrophic
adrenocorticotropic
adrenogenous
adrenogram
adrenokinetic
adrenolytic
adrenomedullotropic
adrenomegaly
adrenopathy
adrenopause
adrenoprival
adynamia
  a. episodica hereditaria
aerophagia
afazea. See *aphasia.*
afibrinogenemia
aftha. See *aphtha.*
agalactia
agalactous
agalorrhea
agammaglobulinemia
aglutition
agranulemia
agranulocytopenia
agranulocytosis
agranulosis
ague

ague *(continued)*
    brass-founders' a.
    catenating a.
    dumb a.
    quartan a.
    quintan a.
    quotidian a.
    shaking a.
    tertian a.
Ahumada-Del Castillo
    syndrome
akalazea. See *achalasia.*
akawlinosis. See *acaulinosis.*
akilahnemea. See *achylanemia.*
akinesia
akondroplazea. See
    achondroplasia.
akroahsitosis. See
    achroacytosis.
akromikrie
alastrim
Albers-Schönberg's syndrome
albinism
Albright's syndrome
albuminemia
albuminuria
albumosuria
alcaptonuria
alcoholic
alcoholism
aldosteronism
aleukemia
aleukia
    a. hemorrhagica
alkalosis
allantiasis
allergy
alopecia

alymphocytosis
alymphoplasia
amanitotoxin
amaurosis
    albuminuric a.
amebiasis
    hepatic a.
ameboma
amenorrhea
aminoaciduria
amnesia
amyloidosis
amylosuria
amyotrophy
    diabetic a.
anafil-. See words beginning
    anaphyl-.
analbuminemia
anaphylactia
anaphylactic
anaphylactoid
anaphylaxis
anaplasia
anaplasmosis
ancylostomiasis
Anders' disease
Andersen's disease
anemia
    aplastic a.
    Bagdad Spring a.
    Biermer-Ehrlich a.
    Chvostek's a.
    Cooley's a.
    Dresbach's a.
    Edelmann's a.
    hemolytic a.
    Herrick's a.
    hypochromic a.

anemia *(continued)*
    hypoplastic a.
    icterohemolytic a.
    Lederer's a.
    Mediterranean a.
    myelophthisic a.
    pernicious a.
    sickle cell a.
    spherocytic a.
    thrombopenic a.
anergy
aneurysm
angiitis
    visceral a.
angina
    a. cordis
    monocytic a.
    a. nervosa
    a. pectoris
    Plaut's a.
    Schultz's a.
    vasomotor a.
angiohemophilia
angiokeratoma
    a. corporis diffusum
angiolupoid
angioma
angiomatosis
    hemorrhagic familial a.
angiomatous
angiomyosarcoma
angioneuralgia
angioneurosis
angiopancreatitis
anhidrosis
anhydremia
anisocytosis
anisuria

anomaly
    Ebstein's a.
    Hegglin's a.
anorexia
    a. nervosa
anorexic
anoxemia
anoxia
ansilostomiasis. See
    ancylostomiasis.
antagonist
    metabolic a.
anthracosis
    a. linguae
anthrax
anthrocosilicosis
anuria
aortitis
apancrea
apancreatic
aparathyrosis
aphasia
aphtha
apnea
apoplexy
appendicitis
arachnodactyly
arachnoiditis
Arakawa-Higashi syndrome
areolitis
arginosuccinicaciduria
Arias' syndrome
ariboflavinosis
Armanni-Ehrlich's degeneration
arrhythmia
arteriosclerosis
arteritis
arthralgia

arthralgia
    a. saturnina
arthritis
    degenerative a.
    gouty a.
    a. hiemalis
    hypertrophic a.
    a. nodosa
    rheumatoid a.
    tuberculous a.
arthrogryposis
arthropathia
    a. ovaripriva
    a. psoriatica
arthrosis
asbestosis
ascariasis
ascites
ascorbemia
Aseli's pancreas
asfiksea. See *asphyxia.*
Asiatic cholera
asiderosis
asinus. See *acinus.*
aspergillosis
asphyxia
astereognosis
asterixis
asthenia
    a. gravis
        hypophyseogenea
asthma
    Heberden's a.
astrocytoma
ataxia
atelectasis
atherosclerosis
athetosis

athyreosis
atrophy
    Sudeck's a.
Australian X disease
autolysis
avitaminosis
Ayerza's syndrome
azmah. See *asthma.*
azotemia
Baber's syndrome
Babinski's sign
bacillemia
bacilluria
bacteremia
bacteriuria
Bagdad Spring anemia
balantidiasis
Balser's fatty necrosis
Banti's
    disease
    syndrome
Bard-Pic syndrome
Bar's syndrome
bartonellosis
Basedow's disease
Bassen-Kornzweig syndrome
bath
    paraffin b.
Bearn-Kunkel syndrome
Begbie's disease
Behcet's disease
Behr's disease
Bell's palsy
beriberi
Bernard's syndrome
berylliosis
Besnier's disease
Biermer-Ehrlich anemia

bilharziasis
bilirubinemia
bisinosis. See *byssinosis.*
blastomycosis
BMR — basal metabolic rate
Boeck's sarcoid
botulism
bradycardia
Brill-Symmer's disease
Brill-Zinsser disease
bromohyperhidrosis
bronchiectasis
bronchiolitis
bronchitis
bronchopneumonia
brucellosis
Bruhl's disease
bruit
    Verstraeten's b.
brwe. See *bruit.*
bubonalgia
bubonulus
Budd-Chiari syndrome
Budd's cirrhosis
Buerger's disease
Burkitt's tumor
bursitis
Busse-Buschke disease
Butter's cancer
byssinosis
cachexia
café au lait spots
Caisson disease
calcemia
calcinosis
    c. interstitialis
    c. universalis
California encephalitis

calor
    c. febrilis
    c. fervens
    c. innatus
    c. internus
cancer
    acinous c.
    adenoid c.
    c. atrophicans
    Butter's c.
    cellular c.
    cerebriform c.
    dendritic c.
    dermoid c.
    endothelial c.
    epidermal c.
    epithelial c.
    fungous c.
    glandular c.
    hematoid c.
    c. in situ
    Lobstein's c.
    medullary c.
    melanotic c.
    retrograde c.
    scirrhous c.
    solanoid c.
    spider c.
    tubular c.
    villous duct c.
    withering c.
canceration
canceremia
cancericidal
cancerous
cancroid
candidiasis
candidosis

Caplan's syndrome
carcinoma
    acinous c.
    c. adenomatosum
    alveolar c.
    anaplastic c.
    basal cell c.
    c. basocellulare
    bronchogenic c.
    chorionic c.
    colloid c.
    comedo c.
    corpus c.
    c. cutaneum
    cylindrical c.
    cylindrical cell c.
    ductal c.
    c. durum
    embryonal c.
    encephaloid c.
    epidermoid c.
    epithelial c.
    c. epitheliale adenoides
    erectile c.
    c. exulcere
    c. fibrosum
    gelatiniform c.
    c. gigantocellulare
    glandular c.
    granulosa cell c.
    hair-matrix c.
    hematoid c.
    hyaline c.
    infiltrating ductal cell c.
    c. in situ
    lenticular c.
    c. lenticulare
    lipomatous c.

carcinoma *(continued)*
    lobular c.
    c. mastitoides
    c. medullare
    c. melanodes
    melanotic c.
    c. molle
    mucinous c.
    c. muciparum
    c. mucocellulare
    c. mucosum
    c. myxomatodes
    c. nigrum
    c. ossificans
    osteoid c.
    periportal c.
    preinvasive c.
    pultaceous c.
    c. sarcomatodes
    schneiderian c.
    scirrhous c.
    c. scroti
    c. simplex
    solanoid c.
    c. spongiosum
    squamous c.
    squamous cell c.
    c. telangiectaticum
    c. telangiectodes
    c. tuberosum
    tuberous c.
    c. villosum
carcinomatoid
carcinomatosis
carcinomatous
carcinosarcoma
carcinosis
cardiac

cardiospasm
cardiothyrotoxicosis
carotenemia
Carrión's disease
catabolism
cataplexy
causalgia
celialgia
celiopathy
cellulitis
cephalalgia
cestodiasis
Chagas' disease
chancre
chancroid
Charcot's cirrhosis
cheilosis
chemotherapy
Cheyne-Stokes respiration
Chiari-Frommel syndrome
chickenpox
chloremia
chlorosis
chloruremia
cholangiogram
cholangiography
cholangiohepatoma
cholangiole
cholangiolitis
cholangioma
cholangitis
    catarrhal c.
    c. lenta
cholecystitis
cholecystolithiasis
choledocholithiasis
cholelithiasis
cholemia

cholemia *(continued)*
    familial c.
    Gilbert's c.
cholepathia
    c. spastica
choleperitoneum
cholera
    Asiatic c.
    bilious c.
    c. morbus
    c. nostras
cholestasis
cholesteremia
cholesterol
cholesteroleresis
cholesterolosis
cholesteroluria
cholesterosis
chondritis
chondromalacia
chondrosarcoma
chordoma
chorea
chorioepithelioma
choriomeningitis
    lymphocytic c.
    pseudolymphocytic c.
Christmas disease
chromoblastomycosis
Chvostek's anemia
Chvostek-Weiss sign
cirrhosis
    alcoholic c.
    atrophic c.
    Budd's c.
    Charcot's c.
    Cruveilhier-Baumgarten c.
    Glisson's c.

cirrhosis *(continued)*
    Hanot's c.
    Laennec's c.
    Maixner's c.
    portal c.
    Todd's c.
claudication
    intermittent c.
climacteric
clonorchiasis
clostridia
coccidioidomas
coccidioidomycosis
coccidiosis
colibacillosis
colic
    renal c.
    ureteral c.
    uterine c.
colisepsis
colitis
Colorado tick fever virus
comedocarcinoma
communicable
Conn's syndrome
constipation
contracture
    Dupuytren's c.
convulsion
Cooley's anemia
COPD – chronic obstructive
    pulmonary disease
coproporphyria
cor
    c. pulmonale
    c. triatriatum
coryza
Coxsackie virus

cretinism
croup
Cruveilhier-Baumgarten
    cirrhosis
cryoglobulinemia
cryptococcosis
Curschmann's disease
Cushing's syndrome
CVA – cerebrovascular
    accident
cyanosis
cyst
cystadenocarcinoma
cystadenoma
cystadenosarcoma
cystathioninuria
cysticercosis
cystinemia
cystinosis
cystinuria
cystitis
cystoadenoma
cystocarcinoma
cystomyoma
cystomyxoadenoma
cystomyxoma
cystosarcoma
    c. phylloides
cytomycosis
dactylolysis
    d. spontanea
Darier-Roussy sarcoid
Debove's disease
degeneration
    amyloid d.
    Armanni-Ehrlich's d.
    hepatolenticular d.
    hyaline d.

Degos' disease
dehydration
Déjerine-Sottas disease
delirium
    d. tremens
De Morgan's spots
dengue
deradenitis
deradenoncus
dermalaxia
dermametropathism
dermamyiasis
dermataneuria
dermatitis
dermatomucosomyositis
dermatomycosis
dermatophytid
dermatophytosis
dermatosis
desequestration
deshydremia
dethyroidism
detoxification
diabetes
    d. alternans
    d. insipidus
    Lancereaux's d.
    latent d.
    d. mellitus
diabetic
    brittle d.
dialysis
diaphoresis
diaphoretic
diaphragm
diaphragma
diarrhea
diaspironecrobiosis

diaspironecrosis
diathermy
diathesis
diet
    Ebstein's d.
difilobothriasis. See
    diphyllobothriasis.
difth-. See words beginning
    diphth-.
digitalization
DiGuglielmo's syndrome
diphtheria
diphtheroid
diphyllobothriasis
diplegia
diplococcemia
dis-. See also words beginning
    dys-.
disease
    Abrami's d.
    Acosta's d.
    Adams-Stokes d.
    Addison's d.
    Anders' d.
    Andersen's d.
    Australian X d.
    Banti's d.
    Basedow's d.
    Begbie's d.
    Behçet's d.
    Behr's d.
    Besnier's d.
    Brill-Symmer's d.
    Brill-Zinsser d.
    Bruhl's d.
    Buerger's d.
    Busse-Buschke d.
    Caisson d.

disease *(continued)*

- Carrión's d.
- cat-scratch d.
- Chagas' d.
- Christmas d.
- Curschmann's d.
- Debove's d.
- Degos' d.
- Déjerine-Sottas d.
- Dressler's d.
- Ebstein's d.
- Fabry's d.
- Flajani's d.
- Friedländer's d.
- Gamna's d.
- Gandy-Nanta d.
- Gaucher's d.
- Gilchrist's d.
- Graves' d.
- Hand-Schüller-Christian d.
- Hanot's d.
- Hansen's d.
- Hartnup's d.
- Hashimoto's d.
- Heberden's d.
- hemolytic d.
- Hers' d.
- Hodgkin's d.
- Huchard's d.
- Hutinel's d.
- Krabbe's d.
- Letterer-Siwe d.
- Lignac's d.
- Marie's d.
- mast cell d.
- Mathieu's d.
- Meleda d.

disease *(continued)*

- Meniere's d.
- Mikulicz's d.
- Möbius' d.
- Monge's d.
- Morquio's d.
- Nicolas-Favre d.
- Niemann-Pick d.
- Niemann's d.
- Osler's d.
- Osler-Vaquez d.
- Paget's d.
- Parkinson's d.
- Parrot's d.
- Parry's d.
- Parsons' d.
- Pavy's d.
- Pick's d.
- Pott's d.
- pulseless d.
- Raynaud's d.
- Refsum's d.
- Reiter's d.
- Rokitansky's d.
- Runneberg's d.
- San Joaquin Valley d.
- Sheehan's d.
- Simmonds' d.
- Sternberg's d.
- Stuart-Bras d.
- Tangier d.
- tsutsugamushi d.
- von Gierke's d.
- von Willebrand's d.
- Weil's d.
- Werner's d.
- Wernicke's d.
- Wilson's d.

distomiasis
    hemic d.
    hepatic d.
diuresis
diverticulitis
diverticulosis
diverticulum
    Meckel's d.
dracunculiasis
Dresbach's
    anemia
    syndrome
Dressler's disease
dropsy
Dupuytren's contracture
dwarfism
    pituitary d.
dysarthria
dyscrasia
    blood d.
    lymphatic d.
dyscrinism
dysdiemorrhysis
dysdipsia
dysendocrisiasis
dysentery
    amebic d.
dysesthesia
dysgammaglobulinemia
dysglobulinemia
dyshepatia
dyshidrosis
dyskeratosis
dyskinesia
dyspancreatism
dysparathyroidism
dyspareunia
dyspepsia

dysphagia
dyspinealism
dyspituitarism
dysplasia
dyspnea
dysponderal
dyspragia
dysproteinemia
dyssebacea
dysthyroidism
dystonia
dysuria
Eastern equine encephalo-
    myelitis
Ebstein's
    anomaly
    diet
    disease
ecchymosis
eccyclomastoma
echinococcosis
echinostomiasis
echovirus
eclampsia
ecphyma
    e. globulus
ectasia
ecthyma
ectodermosis
    e. erosiva pluriorificialis
ectopia
eczema
Edelmann's anemia
edema
    Milroy's e.
    nonpitting e.
    pedal e.
    Pirogoff's e.

edema
   prehepatic e.
edematous
edentulous
Ehlers-Danlos syndrome
ekfima. See *ecphyma.*
ekimosis. See *ecchymosis.*
ekino-. See words beginning
   echino-.
eksanthema. See *exanthema.*
eksiklomastoma. See
   eccyclomastoma.
ekthima. See *ecthyma.*
ekzema. See *eczema.*
elastofibroma
   e. dorsi
elastoma
elastosis
electrolysis
electrolyte
electromyography
electrophoresis
electropyrexia
elephantiasis
ellipsoid
   e. of spleen
elliptocytosis
emaciation
embolemia
embolism
embolomycotic
embolus
EMC – encephalomyocarditis
emetatrophia
emphysema
empyema
encephalitis
   California e.

encephalitis *(continued)*
   Japanese B e.
   Japanese B-West Nile e.
   Murray Valley e.
   Russian spring-summer
      e.
   St. Louis e.
encephalomyelitis
   Eastern equine e.
   Venezuelan equine e.
   Western equine e.
encephalopathy
   hepatic e.
   Wernicke's e.
enchondromatosis
endarteritis
endocarditis
   bacterial e.
endocrine
endocrinosis
endometriosis
endothelioangiitis
endothelioblastoma
endotheliocytosis
endotheliomatosis
endotheliomyoma
endotheliomyxoma
endotoxicosis
enkondromatosis. See
   enchondromatosis.
ensefal-. See words beginning
   encephal-.
entamebiasis
enteritis
   e. necroticans
enterobiasis
enterovirus
eosinophilia

eosinophilia
> Löffler's e.

epidemic
epidermodysplasia
epidermophytosis
epididymis
epididymitis
epilepsy
epiloia
epistaxis
> Gull's renal e.

epithelioblastoma
epithelioma
epituberculosis
Erb's sign
erethism
ergotism
erisipela de la costa
erysipelas
erythema
> e. multiforme
>
> e. nodosum
>
> e. toxicum

erythematous
erythralgia
erythrasma
erythremia
erythroblastoma
erythroblastomatosis
erythroblastopenia
erythroblastosis
erythrocyanosis
erythrocythemia
erythrocytosis
> leukemic e.
>
> e. megalosplenica

erythroderma
erythrogenesis

erythrogenesis
> e. imperfecta

erythroleukemia
erythroleukosis
erythromelalgia
erythromelia
erythroneocytosis
erythropenia
erythropoiesis
eschar
esophagitis
estriasis. See *oestriasis.*
ethanasia
eunuchism
> pituitary e.

euthanasia
euthyroid
euthyroidism
exanthema
> e. subitum

exhaustion
exogenous
exostosis
expectoration
exsanguination
Fabry's disease
facies
> Parkinson's f.

fagositosis. See *phagocytosis.*
Fallot's tetralogy
Falta's triad
Fanconi's syndrome
farinjitis. See *pharyngitis.*
Farre's tubercles
fasciolopsiasis
fatigue
favism
Felty's syndrome

fenetidinurea. See
   phenetidinuria.
fenilketonurea. See
   phenylketonuria.
feno-. See words beginning
   pheno-.
feo-. See words beginning
   pheo-.
fetor
   f. hepaticus
fever
   etiocholanolone f.
   Haverhill f.
   hay f.
   hemorrhagic f.
   Malta f.
   Oroya f.
   phlebotomus f.
   Q f.
   quartan f.
   quinine f.
   quintana f.
   quotidian f.
   rat-bite f.
   rheumatic f.
   Rift Valley f.
   Rocky Mountain
      spotted f.
   San Joaquin f.
   scarlet f.
   South American
      hemorrhagic f.
   Southeast Asian
      mosquito-borne
      hemorrhagic f.
   streptobacillary f.
   typhoid f.
   undulant f.

fever *(continued)*
   West Nile f.
   Yellow f.
fibrillation
fibrinogenemia
fibrinogenopenia
fibrinolysis
fibrinopenia
fibroadamantoblastoma
fibroadenia
fibroadenoma
fibroadenosis
fibroblastoma
fibrocyst
fibrocystic
fibrocystoma
fibroelastosis
fibrolymphoangioblastoma
fibroma
fibromatoid
fibromatosis
fibromyoma
fibromyositis
fibromyxosarcoma
fibrosarcoma
fibrosis
   cystic f.
fibrositis
fikomycosis. See
   phycomycosis.
filariasis
Fitz-Hugh's syndrome
Fitz's
   law
   syndrome
flagellosis
Flajani's disease
flebitis. See *phlebitis.*

flebo-. See words beginning
   phlebo-.
fleckmilz
folliculitis
food poisoning
   Bacillus cereus f. p.
   enterococcal f. p.
fragilitas
   f. sanguinis
fragilocytosis
Friedländer's disease
frostbite
fructosuria
furunculosis
Gaisböck's syndrome
galactorrhea
galactosemia
gallstones
Gamna's disease
Gandy-Gamna
   nodules
   spleen
Gandy-Nanta disease
ganglion
   Troisier's g.
ganglioneuroma
gangrene
   Raynaud's g.
Gardner's syndrome
gargoylism
gastrectasia
Gaucher's
   disease
   splenomegaly
geotrichosis
German measles
giardiasis
gigantism

Gilbert's cholemia
Gilchrist's
   disease
   mycosis
glanders
Glanzmann's syndrome
Glisson's cirrhosis
globulinemia
globus
   g. hystericus
glomangioma
glomerulitis
glomerulonephritis
glomerulosclerosis
   intercapillary g.
glossitis
glucosuria
glycemia
glycopenia
glycopolyuria
glycosuria
goiter
   adenomatous g.
   colloid g.
   exophthalmic g.
   fibrous g.
   follicular g.
   intrathoracic g.
   nodular g.
   papillomatous g.
   parenchymatous g.
   substernal g.
   toxic g.
gongylonemiasis
gonorrhea
Goodpasture's syndrome
gout
   abarticular g.

gout *(continued)*
    articular g.
    calcium g.
    chalky g.
    latent g.
    lead g.
    misplaced g.
    oxalic g.
    polyarticular g.
    retrocedent g.
    rheumatic g.
    saturnine g.
    tophaceous g.
gouty
Graefe's sign
granuloblastosis
granulocytopenia
granulocytosis
granuloma
    amebic g.
    Hodgkin's g.
granulomatosis
    g. siderotica
    Wegener's g.
Graves' disease
grippe
Gubler's icterus
Guillain-Barré syndrome
Gull's renal epistaxis
gumma
Günther's syndrome
gynecomastia
hamartoma
hamartomatosis
Hamman-Rich syndrome
Hand-Schüller-Christian
    disease
Hanger-Rose skin test

Hanot's
    cirrhosis
    disease
Hansen's disease
Harris' syndrome
Hartnup's disease
Hashimoto's
    disease
    struma
Haverhill fever
Hayem's icterus
Hayem-Widal syndrome
headache
    cluster h.
    Horton's h.
    migraine h.
heartburn
Heberden's
    asthma
    disease
    nodes
    rheumatism
Heerfordt's syndrome
Hegglin's anomaly
helminthiasis
    cutaneous h.
    h. elastica
    h. wuchereri
hemangioblastoma
hemangioma
hemarthrosis
hematemesis
hematogenesis
hematoma
    epidural h.
hematomycosis
hematomyelia
hematopenia

hematoporphyria
hematuria
hemiparesis
hemiplegia
hemisporosis
hemobilinuria
hemoblastosis
hemochromatosis
hemocytoblastoma
hemodialysis
hemoglobinemia
hemoglobinuria
hemophilia
hemopneumothorax
hemoptysis
hemosiderosis
hemuresis
hepar
    h. adiposum
    h. lobatum
hepatalgia
hepatargia
hepatatrophia
hepatic
hepatism
hepatitis
    anicteric h.
    infectious h.
    serum h.
    viral h.
hepatocele
hepatocirrhosis
hepatodynia
hepatodystrophy
hepatoglobinemia
hepatohemia
hepatolienal
hepatoma

hepatomalacia
hepatomegaly
hepatomphalos
hepatonephritis
hepatonephromegaly
hepatoperitonitis
hepatophyma
hepatoportal
hepatoptosis
hepatorrhagia
hepatorrhexis
hepatosis
hepatosplenitis
hepatosplenomegaly
hepatotoxicity
heredopathia
    h. atactica
        polyneuritiformis
hermaphroditism
herpangina
herpes
    h. catarrhalis
    h. generalisatus
    h. labialis
    h. meningoencephalitis
    h. simplex
    h. zoster
herpesvirus
Herrick's anemia
Hers' disease
heteradenia
heteropancreatism
heterophyiasis
hibernoma
hiccup
Hickey-Hare test
hidradenitis
    h. suppurativa

hidrorrhea
hidrosadenitis
    h. axillaris
    h. destruens suppurativa
hidrosis
histiocytomatosis
histiocytosis
    h. X
histoplasmosis
Hodgkin's
    disease
    granuloma
Homans' sign
homocystinuria
hookworm
Horton's
    headache
    syndrome
Huchard's disease
Hutchinson's triad
Hutinel's disease
hyaloserositis
hydatid
hydatidoma
hydatidosis
hydremia
hydrocephalus
hydrophobia
hydrops
hydroxyprolinemia
hyloma
hymenolepiasis
hyperaminoaciduria
hyperbilirubinemia
hypercalcemia
hypercalciuria
hypercapnia
hyperchloremia

hypercholesterolemia
hypercholesterolia
hyperchromatism
    macrocytic h.
hyperchromia
hyperemesis
    h. hiemis
hyperemia
hyperesthesia
hypergammaglobulinemia
hypergenesis
hyperglobulinemia
hyperglycemia
hyperglyceridemia
hyperglycinemia
hyperglycinuria
hypergonadism
hyperhidrosis
    h. lateralis
hyperhistidinemia
hyperinsulinemia
hyperinsulinism
hyperkalemia
hyperkeratomycosis
hyperkeratosis
hyperketonemia
hyperketonuria
hyperkinemia
hyperlipemia
hyperlipidemia
hyperlipoproteinemia
hyperliposis
hypernatremia
hypernitremia
hypernormocytosis
hyperoxaluria
hyperoxemia
hyperparathyroidism

hyperpathia
hyperpepsinemia
hyperphosphatemia
hyperphosphaturia
hyperphosphoremia
hyperpituitarism
 basophilic h.
 eosinophilic h.
hyperplasia
hyperpnea
hyperpotassemia
hyperprolinemia
hyperproteinemia
hyperpyrexia
hypersplenism
hypertension
hypertensive
hyperthermia
hyperthrombinemia
hyperthrombocytemia
hyperthyroidism
hypertrichiasis
hypertriglyceridemia
hypertrophy
 Marie's h.
hyperuricemia
hypervalinemia
hyperventilation
hypervitaminosis
hypervolemia
hypoadrenalemia
hypoadrenalism
hypoalbuminemia
hypoalbuminosis
hypoaldosteronemia
hypoaminoacidemia
hypocalcemia
hypocapnia

hypochloremia
hypochromasia
hypochromemia
 idiopathic h.
hypochromia
hypochrosis
hypocrinism
hypocythemia
hypodermoclysis
hypodermolithiasis
hypoendocrinism
hypoestrogenemia
hypofibrinogenemia
hypogammaglobulinemia
hypoglycemia
hypogonadism
hypogonadotrophism
hypogranulocytosis
hypohepatia
hypoinsulinemia
hypoinsulinism
hypokalemia
hypolepidoma
hypoleukocytosis
hypolipidemia
hyponatremia
hyponeocytosis
hyponitremia
hypoparathyroidism
hypophosphatasia
hypophosphatemia
hypopiesia
hypopiesis
hypopituitarism
hypoplasia
hypoproteinemia
hypoprothrombinemia
hyposialadenitis

hyposthenuria
hypotension
  orthostatic h.
hypothermia
  endogenous h.
hypothrombinemia
hypothyroidism
hypotonic
hypoventilation
hypovitaminosis
hypovolemia
hypoxemia
hypoxia
ichthyosarcotoxism
ichthyosis
icteric
icteroanemia
icterohepatitis
icterus
    acholuric hemolytic i.
      with splenomegaly
    bilirubin i.
    i. castrensis gravis
    i. castrensis levis
    i. catarrhalis
    cythemolytic i.
    i. gravis
    Gubler's i.
    Hayem's i.
    i. hemolyticus
    i. infectiosus
    i. praecox
    i. simplex
    spirochetal i.
    i. typhoides
    urobilin i.
    i. viridans
ictus

iksodiasis. See *ixodiasis.*
ikterik. See *icteric.*
iktero-. See words beginning
    ictero-.
ikterus. See *icterus.*
iktheosarkotoksizm. See
    ichthyosarcotoxism.
iktheosis. See *ichthyosis.*
iktus. See *ictus.*
immunity
immunization
impetigo
impotence
incarnatio
    i. unguis
incontinentia
    i. pigmenti
incubation
Indian tick typhus
indoluria
inebriation
infarction
    myocardial i.
infection
infectious
infertility
infestation
inflammation
influenza
infundibuloma
inguinodynia
inoculation
inocystoma
insomnia
insulinemia
insulinogenesis
insulinoma
insuloma

intersexuality
interstitialoma
intertrigo
intestine
intussusception
iritis
    diabetic i.
    gouty i.
ischemia
isonormocytosis
isopathy
isosthenuria
isotope
ixodiasis
Janeway's spots
Japanese B encephalitis
Japanese B-West Nile
    encephalitis
jaundice
    hemolytic j.
    obstructive j.
kahkeksea. See *cachexia.*
kala-azar
kalemia
kaliopenia
Kartagener's syndrome
katzenjammer
Kayser-Fleischer ring
kemotherape. See
    chemotherapy.
keratitis
keratoderma
    k. blennorrhagica
keratoma
keratomalacia
keratosis
kernicterus
ketoacidosis

kifosis. See *kyphosis.*
kilosis. See *cheilosis.*
Kimmelstiel-Wilson syndrome
kinetosis
Kleine-Levin syndrome
Klinefelter's syndrome
klor-. See words beginning
    chlor-.
koksake. See *coxsackie.*
kolange-. See words beginning
    cholangi-.
kole-. See words beginning
    chole-.
kolera. See *cholera.*
koles-. See words beginning
    choles-.
kondritis. See *chondritis.*
kondro-. See words beginning
    chondro-.
kopf-tetanus
kordoma. See *chordoma.*
korea. See *chorea.*
koreo-. See words beginning
    chorio-.
Krabbe's disease
kromoblastomikosis. See
    chromoblastomycosis.
Kundrat's lymphosarcoma
kwashiorkor
kyphosis
Laennec's cirrhosis
la grippe
Lancereaux's diabetes
Landouzy's purpura
laryngitis
law
    Fitz's l.
LE – lupus erythematosus

LED — lupus erythematosus
    disseminatus
Lederer's anemia
leiomyoma
leiomyosarcoma
leishmaniasis
leprosy
leptoprosopia
leptospirosis
    l. icterohemorrhagica
Leriche's syndrome
Letterer-Siwe disease
leukemia
leukocytosis
leukodystrophy
leukolymphosarcoma
leukopenia
leukoplakia
Lignac's disease
Lignac-Fanconi syndrome
line
    Sergent's white l.
liomioma. See *leiomyoma.*
liomiosarkoma. See
    leiomyosarcoma.
lipemia
lipiduria
lipoblastosis
lipochondrodystrophy
lipodystrophia
    l. progressiva
lipodystrophy
lipoma
lipomatosis
lipoproteinemia
    A-beta l.
liver
    amyloid l.

liver *(continued)*
    brimstone l.
    cirrhotic l.
    lardaceous l.
Loa
    L. loa
loaiasis
Lobstein's cancer
Löffler's
    eosinophilia
    syndrome
lordosis
lues
    l. hepatis
Luft's syndrome
lumbago
    ischemic l.
lupus
    l. erythematosus
    l. nephritis
    l. pernio
lymphadenectasis
lymphadenhypertrophy
lymphadenia
    l. ossea
lymphadenitis
    caseous l.
    paratuberculous l.
lymphadenocyst
lymphadenogram
lymphadenography
lymphadenoid
lymphadenoleukopoiesis
lymphadenoma
lymphadenopathy
lymphadenosis
lymphadenovarix
lymphangiectasis

lymphangioendothelio-
 blastoma
lymphangioendothelioma
lymphangiofibroma
lymphangiosarcoma
lymphangitis
lymphatism
lymphedema
 l. praecox
lymphemia
lymphoblastoma
 giant follicular l.
lymphoblastomatosis
lymphocystosis
lymphocythemia
lymphocytoma
lymphocytopenia
lymphocytosis
lymphodermia
lymphogranuloma
lymphogranulomatosis
lymphoidotoxemia
lymphoma
 giant follicular l.
lymphomatosis
lymphopathia
 l. venereum
lymphopenia
lymphosarcoleukemia
lymphosarcoma
 Kundrat's l.
lymphosarcomatosis
lymphotoxemia
lysemia
MacLeod's capsular
 rheumatism
macrodystrophia
 m. lipomatosa progressiva

macrogenitosomia
 m. praecox
macroglobulinemia
 Waldenström's m.
macrosomatia
 m. adiposa congenita
maculation
 pernicious m.
maduromycosis
Maixner's cirrhosis
mal
 m. de mer
malabsorption
maladie
malaise
malaria
malignancy
malignant
mali-mali
malnutrition
Malta fever
mamillary
mamillitis
mamma
mammogram
mammoplasia
marasmus
Marchand's adrenal's
Marchiafava-Micheli syndrome
Marfan's syndrome
Marie's
 disease
 hypertrophy
 sign
mastadenoma
mastalgia
mastatrophy
mastauxe

masthelcosis
mastitis
mastocarcinoma
mastochondroma
mastocytosis
mastoiditis
mastoncus
mastopathia
    m. cystica
mastopathy
mastoplastia
mastoptosis
Mathieu's disease
measles
    German m.
Meckel's diverticulum
mediastinitis
mediastinum
Medications. See Sections on
    specific organ systems.
Mediterranean anemia
medulloblastoma
megacolon
megakaryoblastoma
megakaryocytosis
megalerythema
melanosis
melanuria
melasma
    m. addisonii
    m. suprarenale
Meleda disease
melena
melenemesis
melioidosis
menarche
Meniere's
    disease

Meniere's
    syndrome
meningitis
meningococcemia
meningopneumonitis
meningotyphoid
meniscocytosis
menopause
menstruation
meralgia
    m. paresthetica
Merseburg triad
metabolic
metabolism
metagonimiasis
metamorphosis
    fatty m.
metaplasia
    myeloid m.
metastases
metastasis
metastasize
metastatic
methemoglobinemia
microcephaly
microcythemia
microlithiasis
micturition
mielo-. See words beginning
    myelo-.
migraine
miks-. See words beginning
    myx-.
mikso-. See words beginning
    myxo-.
Mikulicz's disease
miliaria
Milroy's edema

mirinjitis. See *myringitis.*
mittelschmerz
Möbius'
    disease
    sign
Monge's disease
moniliasis
mononucleosis
    infectious m.
morbilliform
Morquio's disease
MS – multiple sclerosis
mucopurulent
mucormycosis
mucosanguineous
mucositis
    m. necroticans
        agranulocytica
mucoviscidosis
mumps
Münchausen's syndrome
murmur
    heart m.
Murray Valley encephalitis
myalgia
myasthenia
    m. gravis
myasthenic
myatonia
    m. congenita
myatrophy
mycethemia
mycetismus
mycobacteriosis
Mycobacterium
    M. tuberculosis
mycosis
    Gilchrist's m.

mycosis
    splenic m.
mycotoxicosis
myelemia
myelitis
myeloblastemia
myeloblastoma
myeloblastomatosis
myeloblastosis
myelocythemia
myelocytoma
myelocytomatosis
myelofibrosis
myeloma
    giant cell m.
myelosarcoma
myelosarcomatosis
myelosclerosis
myelosis
myelotoxicosis
myiasis
myoblastoma
myocardia
myocardiac
myocardial
myocarditis
    acute bacterial m.
myocardosis
myoglobulinuria
myolysis
    m. cardiotoxica
myoma
myositis
myringitis
myxadenitis
myxadenoma
myxangitis
myxasthenia

myxedema
myxoblastoma
myxochondrofibrosarcoma
myxochondroma
myxochondrosarcoma
myxodermia
myxofibrosarcoma
myxoidedema
myxoma
myxomatosis
myxosarcoma
myxovirus
nanism
    Paltauf's n.
narcolepsy
natremia
natriuresis
nausea
necrobiosis
    n. lipoidica
    n. lipoidica diabeticorum
necrosis
    Balser's fatty n.
    decubital n.
    icteric n.
nefritis. See nephritis.
nefro-. See words beginning
    nephro-.
nemathelminthiasis
nematodiasis
neoplasm
nephritis
nephrocalcinosis
nephrocirrhosis
nephrocystitis
nephrocystosis
nephrolithiasis
nephropyelitis

nephrosclerosis
nephrosis
neuralgia
neurasthenia
neuritis
neuroamebiasis
neuroblastoma
neurofibroma
neuroma
    acoustic n.
neuromyositis
neurosyphilis
neutropenia
neutrophilia
Nicolas-Favre disease
Niemann-Pick disease
Niemann's
    disease
    splenomegaly
Nikolsky's sign
nocardiosis
noctalbuminuria
nocturia
node
    Heberden's n's.
    Osler's n's.
    Parrot's n.
nodule
    cold n.
    Gandy-Gamna n's.
numo-. See words beginning
    pneumo-.
nystagmus
obesity
    endogenous o.
    exogenous o.
ochrodermatosis
ochrodermia

ochronosis
odon-eki
odoriferous
oestriasis
ofthal-. See words beginning
    ophthal-.
okro-. See words beginning
    ochro-.
oksalosis. See *oxalosis*.
okseuriasis. See *oxyuriasis*.
oligemia
oligochromemia
oligocythemia
oligophrenia
        phenylpyruvic o.
oligoplasmia
oligoptyalism
oligotrophia
oliguria
onchocerciasis
onyalai
onychomycosis
oophoritis
        o. parotidea
ophthalmia
ophthalmoplegia
opisthorchiasis
opisthotonos
orchitis
        o. parotidea
        o. variolosa
orf
ornithosis
Oroya fever
orthopnea
Osler's
        disease
        nodes

Osler's *(continued)*
    sign
    syndrome
Osler-Vaquez disease
osteitis
osteoarthritis
osteolysis
osteomalacia
osteomyelitis
osteopetrosis
osteoporosis
osteosclerosis
overhydration
oxalosis
oxyuriasis
pachydermoperiostosis
pachymeningitis
Paget's disease
pake-. See words beginning
    pachy-.
palpitation
palsy
        Bell's p.
Paltauf's nanism
pancreas
        Aseli's p.
        p. divisum
        Willis' p.
        Winslow's p.
pancreatalgia
pancreatemphraxis
pancreathelcosis
pancreatitis
pancytopenia
panhypopituitarism
panneuritis
        p. epidemica
panniculus

pansitopenea. See
   pancytopenia.
pantatrophia
pantatrophy
papilla
papillary
papilledema
papillitis
papilloadenocystoma
papillocarcinoma
papilloma
papillomatosis
papillomatous
papillosarcoma
papular
papule
papuloerythematous
papulosquamous
paracentesis
paracoccidioidomycosis
paragonimiasis
paragranuloma
parahemophilia
parakeratosis
paralysis
parascarlatina
parasitemia
parasitic
parathyroid
parathyroidoma
parathyroprival
parathyroprivia
parathyrotoxicosis
paresis
paresthesia
Parkinson's
   disease
   facies

Parkinson's
   syndrome
parkinsonian
parkinsonism
   postencephalitis p.
paroksizm. See *paroxysm.*
paroksizmal. See
   paroxysmal.
parotid
parotidoscirrhus
parotidosclerosis
parotitis
   p. phlegmonosa
paroxysm
paroxysmal
Parrot's
   disease
   node
   ulcer
Parry's disease
Parsons' disease
pasteurellosis
pathoglycemia
Patterson-Brown-Kelly
   syndrome
Paul's treatment
Pautrier's abscess
Pavy's disease
peadra. See *piedra.*
pectenosis
pectoralgia
pediculosis
Pel-Ebstein pyrexia
pellagra
pelohemia
pemfigoid. See *pemphigoid.*
pemfigus. See *pemphigus.*
pemphigoid

pemphigus
    p. erythematosus
    p. foliaceus
    p. neonatorum
    p. vegetans
    p. vulgaris
penicilliosis
pentastomiasis
pentatrichomoniasis
pentosemia
pentosuria
periarteritis
    p. nodosa
pericarditis
peritonitis
perityphlitis
perlingual
pertussis
pestilence
pestis
    p. ambulans
    p. bubonica
    p. siderans
petechia
petechiasis
Pfuhl's sign
phagocytosis
pharyngitis
phenetidinuria
phenolemia
phenoluria
phenomenon
    Raynaud's p.
    Rumpel-Leede p.
phenylketonuria
pheochromoblastoma
pheochromocytoma
phlebitis

phleboclysis
phlebothrombosis
photophobia
photoscan
phototherapy
phycomycosis
pian
    p. bois
piarhemia
pica
Pick's disease
pickwickian syndrome
piedra
pinocytosis
Pirogoff's edema
pituitarism
pituitary
pituitrism
pityriasis
placebo
plague
Plaut's angina
pleochromocytoma
pleocytosis
pleomastia
pleura
pleuralgia
pleurisy
pleurocholecystitis
pleurodynia
plombage
Plummer-Vinson syndrome
PND — paroxysmal nocturnal
    dyspnea
pneumococcemia
pneumococcosis
pneumococcus
pneumoconiosis

pneumonia
    pneumococcal p.
pneumonitis
pneumothorax
podagra
podalgia
poikilocytosis
poikiloderma
poikilodermatomyositis
poisoning
    mushroom p.
polioencephalitis
poliomyelencephalitis
poliomyelitis
    bulbar p.
poliothrix
poliovirus
pollinosis
polyadenitis
polyadenosis
polyarteritis
polyarthritis
polychondritis
polycythemia
    myelopathic p.
    splenomegalic p.
    p. vera
polycytosis
polydipsia
polydysplasia
polyemia
polymyositis
polyneuritis
polyneuropathy
    erythredema p.
polyphagia
polyposis
polypus

polyradiculitis
polyradiculoneuritis
polyrrhea
polysarcia
polyserositis
polyuria
Poncet's rheumatism
porphyria
Pott's disease
preeclampsia
proctalgia
    p. fugax
proctencleisis
proctitis
    epidemic gangrenous p.
proctodynia
proctorrhagia
proctorrhea
proctoscopy
proctosigmoidoscopy
progeria
proteinemia
proteinosis
proteinuria
    orthostatic p.
prothrombin
prothrombinopenia
protocoproporphyria
prurigo
pruritus
psammocarcinoma
psammoma
psammosarcoma
pseudoacanthosis
    p. nigricans
pseudoaldosteronism
pseudohemophilia
    p. hepatica

pseudohermaphrodism
pseudohyperkalemia
pseudohyponatremia
pseudohypoparathyroidism
pseudoleukemia
    p. lymphatica
pseudoproteinuria
pseudo-pseudohypopara-
    thyroidism
pseudoxanthoma
    p. elasticum
psilosis
psittacosis
psoriasis
ptosis
pulpa
    p. lienis
PUO — pyrexia of unknown
    origin
purpura
    p. cachectica
    p. hemorrhagica
    idiopathic p.
    Landouzy's p.
    orthostatic p.
    p. rheumatica
    Schönlein-Henoch p.
    thrombocytopenic p.
    p. variolosa
pyarthrosis
pyelitis
pyelonephritis
pyelonephrosis
pyemia
    cryptogenic p.
pyrexia
    Pel-Ebstein p.
pyrogenic

pyroglobulinemia
pyruvemia
pyuria
Q fever
quarantine
rabdomioma. See
    rhabdomyoma.
rabies
rachitis
radiation
radioactivity
radioiodine
radioisotope
radioneuritis
radiotherapy
RAI — radioactive iodine
rakitis. See *rachitis.*
ranula
    pancreatic r.
Raynaud's
    disease
    gangrene
    phenomenon
recrudescence
Refsum's disease
regimen
regurgitation
    aortic r.
Reifenstein's syndrome
Reiter's
    disease
    syndrome
Rénon-Delille syndrome
respiration
    Cheyne-Stokes r.
resuscitation
reticulocytosis
reticuloendothelioma

reticuloendotheliosis
    leukemic r.
retinitis
rhabdomyoma
rheumapyra
rheumarthritis
rheumatalgia
rheumatic
rheumatid
rheumatism
    Heberden's r.
    MacLeod's capsular r.
    Poncet's r.
rheumatoid
rhinitis
rhinophyma
rhinorrhea
rhinosporidiosis
rhonchi
rickets
rickettsial
rickettsialpox
rickettsiosis
Riedel's struma
Rift Valley fever
ring
    Kayser-Fleischer r.
rinitis. See *rhinitis.*
rino-. See words beginning
    rhino-.
Rocky Mountain spotted fever
Rokitansky's disease
Romaña's sign
Romberg-Paessler syndrome
Romberg's sign
rongki. See *rhonchi.*
rooma-. See words beginning
    rheuma-.

Rosenbach's syndrome
roseola
roseolus
Rotor's syndrome
roundworm
rubella
    r. scarlatinosa
rubeola
    r. scarlatinosa
rubor
rubra
Rumpel-Leede phenomenon
Runeberg's type
Runneberg's disease
rupia
Russian spring-summer
    encephalitis
St. Louis encephalitis
salmonellosis
samokarsinoma. See
    psammocarcinoma.
samoma. See *psammoma.*
samosarkoma. See
    psammosarcoma.
San Joaquin fever
San Joaquin Valley disease
sarcocarcinoma
sarcoid
    s. of Boeck
    Darier-Roussy s.
    Schaumann's s.
    Spiegler-Fendt s.
sarcoidosis
sarcoma
    reticulum cell s.
sarcomphalocele
sarcosepsis
sarcosis

SBE — subacute bacterial
    endocarditis
scabies
scalenus anticus syndrome
scarlatina
Schaumann's sarcoid
schistosomiasis
    cutaneous s.
    hepatic s.
Schmidt's syndrome
Schönlein-Henoch purpura
Schultz's angina
schwannoma
scleredema
sclerodactylia
    s. annularis ainhumoides
scleroderma
scleromalacia
sclerosis
    multiple s.
scoleciasis
scopulariopsosis
scotodinia
scotoma
scrofula
scrofuloderma
scurvy
sefalaljeah. See *cephalalgia.*
seizure
Senear-Usher syndrome
senile
sepsis
    s. lenta
    puerperal s.
septicemia
septicophlebitis
septicopyemia
Sergent's white line

Sézary's syndrome
sferositosis. See *spherocytosis.*
shangker. See *chancre.*
shangkroid. See *chancroid.*
Sheehan's disease
shigellosis
shingles
shock
    insulin s.
sialadenitis
sialoadenitis
sialoangiitis
sialorrhea
    s. pancreatica
sickle cell anemia
sign
    Babinski's s.
    Chvostek-Weiss s.
    Erb's s.
    Graefe's s.
    Homans' s.
    Marie's s.
    Möbius' s.
    Nikolsky's s.
    Osler's s.
    Pfuhl's s.
    Romaña's s.
    Romberg's s.
    Stellwag's s.
    Troisier's s.
    Trousseau's s.
    Unschuld's s.
silicatosis
silicosis
silicotuberculosis
silosis. See *psilosis.*
Simmonds' disease
singultus

sinusitis
sirrosis. See *cirrhosis.*
sitakosis. See *psittacosis.*
Sjögren's syndrome
skistosomiasis. See
schistosomiasis.
SLE — systemic lupus
erythematosus
smallpox
sootsoogamooshe. See
tsutsugamushi.
soriasis. See *psoriasis.*
South African tick typhus
South American hemorrhagic
fever
Southeast Asian mosquito-
borne hemorrhagic fever
spherocytosis
Spiegler-Fendt sarcoid
spina bifida
spirochetosis
spleen
accessory s.
Gandy-Gamna s.
lardaceous s.
splenadenoma
splenalgia
splenatrophy
splenauxe
splenculus
splenectasis
splenectomy
splenectopia
splenelcosis
splenemia
splenemphraxis
spleneolus
splenepatitis

splenetic
splenic
splenicterus
splenitis
spodogenous s.
splenocele
splenocleisis
splenocolic
splenocyte
splenodynia
splenogenous
splenogram
splenogranulomatosis
s. siderotica
splenography
splenohepatomegaly
splenokeratosis
splenolymphatic
splenolysin
splenolysis
splenoma
splenomalacia
splenomedullary
splenomegaly
Gaucher's s.
hemolytic s.
hypercholesterolemic s.
myelophthisic s.
Niemann's s.
siderotic s.
spodogenous s.
splenometry
splenomyelogenous
splenomyelomalacia
splenoncus
splenonephric
splenonephroptosis
splenopancreatic

splenoparectasis
splenopathy
splenopexy
splenophrenic
splenoptosis
splenorrhagia
splenosis
splenotoxin
splenotyphoid
splenulus
spondylitis
    von Bechterew-
      Strumpell s.
spondylosis
sporotrichosis
spot
    café au lait s's.
    De Morgan's s's.
    Janeway's s's.
sprue
staphylococcus
status
    s. asthmaticus
    s. choleraicus
    s. degenerativus
    s. epilepticus
    s. lymphaticus
    s. parathyreoprivus
    s. praesens
    s. thymicolymphaticus
steatorrhea
Stein-Leventhal syndrome
Stellwag's sign
stenosis
    aortic s.
    mitral s.
sterility
Sternberg's disease

sternutatio
    s. convulsiva
Stevens-Johnson syndrome
stomatitis
stomatocytosis
Strachan-Scott syndrome
streptococcus
stridor
strongyloidiasis
struma
    s. basedowificata
    Hashimoto's s.
    s. lymphomatosa
    Riedel's s.
Stuart-Bras disease
stuporous
sucrosemia
Sudeck's atrophy
sudo-. See words beginning
    pseudo-.
sulfhemoglobinemia
sunstroke
Sutton-Rendu-Osler-Weber
    syndrome
syncope
    carotid sinus s.
syndrome
    Abderhalden-Fanconi s.
    Achard-Thiers s.
    Adams-Stokes s.
    adrenogenital s.
    Ahumada-Del Castillo s.
    Albers-Schönberg's s.
    Albright's s.
    aortic arch s.
    Arakawa-Higashi s.
    Arias' s.
    Ayerza's s.

syndrome *(continued)*
- Baber's s.
- Banti's s.
- Bard-Pic s.
- Bar's s.
- Bassen-Kornzweig s.
- Bearn-Kunkel s.
- Bernard's s.
- Budd-Chiari s.
- Caplan's s.
- carpal tunnel s.
- cervical rib s.
- Chiari-Frommel s.
- Conn's s.
- Cushing's s.
- DiGuglielmo's s.
- Dresbach's s.
- Ehlers-Danlos s.
- Fanconi's s.
- Felty's s.
- Fitz-Hugh's s.
- Fitz's s.
- Gaisböck's s.
- Gardner's s.
- Glanzmann's s.
- Goodpasture's s.
- Guillain-Barré s.
- Günther's s.
- Hamman-Rich s.
- Harris' s.
- Hayem-Widal s.
- Heerfordt's s.
- Horton's s.
- Kartagener's s.
- Kimmelstiel-Wilson s.
- Kleine-Levin s.
- Klinefelter's s.
- Leriche's s.

syndrome *(continued)*
- Lignac-Fanconi s.
- Löffler's s.
- Luft's s.
- malabsorption s.
- Marchiafava-Micheli s.
- Marfan's s.
- Meniere's s.
- Munchausen's s.
- Osler's s.
- Parkinson's s.
- Patterson-Brown-
    Kelly s.
- pickwickian s.
- Plummer-Vinson s.
- Reifenstein's s.
- Reiter's s.
- Rénon-Delille s.
- Romberg-Paessler s.
- Rosenbach's s.
- Rotor's s.
- scalenus anticus s.
- Schmidt's s.
- Senear-Usher s.
- Sézary's s.
- Sjögren's s.
- Stein-Leventhal s.
- Stevens-Johnson s.
- Strachan-Scott s.
- Sutton-Rendu-Osler-
    Weber s.
- Takayasu's s.
- Tietze's s.
- Troisier-Hanot-
    Chauffard s.
- Troisier's s.
- Turner's s.
- Wallenberg's s.

syndrome *(continued)*
    Waterhouse-
        Friderichsen s.
    Weil's s.
synovioma
syphilis
tabes
    diabetic t.
    t. dorsalis
tachycardia
Takayasu's syndrome
Tangier disease
telalgia
telangiectasia
telangiectasis
tenesmus
tenosynovitis
test
    Hanger-Rose skin t.
    Hickey-Hare t.
tetanus
tetany
    hyperventilation t.
    parathyroid t.
    parathyroprival t.
    rheumatic t.
    thyroprival t.
tetralogy
    t. of Fallot
thalassemia
thrombasthenia
thromboangiitis
    t. obliterans
thromboarteriosclerosis
    t. obliterans
thrombocytasthenia
thrombocythemia
thrombocytopenia

thrombocytopenic purpura
thrombocytosis
thrombopenia
thrombophlebitis
thrombosis
thrush
thymoma
thymus
thyroid
thyroidism
thyroiditis
thyromegaly
thyrophyma
thyroprival
thyrotoxicosis
tic
    t. douloureux (doo-loo-
        roo)
Tietze's syndrome
tinnitus
Todd's cirrhosis
tonsillitis
tophus
    t. syphiliticus
torticollis
torulosis
tosis. See *ptosis.*
toxemia
toxicity
toxicosis
toxocariasis
toxoplasmosis
tracheitis
trachelagra
trachoma
treatment
    Paul's t.
    Yeo's t.

trematodiasis
treponematosis
treponemiasis
triad
    Falta's t.
    Hutchinson's t.
    Merseburg t.
trichinosis
trichocephaliasis
trichoglossia
trichomoniasis
trichophytosis
trichostrongylosis
trichuriasis
trikinosis. See *trichinosis.*
triko-. See words beginning
    tricho-.
trikuriasis. See *trichuriasis.*
trismus
trisomy 13, 18, 21
trofedema. See *trophedema.*
Troisier-Hanot-Chauffard
    syndrome
Troisier's
    ganglion
    sign
    syndrome
trophedema
Trousseau's sign
trypanosomiasis
tsutsugamushi disease
tubercle
    Farre's t's.
tuberculin
tuberculosis
tularemia
tumor
    Abrikossoff's t.

tumor *(continued)*
    Burkitt's t.
    islet cell t.
    Wilms' t.
Turner's syndrome
type
    Runeberg's t.
typhoid
typhoidette
typhus
    Indian tick t.
    South African tick t.
ulcer
    Parrot's u.
ulceration
uncinariasis
undulant fever
Unschuld's sign
unsinariasis. See *uncinariasis.*
unukizm. See *eunuchism.*
uremia
uremic
urethritis
URI – upper respiratory
    infection
uricosuria
urobilinemia
urobilinuria
urolithiasis
urticaria
uthanazea. See *euthanasia.*
uthiroid. See *euthyroid.*
uthiroidism. See *euthyroidism.*
vaccination
    smallpox v.
vaccine
varicella
variola

varix
Venezuelan equine
    encephalomyelitis
vermiculous
Verstraeten's bruit
vertigo
virus
        Colorado tick fever v.
        Coxsackie v.
vitiligo
vitium
        v. conformationis
        v. primae formationis
von Bechterew-Strumpell
    spondylitis
von Gierke's disease
von Willebrand's disease
vookereriasis. See
    wuchereriasis
Waldenström's
    macroglobulinemia
Wallenberg's syndrome
Waterhouse-Friderichsen
    syndrome
Wegener's granulomatosis
Weil's
        disease
        syndrome
Werner's disease
Wernicke's

Wernicke's *(continued)*
    disease
    encephalopathy
West Nile fever
Western equine
    encephalomyelitis
whooping cough
Willis' pancreas
Wilms' tumor
Wilson's disease
Winslow's pancreas
wuchereriasis
xanthelasma
xanthogranuloma
xanthoma
        x. diabeticorum
xanthomatosis
xanthosis
        x. diabetica
xerophthalmia
xerosis
yaws
yellow fever
Yeo's treatment
zan-. See words beginning *xan-.*
zantho-. See words beginning
    xantho-.
zerofthalmea. See
    xerophthalmia.
zerosis. See *xerosis.*

OBSTETRICS AND GYNECOLOGY

AB — abortion
abactio
abactus venter
abdominal
abdominohysterectomy
abdominohysterotomy
Abell's operation
ablatio
    a. placentae
ABO incompatibility
abort
aborticide
abortifacient
abortion
    afebrile a.
    ampullar a.
    cervical a.
    contagious a.
    criminal a.
    epizootic a.
    habitual a.
    imminent a.
    inevitable a.
    infectious a.
    justifiable a.
    septic a.
    spontaneous a.
    therapeutic a.
    threatened a.
    tubal a.

abortion
    vibrio a.
abortionist
abortive
abortus
abruptio
    a. placentae
    a. placentae marginalis
abscess
acanthosis
accouchement
    a. force
accoucheur
acephalocystis racemosa
Achard-Thiers syndrome
acrocyanosis
acrohysterosalpingectomy
Adair's tenaculum
adenitis
adenoacanthoma
adenocarcinoma
adenofibroma
adenoma
    a. endometrioides ovarii
    a. ovarii testiculare
    a. tubulare testiculare
      ovarii
adenomyofibroma
adenomyoma
adenomyomatosis

adenomyometritis
adenomyosis
adenomyositis
adenopathy
adhesion
    filamentous a.
adnexa
    a. uteri
adnexal
adnexectomy
adnexitis
adnexogenesis
adnexopexy
adnexorganogenic
aerocolpos
afibrinogenemia
after-birth
after-coming head
after-pains
agenitalism
Ahlfeld's sign
Ahumada-Del Castillo
    syndrome
AID — artificial insemination
    donor
aidoiitis
albuginea
    a. ovarii
albumin
Aldrich's operation
Alexander-Adams operation
Alexander's operation
algomenorrhea
Allen-Masters syndrome
Allis'
    clamp
    forceps
alopecia

alopecia
    postpartum a.
amenia
amenorrhea
    absolute a.
    dysponderal a.
    hypothalamic a.
    lactation a.
    ovarian a.
    physiologic a.
    pituitary a.
    premenopausal a.
    primary a.
    relative a.
    secondary a.
amenorrheal
ametria
amniocentesis
amniochorial
amniogenesis
amniogram
amniography
amnioma
amnion
amnionic
amnionitis
amniorrhea
amniorrhexis
amniotic
    a. fluid
amniotin
amniotome
    Baylor's a.
    Beacham's a.
amniotomy
ampule
ampulla
anastomosis

anastomosis
  ureterotubal a.
android
anesthesia
  caudal a.
  chloroform a.
  endotracheal a.
  epidural a.
  ether a.
  general a.
  pentothal a.
  pudendal block a.
  sacral block a.
  saddle block a.
  sodium pentothal a.
  spinal a.
  twilight sleep a.
angle
  costovertebral a.
anisocytosis
ankylocolpos
anovaginal
anovaria
anovarism
anovular
anovulation
anovulatory
anovulia
anovulomenorrhea
anoxia
  a. neonatorum
anteflexed
anteflexio
  a. uteri
anteflexion
antenatal
antepartal
antepartum

anteversion
anteverted
anthropoid
antihypertensive
A & P repair — anterior and
  posterior repair
Apgar
  rating
  score
aplasia
apoplexia
  a. uteri
apoplexy
  uterine a.
  uteroplacental a.
applicator
  Ernst's a.
  Fletcher's loading a.
arcuate
areno-. See words beginning
  arrheno-.
areola
areolar
Arey's rule
Arias-Stella's phenomenon
Arnoux's sign
arrhenoblastoma
arrhenogenic
arrhenoma
arrhenomimetic
artery
  hypogastric a.
  iliac a.
  ilioinguinal a.
  ovarian a.
  pudendal a.
  uterine a.
ascensus

ascensus
    a. uteri
Aschheim-Zondek test
ascites
Asherman's syndrome
aspiration
    vacuum a.
aspirator
    blue tip a.
    red tip a.
    vacuum a.
    yellow tip a.
asynclitism
Atlee's dilator
atony
    uterine a.
atopomenorrhea
atresia
atrium
    a. vaginae
atrophy
atypical
Auerbach's plexus
augmentation
ausculatory
Auvard-Remine speculum
Auvard's
    cranioclast
    weighted speculum
avascular
axillary
Ayerst's knife
AZ test — Aschheim-Zondek test
Babcock's clamp
Backhaus' towel clamp
Baer's vesicle
bag

bag *(continued)*
    Champetier de Ribes b.
    Voorhees' b.
Bailey-Williamson forceps
balanic
Baldwin's operation
Baldy's operation
Baldy-Webster operation
Balfour's retractor
Ballantine's clamp
ballottement
Ball's operation
Bandl's ring
Bard-Parker blade
Barkow
    colliculus of B.
barren
Barrett-Allen forceps
Barrett's
    forceps
    tenaculum
bartholinitis
Bartholin's
    cyst
    gland
Barton's
    forceps
    traction handle
Basedow's disease
basiotripsy (fetal)
Basset's operation
Baudelocque's operation
Baylor's amniotome
Beacham's amniotome
Beatson's operation
Beccaria's sign
Beck. See *Boeck.*
Beclard's sign

Bel-O-Pak
Bellow's pack
Benaron's forceps
benign
Berlind-Auvard speculum
Berry's forceps
Beuttner's method
bicornuate
bifid
bilirubin
Billroth's forceps
Bill's traction handle
bimanual
biopsies
biopsy
  bite b.
  cervical b.
  cold knife conization b.
  cone b.
  endometrial b.
  excisional b.
  four point b.
  multiple b.
  needle b.
  punch b.
  sponge b.
  wedge b.
Birnberg's bow
Bissell's operation
bivalve
Black-Wylie dilator
bladder
  b. blade
  dome of b.
  b. flap
blade
  Bard-Parker b.
  bladder b.

blennorrhea
block
  paracervical b.
  pudendal b.
blood
  cord b.
Blot's perforator
Boeck's sarcoidosis
boggy
Bolt's sign
Bond's forceps
Bonnaire's method
bosselated
Bovie unit
bow
  Birnberg's b.
Bowen's disease
box
  Stockholm b.
Bozeman's forceps
Braasch's forceps
Bracht's maneuver
Brandt's
  technique
  treatment
Brantley-Turner retractor
Braun-Fernwald sign
Braun-Jardine-DeLee hook
Braun's
  cranioclast
  hook
  scissors
  tenaculum
Braune's canal
Braxton-Hicks
  contraction
  sign
  version

breast. See under General
Surgical Terms.
breech
    b. delivery
    b. extraction
    b. presentation
Breisky's
    disease
    pelvimeter
Brenner's tumor
Brentano's syndrome
Breu's mole
Brewer's speculum
Broder's classification
Brouha's test
bruit
brute. See *bruit.*
Buie clamp
bulbus
    b. vestibuli vaginae
Bumm's curet
BUS glands – Bartholin's,
    urethral and Skene's
    glands
Buxton clamp
cachectic
cachexia
    c. ovariopriva
calculation
    Johnson's c.
canal
    Braune's c.
    cervical c.
    endocervical c.
    c. of Nuck
cannula
    Holman-Mathieu c.
    Hudgins' c.

cannula *(continued)*
    Jarcho's c.
    Kahn's c.
    Neal's c.
    Rubin's c.
caput
    c. medusae
    c. succedaneum
carcinoma
    comedo c. See
      comedocarcinoma.
    cylindromatous c.
    ductal c.
    embryonal c.
    epidermoid c.
    granulosa cell c.
    gyriform c.
    infiltrating c.
    c. in situ
    intraepithelial c.
    invasive c.
    macrofolliculoid c.
    microfolliculoid c.
    parenchymatous c.
    squamous cell c.
carcinosarcoma
carina
    c. fornicis
    c. urethralis vaginae
caruncle
    hymenal c's.
    urethral c.
carunculae hymenales
catamenia
catamenial
catamenogenic
catheter
    Foley c.

catheter *(continued)*
    French c.
    Fritsch's c.
    indwelling c.
    Wurd's c.
cauterization
cauterized
cautery
    Percy's c.
cavity
    endometrial c.
cavum
    c. uteri
CDC – calculated date of
   confinement
celiocolpotomy
celiohysterectomy
celiohysterotomy
celiosalpingectomy
celiosalpingotomy
celiotomy
    vaginal c.
cell
    atypical c.
    bank c.
    basket c.
    ciliated c.
    clue c.
    cornified c.
    decidual c.
    endocervical c.
    endometrial c.
    epithelial c.
    epithelioid c.
    hilar c.
    intercalary c.
    keratinized c.
    Langhan's c.

cell *(continued)*
    luteum c.
    mesothelial c.
    navicular c.
    Paget's c.
    parabasal c.
    precornified c.
    superficial c.
    syncytial c.
    "tadpole" c.
    target c.
    tart c.
    theca lutein c.
    Walthard's c.
cephalad
cephalic
cephalometry
cephalopelvic
cerclage
cervical
    c. biopsy
    c. canal
    c. conization
    c. fascia
    c. os
cervicectomy
cervicitis
cervicocolpitis
cervicovaginal
cervicovaginitis
cervicovesical
cervimeter
cervitome
    Milex c.
cervix
    conglutination of c.
    incompetent c.
    c. uteri

cesarean. See under *section*.
CGT – chorionic gonadotropin
Chadwick's sign
Chamberlen's forceps
Champetier de Ribes' bag
chancroid
Chiari-Frommel syndrome
chloasma
    c. gravidarum
    c. uterinum
chlorosis
    c. vulvae
chondromalacia
    c. fetalis
chorioadenoma
    c. destruens
chorioamnionitis
choriocarcinoma
chorioepithelioma
chorion
    c. frondosum
chorionic
    c. gonadotropin
    c. villi
chorioplacental
cicatrix
circumcision
circumoral
clamp
    Allis' c.
    Babcock's c.
    Backhaus' towel c.
    Ballantine's c.
    Buie c.
    Buxton c.
    Heaney's c.
    Kane's c.

clamp *(continued)*
    Kelly's c.
    Kocher's c.
    Lahey's c.
    Oschner's c.
    Willet's c.
    Yellan c.
classification
    Broder's c.
Claudius' fossa
cleidotomy (fetal)
cleidotripsy
climacteric
climacterium
    c. praecox
clitoral
clitoridauxe
clitoridean
clitoridectomy
clitoriditis
clitoridotomy
clitoris
    bifid c.
    crura of c.
    prepuce of c.
clitorism
clitoritis
clitoromania
clitorotomy
cloaca
Cloquet's node
closure
    Latzko's c.
Coffey's operation
coil
    Margulles' c.
coitophobia
coitus

coitus *(continued)*
    c. á la vache
    c. incompletus
    c. interruptus
    c. reservatus
coleocele
coleocystitis
coleoptosis
coleospastia
coleotomy
colliculus
    c. of Barkow
    cervical c. of female
      urethra
Collin's
    forceps
    pelvimeter
    speculum
Collyer's pelvimeter
colostrum
    c. gravidarum
    c. puerperarum
colovaginal
colpalgia
colpatresia
colpectasia
colpectasis
colpectomy
colpeurysis
colpismus
colpitic
colpitis
    c. emphysematosa
    emphysematous c.
    c. granulosa
    c. mycotica
colpocele
colpoceliocentesis

colpoceliotomy
colpocleisis
colpocystitis
colpocystocele
colpocystoplasty
colpocystotomy
colpocystoureterocystotomy
colpocytogram
colpocytology
colpodynia
colpoepisiorrhaphy
colpohyperplasia
colpohysterectomy
colpohysteropexy
colpohysterorrhaphy
colpohysterotomy
colpolaparotomy
colpomicroscope
colpomicroscopic
colpomicroscopy
colpomycosis
colpomyomectomy
colpoperineoplasty
colpoperineorrhaphy
colpopexy
colpoplasty
colpopoiesis
colpopolypus
colpoptosis
colporectopexy
colporrhagia
colporrhaphy
colporrhexis
colposcope
colposcopy
colpospasm
colpostat
colpostenosis

colpostenotomy
colpotherm
colpotomy
colpoureterocystotomy
colpoureterotomy
colpoxerosis
comedocarcinoma
commissura
    c. labiorum anterior
    c. labiorum posterior
    c. labiorum pudendi
commissure
    anterior c. of labia
    posterior c. of labia
compatible
conception
conceptus
conduplicato
    c. corpore
condyloma
    c. acuminatum
    c. latum
    c. subcutaneum
condylomatoid
condylomatosis
condylomatous
condylotomy
configuration
    arcuate c.
confinement
conglutinatio
    c. orificii externi
conglutination
conization
    cold knife c.
conjugata
    c. vera obstetrica
conjugate

conjugate *(continued)*
    diagonal c.
    obstetric c.
contraception
contraceptive
contraction
    Braxton-Hicks c.
    premonitory c's.
Coombs' test
copious
copulation
cord
    medullary c's.
    ovigerous c's.
    umbilical c.
cord blood
Corey's forceps
Corner-Allen test
cornu
cornua
cornual
corpora atretica
corpus
    c. albicans
    c. cavernosum clitoridis
    c. clitoridis
    c. glandulosum
    c. hemorrhagicum
    c. luteum
    c. spongiosum urethrae
      muliebris
    c. uteri
    uterine c.
cortex
costovertebral
cotyledon
Couvelaire's
    syndrome

Couvelaire's
    uterus
cranioclasis (fetal)
cranioclast
    Auvard's c.
    Braun's c.
    Zweifel-DeLee c.
craniotome
craniotomy (fetal)
Crede's method
cretin
cribriform
crista
    c. urethralis femininae
    c. urethralis muliebris
crus
    c. clitoridis
    c. of clitoris
    c. glandis clitoridis
cryostat
cryotherapy
cryptomenorrhea
crystalline
CS – cesarean section
C-section – cesarean section
cul-de-sac
    Douglas' c.d.s.
culdocentesis
culdoscope
    Decker's c.
culdoscopy
Cullen's sign
cumulus
    c. oophorus
    ovarian c.
    c. ovaricus
cuneihysterectomy
curet

curet *(continued)*
    Bumm's c.
    Greene's c.
    Gusberg's c.
    Hannon's c.
    Heaney's c.
    Holden's c.
    Holtz's c.
    Hunter's c.
    Kelly-Gray c.
    Kelly's c.
    Kushner-Tandatnick c.
    Lounsbury's c.
    Novak's c.
    Randall's c.
    Récamier's c.
    Reich-Nechtow c.
    Sims' c.
    Skene's c.
    Thomas' c.
curettage
    fractional c.
    suction c.
curette. See *curet.*
curettement
Curtius' syndrome
Cusco's speculum
CVA – costovertebral angle
CWP – childbirth without
   pain
cyanotic
cycle
    aberrant c.
    anovulatory c.
    endometrial c.
    genesial c.
    gonadotrophic c.
    menstrual c.

cycle *(continued)*
>   myometrial c.
>   oogenetic c.
>   ovarian c.
>   reproductive c.
>   sexual c.

cyclic
cyema
cyesedema
cyesiognosis
cyesiology
cyesis
cyestein
cyogenic
cyonin
cyophoria
cyophoric
cyotrophy
cyst
>   atheromatous c.
>   Bartholin's c.
>   chocolate c.
>   chorionic c.
>   corpus luteum c.
>   dermoid c.
>   embryonal c.
>   endometrial c.
>   epoophoron c.
>   follicular c.
>   gartnerian c.
>   granulosa lutein c.
>   hemorrhagic c.
>   hymenal c.
>   inclusion c.
>   inflammatory c.
>   lutein c.
>   c. of Morgagni
>   morgagnian c.

cyst *(continued)*
>   nabothian c.
>   Naboth's c's.
>   oophoritic c.
>   ovarian c.
>   paroophoritic c.
>   parovarian c.
>   pedicled c.
>   polycystic c.
>   retention c.
>   Sampson's c.
>   sebaceous c.
>   theca-lutein c.
>   tubo-ovarian c.
>   vaginal inclusion c.
>   wolffian c.

cystadenocarcinoma
cystadenoma
>   mucinous c.
>   pseudomucinous c.
>   serous c.

cystocele
cystoelytroplasty
cystolutein
cystoma
>   myxoid c.
>   c. serosum simplex

cystomatitis
cystomatous
cystometrogram
cystosarcoma
>   c. phylloides

cystourethrocele
cytogenic
Dalkon shield
Danforth's
>   method
>   sign

David's disease
Davis' operation
D & C – dilatation and
   curettage
De Alvarez's forceps
Deaver's retractor
decidua
   basal d.
   d. basalis
   capsular d.
   d. capsularis
   menstrual d.
   d. menstrualis
   parietal d.
   d. parietalis
   reflex d.
   d. reflexa
   d. serotina
   d. vera
decidual
decidualitis
deciduate
deciduation
deciduitis
deciduoma
deciduomatosis
decipara
Decker's culdoscope
defervesced
deflection
   vesicouterine d.
defundation
defundectomy
DeLee's
   forceps
   maneuver
   pelvimeter
   retractor

DeLee's
   tenaculum
delivery
   breech d.
   low forceps d.
   mid forceps d.
denidation
depression
   reactive d.
dermoplast spray
descensus
   d. uteri
   uterine d.
desensin
Desjardin's forceps
desultory
detachment
   annular d.
Deventer's
   diameter
   pelvis
Devilbiss' speculum
Devilbiss-Stacey speculum
Dewees' sign
Dewey's forceps
dextroposition
dextrorotation
dextrostix
dextroverted
diameter
   Deventer's d.
   Löhlein's d.
diaphragm
   Ramses' d.
diastasis
   d. recti abdominis
Diday's law
didelphia

didelphic
Dienst's test
dihysteria
dilatation
dilated
dilation
dilator
    Atlee's d.
    Black-Wylie d.
    Goodell's d.
    Hank-Bradley d.
    Hank's d.
    Hegar's d.
    Hurtig's d.
    Jolly's d.
    Kelly's d.
    Palmar's d.
    Pratt's d.
    Reich-Nechtow d.
    Starlinger's d.
    Wylie's d.
diovulatory
diphasia
dis-. See words beginning dys-.
discission
discrete
disease
    Basedow's d.
    Bowen's d.
    Breisky's d.
    David's d.
    fibrocystic d.
    Fox-Fordyce d.
    Halban's d.
    Lignac-Fanconi d.
    Maher's d.
    Niemann-Pick d.
    Paget's d.

disease (continued)
    pelvic inflammatory d.
    Schroeder's d.
    Valsuani's d.
disproportion
    cephalopelvic d.
Doleris' operation
Donald-Fothergill operation
Donald's operation
doptone
douche
Douglas'
    cul-de-sac
    fold
    line
    pouch
douglascele
douglasitis
Doyen's
    operation
    retractor
    scissors
    vaginal hysterectomy
drain
    Penrose d.
drip
    pitocin d.
drugs. See Medications.
Dubovitz's syndrome
duct
    Gartner's d.
    mesonephric d.
    mullerian d.
    Reichel's cloacal d.
    Skene's d.
    wolffian d.
ductuli transversi epoophori
ductus

ductus
    d. epoophori
      longitudinalis
Dudley's
    hook
    operation
Dührssen's
    incision
    operation
    tampon
duipara
Duncan's mechanism
Duplay's
    hook
    tenaculum
D 5 & W – 5% dextrose and
    water
dye
    Indigo carmine d.
dysfunction
dysfunctional
dysgerminoma
dyskinesia
    uterine d.
dysmenorrhea
    d. intermenstrualis
    plethoric d.
    psychogenic d.
dyspareunia
dysplasia
dysponderal
dystocia
Eastman's retractor
easy-pulls
EBL – estimated blood loss
eclampsia
ectocervix
ectopic

EDC – estimated date of
    confinement
    expected date of
    confinement
Eder's forceps
effaced
effacement
electrometrogram
elephantiasis
    e. of vulva
Elliott's
    forceps
    treatment
emansio mensium
embryo
embryoctony
embryogenesis
embryogenetic
embryogenic
embryonal
embryonate
embryonic
embryoniform
embryonism
embryonization
embryonoid
embryopathia
    e. rubeolaris
embryopathology
embryopathy
embryotocia
embryotome
embryotomy
emesis
    e. gravidarum
emmenagogic
emmenagogue
emmenia

emmenic
emmeniopathy
emmenology
Emmert-Gellhorn pessary
Emmet's
    operation
    retractor
Emmett's
    hook
    scissors
en bloc
endocervical
    e. canal
    e. mucosa
    e. polyp
endocervicitis
endocolpitis
endometrectomy
endometria
endometrioid
endometrioma
endometriosis
    e. externa
    e. interna
    ovarian e.
    e. ovarii
    e. uterina
    e. vesicae
endometriotic
endometritis
    bacteriotoxic e.
    decidual e.
    e. dissecans
    exfoliative e.
    glandular e.
    membranous e.
    puerperal e.
    syncytial e.

endometrium
    hyperplastic e.
    secretory e.
    Swiss-cheese e.
endosalpingitis
endosalpingoma
endosalpingosis
endosalpinx
endotoxic
endouterine
engorge
engorgement
entad
ental
enterocele
enucleated
epichorion
epimenorrhagia
epimenorrhea
episioclisia
episioelytrorrhaphy
episioperineoplasty
episioperineorrhaphy
episioplasty
episiorrhaphy
episiostenosis
episiotomy
epithelial
epithelialized
epithelioid
epithelioma
    e. of Malherbe
epoophorectomy
epoophoron
    e. cyst
Ernst's applicator
eroded
erosion

erythroblastosis
    e. fetalis
    e. neonatorum
escutcheon
Estes' operation
esthiomene
estrogen
etrohysterectomy
EUA – examination under
  anesthesia
eutocia
eversion
evert
examination
    bimanual e.
    gynecologic e.
    hanging drop e.
    postpartal e.
    speculum e.
    vaginorectal e.
exenteration
exercise
    Kegel's e.
exfetation
exometritis
exophytic
extraction
    breech e.
extraperitoneal
extrauterine
extravaginal
falciform
Falk's operation
Falk-Shukuris operation
fallectomy
fallopian tube
fallostomy
fallotomy

Farre's line
Farris' test
fascia
    cervical f.
    pubovesicocervical f.
    subvesical f.
fecalith
fenestrated
fenestration
Ferguson's scissors
Fergusson's speculum
Ferris' forceps
fertile
fertility
fertilization
fetal
    f. asphyxia
    f. distress
    f. heart sound
    f. heart tone
    f. hydrops
    f. monitor
    f. oophoritis
fetal position
    LFA – left fronto-
      anterior
    LFP – left fronto-
      posterior
    LFT – left fronto-
      transverse
    LMA – left mento-
      anterior
    LMP – left mento-
      posterior
    LMT – left mento-
      transverse
    LOA – left occipito-
      anterior

fetal position *(continued)*
    LOP — left occipito-
        posterior
    LOT — left occipito-
        transverse
    LSA — left sacroanterior
    L. Sc. A. — left scapulo-
        anterior
    L. Sc. P. — left scapulo-
        posterior
    LSP — left sacroposterior
    LST — left sacro-
        transverse
    RFA — right fronto-
        anterior
    RFP — right fronto-
        posterior
    RFT — right fronto-
        transverse
    RMA — right mento-
        anterior
    RMP — right mento-
        posterior
    RMT — right mento-
        transverse
    ROA — right occipito-
        anterior
    ROP — right occipito-
        posterior
    ROT — right occipito-
        transverse
    RSA — right sacro-
        anterior
    R. Sc. A. — right
        scapuloanterior
    R. Sc. P. — right
        scapuloposterior
    RSP — right sacro-

fetal position *(continued)*
        posterior
    RST — right sacro-
        transverse
fetation
feticide
feticulture
fetogram
fetography
fetometry
fetoplacental
fetus
    f. acardiacus
    f. amorphus
    calcified f.
    f. compressus
    harlequin f.
    f. in fetu
    macerated f.
    mummified f.
    paper-doll f.
    papyraceous f.
    f. papyraceus
    parasitic f.
    f. sanguinolentis
    sireniform f.
Feulgen stain
FHS — fetal heart sound
FHT — fetal heart tone
fibroadenoma
fibrocystic
fibroid
fibroidectomy
fibroma
fibromyoma
fibromyomata
fibromyomectomy
filamentous

fimbria
    ovarian f.
    f. ovarica
fimbriae tubae uterinae
fimbriae of uterine tube
fimbriated
fimbriocele
fistula
    rectolabial f.
    rectovaginal f.
    vulvorectal f.
Fitz-Hugh's syndrome
flebitis. See *phlebitis.*
Fletcher's
    loading applicator
    suit
Fletcher-Van Doren forceps
fluffs
fluid
    amniotic f.
    crystalline f.
fluor
    f. albus
Foerster's forceps
fold
    Douglas' f.
    Pawlik's f's.
Foley catheter
follicle
    graafian f's.
    nabothian f's.
    Naboth's f's.
    ovarian f.
    primordial f.
follicular
folliculoma
forceps
    Allis' f.

forceps *(continued)*
    Bailey-Williamson f.
    Barrett-Allen f.
    Barrett's f.
    Barton's f.
    Benaron's f.
    Berry's f.
    Billroth's f.
    Bond's f.
    Bozeman's f.
    Braasch's f.
    Chamberlen's f.
    Collin's f.
    Corey's f.
    De Alvarez's f.
    DeLee's f.
    Desjardin's f.
    Dewey's f.
    Eder's f.
    Elliott's f.
    Ferris' f.
    Fletcher-Van Doren f.
    Foerster's f.
    Garrigue's f.
    Gaylor's f.
    Gellhorn's f.
    Gelpi-Lowrie f.
    Glenner's f.
    Gordon's f.
    Gutglass' f.
    Hale's f.
    Hartman's f.
    Hawkins' f.
    Hawks-Dennen f.
    Heaney-Ballantine f.
    Heaney-Kanter f.
    Heaney-Rezek f.
    Heaney's f.

forceps *(continued)*

Heise's f.
Henrotin's f.
Hirst-Emmett f.
Hodge's f.
Iowa f.
Jacobs' f.
Jarcho's f.
Kelly's f.
Kennedy's f.
Kielland-Luikart f.
Kielland's f. (Kjelland's f.)
Krause's f.
Laufe-Barton-Kielland f.
Laufe-Piper f.
Laufe's f.
Levret's f.
Long Island f.
Long's f.
Luikart's f.
Luikart-Simpson f.
Maier's f.
Mann's f.
Maryan's f.
McLane's f.
McLane-Tucker f.
McLane-Tucker-Luikart f.
Mitchell-Diamond f.
Mundie's f.
Newman's f.
O'Hanlon's f.
Overstreet's f.
ovum f.
Pean's f.
Phaneuf's f.
Piper's f.

forceps *(continued)*

placental f.
polyp f.
Randall's stone f.
ring f.
Rochester-Carmalt f.
Rochester-Ochsner f.
Rochester-Pean f.
Russell's f.
Schroeder's f.
Schubert's f.
Schwartz's f.
Schweizer's f.
Segond's f.
Senn f.
Simpson's f.
Simpson-Luikart f.
Skene's f.
Smith's f.
Somers' f.
sponge f.
Staude-Moore f.
Staude's f.
stone f.
Tarnier's f.
Teale's f.
Thoms' f.
Thoms-Allis f.
Thoms-Gaylor f.
Tischler's f.
tissue f.
Tucker-McLean f.
Van-Doren f.
vulsellum f.
Walton's f.
Walton-Schubert f.
Weisman's f.
Wertheim-Cullen f.

forceps *(continued)*
>   Wertheim's f.
>   Willett's f.
>   Wittner's f.
>   Yeoman's f.

forewaters
fornices
fornix
fossa
>   Claudius' f.
>   f. navicularis
>   obturator f.
>   ovarian f.
>   f. ovarica
>   f. of vestibule of vagina
>   f. vestibuli vaginae

Fothergill's operation
fourchette
Fox-Fordyce disease
fractional
Frangenheim-Goebell-Stoeckel
>   operation

frenal
French catheter
frenulum
>   f. of clitoris
>   f. labiorum pudendi

frenum
>   f. of labia

Freund's
>   law
>   operation

Friedman-Lapham test
Friedman's retractor
Friedman's test
frigid
frigidity
Fritsch-Asherman syndrome

Fritsch's
>   catheter
>   operation

Frommel's operation
FTLB – full term living birth
FTND – full term normal
>   delivery

fulcrum
fulguration
fundectomy
fundus
>   f. uteri
>   f. of uterus
>   f. of vagina
>   f. vaginae

fungating
funis
Gabastou's hydraulic method
Galli-Mainini test
Gariel's pessary
Garrigue's
>   forceps
>   speculum

Gartner's duct
gastrocolpotomy
Gauss's sign
Gaylor's forceps
GC – gonococcus
>   gonorrhea

Gehrung pessary
Gellhorn's
>   forceps
>   pessary

Gelpi-Lowrie forceps
Gelpi's retractor
genesial
genitalia
genitourinary

gestation
gestational
gestosis
Gigli's operation
Gilliam-Doleris' operation
Gilliam's operation
Giordano's operation
gland
>Bartholin's g.
>BUS g's.
>Naboth's g's.
>Skene's g.
>urethral g.
>vestibular g.
glans
>g. clitoridis
>g. of clitoris
Glenner's
>forceps
>retractor
Goffe's operation
Golden's sign
gonad
gonadotrophic
gonadotropin
gonococcus
gonorrhea
Goodall-Power operation
Goodell's
>dilator
>law
>sign
Gordan-Overstreet syndrome
Gordon's forceps
Gottschalk's operation
graafian
>g. follicle
>g. ovule

Grant-Ward operation
granulosa
>g. lutein
Graves' speculum
gravid
gravida I, II, III, etc.
gravidic
gravidism
graviditas
>g. examnialis
>g. exochorialis
gravidity
gravidocardiac
gravidopuerperal
Grawitz's tumor
Green-Armytage operation
Greene's curet
grip
>Pawlik's g.
Gusberg's curet
Gutglass' forceps
Guttmann's
>retractor
>speculum
GYN — gynecology
gynatresia
gynecoid
>g. pelvis
gynecoil
gynecologic
gynecological
gynecologist
gynecology
gynecopathy
gynecotokology
gyneduct
gynopathic
gynopathy

gynoplastics
gynoplasty
Haase's rule
Halban's
    disease
    sign
Hale's forceps
Hamilton's method
Hank-Bradley dilator
Hank's dilator
Hannon's curet
Harrison's method
Hartman's forceps
Hawkins' forceps
Hawks-Dennen forceps
HCG – human chorionic
    gonadotropin
Heaney-Ballantine forceps
Heaney-Kanter forceps
Heaney-Rezek forceps
Heaney's
    clamp
    curet
    forceps
    needle holder
    retractor
    vaginal hysterectomy
Heaney-Simon retractor
Hegar's
    dilator
    operation
    sign
Heise's forceps
hematocele
    parametric h.
    pudendal h.
    retrouterine h.
    vaginal h.

hematochlorine
hematocolpometra
hematocolpos
hematoma
hematome
hematometra
hematosalpinx
hemelytrometra lateralis
hemorrhage
hemostasis
Henrotin's
    forceps
    speculum
herpes
    h. genitalis
    h. gestationis
    h. menstrualis
    h. progenitalis
Hicks'
    sign
    version
hilar
Hirst-Emmett forceps
Hirst's operation
hirsutism
His' rule
Hodge's
    forceps
    maneuver
    pessary
Hoehne's sign
Hogben's test
Holden's curet
Holman-Mathieu cannula
Holtz's curet
hood
    Rock-Mulligan h.
hook

hook *(continued)*
    Braun-Jardine-DeLee h.
    Braun's h.
    Dudley's h.
    Duplay's h.
    Emmett's h.
    Kelly's h.
    Mayo's h.
    Newman's h.
    Schwartz's h.
hormonal
hormone
hormonotherapy
horn
    h. of clitoris
    h. of uterus
Horrocks' maieutic
Hudgins' cannula
Huffman-Graves speculum
Huhner's test
Hunter's
    curet
    ligament
Hurtig's dilator
hydatid
    h. of Morgagni
hydatidiform
hydramnios
hydrocele
    h. feminae
    h. muliebris
    Nuck's h.
hydrocephalus
hydrocolpos
hydroparasalpinx
hydrops
    h. fetalis
    h. folliculi

hydrorrhea
    h. gravidarum
hydrosalpinx
    h. follicularis
    intermittent h.
    h. simplex
hydrotubation
hydroureter
hydrovarium
hymen
    annular h.
    h. bifenestratus
    h. biforis
    circular h.
    cribriform h.
    denticular h.
    falciform h.
    fenestrated h.
    imperforate h.
    infundibuliform h.
    lunar h.
    septate h.
    h. septus
    h. subseptus
hymenal
    h. band
    h. ring
hymenectomy
hymenitis
hymenorrhaphy
hymenotome
hymenotomy
hyperbilirubinemia
hyperemesis
    h. gravidarum
hyperestrogenism
hyperflexion
hypermenorrhea

hypernephroma
hyperovaria
hyperovarianism
hyperovarism
hyperplasia
    adenomatous h.
    endometrial h.
    postmenopausal h.
    proliferative h.
    stromal h.
hyperthecosis
hypertonic
hypertrophy
hypofibrinogenemia
hypofunction
hypomenorrhea
hypoplasia
hypospadias
    female h.
hypothalamic
hypotonic
hypovaria
hypovarianism
hysteralgia
hysteratresia
hysterectomy
    abdominal h.
    cesarean h.
    chemical h.
    Doyen's vaginal h.
    Heaney's vaginal h.
    Latzko's radical h.
    Mayo-Ward vaginal h.
    paravaginal h.
    Porro's h.
    radical h.
    Ries-Wertheim h.
    Schauta's radical

hysterectomy *(continued)*
    vaginal h.
    Spalding-Richardson h.
    subtotal h.
    supracervical h.
    supravaginal h.
    total abdominal h.
    total h.
    vaginal h.
    Wertheim's radical h.
hystereurynter
hystereurysis
hysterobubonocele
hysterocarcinoma
hysterocele
hysterocervicotomy
hysterocleisis
hysterocolpectomy
hysterocolposcope
hysterocystic
hysterocytocleisis
hysterodynia
hysterogastrorrhaphy
hysterogram
hysterograph
hysterography
hysterolaparotomy
hysterolith
hysterology
hysterolysis
hysterometer
hysterometry
hysteromyoma
hysteromyomectomy
hysteromyotomy
hystero-oophorectomy
hystero-ovariotomy
hysteropathy

hysteropexia
hysteropexy
hysteroptosia
hysteroptosis
hysterorrhaphy
hysterosalpingectomy
hysterosalpingogram
hysterosalpingography
hysterosalpingo-
    oophorectomy
hysterosalpingostomy
hysteroscope
hysteroscopy
hysterospasm
hysterostat
hysterostomatocleisis
hysterostomatome
hysterostomatomy
hysterotome
hysterotomotokia
hysterotomy
hysterotrachelectasia
hysterotrachelectomy
hysterotracheloplasty
hysterotrachelorrhaphy
hysterotrachelotomy
hysterotubography
hysterovaginoenterocele
idiometritis
ileus
I.M. cocktail – intramuscular
    cocktail
implantation
in situ
incision
        circumferential i.
        Dührssen's i.
        infraumbilical i.

incision *(continued)*
        midline i.
        Pfannenstiel's i.
        Schuchardt's i.
        suprapubic i.
        transverse i.
incompatibility
incontinence
        stress i.
index
        Mengert's i.
indices
Indigo carmine dye
induced
induction
inertia
        uterine i.
infertilitas
        i. feminis
infertility
infundibula
infundibular
infundibuliform
infundibulum
        i. of fallopian tube
        i. tubae uterinae
        i. of uterine tube
inguinolabial
insemination
        artificial i. donor
        heterologous i.
        homologous i.
insufflation
        methylene blue i.
        tubal i.
insufflator
        Kidde's tubal i.
intercalary

intercourse
intermenstrual
intermural
interstitial
intracervical
intrafetation
intramural
intranatal
intraovarian
intrapartum
intraplacental
intratubal
intrauterine
intravaginal
introitus
    marital i.
    parous i.
    i. vaginae
in utero
inversion
    i. of uterus
involution
Iowa forceps
IPD — inflammatory pelvic
   disease
Irving's operation
Isaac's differential distortion
   divergent method
ischiopubic
ischiopubiotomy
ischiorectal
ischiovaginal
isoimmunization
isthmica nodosa
isthmus
    i. of fallopian tube
    i. tubae uterinae
    i. uteri

isthmus
    i. of uterus
IU — international unit
IUD — intrauterine device
IV cocktail — intravenous
   cocktail
Jackson's retractor
Jacobs'
    forceps
    tenaculum
Jacquemier's sign
Jarcho's
    cannula
    forceps
Johnson's calculation
Jolly's dilator
Jonas-Graves speculum
Jonge's position
Jungbluth
    vasa propria of J.
Kahn-Graves speculum
Kahn's
    cannula
    tenaculum
kakektic. See *cachectic.*
kakexia. See *cachexia.*
Kane's clamp
Kanter's sign
Kapeller-Adler test
Kegel's exercise
Keith's needle
Kelly's
    clamp
    curet
    dilator
    forceps
    hook
    operation

Kelly's
  scissors
Kelly-Gray curet
Kennedy's
  forceps
  operation
keratinized
Kergaradec's sign
Kerr's cesarean section
Kidde's tubal insufflator
Kielland-Luikart forceps
Kielland's forceps (Kjelland's
  forceps)
Klinefelter's syndrome
Kline's flocculation test
kloasma. See *cloasma.*
Klotz's syndrome
Kluge's method
knife
    Ayerst's k.
    Pace's k.
kocherization
kocherized
Kocher's clamp
Kocks's operation
koleo-. See words beginning
  coleo-.
kolostrum. See *colostrum.*
kolp-, kolpo-. See words
  beginning *colp-, colpo-.*
kondilo-. See words beginning
  condylo-.
kondro-. See words beginning
  chondro-.
korio-. See words beginning
  chorio-.
kotiledon. See *cotyledon.*
kraurosis

kraurosis
    k. vulva
Krause's forceps
Kristeller's method
Kronig's cesarean section
Krukenberg's tumor
krura. See *crura.*
kryo-. See words beginning
  cryo-.
kuldo-. See words beginning
  culdo-.
Kupperman's test
Kushner-Tandatnick curet
Küstner's
    law
    sign
kyphosis
    dorsal k.
kyphotic
labia
    l. majora
    l. majus
    l. minora
labial
labium
labor
    atonic l.
    desultory l.
    dyskinetic l.
    habitual l.
    induced l.
    instrumental l.
    mimetic l.
    obstructed l.
    postponed l.
    precipitate l.
    prodromal l.
    protracted l.

labor
  spontaneous l.
laceration
  fishmouth l.
lactation
lacteal
lactic
lacuna
  intervillous l.
Ladin's sign
Lahey's clamp
lamination
Landou's sign
Langhan's
  cell
  stria
laparocolpohysterotomy
laparocystotomy
laparohysterectomy
laparohystero-oophorectomy
laparohysterosalpingo-
  oophorectomy
laparohysterotomy
laparokelyphotomy
laparomonodidymus
laparomyomectomy
laparosalpingectomy
laparosalpingo-oophorectomy
laparosalpingotomy
laparoscope
laparoscopic
laparoscopy
laparotomy
  exploratory l.
laparotrachelotomy
laparouterotomy
Lash's operation
Latzko's

Latzko's *(continued)*
  cesarean section
  closure
  operation
  radical hysterectomy
Laufe-Barton-Keilland forceps
Laufe-Piper forceps
Laufe's forceps
law
  Diday's l.
  Freund's l.
  Goodell's l.
  Küstner's l.
  Leopold's l.
  Levret's l.
  Pajot's l.
LeFort's operation
leiomyoma
  l. uteri
leiomyomata
  l. uteri
leiomyosarcoma
Leopold's
  law
  maneuver
  operation
Lerous's method
leukocytosis
leukokraurosis
leukophlegmasia
leukoplakia
  l. vulvae
leukorrhea
level
  pregnanediol l.
Levret's
  forceps
  law

LFA — left frontoanterior
LFP — left frontoposterior
LFT — left frontotransverse
libido
ligament
    anterior l.
    broad l.
    cardinal l.
    Hunter's l.
    infundibulopelvic l.
    keystone l.
    lacunar l.
    lateral l.
    Mackenrodt's l.
    ovarian l.
    posterior l.
    rectouterine l.
    round l.
    sacrogenital l.
    sacrouterine l.
    suspensory l.
    uterosacral l.
    vesicouterine l.
ligamenta
    l. ovarii proprium
ligation
    tubal l.
Lignac-Fanconi disease
line
    Douglas' l.
    Farre's l.
linea
    l. nigra
lio-. See words beginning
    leio-.
lipoid
Lippe's loop
liquor

liquor *(continued)*
    l. amnii
    l. chorii
    l. folliculi
lithopedion
littritis
Litzmann's obliquity
LMA — left mentoanterior
      last menstrual period
LMP — left mentoposterior
LMT — left mentotransverse
LNMP — last normal
    menstrual period
LOA — left occipitoanterior
lochia
    l. alba
    l. cruenta
    l. purulenta
    l. rubra
    l. sanguinolenta
lochial
lochiocolpos
lochiocyte
lochiometra
lochiometritis
lochiopyra
lochiorrhagia
lochiorrhea
lochioschesis
lochiostasis
lochometritis
lochoperitonitis
Löhlein's diameter
Long Island forceps
Long's forceps
loop
    Lippe's l.
LOP — left occipitoposterior

LOT – left occipitotrans-
verse
Lounsbury's curet
Lovesett's maneuver
LSA – left sacroanterior
L. Sc. A. – left scapulo-
anterior
L. Sc. P. – left scapulo-
posterior
LSP – left sacroposterior
LST – left sacrotransverse
Lugol's stain
Luikart-Bill traction handle
Luikart's forceps
Luikart-Simpson forceps
lumen
    vaginal l.
luteal
luteectomy
lutein
luteinic
luteinization
luteoid
luteoma
luteum
lying-in
lymphogranuloma
    l. benignum
    Schaumann's benign l.
    venereal l.
    l. venereum
lyo-. See words beginning
   leio-.
lyra
    l. uteri
    l. uterina
    l. vaginae
lyre

lyre *(continued)*
    l. of uterus
    l. of vagina
maceration
Mackenrodt's
    ligament
    operation
macula
    m. gonorrhoeica
    Saenger's m.
Madlener operation
Maher's disease
Maier's forceps
maieusiomania
maieusiophobia
maieutic
    Horrocks' m.
Malherbe
    epithelioma of M.
malposition
malpresentation
mammectomy
mammogram
Manchester
    operation
    ovoid
maneuver
    Bracht's m.
    DeLee's m.
    Hodge's m.
    Leopold's m.
    Lovesett's m.
    Massini's m.
    Mauriceau's m.
    Mauriceau-Smellie m.
    Müller-Hillis m.
    Munro-Kerr m.
    Phaneuf's m.

maneuver *(continued)*
    Pinard's m.
    Prague m.
    Ritgen m.
    Scanzoni's
    Schatz's m.
    Van Hoorn's m.
    Wigand's m.
manner
    Pomeroy's m.
Mann's forceps
Marchetti test
Margulles' coil
Marshall-Marchetti operation
Marshall-Marchetti-Krantz
    operation
marsupialization
Martin's
    operation
    pelvimeter
Maryan's forceps
masculinovoblastoma
Mason-Auvard speculum
Massini's maneuver
mastectomy
mastitis
    cystic m.
maturation
Mauriceau's maneuver
Mauriceau-Smellie maneuver
Mayer-Rokitansky-Küster
    syndrome
Mayer's speculum
Mayo-Harrington scissors
Mayor's sign
Mayo-Sims scissors
Mayo-Ward vaginal
    hysterectomy

Mayo's
    hook
    needle
    scissors
maza
mazic
McCall's operation
McCall-Schuman operation
McDonald's operation
McDowell's operation
McIndoe operation
McLane's forceps
McLane-Tucker forceps
McLane-Tucker-Luikart
    forceps
meatus
    urinary m.
mechanism
    Duncan's m.
    Schultze's m.
meconium
Medications
    Amicar
    aminophylline
    ammonium chloride
    Amnestrogen
    ampicillin
    Amytal
    Ascodeen
    Ascriptin
    Atarax
    AVC cream
    Azo-Gantrisin
    Bendectin
    Benzestrol
    Betadine
    Bonadoxin

Medications *(continued)*
- Bonine
- Carbocaine
- chloramphenicol
- Chloromycetin
- chlorotrianisene
- Clomid
- clomiphene
- Cobalt
- Conestron
- Conjutabs
- C-Quens
- Cyclex
- Cytomel
- Cytoxan
- Daprisal
- Deladumone
- Delalutin
- Delatestryl
- Delestrogen
- Delfin
- Deluteval
- Demerol
- Depo-Testosterone
- Devergan
- Diamox
- dienestrol
- diethylstilbestrol
- Dilaudid
- Diocloquin
- Diuril
- Donnaprin
- Duoprin
- Duosterone
- Duphaston
- Duragesic
- Dysonil
- Edrisal

Medications *(continued)*
- Elase
- Enovid
- Ergoapiol
- ergonovine
- ergotamine
- Ergotrate
- Esidrix
- Estan
- Estinyl
- estradiol
- Estratest
- estrone
- Estrovarin
- Estrugenone
- Estrusol
- Falvin
- Femogen
- Flagyl
- Floraquin
- Furacin
- Gantrisin
- Gelfoam pack
- Gentia-Jel
- Gerandrest
- Gestest
- Glutest
- Gynetone
- Hague solution
- Hasacode
- Hasamal
- Hesper-C
- Hormonin
- HydroDiuril
- hydroxyprogesterone caproate
- Hygroton
- Indigo carmine

Medications *(continued)*

Keflex
Keflin
Koagamin
Largon
Lidaform
Lorfan
Loridine
Lutrexin
lututrin
magnesium sulfate
Mantadil
Menest
Menformin
meperidine
Mercuhydrin
Metandren
methallenestril
Methergine
methylene blue
methylergonovine
  maleate
metronidazole
Miltown
Monsell's solution
Mycostatin
Nembutal
Neosporin
Nisentil hydrochloride
Norinyl
Norlestrin
Norlutin
Norquen
Novocain
Ogen
Oreton
Ortho-Novum
Ovocylin

Medications *(continued)*

Ovulen
oxytocin
Panitol
Paradol
Perandren
Pergonal
Phenergan
piperazine estrone
  sulfate
Pitocin
Pituitrin
Polycillin
potassium permanganate
Preceptin
Premarin
Pre-Mens
Prodox
progesterone
Progestin
Progynon
Proluton
promazine
promethazine
Propion-Gel
Prostigmin
Provera
Provest
Pyridium
Restrol
Ringer's lactate
Salpix
scopolamine
secobarbital
Sigesic
Sparine
sparteine
Spartocin

Medications *(continued)*
    Stilbestrol
    Stilbetin
    Stilphostrol
    Sultrin cream
    Supac
    Surgicel
    Synestrol
    Synirin
    Synthroid
    Syntocinon
    TACE
    Talwin
    Test-Estrin
    testosterone
    Theelin
    thiopental
    Thiosulfil
    thio-tepa
    Thorazine
    Tigan
    Tocosamine
    Tricouron
    Trilene
    Uteracon
    Vallestril
    Vistaril
    Vitron-C
    Wynestron
    Xylocaine
    Zactirin
megaloclitoris
Meigs' syndrome
Meigs-Cass syndrome
melanoma
melasma
    m. gravidarum
menalgia

menarche
menarchial
membrane
    mucous m.
Mengert's index
Menge's
    operation
    pessary
menhidrosis
menolipsis
menometrorrhagia
menopausal
menopause
menophania
menoplania
menorrhagia
menorrhalgia
menorrhea
menorrheal
menoschesis
menosepsis
menostasis
menotaxis
menotoxic
menotoxin
menoxenia
menses
menstrual
menstruant
menstruate
menstruation
    anovular m.
    anovulatory m.
    nonovulational m.
    ovulatory m.
    regurgitant m.
    retrograde m.
    scanty m.

menstruation *(continued)*
    supplementary m.
    suppressed m.
    vicarious m.
menstruous
menstruum
mesenchymal
mesometritis
mesometrium
mesonephric
mesonephroma
mesosalpinx
mesothelial
mesothelioma
mesovarium
metacyesis
metaplasia
    squamous m.
method
    Beuttner's m.
    Bonnaire's m.
    Crede's m.
    Danforth's m.
    Gabastou's hydraulic m.
    Hamilton's m.
    Harrison's m.
    Isaac's differential
        distortion divergent m.
    Kluge's m.
    Kristeller's m.
    Lerous's m.
    Pajot's m.
    Puzo's m.
    rhythm m.
    Schultze's m.
    Schuman's m.
    Smellie's m.
    Watson's m.

methylene blue insufflation
metra
metralgia
metranoikter
metratonia
metratrophia
metrectasia
metrectomy
metrectopia
metreurynter
metreurysis
metria
metritis
    m. dissecans
    dissecting m.
    puerperal m.
metrocampsis
metrocarcinoma
metrocele
metrocolpocele
metrodynia
metroendometritis
metrofibroma
metrogenous
metrogonorrhea
metrography
metromalacoma
metromenorrhagia
metropathia
    m. haemorrhagica
metropathic
metropathy
metroperitoneal
metroperitonitis
metrophlebitis
metroptosis
metrorrhagia
metrorrhea

metrorrhexis
metrosalpingitis
metrosalpingogram
metrosalpingography
metroscope
metrostaxis
metrostenosis
metrotome
metrotomy
metrotoxin
metrotubography
Metzenbaum scissors
MH – marital history
Milex cervitome
Miller's speculum
Mitchell-Diamond forceps
mitotic
mittelschmerz
mole
    Breu's m.
    hydatidiform m.
mongoloid
monilial
monocyesis
mons
    m. pubis
    m. ureteris
    m. veneris
Montgomery strap
morcellated
morcellation
morcellement
Morgagni
    cyst of M.
    hydatid of M.
Moschcowitz's operation
motile
mucinous

mucosa
    endocervical m.
Mueller's needle
Müller-Hillis maneuver
müllerian
müllerianoma
müllerianosis
mülleriosis
Muller's operation
multigravida
multiloculated
multipara
multiparity
multiparous
Mundie's forceps
Munnell's operation
Munro-Kerr maneuver
muscle
    levator ani m.
    pubovaginal m.
    pyramidalis m.
    recti m.
    rectouterine m.
    sphincter ani m.
myoma
myomagenesis
myomata
    m. uteri
myomatectomy
myomatosis
myomatous
myomectomy
myometrial
myometritis
myometrium
myomohysterectomy
myomotomy
myosalpingitis

myosalpinx
myosarcoma
mytotic. See *mitotic.*
nabothian
Naboth's
    cysts
    follicles
    glands
    ovules
    vesicle
Nägele's
    obliquity
    pelvis
    rule
navicular
NB — newborn
Neal's cannula
necrosis
necrotic
needle
    Keith's n.
    Mayo's n.
    Mueller's n.
    Pereyra n.
    Shirodkar n.
    Touhey's n.
    Verres' n.
    Vim-Silverman n.
    Voorhes' n.
needle holder
    Heaney's n. h.
Nelson's scissors
neonatal
neonate
neonatologist
neonatology
nerve
    ilioinguinal n.

nerve *(continued)*
    pudendal n.
    uterine n.
neumo-. See words beginning
    pneumo-.
neurectomy
    presacral n.
Newman's
    forceps
    hook
Nickerson's medium smear
Niemann-Pick disease
node
    Cloquet's n.
nodule
    discrete n.
Norethindrone test
Norethynodrel test
Nott's speculum
Novak's curet
Nuck
    canal of N.
    hydrocele of N.
nulligravida
nullipara
nulliparity
nulliparous
numo-. See words beginning
    pneumo-.
nympha
nymphae
nymphectomy
nymphitis
nymphocaruncular
nymphohymeneal
nymphomania
nymphomaniac
nymphoncus

nymphotomy
OB – obstetrics
OB-GYN – obstetrics and
    gynecology
obliquity
    Litzmann's o.
    Nägele's o.
    Roederer's o.
obliteration
obstetrical
obstetrician
obstetrics
occipital
occipitoanterior
occipitoposterior
octigravida
octipara
O'Hanlon's forceps
oligohydramnios
oligohypermenorrhea
oligohypomenorrhea
oligomenorrhea
oligo-ovulation
Olshausen's
    operation
    sign
oogenesis
oogenetic
oophoralgia
oophorectomize
oophorectomy
oophoritis
oophorocystectomy
oophorocystosis
oophorogenous
oophorohysterectomy
oophoroma
oophoron

oophoropathy
oophoropeliopexy
oophoropexy
oophoroplasty
oophororrhaphy
oophorosalpingectomy
oophorosalpingitis
oophorostomy
oophorotomy
oophorrhagia
operation
    Abell's o.
    Aldrich's o.
    Alexander-Adams o.
    Alexander's o.
    Baldwin's o.
    Baldy's o.
    Baldy-Webster o.
    Ball's o.
    Basset's o.
    Baudelocque's o.
    Beatson's o.
    Bissell's o.
    Coffey's o.
    Davis' o.
    Doleris' o.
    Donald-Fothergill o.
    Donald's o.
    Doyen's o.
    Dudley's o.
    Dührssen's o.
    Emmet's o.
    Estes' o.
    Falk's o.
    Falk-Shukuris o.
    Fothergill's o.
    Frangenheim-Goebell-
       Stoeckel o.

operation *(continued)*
    Freund's o.
    Fritsch's o.
    Frommel's o.
    Gigli's o.
    Gilliam-Doleris' o.
    Gilliam's o.
    Giordano's o.
    Goffe's o.
    Goodall-Power o.
    Gottschalk's o.
    Grant-Ward o.
    Green-Armytage o.
    Hegar's o.
    Hirst's o.
    Irving's o.
    Kelly's o.
    Kennedy's o.
    Kocks's o.
    Lash's o.
    Latzko's o.
    LeFort's o.
    Leopold's o.
    Mackenrodt's o.
    Madlener o.
    Manchester o.
    Marshall-Marchetti o.
    Marshall-Marchetti-
        Krantz o.
    Martin's o.
    McCall's o.
    McCall-Schuman o.
    McDonald's o.
    McDowell's o.
    McIndoe o.
    Menge's o.
    Moschcowitz's o.
    Muller's o.

operation *(continued)*
    Munnell's o.
    Olshausen's o.
    Pean's o.
    Peterson's o.
    Pomeroy's o.
    Porro's o.
    Porro-Veit o.
    Pozzi's o.
    Récamier's o.
    Ries-Wertheim o.
    Rizzoli's o.
    Rubin's o.
    Saenger's o.
    Scanzoni's o.
    Schauffler's o.
    Schauta's o.
    Schauta-Wertheim o.
    Schröder's o.
    Schuchardt's o.
    Shirodkar o.
    Simon's o.
    Spalding-Richardson o.
    Spinelli's o.
    Strassman-Jones o.
    Sturmdorf's o.
    Taussig-Morton o.
    Taussig's o.
    Te Linde o.
    Thomas' o.
    Tuffier's o.
    Twombly's o.
    Twombly-Ulfelder's o.
    Walthardt's o.
    Water's o.
    Watkins' o.
    Watkins-Wertheim o.
    Webster's o.

operation *(continued)*
    Wertheim's o.
    Wertheim-Schauta o.
    Wharton's o.
    Whitacre's o.
    William's o.
    Williams-Richardson o.
    Wylie's o.
orifice
    abdominal o. of uterine
      tube
    hymenal o.
    o. of uterus
os
Oschner's clamp
Osiander's sign
ostium
O'Sullivan-O'Connor
    retractor
    speculum
outlet
    marital o.
ovarian
ovariectomy
ovaries
ovarin
ovariocele
ovariocentesis
ovariocyesis
ovariodysneuria
ovariogenic
ovariohysterectomy
ovarioncus
ovariopathy
ovariorrhexis
ovariosalpingectomy
ovariosteresis
ovariostomy

ovariotestis
ovariotherapy
ovariotomist
ovariotomy
ovariotubal
ovariprival
ovaritis
ovarium
ovarotherapy
ovary
Overstreet's forceps
oviduct
ovoid
    Manchester o.
ovotestis
ovotherapy
ovulation
ovulatory
ovule
    graafian o's.
    Naboth's o's.
    primitive o.
    primordial o.
ovulogenous
ovulum
ovum
    blighted o.
oxytocic
oxytocin
oxyuriasis
Pace's knife
pack
    Bellow's p.
packing
    iodoform gauze p.
Pagano-Levin medium smear
Paget's
    cell

Paget's
    disease
Pajot's
    law
    method
Palmar's dilator
pampiniform
panhysterectomy
panhystero-oophorectomy
panhysterosalpingectomy
panhysterosalpingo-
    oophorectomy
Papanicolaou's
    smear
    stain
papyraceous
para – primipara
para, 0, 1, 2, 3, etc.
paracentesis
paracolpitis
paracolpium
paragomphosis
parametrial
parametric
parametritic
parametritis
parametrium
parasalpingeal
parasalpingitis
paratubal
parauterine
paravaginal
paravaginitis
parenchymatous
parietal
paroophoric
paroophoritis
paroophoron

parous
parovarian
parovariotomy
parovaritis
parovarium
pars
    p. fetalis placentae
    p. uterina placentae
    p. uterina tubae uterinae
partes genitales externae
    muliebres
partes genitales femininae
    externae
parturient
parturifacient
parturiometer
parturition
partus
    p. agrippinus
    p. caesareus
    p. immaturus
    p. maturus
    p. precipitatus
    p. prematurus
    p. serotinus
    p. siccus
patent
Path – pathology
patulous
pavilion
    p. of the oviduct
Pawlik's
    fold
    grip
    triangle
Pean's
    forceps
    operation

Pederson's speculum
pedicle
pediculosis
pedunculated
pelvic
pelvicellulitis
pelvicephalography
pelvicephalometry
pelvicliseometer
pelvifixation
pelvigraph
pelvilithotomy
pelvimeter
    Breisky's p.
    Collin's p.
    Collyer's p.
    DeLee's p.
    Martin's p.
    Thoms' p.
    William's p.
pelvimetry
pelvis
    p. aequabiliter justo
      major
    p. aequabiliter justo
      minor
    android p.
    p. angusta
    anthropoid p.
    beaked p.
    brachypellic p.
    contracted p.
    Deventer's p.
    dolichopellic p.
    funnel-shaped p.
    gynecoid p.
    mesatipellic p.
    Nägele's p.

pelvis *(continued)*
    pithecoid p.
    p. plana
    platypellic p.
    platypelloid p.
    Robert's p.
    rostrate p.
pendulous
Penrose drain
Percy's cautery
Pereyra
    needle
    procedure
perforator
    Blot's p.
    Smellie's p.
pericolpitis
perimetrosalpingitis
perinatal
perineal
perineauxesis
perineocele
perineocolporectomyo-
    mectomy
perineometer
perineoplasty
perineorrhaphy
perineotomy
perineovaginal
perineovaginorectal
perineovulvar
perineum
perioophoritis
perioophorosalpingitis
perioothecitis
perioothecosalpingitis
perisalpingitis
perisalpingo-ovaritis

perisalpinx
peritoneal
peritonealize
peritoneopexy
peritoneum
    parietal p.
peritonitis
periuterine
perivaginal
perivaginitis
per primam
pessary
    cup p.
    diaphragm p.
    doughnut p.
    Emmert-Gellhorn p.
    Gariel's p.
    Gehrung p.
    Gellhorn p.
    gynefold p.
    Hodge's p.
    lever p.
    Menge's p.
    ring p.
    Smith-Hodge p.
    Smith's p.
    stem p.
    Thomas' p.
    Wylie's p.
    Zwanck's p.
Peterson's operation
Pfannenstiel's incision
Phaneuf's
    forceps
    maneuver
phenomenon
    Arias-Stella's p.
    Strassmann's p.

phenylstix
phimosis
    p. vaginalis
phlebitis
phlegmasia
    p. alba dolens
    p. alba dolens
        puerperarum
    cellulitic p.
phototherapy
Picot's speculum
PID — pelvic inflammatory
    disease
pielo-. See words beginning
    pyelo-.
Pinard's
    maneuver
    sign
pio-. See words beginning
    pyo-.
Piper's forceps
Piskacek's sign
pithecoid
pitocin drip
placenta
    accessory p.
    p. accreta
    annular p.
    battledore p.
    bidiscoidal p.
    bilobate p.
    bilobed p.
    p. bipartita
    bipartite p.
    chorioallantoic p.
    choriovitelline p.
    p. circumvallata
    circumvallate p.

placenta *(continued)*
- cirsoid p.
- p. cirsoides
- deciduous p.
- p. diffusa
- p. dimidiata
- dimidiate p.
- discoid p.
- p. discoidea
- duplex p.
- endotheliochorial p.
- epitheliochorial p.
- p. febrilis
- p. fenestrata
- fetal p.
- p. foetalis
- fundal p.
- furcate p.
- hemochorial p.
- hemoendothelial p.
- horseshoe p.
- incarcerated p.
- p. increta
- labyrinthine p.
- lobed p.
- p. marginalis
- p. marginata
- maternal p.
- p. membranacea
- multilobate p.
- multilobed p.
- p. multipartita
- p. nappiformis
- nondeciduous p.
- p. obsoleta
- panduriform p.
- p. panduriformis
- p. percreta

placenta *(continued)*
- p. praevia
- p. praevia centralis
- p. praevia marginalis
- p. praevia partialis
- p. previa
- p. reflexa
- p. reniformis
- retained p.
- Schultze's p.
- p. spuria
- stone p.
- p. succenturiata
- succenturiate p.
- syndesmochorial p.
- p. triloba
- trilobate p.
- p. tripartita
- tripartite p.
- p. triplex
- p. truffée
- p. uterina
- uterine p.
- velamentous p.
- villous p.
- yolk-sac p.
- zonary p.
- zonular p.

placentae
- ablatio p.
- abruptio p.
- abruptio placentae
- marginalis p.

placental

placentation

placentitis

placentocytotoxin

placentogenesis

placentography
placentoid
placentologist
placentology
placentoma
placentopathy
placentotherapy
plaque
platypellic
platypelloid
plethoric
plexus
    Auerbach's p.
    p. cavernosus clitoridis
    cavernous p. of clitoris
    ovarian p.
    p. ovaricus
    pampiniform p.
    p. pampiniformis
    uterine p.
    uterovaginal p.
    p. uterovaginalis
    vaginal p.
    p. venosus vaginalis
    venous p.
plica
    p. rectouterina
plicae ampullares tubae
    uterinae
plicae isthmicae tubae
    uterinae
plicae tubariae tubae
    uterinae
plicae vaginae
plication
PMP — previous menstrual
    period
pneumoamnios

pneumogynecogram
pneumoperitoneum
polycyesis
polycystic
polyhydramnios
polyhypermenorrhea
polyhypomenorrhea
polymenorrhea
polyp
    cervical p.
    endocervical p.
    sessile p.
polypectomy
polypoid
Pomeroy's
    manner
    operation
Porro's
    cesarean section
    hysterectomy
    operation
Porro-Veit operation
portio
    p. supravaginalis cervicis
    p. vaginalis cervicis
position. See also *fetal
   position.*
    dorsal lithotomy p.
    Jonge's p.
    lithotomy p.
    Samuel's p.
    semi-Fowler's p.
    supine p.
    Trendelenburg p.
    Walcher's p.
postabortal
postcoital
post coitum

postmenopausal
postmenstrua
postpartum
Potter's version
pouch
    p. of Douglas
    vesicouterine p.
Pozzi's operation
PPA – phenylpyruvic acid
Prague maneuver
Pratt's dilator
preeclampsia
pregnancy
    afetal p.
    bigeminal p.
    cornual p.
    ectopic p.
    entopic p.
    exochorial p.
    extrauterine p.
    gemellary p.
    heterotopic p.
    hydatid p.
    hysteric p.
    interstitial p.
    intraligamentary p.
    intramural p.
    intraperitoneal p.
    intrauterine p.
    mesenteric p.
    molar p.
    mural p.
    ovarioabdominal p.
    oviducal p.
    parietal p.
    sacrofetal p.
    sacrohysteric p.
    spurious p.

pregnancy *(continued)*
    stump p.
    term p.
    tubal p.
    tuboabdominal p.
    tuboligamentary p.
    tubo-ovarian p.
    tubouterine p.
    uteroabdominal p.
    utero-ovarian p.
    uterotubal p.
pregnanediol level
pregnant
premenarchal
premenstrua
premenstrual
premenstruum
prenatal
prepuce
preputial
preputium
    p. clitoridis
presentation. See also *fetal position.*
    breech p.
    brow p.
    cephalic p.
    compound p.
    face p.
    footling breech p.
    footling p.
    funis p.
    longitudinal p.
    oblique p.
    parietal p.
    pelvic p.
    placental p.
    polar p.

presentation *(continued)*
    shoulder p.
    torso p.
    transverse p.
    trunk p.
    vertex p.
previable
primagravid
primagravida
primipara
primiparity
primiparous
procedure
    Pereyra p.
    Shirodkar p.
    Strap p.
    Temple p.
procidentia
progenital
progestational
progesteroid
progesterone
progestin
progestogen
progestomimetic
progravid
prolapse
    p. of uterus
proliferative
pruritus
Pryor-Pean retractor
pseudocorpus luteum
pseudocyesis
pseudoendometritis
pseudoerosion
pseudomamma
pseudomenstruation
pseudomucin

pseudopregnancy
psoas
psychosis
PU — pregnancy urine
pubocervical
pubovesicocervical
pudendal
pudendum
    p. femininum
    p. muliebre
puerpera
puerperal
puerperalism
puerperant
puerperium
punctiform
Puzo's method
pyelitis
    p. gravidarum
pyelocystitis
pyocolpocele
pyocolpos
pyometra
pyometritis
pyometrium
pyo-ovarium
pyosalpingitis
pyosalpingo-oophoritis
pyosalpingo-oothecitis
pyosalpinx
quadripara
quintipara
rachitic
radium
rakitic. See *rachitic.*
Ramses' diaphragm
Randall's
    curet

Randall's *(continued)*
 sign
 stone forceps
Rasch's sign
rating
 Apgar r.
reaction
 depressive r.
Récamier's
 curet
 operation
rectocele
rectolabial
rectouterine
rectovaginal
regime
 Smith & Smith r.
Reichel's cloacal duct
Reich-Nechtow
 curet
 dilator
retractor
 Balfour's r.
 Brantley-Turner r.
 Deaver's r.
 DeLee's r.
 Doyen's r.
 Eastman's r.
 Emmet's r.
 Friedman's r.
 Gelpi's r.
 Glenner's r.
 Guttmann's r.
 Heaney's r.
 Heaney-Simon r.
 Jackson's r.
 O'Sullivan-O'Connor r.
 Pryor-Pean r.

retractor *(continued)*
 Rigby's r.
 Sims' r.
 Sims-Kelly r.
 Wesson's r.
retrocervical
retrocessed
retrocession
retrodisplacement
retroflexion
retroplacental
retroposition
retrouterine
retroversion
retroverted
Reusner's sign
RFA – right frontoanterior
RFP – right frontoposterior
RFT – right frontotransverse
Rh. factor – Rhesus factor
Rh. neg. – Rhesus factor
 negative
Rh. pos. – Rhesus factor
 positive
Rho-Gam test
Richardson's
 suture
 technique
Ries-Wertheim
 hysterectomy
 operation
Rigby's retractor
ring
 Bandl's r.
 hymenal r.
Ringer's lactate stain
Rinman's sign
Ritgen maneuver

Rizzoli's operation
RMA — right mentoanterior
RMP — right mentoposterior
RMT — right mentotransverse
ROA — right occipitoanterior
Robert's pelvis
Rochester-Carmalt forceps
Rochester-Ochsner forceps
Rochester-Pean forceps
Rock-Mulligan hood
Roederer's obliquity
Rohr's stria
rooming-in
ROP — right occipitoposterior
ROT — right
   occipitotransverse
Rotunda treatment
RSA — right sacroanterior
R. Sc. A. — right
   scapuloanterior
R. Sc. P. — right
   scapuloposterior
RSP — right sacroposterior
RST — right sacrotransverse
rubella
Rubin's
   cannula
   operation
   test
ruga
rugae
   r. of vagina
   r. vaginales
rule
   Arey's r.
   Haase's r.
   His' r.
   Nägele's r.

Russell's forceps
Sabin-Feldman test
sacrouterine
sactosalpinx
Saenger's
   macula
   operation
   suture
Saf-t-coil
saline
Salmon's sign
salpingectomy
salpingemphraxis
salpingian
salpingitic
salpingitis
   chronic interstitial s.
   chronic vegetating s.
   hemorrhagic s.
   hypertrophic s.
   s. isthmica nodosa
   mural s.
   nodular s.
   parenchymatous s.
   s. profluens
   pseudofollicular s.
   purulent s.
   tuberculous s.
salpingocele
salpingocyesis
salpingogram
salpingography
salpingolithiasis
salpingolysis
salpingo-oophorectomy
salpingo-oophoritis
salpingo-oophorocele
salpingo-oothecitis

salpingo-oothecocele
salpingo-ovariectomy
salpingo-ovariotomy
salpingoperitonitis
salpingopexy
salpingoplasty
salpingorrhaphy
salpingostomatomy
salpingostomatoplasty
salpingostomy
salpingotomy
salpinx
Sampson's cyst
Samuel's position
sanguineous
sarcoidosis
    Boeck's s.
sarcoma
Scanzoni's
    maneuver
    operation
Schatz's maneuver
Schauffler's operation
Schaumann's benign
   lymphogranuloma
Schauta's
    operation
    radical vaginal
      hysterectomy
Schauta-Wertheim operation
Schiller's test
Schröder's operation
Schroeder's
    disease
    forceps
    scissors
    syndrome
Schubert's forceps

Schuchardt's
    incision
    operation
Schuller's stain
Schultze's
    mechanism
    method
    placenta
Schuman's method
Schwartz's
    forceps
    hook
Schweizer's forceps
scissors
    Braun's s.
    Doyen's s.
    Emmett's s.
    Ferguson's s.
    Kelly's s.
    Mayo-Harrington s.
    Mayo's s.
    Mayo-Sims s.
    Metzenbaum s.
    Nelson's s.
    Schroeder's s.
    Sims' s.
    umbilical s.
    Waldmann's s.
sclerocystic
sclero-oophoritis
sclero-oothecitis
score
    Apgar s.
    Silverman's s.
Scully's tumor
secretory
section
    cesarean s.

section *(continued)*
>   cesarean s., cervical
>   cesarean s., classic
>   cesarean s., corporeal
>   cesarean s., extraperitoneal
>   cesarean s., Kerr's
>   cesarean s., Kronig's
>   cesarean s., Latzko's
>   cesarean s., low
>   cesarean s., Porro's
>   cesarean s., transperitoneal
>   cesarean s., transverse
>   cesarean s., Water's
>   frozen s.

secundigravida
secundina
secundinae
secundine
secundipara
secundiparity
secundiparous
sefalo-. See words beginning *cephalo-.*
Segond's
>   forceps
>   spatula

semen
semi-Fowler's position
seminoma
>   ovarian s.

Senn forceps
sepsis
>   puerperal s.

septate
septicemia
septigravida

septum
>   s. corporum cavernosorum clitoridis
>   placental s.
>   rectovaginal s.
>   s. rectovesicale

serocystoma
serosa
serosal
serosanguineous
serous
Sertoli-Leydig cell tumor
serviko-. See words beginning *cervico-.*
sessile
sextigravida
sextipara
Sheehan's syndrome
shield
>   dacron s.
>   Dalkon s.

Shirodkar
>   needle
>   operation
>   procedure

Shorr's stain
sign
>   Ahlfeld's s.
>   Arnoux's s.
>   Beccaria's s.
>   Beclard's s.
>   Bolt's s.
>   Braun-Fernwald s.
>   Braxton-Hicks s.
>   Chadwick's s.
>   Cullen's s.
>   Danforth's s.
>   Dewees' s.

sign *(continued)*
  Gauss' s.
  Golden's s.
  Goodell's s.
  Halban's s.
  Hegar's s.
  Hicks' s.
  Hoehne's s.
  Jacquemier's s.
  Kanter's s.
  Kergaradec's s.
  Kustner's s.
  Ladin's s.
  Landou's s.
  Mayor's s.
  Olshausen's s.
  Osiander's s.
  Pinard's s.
  Piskacek's s.
  Randall's s.
  Rasch's s.
  Reusner's s.
  Rinman's s.
  Salmon's s.
  Spalding's s.
  Tarnier's s.
  Von Fernwald's s.
Silverman's score
Simmond's speculum
Simon's operation
Simpson-Luikart forceps
Simpson's
  forceps
  sound
Sims-Huhner test
Sims-Kelly retractor
Sims'
  curet

Sims' *(continued)*
  retractor
  scissors
  sound
  speculum
sinografin
skeletonized
Skene's
  curet
  duct
  forceps
  gland
smear
  buccal s.
  Nickerson's medium s.
  Pagano-Levin medium s.
  Papanicolaou's s.
smegma
  s. clitoridis
  s. embryonum
Smellie's
  method
  perforator
Smith-Hodge pessary
Smith's
  forceps
  pessary
Smith & Smith regime
sois. See *psoas.*
Somers' forceps
sonogram
sound
  Simpson's s.
  Sims' s.
  uterine s.
Spalding-Richardson
  hysterectomy
  operation

Spalding's sign
spatula
 Segond's s.
 Tauber's s.
speculum
 Auvard-Remine s.
 Auvard's weighted s.
 Berlind-Auvard s.
 Brewer's s.
 Collin's s.
 Cusco's s.
 Devilbiss' s.
 Devilbiss-Stacey s.
 duck-billed s.
 Fergusson's s.
 Garrigue's s.
 Graves' s.
 Guttmann's s.
 Henrotin's s.
 Huffman-Graves s.
 Jonas-Graves s.
 Kahn-Graves s.
 Mason-Auvard s.
 Mayer's s.
 Miller's s.
 Nott's s.
 O'Sullivan-O'Connor s.
 Pederson's s.
 Picot's s.
 Simmond's s.
 Sims' s.
 weighted s.
 Weisman-Graves s.
 wire bivalve s.
sphincter
 s. vaginae
Spinelli's operation

spray
 dermoplast s.
squamocolumnar
stain
 Feulgen s.
 Lugol's s.
 Papanicolaou's s.
 Ringer's lactate s.
 Schuller's s.
 Shorr's s.
Starlinger's dilator
Staude-Moore forceps
Staude's forceps
Stein-Leventhal syndrome
stellate
stenosis
stent
 foam rubber vaginal s.
sterility
sterilization
Steri-strips
stick
 sponge s.
stillbirth
stillborn
Stockholm box
strap
 Montgomery s.
Strap procedure
Strassman-Jones operation
Strassmann's phenomenon
stria
 Langhans' s.
 Rohr's s.
striae
striae gravidarum
stricture

Stroganoff's treatment
    (Stroganov's)
stroma
       ovarian s.
       s. ovarii
       s. of ovary
stromal
study
       air s.
       cytogenetic s.
Sturmdorf's
    operation
    suture
stylet
subinvolution
submucous
subserous
subumbilical
subvesical
sudo-. See words beginning
    pseudo-.
suit
       Fletcher's s.
sulcus
Sulkowich's test
supernumerary
suprapubic
surgical procedures. See
    operations.
suspension
suture
       angle s.
       baseball s.
       ethilon s.
       Richardson's s.
       Saenger's s.
       Sturmdorf's s.
Swiss-cheese endometrium

symphysis
    s. pubica
    s. pubis
synchondrosis
syncopal
syncytial
syncytioma
syncytiotoxin
syndrome
       Achard-Thiers s.
       Ahumada-Del Castillo s.
       Allen-Masters s.
       Asherman's s.
       Brentano's s.
       Chiari-Frommel s.
       Couvelaire's s.
       Curtius' s.
       Dubovitz's s.
       Fitz-Hugh's s.
       Fritsch-Asherman s.
       Gordan-Overstreet s.
       Klinefelter's s.
       Klotz's s.
       Mayer-Rokitansky-
         Küster s.
       Meigs' s.
       Meigs-Cass s.
       Schroeder's s.
       Sheehan's s.
       Stein-Leventhal s.
       Turner's s.
       Young's s.
       Youssef's s.
synechia
    s. vulvae
synechiae
syo-. See words beginning
    cyo-

syphilis
tampon
    Dührssen's t.
tandem
Tarnier's
    forceps
    sign
Tauber's spatula
Taussig-Morton operation
Taussig's operation
Teale's forceps
technique
    Brandt's t.
    Richardson's t.
telangiectatic
telangiecteric
Te Linde operation
Temple procedure
tenaculum
    Adair's t.
    Barrett's t.
    Braun's t.
    DeLee's t.
    Duplay's t.
    Jacobs' t.
    Kahn's t.
    marlex atraumatic t.
    sharp toothed t.
teratoma
teratome
tertipara
tertigravida
test
    agglutination inhibition
      t.
    Aschheim-Zondek t.
    benzidine t.
    Brouha's t.

test *(continued)*
    chorionic gonadotropin
      t.
    Coombs' t.
    Corner-Allen t.
    cross-matching t.
    dexamethasone
      suppression t.
    Dienst's t.
    Farris' t.
    fibrindex t.
    Friedman-Lapham t.
    Friedman's t.
    frog t.
    Galli-Mainini t.
    gravindex t.
    Hogben's t.
    Huhner's t.
    immunologic t.
    Kapeller-Adler t.
    Kline's flocculation t.
    Kupperman's t.
    Marchetti t.
    nitrazine t.
    Norethindrone t.
    Norethynodrel t.
    progesterone
      withdrawal t.
    Rho-Gam t.
    Rubin's t.
    Sabin-Feldman t.
    Schiller's t.
    Sims-Huhner t.
    Sulkowich's t.
    Thorn t.
    thymol turbidity t.
    toad t.
    ultrasound t.

test *(continued)*
    Visscher-Bowman t.
    Von-Pohle's t.
    Wampole's t.
    Wilson's t.
    Xenopus laevis t.
testiculoma
    t. ovarii
theca
    t. folliculi
    t. lutein
thecoma
thecomatosin
thecosis
Thomas'
    curet
    operation
    pessary
Thoms'
    forceps
    pelvimeter
Thoms-Allis forceps
Thoms-Gaylor forceps
Thorn test
Tischler's forceps
tissue
    endometrial t.
    interstitial t.
titer
    rubella t.
topography
torsion
tortuosity
Touhey's needle
towel clamp
    Backhaus t. c.
toxemia

trachelectomy
trachelitis
tracheloplasty
trachelorrhaphy
trachelosyringorrhaphy
trachelotomy
traction handle
    Barton's t. h.
    Bill's t. h.
    Luikart-Bill t. h.
transplacental
transvaginal
treatment
    Brandt's t.
    Elliott t.
    Rotunda t.
    Stroganoff's t.
      (Stroganov's)
Trendelenburg position
triangle
    Pawlik's t.
Trichomonas vaginalis
trimester
trisomy
trocar
trophoblast
tube
    fallopian t.
    uterine t.
tuboabdominal
tuboadnexopexy
tuboligamentous
tubo-ovarian
tubo-ovariotomy
tubo-ovaritis
tuboperitoneal
tuboplasty
tubouterine

tubovaginal
Tucker-McLean forceps
Tuffier's operation
tumor
    Brenner's t.
    corticoadrenal t.
    Grawitz's t.
    hypernephroid t.
    Krukenberg's t.
    mesenchymal t.
    Scully's t.
    Sertoli-Leydig cell t.
    theca-cell t.
    Wilms' t.
tunica
    t. mucosa tubae uterinae
    t. mucosa urethrae
      femininae
    t. mucosa urethrae
      muliebris
    t. mucosa uteri
    t. mucosa vaginae
    t. muscularis cervicis
      uteri
    t. muscularis tubae
      uterinae
    t. muscularis urethrae
      femininae
    t. muscularis urethrae
      muliebris
    t. muscularis uteri
    t. muscularis vaginae
    t. serosa tubae uterinae
    t. serosa uteri
Turner's syndrome
Twombly's operation
Twombly-Ulfelder's operation
ulcus

ulcus *(continued)*
    u. phagedaenicum
      corrodens
    u. vulvae acutum
umbilical
umbilicus
    amniotic u.
    decidual u.
unengaged
unicollis
unicornate
unicornis
unit
    Bovie u.
uremia
    puerperal u.
ureter
ureterouterine
ureterovaginal
urethra
    u. feminina
    u. muliebris
urethral
urethrocele
urethrovaginal
urethrovesical
urinary
urogenital
uteralgia
uterectomy
uteri
    fibromyomata u.
uterine
uterismus
uteritis
uteroabdominal
uterocentesis
uterocervical

uterodynia
uterofixation
uterogestation
uterography
uterolith
uteromania
uterometer
uterometry
utero-ovarian
uteropexy
uteroplacental
uteroplasty
uterorectal
uterosacral
uterosalpingography
uteroscope
uterothermometry
uterotomy
uterotonic
uterotropic
uterotubal
uterotubography
uterovaginal
uteroventral
uterovesical
uterus
    u. acollis
    arcuate u.
    u. arcuatus
    u. bicornis
    bicornuate u.
    u. biforis
    u. bilocularis
    u. bipartitus
    bosselated u.
    cochleate u.
    u. cordiformis
    Couvelaire u.

uterus *(continued)*
    u. didelphys
    duplex u.
    u. duplex
    fetal u.
    gravid u.
    u. incudiformis
    u. masculinus
    u. parvicollis
    pubescent u.
    u. septus
    u. simplex
    u. unicornis
utriculoplasty
vagina
vaginal
vaginalectomy
vaginalis
    Trichomonas v.
vaginalitis
vaginapexy
vaginate
vaginectomy
vaginicoline
vaginiperineotomy
vaginismus
vaginitis
    v. adhaesiva
    catarrhal v.
    diphtheritic v.
    emphysematous v.
    glandular v.
    granular v.
    monilial v.
    papulous v.
    senile v.
    Trichomonas v.
vaginoabdominal

vaginocele
vaginocutaneous
vaginodynia
vaginofixation
vaginogenic
vaginogram
vaginography
vaginolabial
vaginometer
vaginomycosis
vaginopathy
vaginoperineal
vaginoperineorrhaphy
vaginoperineotomy
vaginoperitoneal
vaginopexy
vaginoplasty
vaginoscope
vaginoscopy
vaginotome
vaginotomy
vaginovesical
vaginovulvar
vagitus
    v. uterinus
    v. vaginalis
Valsuani's disease
Van-Doren forceps
Van Hoorn's maneuver
varicocele
    ovarian v.
    utero-ovarian v.
vasa praevia
vasa propria of Jungbluth
vault
    vaginal v.
vectis
vein

vein
    ovarian v.
velamentous
velamentum
ventrofixation
ventrohysteropexy
ventrovesicofixation
vernix
Verres' needle
verruca
    v. acuminata
version
    bipolar v.
    Braxton-Hicks v.
    cephalic v.
    Hicks' v.
    podalic v.
    Potter's v.
    Wigand's v.
    Wright's v.
vertex
vesicle
    Baer's v.
    chorionic v.
    graafian v's.
    Naboth's v's.
vesicocervical
vesicouterine
vesicouterovaginal
vesicovaginal
vesicovaginorectal
vesiculae graafianae
vesiculae nabothi
vestibule
    urogenital v.
    v. of vagina
vestibuli vaginae
vestibulourethral

vestibulum
    v. vaginae
viability
viable
vibrio
vibrodilator
villi
villus
Vim-Silverman needle
visceral
Visscher-Bowman test
vitiligo
Von Fernwald's sign
Von-Pohle's test
Voorhees' bag
Voorhes' needle
vulva
    v. clausa
    v. conivens
    v. hians
vulval
vulvar
vulvectomy
vulvismus
vulvitis
    v. blenorrhagica
    creamy v.
    diabetic v.
    diphtheric v.
    diphtheritic v.
    eczematiform v.
    follicular v.
    leukoplakic v.
    pseudoleukoplakic v.
    ulcerative v.
vulvocrural
vulvopathy
vulvorectal

vulvouterine
vulvovaginal
vulvovaginitis
Walcher's position
Waldmann's scissors
Walthard's cell
Walthardt's operation
Walton's forceps
Walton-Schubert forceps
Wampole's test
Water's
    cesarean section
    operation
Watkins' operation
Watkins-Wertheim operation
Watson's method
Webster's operation
Weisman-Graves speculum
Weisman's forceps
Wertheim-Cullen forceps
Wertheim's
    forceps
    operation
    radical hysterectomy
Wertheim-Schauta operation
Wesson's retractor
WF — white female
Wharton's operation
Whitacre's operation
Wigand's
    maneuver
    version
Willet's clamp
Willett's forceps
William's
    operation
    pelvimeter
Williams-Richardson operation

Wilms' tumor
Wilson's test
Wittner's forceps
wolffian
> w. cyst
> w. duct

Wright's version
Wurd's catheter
Wylie's
> dilator
> operation
> pessary

Xenopus laevis test
xeromenia
Yellan clamp
Yeoman's forceps
Young's syndrome
Youssef's syndrome
zeromeneah. See
> *xeromenia.*

Zwanck's pessary
Zweifel-DeLee cranioclast
zygosity

OPHTHALMOLOGY

Abadie's sign
abducens
abduction
ab externus
abiotrophy
    retinal a.
ablatio
    a. retinae
ablepharia
ablepharon
ablepharous
ablephary
ablepsia
ablepsy
abrader
    Howard's a.
abrasio
    a. corneae
abscessus
    a. siccus corneae
abscission
    corneal a.
Acc. — accommodation
accommodation
    absolute a.
    binocular a.
    excessive a.
    negative a.
    positive a.
    relative a.

accommodation
    subnormal a.
achlys
achroacytosis
achromatopia
achromatopic
achromatopsia
achromatosis
acne
    a. ciliaris
acorea
acuity
adaptation
    retinal a.
adaptometer
adduction
adenocarcinoma
adenologaditis
adenophthalmia
Adie's syndrome
aditus
    a. orbitae
adnexa
    a. oculi
Aebli's scissors
affakia. See *aphakia.*
Agamodistomum
    A. ophthalmobium
Agnew's
    keratome

Agnew's
    operation
agnosia
    visual a.
Agrikola's retractor
akinesia
    O'Brien a.
    Van-Lint a.
akinesis
akinetic
aklis. See *achlys.*
aknephascopia
akro-. See words beginning
    achro-.
alacrima
albedo
    a. retinae
albinism
albuginea
    a. oculi
albugo
alexia
    optical a.
alopecia
    a. orbicularis
Alström-Olsen syndrome
amaurosis
    albuminuric a.
    Burns's a.
    cat's eye a.
    central a.
    a. centralis
    cerebral a.
    congenital a.
    diabetic a.
    a. fugax
    hysteric a.
    intoxication a.

amaurosis *(continued)*
    Leber's a.
    saburral a.
    uremic a.
amaurotic
ambiopia
amblyopia
    a. alcoholica
    arsenic a.
    astigmatic a.
    a. crapulosa
    a. cruciata
    a. ex anopsia
    nocturnal a.
    postmarital a.
    quinine a.
    traumatic a.
    uremic a.
amblyopiatrics
amblyoscope
ametrometer
ametropia
    axial a.
    curvature a.
    index a.
    position a.
    refractive a.
ametropic
Amh. − mixed astigmatism
    with myopia
    predominating
Ammon's operation
amotio
    a. retinae
amphamphoterodiplopia
amplitude
    a. of accommodation
    a. of convergence

ampulla
    a. canaliculi lacrimalis
    a. ductus lacrimalis
ampullae
Amsler's needle
Anagnostakis' operation
anaphoria
Andogsky's syndrome
anesthesia
    carbocaine a.
    general a.
    holocaine a.
    intubation a.
    ophthaine a.
Angelucci's syndrome
angiodiathermy
angioma
angiomatosis
    a. of retina
angiophakomatosis
angle
    kappa a.
anhidrosis
aniridia
aniseikonia
aniseikonic
anisoaccommodation
anisocoria
anisometrope
anisometropia
anisometropic
anisophoria
anisopia
ankyloblepharon
    a. filiforme adnatum
annular
    a. plexus
annulus

annulus *(continued)*
    a. ciliaris
    a. zinnii
anomalopia
anomaloscope
anomaly
    Peters' a.
anoopsia
anophoria
anophthalmia
anophthalmos
anophthalmus
anopia
anopsia
anorthopia
anotropia
Anthony's compressor
anthrax
Anton-Babinski syndrome
anulus
    a. of conjunctiva
    a. conjunctivae
    a. iridis major
    a. iridis minor
    a. tendineus communis
aphakia
aphakic
aphasia
    visual a.
aplasia
    retinal a.
applanation
applicator
    Gifford's a.
aqueous
    a. humor
aquocapsulitis
arachnodactyly

arachnoiditis
    optochiasmatic a.
ARC — anomalous retinal
  correspondence
arch
    Salus' a.
arcus
    a. juvenilis
    a. lipoides corneae
    a. palpebralis inferior
    a. palpebralis superior
    a. parieto-occipitalis
    a. senilis
    a. superciliaris
argamblyopia
argema
Argyll-Robertson pupil
argyria
argyrosis
Arlt-Jaesche operation
Arlt's
    disease
    operation
    scoop
    trachoma
Arruga's
    expressor
    forceps
    operation
    protector
    trephine
arteriola
    a. macularis inferior
    a. macularis superior
    a. medialis retinae
    a. nasalis retinae inferior
    a. nasalis retinae
      superior

arteriola *(continued)*
    a. temporalis retinae
      inferior
    a. temporalis retinae
      superior
arteriole
    medial a. of retina
    nasal a. of retina
    temporal a. of retina
artery
    cilioretinal a.
    hyaloid a.
    long posterior ciliary a.
    posterior conjunctival a.
    short posterior ciliary a.
As. H. — hypermetropic
  astigmatism
As. M. — myopic astigmatism
Ast. — astigmatism
asthenocoria
asthenometer
asthenope
asthenopia
    accommodative a.
    muscular a.
    nervous a.
    retinal a.
    tarsal a.
asthenopic
astigmagraph
astigmatic
astigmatism
    a. against the rule
    corneal a.
    hypermetropic a.
    hyperopic a.
    lenticular a.
    myopic a.

astigmatism *(continued)*
    oblique a.
      a. with the rule
astigmatometer
astigmatoscope
astigmatoscopy
astigmia
astigmic
astigmometer
astigmometry
astigmoscope
Atkinson's technique
atresia
    a. iridis
atrophy
    Behr's a.
    Fuchs' a.
    Schnabel's a.
atropia
    a. choroideae et retinae
    a. dolorosa
    a. gyrata of choroid
atropinism
atropinization
autokeratoplasty
axanthopsia
Axenfeld's syndrome
axis
    optic a.
    visual a.
bacillus
    Koch-Weeks b.
Badal's operation
Baer's nystagmus
Bahr's spud
Ballet's disease
Bamatter's syndrome

Barany's sign
Bardelli's operation
Bard-Parker
    blade
    knife
Barkan's
    knife
    operation
Barraquer-DeWecker scissors
Barraquer's
    brush
    erysiphake
    forceps
    needle holder
    operation
    speculum
Barrio's operation
Bassen-Kornzweig syndrome
Basterra's operation
Batten-Mayou disease
Beal's
    conjunctivitis
    syndrome
Beaupre's forceps
Beaver's
    blade
    handle
    keratome
    knife
Beer's collyrium
Behçet's syndrome
Behr's
    atrophy
    disease
    syndrome
Bekhterev's nystagmus
Bellows' cryoextractor

Bell's
    erysiphake
    palsy
    phenomenon
Benedikt's syndrome
Bennett's forceps
Benson's disease
Berens'
    dilator
    forceps
    implant
    keratome
    operation
    punch
    retractor
    scissors
    spatula
    speculum
Bergemeister's papilla
Berke's forceps
Berlin's
    disease
    edema
Berneheimer's fibers
Biber-Haab-Dimmer
  degeneration
Bielschowsky-Lutz-Cogan
  syndrome
Bielschowsky's
    disease
    operation
    test
Bietti's
    dystrophy
    syndrome
bifocal
binocular
binoculus

binophthalmoscope
binoscope
biomicroscopy
Birch-Hirschfeld lamp
Bishop-Harmon
    cannula
    forceps
Bitot's spots
Bjerrum's
    scotoma
    scotometer
    screen
blade
    Bard-Parker b.
    Beaver's b.
    McPherson-Wheeler b.
Blasius' operation
Blaskovics' operation
Blatt's operation
blef-. See words beginning
   bleph-.
blennorrhea
    b. neonatorum
blepharadenitis
blepharal
blepharectomy
blepharelosis
blepharism
blepharitis
    b. angularis
    b. ciliaris
    b. marginalis
    b. squamosa
    b. ulcerosa
blepharoadenitis
blepharoadenoma
blepharoatheroma
blepharochalasis

blepharochromidrosis
blepharoclonus
blepharoconjunctivitis
blepharodiastasis
blepharoncus
blepharopachynsis
blepharophimosis
blepharophryplasty
blepharoplast
blepharoplasty
blepharoplegia
blepharoptosis
blepharopyorrhea
blepharorrhaphy
blepharospasm
blepharosphincterectomy
blepharostat
blepharostenosis
blepharosynechia
blepharotomy
blepharoxysis
Blessig-Iwanoff cyst
Blessig's cyst
blind
    color b.
blindness
    amnesic color b.
    Bright's b.
    color b.
    cortical psychic b.
    snow b.
    twilight b.
block
    O'Brien b.
    retrobulbar b.
    Van-Lint b.
blow-out fracture
body

body *(continued)*
    ciliary b.
    Landolt's b's.
    Prowazek-Greeff b's.
Bohm's operation
Bonaccolto's
    forceps
    scleral ring
Bonnet-Dechaume-Blanc
  syndrome
Bonn's forceps
Bonzel's operation
Borthen's operation
Bossalino's operation
Bourneville's disease
Bovie unit
Bowen's disease
Bowman's
    membrane
    needle
    probe
Boynton's needle holder
Bracken's forceps
Braid's strabismus
Brailey's operation
Brawley's retractor
Briggs' operation
Bright's
    blindness
    eye
Bruch's membrane
Brucke's
    fibers
    lens
    muscle
Bruecke
    tunica nervea of B.
brush

brush *(continued)*
>Barraquer's b.
>Haidinger's b's.

Brushfield's spot
Budinger's operation
bulbus
>b. oculi

Buller's shield
Bumke's pupil
bundle
>b. of Drualt

Bunge's spoon
buphthalmia
buphthalmos
buphthalmus
bur
>Burwell's b.

Burch-Greenwood tucker
Burch's
>caliper
>pick

Burns's amaurosis
Burwell's bur
Buzzi's operation
byerrum. See *Bjerrum.*
Calhoun-Merz needle
Calhoun's needle
caliculus
>c. ophthalmicus

caligo
>c. corneae
>c. lentis
>c. pupillae

caliper
>Burch's c.
>Castroviejo's c.
>Green's c.
>Jameson's c.

caliper
>Thorpe's c.

Campbell's retractor
campimeter
campimetry
canal
>Ferrein's c.
>hyaloid c.
>Petit's c.
>c. of Schlemm

canaliculi
canaliculitis
canaliculus
>c. lacrimalis

cannula
>Bishop-Harmon c.
>Castroviejo's c.
>Goldstein's c.
>Moncrieff's c.
>Randolph's c.
>Roper's c.
>Tenner's c.

canthectomy
canthi
canthitis
cantholysis
canthoplasty
canthorrhaphy
canthotomy
canthus
capsitis
capsula
>c. lentis

capsule
>c. of Tenon

capsulectomy
capsulitis
capsulolenticular

capsulotome
    Darling's c.
capsulotomy
Carter's
    introducer
    operation
caruncle
    lacrimal c.
caruncula
    c. lacrimalis
Casanellas' operation
Caspar's ring opacity
Castallo's retractor
Castroviejo-Arruga forceps
Castroviejo-Kalt needle holder
Castroviejo's
    caliper
    cannula
    dilator
    forceps
    keratome
    knife
    needle holder
    operation
    punch
    retractor
    scissors
    spatula
    speculum
    trephine
cataphoria
cataract
    adherent c.
    adolescent c.
    after c.
    arborescent c.
    aridosiliculose c.
    aridosiliquate c.

cataract *(continued)*
    axial c.
    blue dot c.
    bony c.
    bottlemakers' c.
    calcareous c.
    capsular c.
    capsulolenticular c.
    caseous c.
    cerulean c.
    cheesy c.
    choroidal c.
    congenital c.
    contusion c.
    coralliform c.
    coronary c.
    cortical c.
    cupuloform c.
    discission c.
    dry-shelled c.
    embryonal nuclear c.
    fibroid c.
    floriform c.
    fusiform c.
    glassblowers' c.
    glaucomatous c.
    heat-ray c.
    hedger's c.
    heterochromic c.
    hypermature c.
    immature c.
    incipient c.
    infantile c.
    intumescent c.
    irradiation c.
    juvenile c.
    Koby's c.
    lacteal c.

cataract *(continued)*
    lamellar c.
    lenticular c.
    lightning c.
    mature c.
    membranous c.
    morgagnian c.
    myotonic c.
    naphthalinic c.
    nuclear c.
    O'Brien's c.
    overripe c.
    perinuclear c.
    peripheral c.
    polar c.
    puddler's c.
    punctate c.
    pyramidal c.
    reduplication c.
    ripe c.
    sanguineous c.
    sedimentary c.
    senile c.
    siliculose c.
    siliquose c.
    snowflake c.
    snowstorm c.
    spindle c.
    stationary c.
    stellate c.
    subcapsular c.
    sunflower c.
    sutural c.
    syphilitic c.
    traumatic c.
    tremulous c.
    unripe c.
    Vogt's c.

cataract
    zonular c.
cataracta
    c. accreta
    c. brunescens
    c. cerulea
    c. complicata
    c. congenita
        membranacea
    c. coronaria
    c. electrica
    c. membranacea accreta
    c. neurodermatica
    c. nigra
    c. ossea
    c. syndermotica
cataractous
catarrh
    vernal c.
cautery
    Hildreth's c.
    Mueller's c.
    Rommel-Hildreth c.
    Rommel's c.
    Scheie's c.
    von-Graefe's c.
    Wadsworth-Todd c.
    Ziegler's c.
cecocentral
Celsus' operation
centrocecal
cerebro-ocular
CF – counting fingers
chalazia
chalazion
chalcosis
    c. lentis
chamber

chamber *(continued)*
    anterior c.
    aqueous c.
    posterior c. of eye
    vitreous c.
Chandler's forceps
chart
    Reuss's color c's.
    Snellen's c.
chemosis
Cheyne's nystagmus
chiasma
    c. opticum
chiasma syndrome
chiasmal
    c. arachnoiditis
chloropsia
choriocapillaris
choriocele
chorioid
chorioidea
chorioretinal
chorioretinitis
chorioretinopathy
choroid
choroidal
choroidea
choroideremia
choroiditis
    areolar c.
    Doyne's c.
    Förster's c.
    c. guttata senilis
    juxtapapillitic c.
    c. myopica
    c. serosa
    syphilitic c.
    Tay's c.

choroiditis
    toxoplasmic c.
choroidocyclitis
choroidoiritis
choroidopathy
choroidoretinitis
chromatopsia
chromatoptometer
cibisotome
cicatricial
cicatrix
cilia
ciliariscope
ciliarotomy
ciliary
    c. body
    c. muscle
    c. process
    c. vein
    c. zonule
ciliectomy
cilioretinal
    c. artery
    c. vein
cilioscleral
cilium
cillosis
circle
    Willis' c.
circlet
    Zinn's c.
Claude's syndrome
Coat's
    disease
    retinitis
    ring
Cogan's
    dystrophy

Cogan's
    syndrome
collarette
collyria
collyrium
    Beer's c.
coloboma
    c. of choroid
    Fuchs's c.
    c. iridis
    c. of iris
    c. lentis
    c. lobuli
    c. of optic nerve
    c. palpebrale
    c. retinae
    c. of vitreous
commissura
    c. palpebrarum lateralis
    c. palpebrarum medialis
    c. superior Meynerti
commissurae supraopticae
commissure
    arcuate c.
    Gudden's c.
    interthalamic c.
    Meynert's c.
    optic c.
    palpebral c.
    posterior c., chiasmatic
    supraoptic c's.
commotio
    c. retinae
compressor
    Anthony's c.
conclination
conformer
    Fox's c.

conjugate
conjunctiva
conjunctival
conjunctiviplasty
conjunctivitis
    actinic c.
    anaphylactic c.
    arc-flash c.
    Beal's c.
    blennorrheal c.
    calcareous c.
    croupous c.
    diphtheritic c.
    diplobacillary c.
    Egyptian c.
    Elschnig's c.
    c. medicamentosa
    meningococcus c.
    molluscum c.
    Morax-Axenfeld c.
    c. necroticans infectiosus
    Parinaud's c.
    Pascheff's c.
    c. petrificans
    phlyctenular c.
    prairie c.
    pseudomembranous c.
    Samoan c.
    Sanyal's c.
    Scrofular c.
    squirrel plague c.
    trachomatous c.
    c. tularensis
    uratic c.
    vernal c.
    welder's c.
    Widmark's c.
    Wucherer's c.

conjunctivoma
conjunctivoplasty
conoid
    Sturm's c.
conophthalmus
consensual
Contino's
    epithelioma
    glaucoma
conus
convergence
convergent
convergiometer
copiopia
Coquille plano lens
Corbett's spud
coreclisis
corectasis
corectome
corectomedialysis
corectomy
corectopia
coredialysis
corediastasis
corelysis
coremorphosis
corenclisis
coreometer
coreometry
coreoplasty
corestenoma
coretomedialysis
coretomy
cornea
    conical c.
    c. farinata
    c. globosa
    c. guttata

cornea *(continued)*
    c. opaca
    c. plana
    sugar-loaf c.
    Vogt's c.
corneal
corneitis
corneoblepharon
corneoiritis
corneosclera
corneoscleral
corona
    c. ciliaris
    Zinn's c.
coroparelcysis
coroplasty
coroscopy
corotomy
corpus
    c. adiposum orbitae
    c. ciliaris
    c. vitreum
correspondence
    anomalous retinal c.
    harmonious retinal c.
    retinal c.
cortex
    c. lentis
couching
Crede's prophylaxis
crises
    Pel's c's.
Critchett's operation
Crookes' lens
Crouzon's disease
cryoextraction
cryoextractor
    Bellows' c.

cryogenic
cryophake
cryoptor
> Thomas' c.

cryostat
cryosurgery
cryptoglioma
cryptophthalmia
cryptophthalmos
cryptophthalmus
crystalline
Csapody's operation
cul-de-sac
> conjunctival c.

Curdy's sclerotome
curette
> Gifford's c.
> Green's c.
> Heath's c.
> Meyhoeffer's c.
> Skeele's c.

cyanosis
> c. bulbi
> c. retinae

cyclectomy
cyclicotomy
cyclitis
> heterochromic c.
> purulent c.
> serous c.

cycloanemization
cycloceratitis
cyclochoroiditis
cyclodamia
cyclodialysis
cyclodiathermy
cycloduction
cycloelectrolysis

cyclogram
cyclokeratitis
cyclopentolate
cyclophoria
cyclophorometer
cyclopia
cycloplegia
cycloplegic
cycloscope
cyclotome
cyclotomy
cyclotropia
cylicotomy
cylindrical
cyst
> Blessig-Iwanoff c's.
> Blessig's c's.
> meibomian c.

cystitome
cystitomy
cystotome
> von Graefe's c.
> Wheeler's c.

Czermak's operation
dacryadenalgia
dacryadenitis
dacryadenoscirrhus
dacryagogatresia
dacryagogic
dacryagogue
dacrycystalgia
dacrycystitis
dacryelcosis
dacryoadenalgia
dacryoadenectomy
dacryoadenitis
dacryoblennorrhea
dacryocanaliculitis

dacryocele
dacryocyst
dacryocystalgia
dacryocystectasia
dacryocystectomy
dacryocystis
    phlegmonous d.
    syphilitic d.
    trachomatous d.
    tuberculous d.
dacryocystitis
dacryocystitome
dacryocystoblennorrhea
dacryocystocele
dacryocystoptosis
dacryocystorhinostenosis
dacryocystorhinostomy
dacryocystorhinotomy
dacryocystostenosis
dacryocystostomy
dacryocystosyringotomy
dacryocystotome
dacryocystotomy
dacryogenic
dacryohelcosis
dacryohemorrhea
dacryolin
dacryolith
    Desmarres' d.
dacryolithiasis
dacryoma
dacryon
dacryops
dacryopyorrhea
dacryopyosis
dacryorhinocystotomy
dacryorrhea
dacryosinusitis

dacryosolenitis
dacryostenosis
dacryosyrinx
Dalrymple's
    disease
    sign
Darling's capsulotome
Daviel's
    operation
    scoop
    spoon
Davis'
    forceps
    knife needle
    spud
debrider
    Sauer's d.
declination
degeneration
    Biber-Haab-Dimmer d.
    Kozlowski's d.
    Vogt's d.
de Grandmont's operation
dehiscence
    iris d.
Dejean's syndrome
delacrimation
Del Toro's operation
Demours' membrane
deorsumduction
deorsumvergence
deorsumversion
Derf's needle holder
dermolipoma
Descartes' law
Descemet's membrane
descemetitis
descemetocele

Desmarres'
   dacryolith
   forceps
   law
   lid elevator
   retractor
   scarifier
detachment
   d. of retina
   retinal d.
deutan
deuteranomalopia
deuteranopia
deviation
   primary d.
   secondary d.
   Skew's d.
Devic's disease
DeVilbiss' irrigator
DeWecker-Pritikin scissors
DeWecker's
   operation
   scissors
dextroclination
dextrocular
dextrocularity
dextrocycloduction
dextrocycloversion
dextroduction
dextrotorsion
dextroversion
dialysis
   d. retinae
diastasis
   iris d.
dichromatopsia
diktyoma
dilator

dilator *(continued)*
   Berens' d.
   Castroviejo's d.
   Heath's d.
   Jones' d.
   Muldoon's d.
   Nettleship-Wilder d.
Dimitry-Bell erysiphake
Dimitry's erysiphake
Dimitry-Thomas erysiphake
Dimmer's keratitis
dimple
   Fuchs' d's.
diopsimeter
diopter
   prism d.
dioptometer
dioptometry
dioptoscopy
dioptre
dioptric
dioptrics
dioptrometer
dioptrometry
dioptroscopy
dioptry
diplopia
   binocular d.
   heteronymous d.
   homonymous d.
   monocular d.
   paradoxical d.
   torsional d.
diplopiometer
diploscope
discission
disclination
disease

disease *(continued)*
- Arlt's d.
- Ballet's d.
- Batten-Mayou d.
- Behr's d.
- Benson's d.
- Berlin's d.
- Bielschowsky's d.
- Bourneville's d.
- Bowen's d.
- Coats' d.
- Crouzon's d.
- Dalrymple's d.
- Devic's d.
- Eales' d.
- Favre's d.
- Franceschetti's d.
- Gaucher's d.
- Graefe's d.
- Graves' d.
- Hand-Schüller-Christian d.
- Harada's d.
- Heerfordt's d.
- Hippel's d.
- Jensen's d.
- Kimmelstiel-Wilson d.
- Koeppe's d.
- Kuhnt-Junius d.
- Lauber's d.
- Leber's d.
- Lindau-Von Hippel d.
- Masuda-Kitahara d.
- Mikulicz's d.
- Mobius' d.
- Niemann-Pick d.
- Norrie's d.
- Purtscher's d.

disease *(continued)*
- Recklinghausen's d.
- Reis-Bücklers d.
- Reiter's d.
- Schilder's d.
- Sichel's d.
- Sjögren's d.
- Vogt-Spielmeyer d.
- Vogt's d.
- von Hippel-Lindau d.
- von Recklinghausen's d.
- Wagner's d.
- Weil's d.
- Westphal-Strumpell d.
- Wilson's d.

disjugate

disk
- anangioid d.
- ciliary d.
- Placido's d.
- Rekoss' d.
- stroboscopic d.

dissector
- Green's d.

distichia

distichiasis

divergence

divergent

Dix's spud

Doherty's implant

Donders'
- glaucoma
- law

dot
- Trantas' d's.

Dougherty's irrigator

Doyne's
- choroiditis

Doyne's
  iritis
dropper
  Undine's d.
Drualt
  bundle of D.
drugs. See *Medications.*
drusen
Duane's syndrome
duct
  lacrimal d.
  nasolacrimal d.
duction
ductus
  d. lacrimales
Duke-Elder lamp
Dupuy-Dutemps' operation
Durr's operation
Duverger and Velter's
  operation
DVA – distance visual acuity
dyscoria
dysmegalopsia
dysopia
  d. algera
dysopsia
dystrophy
  Bietti's d.
  Cogan's d.
  Fehr's d.
  Fleischer's d.
  Franceschetti's d.
  Francois' d.
  Fuchs' d.
  Groenouw's d.
  Maeder-Danis d.
  Meesmann's d.
  Pillat's d.

dystrophy *(continued)*
  Salzmann's d.
  Schlichting's d.
  Schnyder's d.
Eales' disease
Eber's forceps
echinophthalmia
ectasia
  e. iridis
ectiris
ectochoroidea
ectocornea
ectopia
  e. lentis
  e. pupillae congenita
ectropion
  e. cicatriceum
  cicatricial e.
  flaccid e.
  e. luxurians
  e. paralyticum
  e. sarcomatosum
  e. senilis
  e. spasticum
  e. uveae
ectropium
edema
  Berlin's e.
  Iwanoff's retinal e.
  Stellwag's brawny e.
Edinger-Westphal nucleus
edipism
egilops
Egyptian
  conjunctivitis
  ophthalmia
Ehrhardt's forceps
eikonometer

elastosis
  e. dystrophica
Eldridge-Green lamp
electrode
  Gradle's e.
  Kronfeld's e.
  Pischel's e.
  Weve's e.
electrocoagulation
electronystagmograph
electroparacentesis
electroretinogram
electroretinography
elevator
  Desmarres' lid e.
Elliot's
  operation
  trephine
Ellis' needle holder
Elschnig-O'Brien forceps
Elschnig's
  conjunctivitis
  forceps
  knife
  operation
  retractor
  spatula
  spoon
  spot
  syndrome
Ely's operation
Em. – emmetropia
embolism
  retinal e.
embryotoxon
emmetrope
emmetropia
emmetropic

endophthalmitis
  e. phakoanaphylactica
endothelioma
  Sidler-Huguenin's e.
ENG – electronystagmograph
enophthalmos
enophthalmus
enstrophe
entophthalmia
entoptic
entoptoscope
entoptoscopy
entoretina
entropion
  e. cicatriceum
  cicatricial e.
  e. spasticum
  e. uveae
entropium
enucleate
enucleation
enzymatic
EOM – extraocular
  movements
epiblepharon
epibulbar
epicanthal
epicanthus
epicauma
epiphora
episclera
episcleral
episcleritis
  e. partialis fugax
episclerotitis
epitarsus
epithelioma
  Contino's e.

epitheliosis
  e. desquamativa
    conjunctivae
epithelium
  e. anterius corneae
  e. corneae
  corneal e.
  e. of lens
  e. lentis
equator
  e. bulbi oculi
  e. of crystalline lens
  e. of eyeball
  e. of lens
  e. lentis
erysiphake
    Barraquer's e.
    Bell's e.
    Dimitry-Bell e.
    Dimitry's e.
    Dimitry-Thomas e.
    Harrington's e.
    Kara's e.
    L'Esperance's e.
    Maumenee's e.
    Nugent-Green-Dimitry e.
    Post-Harrington e.
    Sakler's e.
    Searcy's e.
    Viers' e.
erysipelas
erythropia
erythropsia
esodeviation
esophoria
esophoric
esotropia
esotropic

Ethicon silk suture
euchromatopsy
euryopia
euthyphoria
Eversbusch's operation
eversion
evisceration
evulsio
    e. nervi optici
Ewald's law
exanthematous
excycloduction
excyclophoria
excyclotropia
exenteration
exodeviation
exophoria
exophoric
exophthalmic
exophthalmogenic
exophthalmometer
    Hertel's e.
    Luedde's e.
exophthalmometric
exophthalmometry
exophthalmos
    endocrine e.
    pulsating e.
exophthalmus
exorbitism
exotropia
exotropic
expressor
    Arruga's e.
    Heath's e.
    Smith's e.
externus
extorsion

extracapsular
extraocular
eye
    blear e.
    Bright's e.
    cinema e.
    dark-adapted e.
    epiphyseal e.
    exciting e.
    hare's e.
    Klieg e.
    lazy e.
    light-adapted e.
    monochromatic e.
    Nairobi e.
    parietal e.
    pineal e.
    pink e.
    schematic e.
    Snellen's reform e.
    squinting e.
    sympathizing e.
eyeball
eyebrow
eyecup
eyeground
eyelash
eyelid
eyestrain
facies
    Hutchinson's f.
fako-. See words beginning
    phaco-.
farsighted
farsightedness
fascia
    f. bulbi
    Tenon's f.

Favre's disease
FB — foreign body
f.c. — foot candles
Fehr's dystrophy
Ferree-Rand perimeter
Ferrein's canal
Ferris-Smith retractor
Ferris-Smith-Sewall retractor
fiber
    Berneheimer's f's.
    Brucke's f's.
    Muller's f's.
    Sappey's f's.
    von Monakow's f's.
fibroplasia
    retrolental f.
Fick's halo
Filatov's operation
Filatov-Marzinkowsky
    operation
Fink's retractor
Fisher's spud
fissure
    palpebral f.
fixation
    binocular f.
Flajani's operation
Fleischer's
    dystrophy
    ring
flikten-. See words beginning
    phlycten-.
floaters
Florentine iris
Flouren's law
fluorescein
focus
Foerster's forceps

Foix's syndrome
fold
    epicanthal f.
    semilunar f. of
      conjunctiva
Foltz's valve
Fontana's space
foot-candle
foramen
    optic f. of sclera
forceps
    Arruga's f.
    Barraquer's f.
    Beaupre's f.
    Bennett's f.
    Berens' f.
    Berke's f.
    Bishop-Harmon f.
    Bonaccolto's f.
    Bonn's f.
    Bracken's f.
    capsule f.
    Castroviejo-Arruga f.
    Castroviejo's f.
    chalazion f.
    Chandler's f.
    Davis' f.
    Desmarres' f.
    Eber's f.
    Ehrhardt's f.
    Elschnig-O'Brien f.
    Elschnig's f.
    fixation f.
    Foerster's f.
    Fuchs' f.
    Gifford's f.
    Green's f.
    Hartman's f.

forceps *(continued)*
    Heath's f.
    Hess' f.
    Hess-Barraquer f.
    Hess-Horwitz f.
    Holth's f.
    Hunt's f.
    Jameson's f.
    Judd's f.
    Kalt's f.
    Katzin-Barraquer f.
    Kerrison's f.
    Kirby's f.
    Knapp's f.
    Kronfeld's f.
    Kuhnt's f.
    Kulvin-Kalt f.
    Lambert's f.
    Lister's f.
    Littauer's f.
    McCullough's f.
    McPherson's f.
    mosquito f.
    Noble's f.
    Noyes' f.
    Nugent's f.
    O'Brien's f.
    Perritt's f.
    Pley's f.
    Prince's f.
    Quevedo's f.
    Reese's f.
    Rolf's f.
    Sauer's f.
    Schweigger's f.
    Shaaf's f.
    Smart's f.
    Spero's f.

forceps *(continued)*
    Stevens' f.
    Thorpe's f.
    Verhoeff's f.
    von Graefe's f.
    Von Mondak's f.
    Waldeau's f.
    Ziegler's f.
fornix
    inferior f.
foro-. See words beginning
    phoro-.
Forster-Fuchs black spot
Förster's
    choroiditis
    operation
    uveitis
Foster-Kennedy syndrome
fovea
    f. centralis
    f. trochlearis
Foville's syndrome
Foville-Wilson syndrome
Fox's
    conformer
    implant
    irrigator
    shield
fracture
    blow-out f.
Franceschetti's
    disease
    dystrophy
    operation
    syndrome
Francis' spud
Francois' dystrophy
Franklin glasses

Fricke's operation
Friede's operation
Friedenwald's
    operation
    ophthalmoscope
    syndrome
Frost-Lang operation
Frost's suture
Fuchs'
    atrophy
    coloboma
    dimples
    dystrophy
    forceps
    heterochromia
    keratitis
    operation
    spot
    syndrome
Fuchs-Kraupa syndrome
Fukala's operation
fundus
    albinotic f.
    f. oculi
    tessellated f.
    f. tigre
funduscope
funduscopic
funduscopy
fusion
galactosemia
gargoylism
Gaucher's disease
Gaule's spots
Gayet's operation
gaze
    conjugate g.
Georgariou's operation

gerontotoxon, gerontoxon
  g. lentis
Gerstmann's syndrome
Gibson's irrigator
Gifford-Galassi reflex
Gifford's
  applicator
  curette
  forceps
  operation
  reflex
  sign
Gillies' operation
Gill's knife
Giraud-Teulon law
glabella
gland
  inferior lacrimal g.
  Krause's g.
  lacrimal g.
  Manz's g's.
  meibomian g.
  Moll's g.
  Rosenmuller's g.
  superior lacrimal g.
  tarsal g.
  Wolfring's g.
  zeisian g.
glanders
glands of Zeis
glasses
  Franklin g.
  Hallauer's g's.
glaucoma
  g. absolutum
  apoplectic g.
  auricular g.
  g. consummatum

glaucoma *(continued)*
  Contino's g.
  Donders' g.
  fulminant g.
  g. imminens
  narrow angle g.
  open angle g.
  g. simplex
glaucomatous
glaucosis
glioma
  g. endophytum
  g. exophytum
  g. retinae
globe
Goldman's applanation
  tonometer
Goldstein's
  cannula
  retractor
Gomez-Marquez's operation
Gonin's operation
goniophotography
goniopuncture
gonioscope
gonioscopy
goniotomy
Gonnin-Amsler marker
gonoblennorrhea
gouge
  Todd's g.
Gradenigo's syndrome
Gradle's
  electrode
  operation
  retractor
Graefe's
  disease

Graefe's *(continued)*
    incision
    knife
    sign
    syndrome
granuloma
    g. iridis
Graves' disease
Green's
    caliper
    curette
    dissector
    forceps
    hook
    knife
    needle holder
    replacer
Gregg's syndrome
Greig's syndrome
Grieshaber's
    keratome
    needle
    needle holder
    trephine
Groenholm's retractor
Groenouw's dystrophy
Grossmann's operation
Gruning's magnet
Gudden's commissure
Guillain-Barre syndrome
Gullstrand's
    law
    slit lamp
gumma
Gunn's syndrome
Gutzeit's operation
Guyton-Maumenee speculum
Guyton-Park speculum

Guyton's operation
Haab's magnet
Haag-Streit slit lamp
Haidinger's brushes
Hallauer's glasses
Hallermann-Streiff syndrome
halo
    Fick's h.
    h. glaucomatosus
    glaucomatous h.
    h. saturninus
Halpin's operation
Halsey's needle holder
Hand-Schüller-Christian
    disease
handle
    Beaver's h.
Harada's
    disease
    syndrome
Harrington's erysiphake
Harrison's scissors
Hartman's forceps
Hartstein's retractor
Hasner's operation
Hassall-Henle warts
head-tilt test
Heath's
    curette
    dilator
    expressor
    forceps
Heerfordt's disease
Heine's operation
hemangioma
hemangiomatosis
hemeralopia
hemianopia

hemianopia *(continued)*
    bitemporal h.
    h. bitemporalis fugax
    congruous h.
    heteronymous h.
    homonymous h.
    uniocular h.
hemianopic
hemianopsia
hemianoptic
hemiopalgia
hemiopia
hemiopic
hemovac
Herbert's operation
Hering's
    law
    test
    theory
herpes
    h. corneae
    h. ophthalmicus
    h. simplex
    h. zoster
Hertel's exophthalmometer
Hertwig-Magendie syndrome
Hess'
    forceps
    operation
    spoon
Hess-Barraquer forceps
Hess-Horwitz forceps
heterochromia
    Fuchs' h.
    h. iridis
heterophoralgia
heterophoria
heterophoric

heterophthalmia
heterophthalmos
heteropsia
heteroptics
heteroscopy
heterotropia
hexachromic
Hildreth's cautery
Hillis' retractor
Hippel-Lindau syndrome
Hippel's
    disease
    operation
hippus
Hirschberg's
    magnet
    method
Hogan's operation
Holmgren's test
Holth's
    forceps
    operation
    punch
homokeratoplasty
hook
    fixation h.
    Green's h.
    Jameson's h.
    Kirby's h.
    Nugent's h.
    O'Connor's h.
    Smith's h.
    Stevens' h.
    Tyrell's h.
    von Graefe's h.
    Wiener's h.
Horay's operation
hordeolum

Horner-Bernard syndrome
Horner's
    law
    muscle
    ptosis
    syndrome
Horner-Trantas spots
horopter
    Vieth-Muller h.
horror
    h. fusionis
Horvath's operation
Hosford's spud
Hotz's operation
Howard's abrader
Hudson's line
Huey's scissors
Hughes' operation
humor
    aqueous h.
    h. aquosus
    h. cristallinus
    crystalline h.
    ocular h.
    vitreous h.
    h. vitreus
Hunt's forceps
Hutchinson's
    facies
    pupil
    syndrome
hyaline
hyalinization
hyalitis
    asteroid h.
    h. punctata
    h. suppurativa
hyaloid

hyaloid *(continued)*
    h. canal
    h. membrane
hyalomucoid
hyalonyxis
hydrophthalmia
hydrophthalmos
hydrophthalmus
hyperhidrosis
hyperkeratosis
hypermetropia
hyperopia
    facultative h.
    manifest h.
hyperopic
hyperphoria
hypertelorism
    ocular h.
    orbital h.
hypertonia
    h. oculi
hypertropia
hyphema
hypophoria
hypopyon
hypotonia
    h. oculi
hypotonus
hypotony
hypotropia
ianthinopsia
ichthyosis
icteric
icterus
illusion
    Kuhnt's i.
image
    Purkinje's i.

image
 Purkinje-Sanson i's.
implant
 Berens' i.
 Doherty's i.
 Fox's i.
 Mules' i.
 polyethylene i.
 silastic i.
 silicone i.
 Wheeler's i.
Imre's
 operation
 treatment
incision
 ab-externo i.
 buttonhole i.
 circumcorneal i.
 circumlimbar i.
 conjunctival i.
 corneoscleral i.
 cruciate i.
 elliptical i.
 Graefe's i.
 intracapsular i.
 keratome i.
 limbal i.
 longitudinal i.
 perilimbal i.
 scratch type i.
 semilunar i.
incycloduction
incyclophoria
incyclotropia
infraduction
infraorbital
infraversion
interpalpebral

interpupillary
intorsion
intracapsular
intraocular
intraorbital
introducer
 Carter's i.
IOP – intraocular pressure
iridal
iridauxesis
iridectasis
iridectome
iridectomesodialysis
iridectomize
iridectomy
 basal i.
 optic i.
 peripheral i.
 sector i.
 stenopeic i.
iridectopia
iridectropium
iridemia
iridencleisis
iridentropium
irideremia
irides
iridesis
iridiagnosis
iridial
iridian
iridic
iridization
iridoavulsion
iridocapsulitis
iridocele
iridochoroiditis
iridocoloboma

iridoconstrictor
iridocorneosclerectomy
iridocyclectomy
iridocyclitis
iridocyclochoroiditis
iridocystectomy
iridodesis
iridodiagnosis
iridodialysis
iridodiastasis
iridodilator
iridodonesis
iridokeratitis
iridokinesia
iridokinesis
iridokinetic
iridoleptynsis
iridology
iridolysis
iridomalacia
iridomesodialysis
iridomotor
iridoncus
iridoparalysis
iridopathy
iridoperiphakitis
iridoplegia
iridoptosis
iridopupillary
iridorhexis
iridoschisis
iridosclerotomy
iridosteresis
iridotasis
iridotomy
iris
    bombé i.
    Florentine i.

iris *(continued)*
    tremulous i.
    umbrella i.
irisopsia
iritic
iritis
    i. blennorrhagique à
      rechutes
    i. catamenialis
    Doyne's i.
    i. papulosa
    i. recidivans staphylo-
      cocco-allergica
    uratic i.
iritoectomy
iritomy
irrigator
    DeVilbiss' i.
    Dougherty's i.
    Fox's i.
    Gibson's i.
    Rollett's i.
    Sylva's i.
Irvine's scissors
ischemia
    i. retinae
Ishihara's
    plate
    test
isocoria
isophoria
isopia
isopter
isoscope
Iwanoff's retinal edema
Jacob's membrane
Jacobson's retinitis
Jaeger's

Jaeger's
    keratome
    lid plate
Jaesche-Arlt operation
Jameson's
    caliper
    forceps
    hook
    operation
jaundice
Javal's ophthalmometer
jaw-winking
Jensen's
    disease
    retinitis
Jones' dilator
Judd's forceps
kahla-. See words beginning
    chala-.
kalko-. See words beginning
    chalco-.
Kalt's
    forceps
    needle holder
kappa angle
Kara's erysiphake
Katzin-Barraquer forceps
Katzin's scissors
Kayser-Fleischer ring
kemosis. See *chemosis.*
Kennedy's syndrome
keratalgia
keratectasia
keratectomy
keratic
keratitis
    acne rosacea k.
    actinic k.

keratitis *(continued)*
    alphabet k.
    artificial silk k.
    band k.
    k. bandelette
    k. bullosa
    dendriform k.
    dendritic k.
    Dimmer's k.
    k. disciformis
    fascicular k.
    k. filamentosa
    Fuchs' k.
    herpetic k.
    hypopyon k.
    lagophthalmic k.
    mycotic k.
    k. nummularis
    oyster shuckers' k.
    parenchymatous k.
    k. petrificans
    phlyctenular k.
    k. profunda
    k. punctata
    k. punctata
      subepithelialis
    k. pustuliformis
      profunda
    k. ramificata
      superficialis
    reticular k.
    ribbon-like k.
    rosacea k.
    Schmidt's k.
    scrofulus k.
    serpiginous k.
    k. sicca
    striate k.

keratitis *(continued)*
    Thygeson's k.
    vasculonebulous k.
    xerotic k.
keratocele
keratocentesis
keratoconjunctivitis
    epidemic k.
    epizootic k.
    flash k.
    k. sicca
    welder's k.
keratoconus
keratoderma
keratoectasia
keratoglobus
keratohelcosis
keratohemia
keratoid
keratoiridocyclitis
keratoiridoscope
keratoiritis
keratoleptynsis
keratoleukoma
keratoma
keratomalacia
keratome
    Agnew's k.
    Beaver's k.
    Berens' k.
    Castroviejo's k.
    Grieshaber's k.
    Jaeger's k.
    Kirby's k.
keratometer
keratometric
keratometry
keratomycosis

keratonosus
keratonyxis
keratopathy
    band k.
keratoplasty
    optic k.
    tectonic k.
keratorhexis
keratoscleritis
keratoscope
keratoscopy
keratotomy
    delimiting k.
kerectasis
kerectomy
keroid
Kerrison's forceps
Key's operation
kias-. See words beginning
    chias-.
Kiloh-Nevin syndrome
Kimmelstiel-Wilson
    disease
    syndrome
kinescope
Kirby's
    forceps
    hook
    keratome
    knife
    operation
    retractor
    scissors
    spoon
    suture
Klieg eye
Knapp-Imre operation
Knapp's

Knapp's *(continued)*
  forceps
  knife
  knife needle
  operation
  retractor
  scissors
  scoop
  spatula
  speculum
  spoon
  streak's
  striae
knife
  Bard-Parker k.
  Barkan's k.
  Beaver's k.
  Castroviejo's k.
  Elschnig's k.
  Gill's k.
  Graefe's k.
  Green's k.
  Kirby's k.
  Knapp's k.
  Lancaster's k.
  Lundsgaard's k.
  McPherson-Wheeler k.
  McPherson-Ziegler k.
  McReynolds' k.
  Parker's k.
  Scheie's k.
  Smith-Green k.
  Tooke's k.
  von Graefe's k.
  Weber's k.
  Wheeler's k.
  Ziegler's k.
knife needle

knife needle *(continued)*
  Davis' k.n.
  Knapp's k.n.
  von Graefe's k.n.
Koby's cataract
Koch-Weeks bacillus
Koeppe's
  disease
  nodule
Koerber-Salus-Elschnig
  syndrome
Kofler's operation
kor-. See words beginning
  chor-.
korio-. See words beginning
  chorio-.
Kozlowski's degeneration
KP — keratic precipitates
Kraupa's operation
Krause's
  gland
  syndrome
Kreibig's opticomalacia
Kreiker's operation
Kriebig's operation
Kronfeld's
  electrode
  forceps
  retractor
Kronlein's operation
Krukenberg's spindle
Kuhnt-Junius disease
Kuhnt's
  forceps
  illusion
  operation
Kuhnt-Szymanowski
  operation

Kulvin-Kalt forceps
Kurz's syndrome
L & A — light and accommodation
Lacarrere's operation
lacrima
lacrimal
lacrimalin
lacrimase
lacrimation
lacrimator
lacrimatory
lacrimonasal
lacrimotome
lacrimotomy
lacus
   l. lacrimalis
LaForce's spud
Lagleyze's operation
lagophthalmos
lagophthalmus
Lagrange's
   operation
   scissors
lake
   lacrimal l.
Lambert's forceps
lamella
lamellar
lamina
   l. basalis
   l. basalis choroideae
   l. basalis corporis ciliaris
   l. choriocapillaris
   l. cribrosa sclerae
   l. elastica anterior
   l. elastica posterior
   episcleral l.

lamina *(continued)*
   l. episcleralis
   l. fusca sclerae
   l. limitans anterior
      corneae
   l. limitans posterior
      corneae
   orbital l.
   l. orbitalis ossis ethmoi-
      dalis
   l. papyracea
   l. superficialis musculi
      levatoris palpebrae
      superioris
   l. suprachorioidea
   suprachoroid l.
   l. suprachoroidea
   l. vasculosa chorioideae
   l. vasculosa choroideae
lamp
   Birch-Hirschfeld l.
   Duke-Elder l.
   Eldridge-Green l.
   Gullstrand's slit l.
   Haag-Streit slit l.
   slit l.
Lancaster's
   knife
   magnet
   speculum
lance
   Rolf's l.
Landolt's
   bodies
   operation
Langenbeck's operation
Lange's speculum
laser

laser *(continued)*
    argon l.
    ruby l.
Lauber's disease
Laurence-Moon-Biedl
  syndrome
law
    Descartes' l.
    Desmarres' l.
    Donders' l.
    Ewald's l.
    Flouren's l.
    Giraud-Teulon l.
    Gullstrand's l.
    Hering's l.
    Horner's l.
    Listing's l.
    Sherrington's l.
    Snell's l.
LE — left eye
Leber's
    amaurosis
    disease
leiomyoma
leiomyosarcoma
lens
    achromatic l.
    acrylic l.
    adherent l.
    aplanatic l.
    apochromatic l.
    biconcave l.
    biconvex l.
    bicylindrical l.
    bifocal l.
    bispherical l.
    Brucke's l.
    cataract l.

lens *(continued)*
    concave l.
    concavoconcave l.
    contact l.
    converging l.
    convex l.
    convexoconcave l.
    Coquille plano l.
    Crookes' l.
    crystalline l.
    cylindrical l.
    decentered l.
    dispersing l.
    immersion l.
    iseikonic l.
    meniscus l.
    omnifocal l.
    orthoscopic l.
    periscopic l.
    planoconcave l.
    planoconvex l.
    prosthetic l.
    punktal l.
    retroscopic l.
    spherical l.
    Stokes' l.
    toric l.
    trifocal l.
lentectomize
lentectomy
lenticonus
lenticular
lenticulo-optic
lenticulostriate
lenticulothalamic
lentiform
lentiglobus
leptotrichosis

leptotrichosis
　　l. conjunctivae
L'Esperance's erysiphake
leukokoria
leukoma
　　l. adhaerens
levoclination
levocycloduction
levocycloversion
levoduction
levotorsion
levoversion
Lewis' scoop
lid everter
　　Walker's l.e.
lid plate
　　Jaeger's l.p.
ligament
　　ciliary l.
　　pectinate l.
　　suspensory l. of lens
　　Zinn's l.
limbal
　　l. groove
limbi palpebrales anteriores
limbi palpebrales posteriores
limbus
　　l. conjunctivae
　　l. of cornea
　　l. corneae
　　l. luteus retinae
Lindau-Von Hippel disease
Lindner's
　　operation
　　spatula
line
　　Hudson's l.
　　Schwalbe's l.

line
　　Stahli's l.
linea
　　l. corneae senilis
lipemia
　　l. retinalis
lipoma
liposarcoma
liquor
　　l. corneae
　　Morgagni's l.
Lister-Burch speculum
Lister's forceps
Listing's law
lithiasis
　　l. conjunctivae
Littauer's forceps
Lockwood's tendon
Lohlein's operation
Londermann's operation
loop
　　Meyer's l.
Lopez-Enriquez operation
Loring's ophthalmoscope
louchettes
Louis-Bar's syndrome
loupe
　　corneal l.
Lowenstein's operation
Lowe's
　　ring
　　syndrome
Luedde's exophthalmometer
Lundsgaard-Burch sclerotome
Lundsgaard's knife
Lyle's syndrome
lymphangiectasis
lymphangioma

lymphoma
lymphosarcoma
Machek's operation
macrophthalmia
macrophthalmous
macropsia
macula
    m. corneae
    m. lutea retinae
    m. retinae
Maddox
    prism
    rod
Maeder-Danis dystrophy
Magitot's operation
magnet
    Gruning's m.
    Haab's m.
    Hirschberg's m.
    Lancaster's m.
    Storz' m.
Majewsky's operation
manner
    McLean's m.
Manz's gland
Marcus-Gunn phenomenon
Marfan's syndrome
Mariotte's spot
marker
    Gonnin-Amsler m.
Marlow's test
maser
Masselon's spectacles
Masuda-Kitahara disease
Mauksch's operation
Maumenee's erysiphake
Mauthner's test
Maxwell's

Maxwell's *(continued)*
    ring
    spot
May's sign
McClure's scissors
McCullough's forceps
McGannon's retractor
McGuire's
    operation
    scissors
McLaughlin's operation
McLean's
    manner
    scissors
    tonometer
McPherson-Castroviejo scissors
McPherson's
    forceps
    needle holder
    scissors
    spatula
    speculum
McPherson-Vannas scissors
McPherson-Wheeler
    blade
    knife
McPherson-Ziegler knife
McReynolds'
    knife
    operation
Medications
    acetazolamide
    Acetonide
    acetylcholine chloride
    Achromycin
    Adrenalin
    Aerosporin Sulfate
    Alcon-Efrin

Medications *(continued)*
    hydrochloride
    Almocetamide
    alpha-Chymar
    alpha-chymotrypsin
    ammonium tartrate
    Argyrol
    Aristocort
    atropine
    Aureomycin
    Bacimycin
    bacitracin
    benoxinate
    benzalkonium
    Biomydrin
    bis-Tropamide
    Blefcon
    Blephamide
    Boracic acid
    boric acid
    Borofax
    butacaine
    Butyn
    carbachol
    Carcholin
    Cetapred
    chloramphenicol
    Chloromycetin
    Chloroptic-P
    chlortetracycline
    Chymar
    chymotrypsin
    cocaine
    Coly-Mycin
    Conjunctilone
    Conjunctin
    Cort-Dome
    Cortef

Medications *(continued)*
    Cortisol
    cortisone
    Cortisporin
    Cortogen
    Cortone
    Cortril
    Cyclogyl
    Cyclomydril
    cyclopentolate
    Dacriose
    Daranide
    Decadron
    Delta-Cortef
    demecarium
    Dendrid
    dexamethasone
    Diamox
    dibucaine
    dichlorphenamide
    Diisopropyl Flurophos-
       phate
    Dorsacaine
    echothiophate
    E-Pilo
    epinephrine
    Epinephryl Borate
    Eppy
    Erythrocin
    erythromycin
    Eserine
    Estivin
    eucatropine
    F-Cortef
    Feldman buffer solution
    Florinef
    Floropryl
    fludrocortisone

Medications *(continued)*

Fludrohydrocortisone
fluorescein
Furacin
Gantrisin
Garamycin
gentamicin
Germa-Medica
Gifford and Smith
  buffer solution
Glaucon
Glyrol
Herplex
homatropine
Humorsol
Hydeltrasol
hydrocortisone
Hydrocortone
hydroxyamphetamine
Hydroxymesterone
Hyoscine
idoxuridine
Ilotycin
Innovar
isoflurophate
Isohist
Isopto Cetapred
Isopto Hydrocortisone
Isopto Mydrapred
Isopto P-H-N
Isopto Prednisolone
Isopto Sterofrin
Kenacort
Kenalog
Kenalog-S
Lacril
Lassar's zinc paste
lidocaine

Medications *(continued)*

Lyteers
mannitol
Maxidex
Maxitrol
Medrol
medrysone
merbromin
Mercurochrome
Merthiolate
methazolamide
methicillin sodium
methylparaben
methylprednisolone
Meticortelone
Metimyd
Metreton
Metycaine
Miochol
Mycifradin
Mycitracin
Mycostatin
Mydriacyl
naphazoline
Neo-Aristocort
Neo-Cortef
NeoDecadron
Neo-Delta-Cortef
Neo-Deltef
Neo-Hydeltrasol
Neo-Medrol
neomycin
Neo-Polycin
Neosone
Neosporin
Neo-Synephrine
Neptazane
Nupercaine

Medications *(continued)*
    nystatin
    Ocu-Cort
    Ophthaine
    Ophthalgan
    Ophthetic
    Ophthocort
    Optef
    Oratrol
    Orthoboric acid
    Osmoglyn
    oxytetracycline
    Panmycin
    Paredrine
    penicillin
    phenylephrine
    pHisoHex
    Phospholine
    physostigmine
    pilocarpine
    piperocaine
    Polycycline
    polymyxin
    Pontocaine
    Predmycin
    Prednefrin
    prednisolone
    prednisone
    Privine
    procaine
    proparacaine
    Propion
    Propylparaben
    rose bengal sodium
    scopolamine
    silver nitrate
    sodium bicarbonate
    Sodium Ethylmercuri-

Medications *(continued)*
    thiosalicylate
    Sodium Sulamyd
    Spectrocin
    Staphcillin
    Statrol
    Steclin
    Stoxil
    streptomycin
    Suladrin
    Sulamyd
    sulfacetamide sodium
    sulfadiazine
    sulfisoxazole
    Terra-Cortil
    Terramycin
    tetracaine
    tetracycline
    Tetracyn
    tetrahydrozoline
    thimerosal
    Thiosulfil
    triamcinolone
    tropicamide
    Tyzine
    Vasocidin
    Vasopred
    Visine
    Xylocaine
    Zephiran
    zinc sulfate
    Zolyse
Meesmann's dystrophy
megalocornea
megalophthalmos
megalophthalmus
megophthalmos
meibomian cyst

meibomian gland
meibomianitis
meibomitis
melanoma
melanosis
 m. sclerae
Meller's
 operation
 retractor
Mellinger's speculum
membrana
 m. capsularis lentis
  posterior
 m. epipapillaris
membrane
 Bowman's m.
 Bruch's m.
 Demours' m.
 Descemet's m.
 hyaloid m.
 Jacob's m.
meridian
meridiani bulbi oculi
meridional
mesh
 marlex m.
 tantalum m.
mesiris
mesoretina
metamorphopsia
 m. varians
method
 Hirschberg's m.
metronoscope
Meyer's loop
Meyhoeffer's curette
Meynert's commissure
microblepharia

microblepharon
microcoria
microcornea
microgonioscope
microphakia
microphthalmia
microphthalmoscope
microphthalmus
micropsia
microptic
Mikulicz's
 disease
 syndrome
Millard-Gubler syndrome
Miller's syndrome
miosis
miotic
Möbius'
 disease
 sign
 syndrome
Moll's gland
Moncrieff's cannula
monocular
monoculus
Mooren's ulcer
Morax-Axenfeld conjunctivitis
Morax's operation
Morgagni's liquor
Mosher-Toti's operation
Motais' operation
movement
 conjugate m.
Mueller's
 cautery
 retractor
 speculum
Muldoon's dilator

Mules'
 implant
 operation
 scoop
Müller's
 fibers
 muscle
 trigone
Murdock-Wiener speculum
muscae volitantes
muscle
 Brücke's m.
 ciliaris m.
 ciliary m.
 Horner's m.
 inferior oblique m.
 inferior rectus m.
 lateral rectus m.
 levator m.
 levator palperbrae
  superior m.
 medial rectus m.
 Müller's m.
 obliquus inferior m.
 obliquus superior m.
 orbicular m. of eye
 orbital m.
 rectus inferior m.
 rectus lateralis m.
 rectus medialis m.
 rectus superior m.
 superior oblique m.
 superior rectus m.
My. – myopia
mydriasis
mydriatic
myectomy
myiodesopsia

myopia
 axial m.
 indicial m.
 pernicious m.
 prodromal m.
myopic
 m. crescent
myotomy
Naffziger's operation
Nairobi eye
nasociliary
nasolacrimal
near-sight
nearsighted
nearsightedness
nebula
needle
 Amsler's n.
 Bowman's n.
 Calhoun-Merz n.
 Calhoun's n.
 Grieshaber's n.
 Stocker's n.
 Weeks' n.
needle holder
 Barraquer's n. h.
 Boynton's n. h.
 Castroviejo-Kalt n. h.
 Castroviejo's n. h.
 Derf's n. h.
 Ellis' n. h.
 Green's n. h.
 Grieshaber's n. h.
 Halsey's n. h.
 Kalt's n. h.
 McPherson's n. h.
 Paton's n. h.
nerve

nerve *(continued)*
    abducens n.
    infratrochlear n.
    optic n.
Nettleship-Wilder dilator
neurectomy
    opticociliary n.
neurochorioretinitis
neurochoroiditis
neurodeatrophia
neuroepithelioma
neurofibroma
neuroretinitis
neuroretinopathy
    hypertensive n.
neurotomy
    opticociliary n.
nicking
Nida's operation
Niemann-Pick disease
Nizetic's operation
Noble's forceps
nodal
nodule
    Koeppe's n.
Norrie's disease
Noyes' forceps
NPC – near point of conver-
    gence
nucleus
    Edinger-Westphal n.
    Perlia's n.
Nugent-Gradle scissors
Nugent-Green-Dimitry
    erysiphake
Nugent's
    forceps
    hook

Nv. – naked vision
NVA – near visual acuity
nyctalopia
nystagmic
nystagmiform
nystagmograph
nystagmoid
nystagmus
    aural n.
    Baer's n.
    Bekhterev's n.
    Cheyne's n.
    disjunctive n.
    end position n.
    labyrinthine n.
    miner's n.
    optokinetic n.
    oscillating n.
    paretic n.
    pendular n.
    undulatory n.
    vestibular n.
    vibratory n.
nystagmusmyoclonus
nystaxis
O'Brien's
    akinesia
    block
    cataract
    forceps
O'Connor-Peter operation
O'Connor's
    hook
    operation
ocular
oculentum
oculi
oculist

oculistics
oculocephalogyric
oculofacial
oculogyration
oculogyria
oculogyric
oculometroscope
oculomotor
oculomotorius
oculomycosis
oculonasal
oculopathy
    pituitarigenic o.
oculopupillary
oculoreaction
oculospinal
oculozygomatic
oculus
OD – oculus dexter – right
  eye
ofthal-. See words beginning
  ophthal-.
opacification
opacity
    Caspar's ring o.
operation
    Agnew's o.
    Ammon's o.
    Anagnostakis' o.
    Arlt-Jaesche o.
    Arlt's o.
    Arruga's o.
    Badal's o.
    Bardelli's o.
    Barkan's o.
    Barraquer's o.
    Barrio's o.
    Basterra's o.

operation *(continued)*
    Berens' o.
    Bielschowsky's o.
    Blasius' o.
    Blaskovics' o.
    Blatt's o.
    Bohm's o.
    Bonzel's o.
    Borthen's o.
    Bossalino's o.
    Brailey's o.
    Briggs' o.
    Budinger's o.
    Buzzi's o.
    Carter's o.
    Casanellas' o.
    Castroviejo's o.
    Celsus' o.
    Critchett's o.
    Csapody's o.
    Czermak's o.
    Daviel's o.
    de Grandmont's o.
    de Wecker's o.
    Del Toro's o.
    Dupuy-Dutemps' o.
    Durr's o.
    Duverger and Velter's o.
    Elliot's o.
    Elschnig's o.
    Ely's o.
    equilibrating o.
    Eversbusch's o.
    Filatov-Marzinkowsky o.
    Filatov's o.
    Flajani's o.
    Forster's o.
    Franceschetti's o.

operation *(continued)*
  Fricke's o.
  Friede's o.
  Friedenwald's o.
  Frost-Lang o.
  Fuchs's o.
  Fukala's o.
  Gayet's o.
  Georgariou's o.
  Gifford's o.
  Gillies' o.
  Gomez-Marquez's o.
  Gonin's o.
  Gradle's o.
  Grossmann's o.
  Gutzeit's o.
  Guyton's o.
  Halpin's o.
  Hasner's o.
  Heine's o.
  Herbert's o.
  Hess' o.
  Hippel's o.
  Hogan's o.
  Holth's o.
  Horay's o.
  Horvath's o.
  Hotz's o.
  Hughes' o.
  Imre's o.
  Jaesche-Arlt o.
  Jameson's o.
  Key's o.
  Kirby's o.
  Knapp-Imre o.
  Knapp's o.
  Kofler's o.
  Kraupa's o.

operation *(continued)*
  Kreiker's o.
  Kriebig's o.
  Kronlein's o.
  Kuhnt's o.
  Kuhnt-Szymanowski o.
  Lacarrere's o.
  Lagleyze's o.
  Lagrange's o.
  Landolt's o.
  Langenbeck's o.
  Lindner's o.
  Lohlein's o.
  Londermann's o.
  Lopez-Enriquez o.
  Lowenstein's o.
  Machek's o.
  Magitot's o.
  magnet o.
  Majewsky's o.
  Mauksch's o
  McGuire's o.
  McLaughlin's o.
  McReynolds' o.
  Meller's o.
  Morax's o.
  Mosher-Toti's o.
  Motais' o.
  Mules' o.
  Naffziger's o.
  Nida's o.
  Nizetic's o.
  O'Connor-Peter o.
  O'Connor's o.
  Panas' o.
  Paufique's o.
  Peter's o.
  Physick's o.

operation *(continued)*
    Polyak's o.
    Poulard's o.
    Quaglino's o.
    Raverdino's o.
    Richet's o.
    Rowinski's o.
    Rubbrecht's o.
    Saemisch's o.
    Schmalz's o.
    Silva-Costa o.
    Smith-Kuhnt-Szyma-
      nowski o.
    Smith's o.
    Snellen's o.
    Soria's o.
    Sourdille's o.
    Spaeth's o.
    Speas' o.
    Spencer-Watson o.
    Stock's o.
    Suarez-Villafranca o.
    Szymanowski-Kuhnt o.
    Szymanowski's o.
    Terson's o.
    Thomas' o.
    Toti-Mosher o.
    Toti's o.
    Trantas' o.
    Verhoeff's o.
    Verwey's o.
    von Graefe's o.
    Waldhauer's o.
    Weekers' o.
    West's o.
    Weve's o.
    Wheeler's o.
    Wiener's o.

operation *(continued)*
    Wilmer's o.
    Wolfe's o.
    Worth's o.
    Ziegler's o.
ophthalmagra
ophthalmalgia
ophthalmatrophia
ophthalmectomy
ophthalmencephalon
ophthalmia
    actinic ray o.
    catarrhal o.
    caterpillar o.
    o. eczematosa
    Egyptian o.
    o. hivialis
    jequirity o.
    o. neonatorum
    o. nodosa
    phlyctenular o.
    scrofulous o.
    strumous o.
    ultraviolet ray o.
ophthalmiatrics
ophthalmic
ophthalmin
ophthalmitic
ophthalmitis
ophthalmoblennorrhea
ophthalmocarcinoma
ophthalmocele
ophthalmocopia
ophthalmodesmitis
ophthalmodiagnosis
ophthalmodiaphanoscope
ophthalmodiastimeter
ophthalmodonesis

ophthalmodynamometer
ophthalmodynamometry
ophthalmodynia
ophthalmoeikonometer
ophthalmofundoscope
ophthalmograph
ophthalmography
ophthalmogyric
ophthalmoleukoscope
ophthalmolith
ophthalmologic
ophthalmologist
ophthalmology
ophthalmomalacia
ophthalmometer
    Javal's o.
ophthalmometroscope
ophthalmometry
ophthalmomycosis
ophthalmomyiasis
ophthalmomyitis
ophthalmomyositis
ophthalmomyotomy
ophthalmoneuritis
ophthalmoneuromyelitis
ophthalmopathy
ophthalmophacometer
ophthalmophantom
ophthalmophlebotomy
ophthalmophthisis
ophthalmoplasty
ophthalmoplegia
    exophthalmic o.
    o. externa
    fascicular o.
    o. interna
    nuclear o.
    Parinaud's o.

ophthalmoplegia *(continued)*
    o. partialis
    o. progressiva
    Sauvineau's o.
    o. totalis
ophthalmoplegic
ophthalmoptosis
ophthalmoreaction
ophthalmorrhagia
ophthalmorrhea
ophthalmorrhexis
ophthalmoscope
    Friedenwald's o.
    ghost o.
    Loring's o.
ophthalmoscopy
ophthalmostasis
ophthalmostat
ophthalmostatometer
ophthalmosteresis
ophthalmosynchysis
ophthalmothermometer
ophthalmotomy
ophthalmotonometer
ophthalmotonometry
ophthalmotoxin
ophthalmotrope
ophthalmotropometer
ophthalmovascular
ophthalmoxerosis
ophthalmoxyster
optesthesia
optic
    o. axis
    o. chiasm
    o. disk
    o. nerve
optical

optician
opticianry
opticist
opticociliary
opticocinerea
opticokinetic
opticomalacia
    Kreibig's o.
opticonasion
opticopupillary
optics
optist
optoblast
optogram
optomeninx
optometer
optometrist
optometry
optomyometer
optophone
optostriate
optotype
ora
    o. serrata
    o. serrata retinae
orbicularis
    o. ciliaris
    o. oculi
orbiculus
    o. ciliaris
orbit
orbita
orbitae
orbital
orbitale
orbitalis
orbitonasal
orbitonometer

orbitonometry
orbitostat
orbitotemporal
orbitotomy
orthometer
orthophoria
    asthenic o.
orthophoric
orthoptic
orthoptics
orthoptist
orthoptoscope
orthoscope
orthoscopy
OS — oculus sinister — left
    eye
OU — oculus unitas — both
    eyes
    oculus uterque — each
    eye
pachyblepharon
pachyblepharosis
palpebra
    tertius p.
palpebrae
palpebral
palpebralis
palpebrate
palpebration
palpebritis
palsy
    Bell's p.
Panas' operation
pannus
    p. carnosus
    p. crassus
    p. degenerativus
    p. eczematosus

pannus *(continued)*
    phlyctenular p.
    p. siccus
    p. tenuis
    p. trachomatosus
panophthalmia
panophthalmitis
panoptic
pantankyloblepharon
papilla
    Bergemeister's p.
    lacrimal p.
    optic p.
papillary
papilledema
papillitis
papilloretinitis
parenchyma
    p. of lens
paresis
Parinaud's
    conjunctivitis
    ophthalmoplegia
    syndrome
Parker's knife
Park's speculum
parophthalmia
parophthalmoncus
paropsis
pars
    p. caeca retinae
    p. ciliaris retinae
    p. iridica retinae
    p. marginalis musculi
        orbicularis oris
    p. optica retinae
    p. orbitalis glandulae
        lacrimalis

pars *(continued)*
    p. orbitalis musculi
        orbicularis oculi
    p. palpebralis glandulae
        lacrimalis
    p. palpebralis musculi
        orbicularis oculi
    p. plana corporis ciliaris
    p. plicata corporis
        ciliaris
Pascheff's conjunctivitis
Paton's needle holder
Paufique's
    operation
    trephine
PD – prism diopter
pectinate
Pel's crises
peribulbar
perimeter
    Ferree-Rand p.
periophthalmitis
periorbita
periorbital
periorbititis
periosteum
peripapillary
periphacitis
peripheral
peripheraphose
periscleral
peritectomy
peritomize
peritomy
PERLA – pupils equal, react
    to light and accommoda-
    tion
Perlia's nucleus

Perritt's forceps
PERRLA – pupils equal,
    round, regular, react to
    light and accommodation
Peter's
    anomaly
    operation
Petit's canal
Petzetakis-Takos syndrome
phacoanaphylaxis
phacocele
phacocyst
phacocystectomy
phacocystitis
phacoerysis
phacoglaucoma
phacohymenitis
phacoiditis
phacoidoscope
phacolysis
phacolytic
phacomalacia
phacometachoresis
phacometer
phacopalingenesis
phacoplanesis
phacosclerosis
phacoscope
phacoscopy
phacoscotasmus
phacotoxic
phacozymase
phakitis
phakoma
phakomatosis
phenomenon
    Bell's p.
    Marcus-Gunn p.

phlyctena
phlyctenular
phlyctenule
phoria
phoriascope
phorometer
phorometry
phoropter
phoroscope
phorotone
photocoagulation
photocoagulator
    Zeiss' p.
photo-ophthalmia
photophobia
photophthalmia
photopia
photopic
photopsia
photoptometer
photoptometry
phthiriasis
phthisis
    p. bulbi
    p. corneae
    ocular p.
Physick's operation
pick
    Burch's p.
Pick's
    retinitis
    vision
pigmentum
    p. nigrum
Pillat's dystrophy
pin
    Pischel's p.
    Walker's p.

pinguecula
Pischel's
    electrode
    pin
Placido's disk
pladarosis
plate
    Ishihara's p.
plexus
    annular p.
    intraepithelial p.
    ophthalmic p.
    p. ophthalmicus
    subepithelial p.
Pley's forceps
plica
    p. lacrimalis
    p. palpebronasalis
    p. semilunaris conjunc-
      tivae
plicae ciliares
plicae iridis
poliosis
Polyak's operation
polycoria
    p. spuria
    p. vera
polyopia, polyopsia
    binocular p.
    p. monophthalmica
Posner-Schlossman syndrome
Post-Harrington erysiphake
Poulard's operation
preretinal
presbyope
presbyopia
presbyopic
Prince's forceps

prism
    p. diopter
    Maddox p.
    Risley's p.
Pritikin's punch
probe
    Bowman's p.
    Theobald's p.
    Williams' p.
    Ziegler's p.
prophylaxis
    Crede's p.
proptometer
proptosis
prosthesis
protector
    Arruga's p.
Prowazek-Greeff bodies
pseudoglioma
pseudonystagmus
pseudopterygium
pseudoptosis
pterion
pterygium
ptosis
    p. adiposa
    Horner's p.
    p. lipomatosis
    p. sympathica
ptotic
punch
    Berens' p.
    Castroviejo's p.
    Holth's p.
    Pritikin's p.
    Rubin-Holth p.
    Walton's p.
punctum

punctum *(continued)*
    p. caecum
    lacrimal p.
    p. lacrimale
pupil
    Argyll-Robertson p.
    Bumke's p.
    cat's eye p.
    Hutchinson's p.
    keyhole p.
    pinhole p.
    skew p's.
pupilla
pupillary
pupillatonia
pupillometer
pupillometry
pupillomotor
pupilloplegia
pupilloscope
pupilloscopy
pupillostatometer
pupillotonia
Purkinje's image
Purkinje-Sanson images
Purtscher's
    angiopathic retinopathy
    disease
quadrantanopia
quadrantanopsia
Quaglino's operation
Quevedo's forceps
rabdomiomah. See
    rhabdomyoma.
ramollitio
    r. retinae
Randolph's cannula
Raverdino's operation
recession

Recklinghausen's disease
reclination
Reese's
    forceps
    syndrome
reflex
    Gifford-Galassi r.
    Gifford's r.
    Weiss's r.
refract
refraction
    homatropine r.
refractometer
Reis-Bückler's disease
Reiter's
    disease
    syndrome
Rekoss' disk
replacer
    Green's r.
resection
retina
    coarctate r.
    leopard r.
    physiological r.
    shot silk r.
    tigroid r.
    watered silk r.
retinal
    r. detachment
retinitis
    actinic r.
    r. albuminurica
    apoplectic r.
    central angiospastic r.
    r. centralis serosa
    r. circinata
    circinate r.

retinitis *(continued)*
>   Coats' r.
>   r. disciformans
>   exudative r.
>   r. gravidarum
>   gravidic r.
>   r. haemorrhagica
>   Jacobson's r.
>   Jensen's r.
>   leukemic r.
>   r. nephritica
>   Pick's r.
>   r. pigmentosa
>   r. proliferans
>   r. punctata albescens
>   punctate r.
>   splenic r.
>   r. stellata
>   striate r.
>   r. syphilitica
>   uremic r.
>   Wagener's r.

retinoblastoma
retinochoroid
retinochoroiditis
>   r. juxtapapillaris

retinocytoma
retinodialysis
retinograph
retinography
retinoid
retinomalacia
retinopapillitis
retinopathy
>   central disk-shaped r.
>   circinate r.
>   diabetic r.
>   exudative r.

retinopathy *(continued)*
>   leukemic r.
>   Purtscher's angiopathic
>   r.

retinoschisis
retinoscope
retinoscopy
retinosis
retinotoxic
retractor
>   Agrikola's r.
>   Berens' r.
>   Brawley's r.
>   Campbell's r.
>   Castallo's r.
>   Castroviejo's r.
>   Desmarres' r.
>   Elschnig's r.
>   Ferris-Smith r.
>   Ferris-Smith-Sewall r.
>   Fink's r.
>   Goldstein's r.
>   Gradle's r.
>   Groenholm's r.
>   Hartstein's r.
>   Hillis' r.
>   Kirby's r.
>   Knapp's r.
>   Kronfeld's r.
>   McGannon's r.
>   Meller's r.
>   Mueller's r.
>   Rizzuti's r.
>   Rollet's r.
>   Stevenson's r.

retrobulbar
retroiridian
retro-ocular

retro-orbital
retrotarsal
Reuss's color charts
Reuss's tables
rhabdomyoma
rhinommectomy
rhinoptia
rhytidosis
Richet's operation
Riddoch's syndrome
Rieger's syndrome
Rifkind's sign
Riley-Day syndrome
ring
    Bonaccolto's scleral r.
    Coats' r.
    common tendinous r.
    Fleischer's r.
    Kayser-Fleischer r.
    Lowe's r.
    Maxwell's r.
    Soemmerring's r.
    Vossius' lenticular r.
rinommektome. See
    rhinommectomy.
Risley's prism
ritidosis. See *rhytidosis.*
rivus
    r. lacrimalis
Rizzuti's retractor
RLF – retrolental fibroplasia
rod
    Maddox r.
    retinal r's.
Rolf's
    forceps
    lance
Rollet's syndrome

Rollett's
    irrigator
    retractor
Romana's sign
Rommel-Hildreth cautery
Rommel's cautery
Rönne's nasal step
Roper's cannula
Rosenmüller's gland
Rot-Bielschowsky syndrome
Rothmund's syndrome
Roth's spot
Rowinski's operation
Rubbrecht's operation
rubeosis
    r. iridis
    r. retinae
Rubin-Holth punch
Rutherfurd's syndrome
sac
    lacrimal s.
sacculus
    s. lacrimalis
Saemisch's
    operation
    ulcer
Sakler's erysiphake
Salus' arch
Salzmann's dystrophy
Samoan conjunctivitis
Sanyal's conjunctivitis
Sappey's fibers
sarcoma
Sattler's veil
Sauer's
    debrider
    forceps
    speculum

Sauvineau's ophthalmoplegia
scalpel
scarifier
    Desmarres' s.
Scarpa's staphyloma
Schäfer's syndrome
Scheie's
    cautery
    knife
Schilder's disease
Schiøtz' tonometer
Schirmer's test
Schlemm's canal
Schlichting's dystrophy
Schmalz's operation
Schmidt's keratitis
Schnabel's atrophy
Schnyder's dystrophy
Schöbl's scleritis
Schöler's treatment
Schön's theory
Schwalbe's line
Schweigger's forceps
scirrhoblepharoncus
scirrhophthalmia
scissors
    Aebli's s.
    Barraquer-DeWecker s.
    Berens' s.
    canalicular s.
    Castroviejo's s.
    corneoscleral s.
    DeWecker-Pritikin s.
    DeWecker's s.
    Harrison's s.
    Huey's s.
    iris s.
    Irvine's s.

scissors *(continued)*
    Katzin's s.
    Kirby's s.
    Knapp's s.
    LaGrange's s.
    McClure's s.
    McGuire's s.
    McLean's s.
    McPherson-Castroviejo s.
    McPherson's s.
    McPherson-Vannas s.
    Nugent-Gradle s.
    Smart's s.
    Spencer's s.
    Stevens' s.
    Thorpe-Castroviejo s.
    Thorpe's s.
    Thorpe-Wescott s.
    Vannas' s.
    Verhoeff's s.
    Walker's s.
    Westcott's s.
    Wilmer's s.
sclera
scleral
    s. crescent
    s. spur
scleratitis
sclerectasia
sclerectasis
sclerectoiridectomy
sclerectoiridodialysis
sclerectome
sclerectomy
scleriasis
scleriritomy
scleritis
    Schöbl's s.

sclerocataracta
sclerochoroiditis
scleroconjunctival
scleroconjunctivitis
sclerocornea
sclerocorneal
scleroiritis
sclerokeratitis
sclerokeratoiritis
sclerokeratosis
scleromalacia
    s. perforans
scleronyxis
sclero-optic
sclerophthalmia
scleroplasty
sclerostomy
scleroticectomy
scleroticochoroiditis
scleroticonyxis
scleroticopuncture
scleroticotomy
sclerotitis
sclerotome
    Curdy's s.
    Lundsgaard-Burch s.
sclerotomy
scoop
    Arlt's s.
    Daviel's s.
    Knapp's s.
    Lewis' s.
    Mules' s.
    Wilder's s.
scotoma
    arcuate s.
    Bjerrum's s.
    centrocecal s.

scotoma *(continued)*
    paracentral s.
    peripapillary s.
    scintillating s.
    Seidel's s.
scotomagraph
scotomameter
scotomatous
scotometer
    Bjerrum's s.
scotometry
screen
    Bjerrum's s.
    tangent s.
Searcy's erysiphake
Seidel's scotoma
septum
    orbital s.
    s. orbitale
Shaaf's forceps
Sherrington's law
shield
    Buller's s.
    Fox's s.
shogrenz. See Sjogren's.
Sichel's disease
siderosis
    s. bulbi
    s. conjunctivae
Sidler-Huguenin's endotheli-
    oma
Siegrist-Hutchinson
    syndrome
sign
    Abadie's s.
    Barany's s.
    Dalrymple's s.
    Gifford's s.

sign *(continued)*
    Graefe's s.
    May's s.
    Mobius' s.
    Rifkind's s.
    Romana's s.
    Stellwag's s.
    von Graefe's s.
    Wilder's s.
Silva-Costa operation
sinus
    s. venosus sclerae
    venous s. of sclera
Sjögren's
    disease
    syndrome
Skeele's curette
Skew's deviation
skiametry
skiascopy
Sklar-Schiøtz' tonometer
slit lamp
Smart's
    forceps
    scissors
Smith-Green knife
Smith-Kuhnt-Szymanowski
    operation
Smith's
    expressor
    hook
    operation
Snellen's
    chart
    operation
    reform eye
Snell's law
Soemmerring's ring

Soria's operation
Sourdille's operation
space
    Fontana's s.
    periscleral s.
    Tenon's s.
    zonular s's.
Spaeth's operation
Spanlang-Tappeiner syndrome
spatia zonularia
spatula
    Berens' s.
    Castroviejo's s.
    Elschnig's s.
    Knapp's s.
    Lindner's s.
    McPherson's s.
    Wheeler's s.
Speas' operation
spectacles
    Masselon's s.
speculum
    Barraquer's s.
    Berens' s.
    Castroviejo's s.
    Guyton-Maumenee s.
    Guyton-Park s.
    Knapp's s.
    Lancaster's s.
    Lange's s.
    lid s.
    Lister-Burch s.
    McPherson's s.
    Mellinger's s.
    Mueller's s.
    Murdock-Wiener s.
    Park's s.
    Sauer's s.

speculum *(continued)*
    Weeks' s.
    Wiener's s.
    Williams' s.
Spencer's scissors
Spencer-Watson operation
Spero's forceps
sphere
spherical
sphincter
    s. iridis
    s. oculi
    s. oris
    s. pupillae
sphincterectomy
sphincterolysis
spindle
    Krukenberg's s.
spoon
    Bunge's s.
    Daviel's s.
    Elschnig's s.
    Hess' s.
    Kirby's s.
    Knapp's s.
sporotrichosis
spot
    Bitot's s.
    blind s.
    Brushfield's s.
    Elschnig's s's.
    Forster-Fuchs black s.
    Fuchs' s.
    Gaule's s's.
    Horner-Trantas s's.
    Mariotte's s.
    Maxwell's s.
    Roth's s.

spud
    Bahn's s.
    Corbett's s.
    Davis' s.
    Dix's s.
    Fisher's s.
    Francis' s.
    Hosford's s.
    LaForce's s.
    Walter's s.
squint
    comitant s.
    convergent s.
    divergent s.
    noncomitant s.
    upward and downward
        s.
Stahli's line
staphyloma
    s. corneae
    s. cornea racemosum
    equatorial s.
    intercalary s.
    s. posticum
    Scarpa's s.
    scleral s.
    uveal s.
staphylomatous
Stargardt's syndrome
Stellwag's
    edema
    sign
stenocoriasis
step
    Rönne's nasal s.
stereocampimeter
stereopsis
Stevens'

Stevens'
  forceps
  hook
  scissors
Stevens-Johnson syndrome
Stevenson's retractor
Stilling-Türk-Duane syndrome
Stocker's needle
Stock's operation
Stokes' lens
Storz' magnet
strabismic
strabismometer
strabismus
    Braid's s.
    s. deorsum vergens
    kinetic s.
    s. sursum vergens
strabometer
strabometry
strabotome
strabotomy
streak
    Knapp's s's.
streptotrichosis
striae
    s. ciliares
    Knapp's s.
striascope
striated
stroma
    s. of cornea
    s. iridis
    s. of iris
    vitreous s.
    s. vitreum
Sturge-Weber syndrome
Sturm's conoid

sty
    meibomian s.
    zeisian s.
Suarez-Villafranca operation
subcapsular
subconjunctival
subepithelial
    s. plexus
sublatio
    s. retinae
substantia
    s. propria corneae
sulcus
superciliary
supercilium
supraduction
supraocular
supraorbital
supratrochlear
surgical procedures. See
    operations.
sursumduction
sursumvergence
sursumversion
suture
    bridle s.
    collagen s.
    corneoscleral s.
    cuticular s.
    dermalon s.
    Ethicon silk s.
    far s.
    Frost's s.
    Kirby's s.
    limbal s.
    mattress s.
    preplaced s.
    postplaced s.

suture *(continued)*
    silk stay s.
    superior rectus traction
      s.
    supramid s.
    Verhoeff's s.
    y-suture
Swan's syndrome
Sylva's irrigator
symblepharon
symblepharopterygium
synchesis
synchysis
    s. scintillans
syndectomy
syndrome
    Adie's s.
    Alström-Olsen s.
    Andogsky's s.
    Angelucci's s.
    Anton-Babinski s.
    Axenfeld's s.
    Bamatter's s.
    Bassen-Kornzweig s.
    Beal's s.
    Behçet's s.
    Behr's s.
    Benedikt's s.
    Bielschowsky-Lutz-
      Cogan s.
    Bietti's s.
    Bonnet-Dechaume-
      Blanc s.
    chiasma s.
    Claude's s.
    Cogan's s.
    Dejean's s.
    Duane's s.

syndrome *(continued)*
    Elschnig's s.
    Foix's s.
    Foster-Kennedy s.
    Foville's s.
    Foville-Wilson s.
    Franceschetti's s.
    Friedenwald's s.
    Fuchs' s.
    Fuchs-Kraupa s.
    Gerstmann's s.
    Gradenigo's s.
    Graefe's s.
    Gregg's s.
    Greig's s.
    Guillain-Barré s.
    Gunn's s.
    Hallermann-Streiff s.
    Harada's s.
    Hertwig-Magendie s.
    Hippel-Lindau s.
    Horner-Bernard s.
    Horner's s.
    Hutchinson's s.
    Kennedy's s.
    Kiloh-Nevin s.
    Kimmelstiel-Wilson s.
    Koerber-Salus-Elschnig
      s.
    Krause's s.
    Kurz's s.
    Laurence-Moon-Biedl s.
    Louis-Bar's s.
    Lowe's s.
    Lyle's s.
    Marfan's s.
    Mikulicz's s.
    Millard-Gubler s.

syndrome *(continued)*
    Miller's s.
    Möbius' s.
    Parinaud's s.
    Petzetakis-Takos s.
    Posner-Schlossman s.
    Reese's s.
    Reiter's s.
    Riddoch's s.
    Rieger's s.
    Riley-Day s.
    Rollet's s.
    Rot-Bielschowsky s.
    Rothmund's s.
    Rutherfurd's s.
    Schäfer's s.
    Siegrist-Hutchinson s.
    Sjögren's s.
    Spanlang-Tappeiner s.
    Stargardt's s.
    Stevens-Johnson s.
    Stilling-Türk-Duane s.
    Sturge-Weber s.
    Swan's s.
    Terry's s.
    Thompson's s.
    Tolosa-Hunt s.
    Touraine's s.
    Uyemura's s.
    Vogt's s.
    Vogt-Koyanagi s.
    Weber's s.
    Werner's s.
    Wernicke's s.
    Wolf's s.
synechia
synechotome
synechotomy

synophrys
synophthalmia
synoptophore
synoptoscope
Szymanowski-Kuhnt operation
Szymanowski's operation
table
    Reuss's t's.
tapetum
    t. choroideae
    t. lucidum
    t. nigrum
    t. oculi
tarsadenitis
tarsal
tarsectomy
tarsitis
tarsocheiloplasty
tarsomalacia
tarsoplasty
tarsorrhaphy
tarsotomy
tarsus
    t. inferior palpebrae
    t. superior palpebrae
Tay's choroiditis
technique
    Atkinson's t.
    Van Lint's t.
teichopsia
telangiectases
telebinocular
tendon
    Lockwood's t.
    superior oblique t.
    Zinn's t.
tendotomy

Tenner's cannula
Tenon's
    capsule
    fascia
    space
tenonitis
tenonometer
tenontotomy
tenotome
tenotomist
tenotomize
tenotomy
tension
    intraocular t.
tereon. See *pterion.*
terijeum. See *pterygium.*
Terry's syndrome
Terson's operation
test
    Bielschowsky's t.
    confrontation field t.
    cover t.
    "E" t.
    head-tilt t.
    Hering's t.
    Holmgren's t.
    Ishihara's t.
    Marlow's t.
    Mauthner's t.
    Schirmer's t.
    shadow t.
tetrastichiasis
Theobald's probe
theory
    Hering's t.
    Schön's t.
    Young-Helmholtz t.
thermosector

thiriahsis. See *phthiriasis.*
Thomas'
    cryoptor
    operation
Thompson's syndrome
Thorpe's
    caliper
    forceps
    scissors
Thorpe-Castroviejo scissors
Thorpe-Wescott scissors
Thygeson's keratitis
tikopseah. See *teichopsia.*
tisis. See *phthisis.*
Todd's gouge
Tolosa-Hunt syndrome
tonogram
tonograph
tonographer
tonography
tonometer
    Goldman's applanation
        t.
    McLean's t.
    Schiøtz' t.
    Sklar-Schiøtz' t.
tonometry
Tooke's knife
torpor
    t. retinae
torsion
tortuous
tosis. See *ptosis.*
Toti-Mosher operation
Toti's operation
Touraine's syndrome
trachoma
    Arlt's t.

trachoma
  brawny t.
trachomatous
transillumination
Trantas'
  dots
  operation
treatment
  Imre's t.
  Schöler's t.
trepanation
  corneal t.
trephination
trephine
  Arruga's t.
  Castroviejo's t.
  Elliott's t.
  Grieshaber's t.
  Paufique's t.
trichiasis
trichromat
trichromatopsia
trifocal
trigone
  Müller's t.
triplokoria
trochlea
tropometer
tucker
  Burch-Greenwood t.
tunica
  t. adnata oculi
  t. conjunctiva
  t. conjunctiva bulbi
  t. conjunctiva bulbi oculi
  t. conjunctiva palpebra-
    rum
  t. fibrosa oculi

tunica *(continued)*
  t. interna bulbi
  t. nervea of Bruecke
  t. vasculosa bulbi
  t. vasculosa oculi
tunicary
Tyrell's hook
ulcer
  Mooren's u.
  Saemisch's u.
ulcus
  u. serpens corneae
ulectomy
Undine's dropper
unit
  Bovie u.
uvea
uveal
uveitic
uveitis
  Förster's u.
  heterochromic u.
  sympathetic u.
uveoparotid
uveoparotitis
uveoplasty
uveoscleritis
Uyemura's syndrome
vaginae bulbi
valve
  Foltz's v.
Van Lint
  akinesia
  block
  technique
Vannas' scissors
varicoblepharon
vasa sanguinea retinae

vascular
vascularization
veil
    Sattler's v.
vein
    ciliary v.
    cilioretinal v.
    posterior conjunctival v.
    vorticose v.
venae
    v. centralis retinae
    vorticosae
venula
    v. macularis inferior
    v. macularis superior
    v. medialis retinae
    v. nasalis retinae inferior
    v. nasalis retinae super-
      ior
    v. retinae medialis
    v. temporalis retinae in-
      ferior
    v. temporalis retinae
      superior
venule
    medial v. of retina
    nasal v. of retina,
      inferior and superior
    temporal v. of retina,
      inferior and superior
vergence
Verhoeff's
    forceps
    operation
    scissors
    suture
version
vertex

Verwey's operation
vesicle
    ocular v.
    ophthalmic v.
    optic v.
vesicula
    v. ophthalmica
Viers' erysiphake
Vieth-Muller horopter
vision
    achromatic v.
    binocular v.
    chromatic v.
    dichromatic v.
    fovial v.
    halo v.
    haploscopic v.
    iridescent v.
    monocular v.
    v. nul
    oscillating v.
    peripheral v.
    photopic v.
    Pick's v.
    pseudoscopic v.
    rod v.
    scoterythrous v.
    scotopic v.
    stereoscopic v.
    tunnel v.
visual
    v. acuity
    v. axis
    v. fields
    v. purple
visualization
visualize
visuometer

vitreous
>v. body
>v. floater
>v. humor

vitreum

VOD – visio oculus dextra –
vision, right eye

Vogt-Koyanagi syndrome

Vogt's
>cataract
>cornea
>degeneration
>disease
>syndrome

Vogt-Spielmeyer disease

von Graefe's
>cautery
>cystotome
>forceps
>hook
>knife
>knife needle
>operation
>sign

von Hippel-Lindau disease

von Monakow's fibers

von Mondak's forceps

von Recklinghausen's disease

VOS – visio oculus sinister –
vision, left eye

Vossius' lenticular ring

VOU – visio oculus uterque –
vision of each eye

Wadsworth-Todd cautery

Wagener's retinitis

Wagner's disease

Waldeau's forceps

Waldhauer's operation

Walker's
>lid everter
>pin
>scissors

walleye

Walter's spud

Walton's punch

wart
>Hassall-Henle w's.

Weber's
>knife
>syndrome

Weekers' operation

Weeks'
>needle
>speculum

Weil's disease

Weiss's reflex

Werner's syndrome

Wernicke's syndrome

Westcott's scissors

Westphal-Strumpell disease

West's operation

Weve's
>electrode
>operation

Wheeler's
>cystotome
>implant
>knife
>operation
>spatula

Widmark's conjunctivitis

Wiener's
>hook
>operation
>speculum

Wilder's

Wilder's *(continued)*
 scoop
 sign
Williams'
 probe
 speculum
Willis' circle
Wilmer's
 operation
 scissors
Wilson's disease
Wolfe's operation
Wolfring's gland
Wolf's syndrome
Worth's operation
Wucherer's conjunctivitis
xanthelasma
 x. palpebrarum
xanthelasmatosis
xanthoma
 x. palpebrarum
xanthomatosis
 x. bulbi
 x. iridis
xanthophane
xanthopia
xanthopsia
xeroma
xerophthalmia
xerophthalmus
xerosis
 x. conjunctivae
 x. superficialis
Young-Helmholtz theory
Y.S. — yellow spot of the
 retina

zan-. See words beginning
 Xan-.
Zeis
 glands of Z.
zeisian gland
Zeiss' photocoagulator
zero-. See words beginning
 Xero-.
zeromah. See *xeroma.*
Ziegler's
 cautery
 forceps
 knife
 operation
 probe
Zinn's
 circlet
 corona
 ligament
 tendon
 zonule
zonula
 z. ciliaris
zonulae
zonular
 z. fibers
 z. space
zonule
 ciliary z.
 z. of Zinn
zonulitis
zonulolysis
 enzymatic z.
zonulotomy
zonulysis

ORTHOPEDICS

abarticular
abarticulation
Abbott-Lucas operation
Abbott's operation
abduction
abductor
abscess
    Brodie's a.
absconsio
AC — acromioclavicular
acantha
acetabular
acetabulectomy
acetabuloplasty
acetabulum
Achilles'
    bursa
    bursitis
    jerk
    tendon
achillobursitis
achillodynia
achillorrhaphy
achillotenotomy
    plastic a.
achondroplasia
aclasis
    diaphyseal a.
    tarsoepiphyseal a.
acoustogram

acrocontracture
acromioclavicular
acromiocoracoid
acromiohumeral
acromion
acromionectomy
acromioscapular
acromiothoracic
acromyotonia
acrostealgia
acrosyndactyly
actinomycosis
Adams'
    operation
    saw
adapter
    McReynolds' a.
adduction
adductor
Adelmann's operation
adventitious
Agnew's splint
AJ — ankle jerk
AK — above knee
akilez. See *Achilles.*
akilo-. See words beginning
    achillo-.
akondroplazea. See
    achondroplasia.
ala

ala *(continued)*
    a. ilii
    a. ossis ilii
    a. ossis ilium
Albee-Delbet operation
Albee's
    operation
    osteotome
Albers-Schönberg
    bone
    disease
Albert's operation
Albright's
    disease
    syndrome
Alexander-Farabeuf periosteo-
    tome
Alexander's
    osteotome
    periosteotome
Allis' sign
Alouette's amputation
ambulation
ambulatory
amputation
    Alouette's a.
    aperiosteal a.
    Béclard's a.
    Bier's a.
    Bunge's a.
    Callander's a.
    Carden's a.
    Chopart's a.
    cineplastic a.
    Dupuytren's a.
    Farabeuf's a.
    Forbe's a.
    Gritti's a.

amputation *(continued)*
    Gritti-Stokes a.
    guillotine a.
    Guyon's a.
    Hancock's a.
    Hey's a.
    Kirk's a.
    Larrey's a.
    Le Fort's a.
    Lisfranc's a.
    MacKenzie's a.
    Maisonneuve's a.
    periosteoplastic a.
    phalangophalangeal a.
    Pirogoff's a.
    Ricard's a.
    Stokes' a.
    Syme's a.
    Teale's a.
    Tripier's a.
    Vladimiroff-Mikulicz a.
amyloid
amyotonia
anapophysis
anarrhexis
Anderson's
    operation
    splint
Angle's splint
angulation
ankle
    tailors' a.
ankylosis
Annandale's operation
anosteoplasia
anostosis
antebrachium
antecubital

anvil
>Bunnell's a.

apofi-. See words beginning
>*apophy-*.

aponeurectomy
aponeurorrhaphy
aponeurosis
aponeurotomy
apophyseal
apophysis
apophysitis
>a. tibialis adolescentium

apparatus
>Kirschner's a.
>Sayre's a.

arachnoid
arachnoidal
arch
>neural a.

areflexia
areten-. See words beginning
>*aryten-*.

artery
>basilic a.
>brachial a.
>cephalic a.
>femoral a.
>genicular a.
>gluteal a.
>interosseous a.
>obturator a.
>peroneal a.
>popliteal a.
>princeps pollicis a.
>profunda brachii a.
>pudendal a.
>radial a.
>radialis indicis a.

artery *(continued)*
>saphenous a.
>vesical a.

arthralgia
arthrectomy
arthritic
arthritis
>rheumatoid a.

arthrocentesis
arthrochalasis
arthrochondritis
arthroclasia
arthrodesis
>Charnley's a.

arthrodynia
arthroereisis
arthrogryposis
arthrokatadysis
arthrolysis
arthroncus
arthronosos
arthro-onychodysplasia
arthropathy
arthrophyma
arthroplasty
>Charnley-Mueller a.

arthrosis
>Charcot's a.
>a. deformans

arthrosteitis
arthrostomy
arthrosynovitis
arthrotomy
articular
articulated
articulatio
articulation
arytenoidectomy

arytenoidopexy
Ashhurst's splint
aspiration
astragalar
astragalectomy
astragalocalcanean
astragalocrural
astragaloscaphoid
astragalotibial
astragalus
ataxia
atrophy
    Sudeck's a.
Augustine's nail
Austin-Moore prosthesis
Avila's operation
avulsion
awl
    Wilson's a.
Baastrup's syndrome
Badgley's
    operation
    plate
Baker's cyst
Bakwin-Eiger syndrome
Balkan splint
bandage
    Desault's b.
    figure-of-8 b.
    Gibney's b.
    Gibson's b.
    Sayre's b.
    scultetus b.
    spica b.
    Velpeau's b.
Bankart's operation
Bardenheuer's extension
Barker's operation

Barré-Liéou syndrome
Barton's
    fracture
    operation
    tong
Barwell's operation
Basile's screw
Bateman's
    operation
    prosthesis
Baylor's splint
Bechterew-Mendel reflex
Bechterew's reflex
Beckman-Adson retractor
Béclard's amputation
bed
    circOlectric b.
belly
Bennett's
    elevator
    fracture
Bent's operation
Bertin's bone
Besnier's rheumatism
biceps
    b. brachii
    b. femoris
Bier's amputation
Bishop's tendon tucker
Bishop-Black tendon tucker
Bishop-DeWitt tendon tucker
Bishop-Peter tendon tucker
BK — below knee
Blount's
    disease
    operation
    osteotome
    plate

Blount's
    retractor
Blundell-Jones operation
Bobroff's operation
body
    Schmorl's b.
Böhler's splint
Böhler-Braun splint
Bohlman's pin
bolt
    Wilson's b.
Bond's splint
bone
    acetabular b.
    acromial b.
    alar b.
    Albers-Schönberg b.
    alisphenoid b.
    astragaloid b.
    astragaloscaphoid b.
    basihyal b.
    basilar b.
    Bertin's b.
    bregmatic b.
    calcaneal b.
    capitate b.
    carpal b's.
    chalky b's.
    coccygeal b.
    collar b.
    cortical b.
    costal b.
    cuneiform b.
    ectethmoid b's.
    endochondral b.
    entocuneiform b.
    epactal b's.
    ethmoid b.

bone *(continued)*
    femoral b.
    fibular b.
    hamate b.
    humeral b.
    hyoid b.
    iliac b.
    intermaxillary b.
    intrachondrial b.
    ischial b.
    lenticular b.
    lunate b.
    mesocuneiform b.
    metacarpal b's.
    metatarsal b's.
    multangular b.
    navicular b.
    occipital b.
    orbitosphenoidal b.
    pelvic b.
    periosteal b.
    petrous b.
    phalangeal b's.
    Pirie's b.
    pisiform b.
    radial b.
    sacral b.
    scaphoid b.
    sesamoid b's.
    supernumerary b.
    tarsal b's.
    temporal b.
    tibia b.
    trapezium b.
    trapezoid b.
    triquetrol b.
    turbinate b.
    ulna b.

bone *(continued)*
    ulnar styloid b.
    unciform b.
    uncinate b.
    vomer b.
    xiphoid b.
    zygomatic b.
bone graft
    diamond inlay b.g.
    hemicylindrical b.g.
    inlay b.g.
    intramedullary b.g.
    medullary b.g.
    onlay b.g.
    osteoperiosteal b.g.
    peg b.g.
Bonner's position
bootonyar. See *boutonnière.*
Bosworth's
    operation
    screw
boutonnière
Bowen's osteotome
Bowlby's splint
bowleg
Boyd's operation
Boyes-Goodfellow hook
brace
    ischial weight-bearing b.
    Lyman-Smith b.
    Taylor's b.
brachial
brachiocrural
brachiocubital
brachiocyllosis
brachium
Bradford's frame
Brant's splint

Brett's operation
Brickner position
Brissaud's scoliosis
Brittain's operation
Brockman's operation
Brodie's
    abscess
    disease
    knee
    ligament
Buck's
    extension
    hook
    operation
    splint
    traction
Büdinger-Ludloff-Laewen
    disease
Bunge's amputation
bunion
bunionectomy
    Keller's b.
bunionette
Bunnell's
    anvil
    drill
    needle
    operation
    probe
bur
    Jordan-Day b.
    Lempert's b.
Burch-Greenwood tendon
    tucker
bursa
    Achilles' b.
    olecranon b.
bursectomy

bursitis
    Achilles' b.
    Duplay's b.
    radiohumeral b.
bursotomy
Butcher's saw
Cabot's splint
calcaneitis
calcaneoapophysitis
calcaneoastragaloid
calceneocavus
calcaneocuboid
calcaneodynia
calcaneofibular
calcaneonavicular
calcaneoplantar
calcaneotibial
calcaneovalgocavus
calcaneus
calcar
    c. pedis
calcification
Callahan's operation
Callander's amputation
callus
    definitive c.
    ensheathing c.
    intermediate c.
    medullary c.
    myelogenous c.
    permanent c.
    provisional c.
Calvé-Perthes disease
Campbell's
    operation
    osteotome
Canadian crutch
canal

canal
    Hunter's c.
cancellated
cancelli
cancellous
cancellus
capeline
capitellum
capitulum
capsule
    articular c.
capsulectomy
capsulitis
    adhesive c.
capsuloplasty
capsulorrhaphy
capsulotomy
Carden's amputation
Carleton's spots
caro
    c. quadrata manus
    c. quadrata sylvii
carpal
carpectomy
carpometacarpal
carpopedal
carpophalangeal
carpoptosis
carpus
    c. curvus
Carrell's operation
Carroll-Legg osteotome
Carroll's osteotome
Carroll-Smith-Petersen
    osteotome
cartilage
cartilaginous
cast

cast *(continued)*
    long-arm c.
    long-leg c.
    short-arm c.
    short-leg c.
Cave-Rowe operation
Cave's operation
cavus
cervical
cervicalis
cervicobrachial
cervicodorsal
cervicodynia
cervico-occipital
cervicoscapular
cervicothoracic
Chandler's
    disease
    elevator
    splint
Chaput's method
Charcot's
    arthrosis
    joint
charleyhorse
Charnley-Mueller arthroplasty
Charnley's arthrodesis
Charriere's saw
cheirospasm
Cherry's osteotome
Chiene's operation
chisel
    Moore's c.
chondral
chondrectomy
chondritis
    c. intervertebralis
      calcanea

chondroblastoma
chondrocarcinoma
chondrocostal
chondrodynia
chondrodysplasia
chondrodystrophia
chondrodystrophy
    c. malacia
chondroepiphyseal
chondroepiphysitis
chondrolysis
chondroma
chondromalacia
chondromatosis
    Reichel's c.
    synovial c.
chondrophyte
chondroplasty
chondroporosis
chondrosarcomatosis
chondrosternal
chondrosternoplasty
chondrotome
chondrotomy
chonechondrosternon
Chopart's
    amputation
    joint
clamp
    Forrester's c.
    Humphries' c.
    Jackson's c.
    Lambotte's c.
    Lowman's c.
    Wester's c.
    Williams' c.
    Wilman's c.
    Wilson's c.

claudication
clavicle
clavicotomy
clavicula
clavicular
claviculus
clavus
clawfoot
clawhand
Clayton's osteotome
clonus
Cloward's osteotome
clubfoot
clubhand
Clutton's joint
Cobb's
    elevator
    gouge
    osteotome
coccygeal
coccygectomy
coccygerector
coccygeus
coccygodynia
coccygotomy
coccyx
Codivilla's
    extension
    operation
Cole's operation
collar
    Thomas' c.
Colles'
    fracture
    splint
Collin's osteoclast
collum
    c. anatomicum humeri

collum *(continued)*
    c. chirurgicum humeri
    c. costae
    c. distortum
    c. femoris
    c. mallei
    c. processus condyloidei
        mandibulae
    c. radii
    c. scapulae
    c. tali
    c. valgum
Colonna's operation
comminuted
comminution
Compere's
    operation
    pin
compression
concavity
condylar
condyle
condylectomy
condylion
condylotomy
condylus
congenerous
connexus
    c. intertendineus
Conn's operation
contractility
    idiomuscular c.
contraction
contracture
    Dupuytren's c.
    ischemic c.
    Volkmann's c.
Converse's osteotome

convexity
Conzett's goniometer
Coopernail's sign
coracoacromial
coracoclavicular
coracohumeral
coracoid
coracoiditis
coracoradialis
coracoulnaris
Corbett's forceps
coronoid
costa
    c. fluctuans
    c. fluctuans decima
costae
    c. spuriae
    c. verae
costal
costalgia
costalis
costectomy
costicartilage
costicervical
costochondral
costochondritis
costoclavicular
costoscapular
costoscapularis
costosternal
costosternoplasty
costotome
costotomy
costotransversectomy
costovertebral
costoxiphoid
Cottle's osteotome
Cotton's fracture

counterextension
countertraction
coxa
    c. adducta
    c. flexa
    c. magna
    c. plana
    c. valga
    c. vara
    c. vara luxans
coxalgia
coxankylometer
coxarthria
coxarthritis
coxarthrocace
coxarthropathy
coxitis
    c. fugax
    senile c.
coxodynia
coxofemoral
coxotomy
coxotuberculosis
Crane's
    mallet
    osteotome
Credo's operation
crena
    c. ani
crepitation
crepitus
cricoid
cricoidectomy
cruciate
crutch
    Canadian c.
Crutchfield's
    operation

Crutchfield's
    tong
Cruveilhier's joint
Cubbins' operation
cubital
cubitocarpal
cubitoradial
cubitus
    c. valgus
    c. varus
curet
    Spratt's c.
Curry's splint
CVA – costovertebral angle
cyst
    Baker's c.
Czerny's disease
dactylolysis
Darrach's operation
Davies-Colley operation
Davis' splint
débridement
decapitation
decompression
deformity
    Ilfeld-Holder d.
    lobster-claw d.
    Madelung's d.
    silver fork d.
    Sprengel's d.
    valgus d.
    varus d.
    Velpeau's d.
    Volkmann's d.
degeneration
    Zenker's d.
degenerative
Delore's method

Denis-Browne club foot
    splint
Denuse's operation
DePalma's prosthesis
DePuy's
    prosthesis
    splint
derangement
    Hey's internal d.
dermatomyositis
Desault's bandage
Deutschländer's disease
Deyerle's
    drill
    plate
    punch
diaclasis
diaphyseal
diaphysectomy
diaphysis
diaphysitis
    tuberculous d.
diaplasis
diaplastic
diapophysis
diarthric
diarthrosis
diastasis
Dickson-Diveley operation
Dickson's operation
Dieffenbach's operation
digit
digital
digitation
Dingman's
    forceps
    osteotome
DIP – distal interphalangeal

DIPJ – distal interphalangeal
   joint
diplegia
dis-. See also words beginning
   dys-.
disarticulation
discogenic
discoid
discoidectomy
disease
   Albers-Schönberg d.
   Albright's d.
   Blount's d.
   Brodie's d.
   Büdinger-Ludloff-
     Laewen d.
   Calvé-Perthes d.
   Chandler's d.
   Czerny's d.
   Deutschländer's d.
   Duplay's d.
   Erichsen's d.
   Freiberg's d.
   Hand-Schüller-
     Christian d.
   Inman's d.
   Jüngling's d.
   Kashin-Bek d.
   Köhler's d.
   Kümmell's d.
   Kümmell-Verneuil d.
   Larsen-Johansson d.
   Legg-Calvé-Waldenström
     d.
   Marie-Strümpell d.
   Marie-Tooth d.
   McArdle's d.
   Morquio's d.

disease *(continued)*
   Ollier's d.
   Osgood-Schlatter d.
   Otto's d.
   Paget's d.
   Pauzat's d.
   Pellegrini-Stieda d.
   Perrin-Ferraton d.
   Perthes' d.
   Pott's d.
   Poulet's d.
   Preiser's d.
   Quervain's d.
   Recklinghausen's d.
   Schanz's d.
   Scheuermann's d.
   Schlatter's d.
   Schmorl's d.
   Sever's d.
   Steinert's d.
   Swediaur's d.
   Talma's d.
   Volkmann's d.
   von Recklinghausen's d.
   Waldenström's d.
disk
   intervertebral d's.
diskectomy
diskitis
diskogram
diskography
dislocatio
   d. erecta
dislocation
   divergent d.
   Kienböck's d.
   Monteggia's d.
   Nélaton's d.

dislocation *(continued)*
    Smith's d.
    subastragalar d.
    subcoracoid d.
    subglenoid d.
dissector
    Lewin's d.
distraction
DJD – degenerative joint disease
dorsalis
dorsiflexion
dorsispinal
dorsolumbar
dorsoscapular
dorsum
Downing's knife
drill
    Bunnell's d.
    Deyerle's d.
    Hall's air d.
    intramedullary d.
    Smedberg's d.
    vitallium d.
driver
    Küntscher's d.
drugs. See *Medications.*
Dunn-Brittain operation
Duplay's
    bursitis
    disease
Dupuytren's
    amputation
    contracture
    splint
dura
dura mater
    d.m. spinalis

Durman's operation
Duverney's fracture
dynamometer
    squeeze d.
dysarthrosis
dyschondroplasia
    Ollier's d.
dysesthesia
dysostosis
dysplasia
    diaphyseal d.
    metaphyseal d.
dystrophy
    muscular d.
ebonation
eburnation
ecchondrotome
ectocondyle
ectromelia
ectrometacarpia
ectrometatarsia
ectrophalangia
Eden-Hybbinette operation
Eggers'
    operation
    plate
    screw
    splint
Eicher's prosthesis
elbow
    capped e.
    tennis e.
electromyography
elevator
    Bennett's e.
    Chandler's e.
    Cobb's e.
    Farabeuf's e.

elevator *(continued)*
      Lane's e.
      Langenbeck's e.
Elliott's plate
Ellis-Jones operation
Elmslie-Cholmeley operation
eminence
      thenar e.
enarthrosis
enchondroma
enchondromatosis
enchondrosarcoma
endochondral
endosteoma
endosteum
Engelmann's splint
enostosis
entepicondyle
epicondylalgia
epicondyle
epicondylitis
epicondylus
epifizee-. See words beginning
      epiphysi-.
epifizeal. See *epiphyseal,* and
      epiphysial.
epimysium
epiphyseal
epiphyses
      stippled e.
epiphysial
epiphysiodesis
epiphysioid
epiphysiolysis
epiphysiopathy
epiphysis
      e. cerebri
      slipped e.

epiphysitis
      vertebral e.
epipyramis
epirotulian
epistropheus
epitendineum
epitenon
epithesis
epitrochlea
Epstein's osteotome
equinovarus
equinus
erasion
      e. of a joint
ergogram
ergograph
      Mosso's e.
Erichsen's
      disease
      sign
Essex-Lopresti method
ethmofrontal
ethmoid
ethmomaxillary
Evans' operation
Ewing's tumor
exarticulation
exercise
      Williams' e.
exostosectomy
exostosis
      e. bursata
      e. cartilaginea
extension
      Bardenheuer's e.
      Buck's e.
      Codivilla's e.
extensor

extractor
  Jewett's e.
  Moore's e.
extremity
Eyler's operation
facet
facetectomy
Fahey's operation
falan-. See words beginning
  phalan-.
falanks. See *phalanx*.
falx
  f. inguinalis
  f. ligamentosa
Farabeuf-Lambotte forceps
Farabeuf's
  amputation
  elevator
  forceps
faradization
  galvanic f.
fascia
  f. lata femoris
fascial
fasciatome
  Luck's f.
fasciculation
fasciculus
fasciectomy
fasciitis
  pseudosarcomatous f.
fasciodesis
fascioplasty
fasciorrhaphy
fasciotomy
femoral
femoroiliac
femorotibial

femur
Ferguson's forceps
fibrocartilage
fibrocartilaginous
fibromatosis
fibrosarcoma
fibrositis
fibula
fibular
fibularis
fibulocalcaneal
finger
  baseball f.
  mallet f.
  trigger f.
Finklestein's test
Fink's tendon tucker
fixation
fizeotherape. See
  physiotherapy.
flatfoot
  spastic f.
flex
flexion
flexor
  f. retinaculum
foramen
foramina
foraminotomy
Forbe's amputation
forceps
  Corbett's f.
  Dingman's f.
  Farabeuf-Lambotte f.
  Farabeuf's f.
  Ferguson's f.
  Hibbs' f.
  Horsley's f.

forceps *(continued)*
    Kern's f.
    Lambotte's f.
    Lane's f.
    Liston-Stille f.
    Littauer-Liston f.
    Martin's f.
    Van Buren's f.
forearm
forefoot
Forrester's clamp
Fowler's
    operation
    position
Fox's splint
fracture
    Barton's f.
    Bennett's f.
    bimalleolar f.
    bucket-handle f.
    closed f.
    Colles' f.
    comminuted f.
    compound f.
    compression f.
    Cotton's f.
    depressed f.
    displaced f.
    Duverney's f.
    epiphysial f.
    Galeazzi's f.
    Gosselin's f.
    greenstick f.
    Guerin's f.
    impacted f.
    intercondylar f.
    intertrochanteric f.
    LeFort's f.

fracture *(continued)*
    linear f.
    march f.
    Monteggia's f.
    Moore's f.
    pathologic f.
    pertrochanteric f.
    pillion f.
    Pott's f.
    Quervain's f.
    Shepherd's f.
    silver-fork f.
    Skillern's f.
    Smith's f.
    spiral f.
    stellate f.
    Stieda's f.
    subcapital f.
    supracondylar f.
    transcervical f.
    transverse f.
    trimalleolar f.
    Wagstaffe's f.
fracture-dislocation
fragilitas
    f. ossium
frame
    Bradford's f.
    Hibbs' f.
    Stryker's f.
Frazier's osteotome
Freiberg's
    disease
    infraction
    knife
Fritz-Lange operation
fusion
    diaphyseal-epiphyseal f.

Gaenslen's sign
gait
    antalgic g.
Galeazzi's
    fracture
    sign
galvanic
galvanization
gampsodactylia
ganglion
ganglionectomy
gangrene
    Pott's g.
Gant's operation
Garré's osteomyelitis
Gatellier's operation
Gelfoam packing
genu
    g. impressum
    g. recurvatum
    g. valgum
    g. varum
Ghormley's operation
Gibney's
    bandage
    perispondylitis
Gibson's
    bandage
    operation
Gillespie's operation
Gill's operation
Girdlestone's operation
glenohumeral
glenoid
Glisson's sling
gluteal
gluteofemoral
gonarthritis

gonarthromeningitis
gonarthrotomy
goniometer
    Conzett's g.
gonitis
    fungous g.
    g. tuberculosa
gonocampsis
Gordon's splint
Gosselin's fracture
gouge
    Cobb's g.
    Moore's g.
Graber-Duvernay operation
Grice-Green operation
Gritti's amputation
Gritti-Stokes amputation
Guerin's fracture
Guillain-Barré syndrome
Guleke-Stookey operation
Guyon's amputation
Haas' operation
Hagie's pin
Hall's air drill
hallux
    h. dolorosa
    h. malleus
    h. rigidus
    h. valgus
    h. varus
hammer toe
Hammond's operation
Hancock's amputation
hand
    Krukenberg's h.
Hand-Schüller-Christian
    disease
Hansen-Street nail

Hansen-Street
    pin
Hark's operation
Harmons' operation
Harris-Beath operation
Hart's splint
Hatcher's pin
Hauser's operation
Heberden's nodes
Heifitz's operation
hemapophysis
hemarthrosis
hemilaminectomy
hemiphalangectomy
hemiplegia
hemivertebra
Henderson's operation
Hendry's operation
Henry-Geist operation
herniated
herniation
       h. of nucleus pulposus
hetero-osteoplasty
Heuter's operation
Heyman's operation
Hey's
    amputation
    internal derangement
Hibbs'
    forceps
    frame
    operation
    osteotome
hip
    snapping h.
Hodgen's splint
Hoen's plate
Hohmann's operation

Hoke's osteotome
Homans' sign
hook
    Boyes-Goodfellow h.
    Buck's h.
Horsley's forceps
Horwitz-Adams operation
Howorth's
    operation
    osteotome
humeral
humeroradial
humeroscapular
humeroulnar
humerus
Humphries' clamp
Hunter's canal
hydrarthrosis
hypalgesia
hyperesthesia
hyperextension
hyperostosis
hypertrophy
    Marie's h.
hypesthesia
hypolemmal
hypothenar
idiomuscular
iksomielitis. See *ixomyelitis.*
Ilfeld-Holder deformity
iliac
iliofemoral
iliofemoroplasty
iliopectineal
iliosacral
iliosciatic
iliospinal
iliotibial

iliotrochanteric
ilioxiphopagus
ilium
immobilization
incision
    deltopectoral i.
infraction
    Freiberg's i.
infrapatellar
Inman's disease
innervation
inochondritis
instability
    lumbosacral i.
instep
insufficientia
    i. vertebrae
interarticular
interdigital
interosseous
interphalangeal
interspace
intertrochanteric
intervertebral
intramedullary
ischial
ischialgia
ischiocapsular
ischiococcygeal
ischiococcygeus
ischiofemoral
ischiofibular
ischiohebotomy
ischiopubic
ischiopubiotomy
ischiosacral
ischiovertebral
ischium

iskeal. See *ischial.*
iskealjea. See *ischialgia.*
iskeo-. See words beginning
   ischio-.
iskeum. See *ischium.*
ithyokyphosis
ixomyelitis
jacket
    Minerva's j.
    plaster-of-paris j.
    Sayre's j.
Jackson's clamp
jerk
    Achilles' j.
    ankle j.
    quadriceps j.
    triceps surae j.
Jewett's
    extractor
    nail
    plate
joint
    apophyseal j's.
    ball-and-socket j.
    biaxial j.
    bilocular j.
    cartilaginous j.
    Charcot's j.
    Chopart's j.
    Clutton's j.
    cochlear j.
    condyloid j.
    Cruveilhier's j.
    diarthrodial j.
    ellipsoidal j.
    fibrocartilaginous j.
    flail j.
    freely movable j.

joint *(continued)*
    hysteric j.
    immovable j.
    intercarpal j's.
    ligamentous j.
    Lisfranc's j.
    Luschka's j's.
    midcarpal j.
    multiaxial j.
    pivot j.
    polyaxial j.
    sacrococcygeal j.
    saddle j.
    scapuloclavicular j.
    spheroidal j.
    spiral j.
    synovial j.
    uniaxial j.
    unilocular j.
    von Gies' j.
joint mice
Jones'
    position
    splint
Jordan-Day bur
Judet's prosthesis
Jüngling's disease
Jung's muscle
juxta-articular
juxtaepiphyseal
Kanavel's splint
Kapel's operation
Kashin-Bek disease
Keith's needle
Keller-Blake splint
Keller's bunionectomy
Kellogg-Speed operation
Kern's forceps

Kessel's plate
Kezerian's osteotome
Kienböck's dislocation
kifo-. See words beginning
    kypho-.
kineplasty
kinesalgia
King-Richards operation
Kirkaldy-Willis operation
Kirk's amputation
Kirmission's raspatory
kirospazm. See *cheirospasm.*
Kirschner's
    apparatus
    wire
KJ – knee jerk
Klippel-Feil syndrome
knee
    Brodie's k.
knife
    Downing's k.
    Freiberg's k.
    Liston's k.
    Lowe-Breck k.
    Smillie's k.
Knowles' pin
knuckle
Koenig-Wittek operation
Köhler's disease
kokse-. See words beginning
    coccy-.
kon-. See words beginning
    chon-.
König's operation
Kreuscher's scissors
Kristiansen's screw
Krukenberg's hand
Kümmell's

Kümmell's *(continued)*
    disease
    spondylitis
Kümmell-Verneuil disease
Küntscher's
    driver
    nail
    reamer
kyphoscoliosis
kyphosis
    Scheuermann's k.
labrum
    l. acetabulare
    l. glenoidale
Laing's plate
Lambotte-Henderson osteo-
    tome
Lambotte's
    clamp
    forceps
    osteotome
lamella
lamina
laminae
laminectomy
    lumbar l.
    thoracic l.
laminotomy
Lane's
    elevator
    forceps
    plate
Langenbeck's
    elevator
    saw
Lange's operation
Larrey's amputation
Larsen-Johansson disease

Lasègue's sign
Lawson-Thornton plate
Le Fort's
    amputation
    fracture
Legg-Calvé-Waldenström
    disease
Legg's osteotome
Leinbach's osteotome
Lempert's bur
L'Episcopo's operation
Levine's operation
Lewin's
    dissector
    splint
Lewin-Stern splint
ligament
    acromioclavicular l.
    Brodie's l.
    calcaneofibular l.
    calcaneonavicular l.
    carpometacarpal l.
    coracoacromial l.
    coracoclavicular l.
    coracohumeral l.
    costoclavicular l.
    cruciate l's.
    cuboideonavicular l.
    cuneonavicular l.
    deltoid l.
    hamatometacarpal l.
    iliofemoral l.
    inguinal l.
    laciniate l.
    olecranon l.
    patellar l.
    pisohamate l.
    pisometacarpal l.

ligament *(continued)*
    radiocarpal l.
    sacrospinous l.
    sternoclavicular l.
    sternocostal l.
    talocalcaneal l.
    talonavicular l.
ligamentous
ligamentum
    l. flavum
    l. teres femoris
line
    Ogston's l.
    Ullmann's l.
linea
    l. alba cervicalis
    l. arcuata ossis ilii
    l. aspera femoris
    l. epiphysialis
    l. glutea
    l. pectinea femoris
    l. terminalis pelvis
    l. trapezoidea
Lippman's prosthesis
Lisfranc's
    amputation
    joint
Liston's knife
Liston-Stille forceps
Littauer-Liston forceps
Littlewood's operation
LOM – limitation of motion
longitudinal
lordoscoliosis
lordosis
lordotic
Lorenz's osteotomy
Lottes' operation

Lowe-Breck knife
Lowman's clamp
LS – lumbosacral
Lucae's mallet
Lucas-Cottrell operation
Luck's
    fasciatome
    operation
Ludloff's operation
lumbago
lumbar
lumbarization
lumbodorsal
lumbosacral
Luschka's joints
luxatio
    l. coxae congenita
    l. erecta
    l. imperfecta
    l. perinealis
luxation
    Malgaigne's l.
Lyman-Smith brace
Lytle's splint
MacAusland's operation
Macewen's osteotomy
MacIntosh's prosthesis
MacKenzie's amputation
MacLeod's capsular rheuma-
    tism
Madelung's deformity
Magnuson's operation
Magnuson-Stack operation
Mahorner-Mead operation
Maisonneuve's amputation
Malgaigne's luxation
malleolar
malleoli

malleolus
malleotomy
mallet
    Crane's m.
    Lucae's m.
    Meyerding's m.
    Rush's m.
malum
    m. articulorum senilis
    m. coxae senilis
malunion
manipulation
Marie's hypertrophy
Marie-Strümpell
    disease
    spondylitis
Marie-Tooth disease
Martin's forceps
Mason-Allen splint
Matchett-Brown prosthesis
Mayer's reflex
Mayfield's osteotome
Mayo's operation
Mazur's operation
McArdle's disease
McBride's operation
McCarroll's operation
McKeever's prosthesis
McLaughlin's
    operation
    plate
    screw
McMurray's
    sign
    test
McReynolds' adapter
mediastinum
Medications

Medications *(continued)*
    acetaminophen
    alphaprodine
    anileridine
    Butazolidin
    codeine
    Darvon
    Demerol
    diazepam
    Dihydrohydroxy-
        codeinone
    epinephrine
    hydrocortisone
    14-Hydroxydihydro-
        codeinane
    Indocin
    indomethacin
    Leritine
    lidocaine
    mefenamic acid
    meperidine
    Nisentil
    Novocain
    oxycodone
    oxyphenbutazone
    pentazocine
    phenylbutazone
    Ponstel
    procaine
    propoxyphene
    Talwin
    Tandearil
    Tylenol
    Valium
    Xylocaine
medulla
    m. ossium
    m. spinalis

medullary
melorheostosis
meningosis
meniscectomy
    medial m.
meniscitis
meniscus
    m. of acromioclavicular
      joint
    m. articularis
    m. articulationis genus,
      laterialis, medialis
    medial m. of knee joint
    m. of temporomaxillary
      joint
mesomelic
mesomorphic
mesomorphy
mesotendineum
metacarpal
metacarpectomy
metacarpophalangeal
metacarpus
metaphysis
metaphysitis
metapophysis
metatarsal
metatarsalgia
metatarsectomy
metatarsophalangeal
metatarsus
    m. adductocavus
    m. adductovarus
    m. adductus
    m. atavicus
    m. latus
    m. primus varus
    m. varus

method
    Chaput's m.
    Delore's m.
    Essex-Lopresti m.
Meyerding's
    mallet
    osteotome
    retractor
Michaelis's rhomboid
Michele's trephine
mielo-. See words beginning
    myelo-.
Mikulicz's operation
Milch's operation
Miner's osteotome
Minerva's jacket
mobilization
Moe's plate
monostotic
Monteggia's
    dislocation
    fracture
Moore's
    chisel
    extractor
    fracture
    gouge
    nail
    osteotome
    pin
    prosthesis
    reamer
    template
Morestin's operation
Morquio's disease
Morton's
    neuralgia
    neuroma

Morton's
    toe
Mosso's ergograph
MP – metacarpophalangeal
MPJ – metacarpophalangeal
    joint
Mumford-Gurd operation
muscle
    abductor digiti quinti m.
    abductor pollicis brevis
      m.
    abductor pollicis longus
      m.
    adductor hallucis m.
    adductor longus m.
    adductor magnus m.
    adductor pollicis m.
    anconeus m.
    biceps brachii m.
    biceps femoris m.
    brachialis m.
    brachioradialis m.
    coracobrachialis m.
    deltoid m.
    extensor carpi radialis
      brevis m.
    extensor carpi radialis
      longus m.
    extensor carpi ulnaris m.
    extensor digiti minimi
      m.
    extensor digiti quinti
      proprius m.
    extensor digitorum
      brevis m.
    extensor digitorum
      communis m.
    extensor digitorum

muscle *(continued)*
    longus m.
    extensor hallucis brevis
      m.
    extensor hallucis longus
      m.
    extensor indicis m.
    extensor pollicis brevis
      m.
    extensor pollicis longus
      m.
    flexor carpi radialis m.
    flexor carpi ulnaris m.
    flexor digitorum brevis
      m.
    flexor digitorum longus
      m.
    flexor digitorum pro-
      fundus m.
    flexor digitorum sub-
      limis m.
    flexor digitorum super-
      ficialis m.
    flexor hallucis brevis m.
    flexor hallucis longus m.
    flexor pollicis brevis m.
    flexor pollicis longus m.
    gastrocnemius m.
    gemellus m.
    gluteus maximus m.
    gluteus medius m.
    gluteus minimus m.
    gracilis m.
    greater trochanter m.
    iliocostalis cervicis m.
    iliocostalis lumborum
      m.
    iliocostalis thoracis m.

muscle *(continued)*
    iliopsoas m.
    interosseous m.
    Jung's m.
    lateral malleolus m.
    palmaris brevis m.
    palmaris longus m.
    paraspinal m.
    pectineus m.
    pectoralis major m.
    pectoralis minor m.
    peroneus brevis m.
    peroneus longus m.
    peroneus tertius m.
    plantar m.
    popliteal m.
    pronator quadratus m.
    pronator teres m.
    psoas m.
    quadriceps femoris m.
    rectus m.
    sartorius m.
    scalenus m.
    semimembranosus m.
    semispinalis m.
    semitendinosus m.
    serratus m.
    soleus m.
    spinalis m.
    sternocleidomastoid m.
    subscapular m.
    supinator m.
    tensor fasciae latae m.
    teres m.
    tibialis m.
    trapezius m.
    triceps brachii m.
    triceps surae m.

muscle *(continued)*
    vastus intermedius m.
    vastus lateralis m.
    vastus medialis m.
muscular
muscularis
musculature
musculoskeletal
musculotendinous
musculus
myalgia
myatonia
myectomy
myelitis
myelocystomeningocele
myelogram
myelography
myelomalacia
myelomeningocele
myeloneuritis
myeloparalysis
myesthesia
myocele
myoclonus
myocrismus
myodemia
myodiastasis
myodynia
myofascitis
myofibril
myofibroma
myofibrosis
myogelosis
myogenic
myohypertrophia
myokerosis
myokinesis
myokymia

myolysis
myoma
myomalacia
myoneurectomy
myopathia
    m. infraspinata
myopathy
myoplasty
myorrhaphy
myorrhexis
myosarcoma
myoscope
myoseism
myositis
myospasm
myosteoma
myosthenometer
myotasis
myotatic
myotenositis
myotenotomy
myotome
myotomy
myotonia
    m. acquisita
    m. atrophica
myotonus
Naffziger's syndrome
nail
    Augustine's n.
    Hansen-Street n.
    Jewett's n.
    Küntscher n.
    Moore's n.
    Neufeld's n.
    Pugh's n.
    Smillie's n.
    Smith-Petersen n.

nail *(continued)*
    Thornton's n.
    Venable-Stuck n.
nailing
    intramedullary n.
nates
navicula
navicular
nearthrosis
neck
    surgical n.
necrosis
    aseptic n.
    Paget's quiet n.
    Zenker's n.
needle
    Bunnell's n.
    Keith's n.
    Turkel's n.
Neer's prosthesis
Nélaton's
    dislocation
    operation
nerve
    peroneal n.
Neufeld's nail
neuralgia
    Morton's n.
neurofibromatosis
neurofibrositis
neurolysis
neuroma
    Morton's n.
neuropathy
neuroskeletal
Nicola's operation
node
    Heberden's n's.

nodule
>Schmorl's n.

nonunion

nucleus
>n. pulposus

Ober's
>operation
>sign
>test

Ogston's
>line
>operation

olecranarthritis

olecranarthropathy

olecranon

olisthy

Ollier's
>disease
>dyschondroplasia
>operation

operation
>Abbott-Lucas o.
>Abbott's o.
>Adams' o.
>Adelmann's o.
>Albee-Delbet o.
>Albee's o.
>Albert's o.
>Anderson's o.
>Annandale's o.
>Avila's o.
>Badgley's o.
>Bankart's o.
>Barker's o.
>Barton's o.
>Barwell's o.
>Bateman's o.
>Bent's o.

operation *(continued)*
>Blount's o.
>Blundell-Jones o.
>Bobroff's o.
>Bosworth's o.
>Boyd's o.
>Brett's o.
>Brittain's o.
>Brockman's o.
>Buck's o.
>Bunnell's o.
>Callahan's o.
>Campbell's o.
>Carrell's o.
>Cave-Rowe o.
>Cave's o.
>Chiene's o.
>Codivilla's o.
>Cole's o.
>Colonna's o.
>Compere's o.
>Conn's o.
>Credo's o.
>Crutchfield's o.
>Cubbins' o.
>Darrach's o.
>Davies-Colley o.
>Denuse's o.
>Dickson-Diveley o.
>Dickson's o.
>Dieffenbach's o.
>Dunn-Brittain o.
>Durman's o.
>Eden-Hybbinette o.
>Eggers' o.
>Ellis-Jones o.
>Elmslie-Cholmeley o.
>Evans' o.

operation *(continued)*
- Eyler's o.
- Fahey's o.
- Fowler's o.
- Fritz-Lange o.
- Gant's o.
- Gatellier's o.
- Ghormley's o.
- Gibson's o.
- Gillespie's o.
- Gill's o.
- Girdlestone's o.
- Graber-Duvernay o.
- Grice-Green o.
- Guleke-Stookey o.
- Haas' o.
- Hammond's o.
- Hark's o.
- Harmon's o.
- Harris-Beath o.
- Hauser's o.
- Heifitz' o.
- Henderson's o.
- Hendry's o.
- Henry-Geist o.
- Heuter's o.
- Heyman's o.
- Hibbs' o.
- Hohmann's o.
- Horwitz-Adams o.
- Howorth's o.
- Kapel's o.
- Kellogg-Speed o.
- King-Richards o.
- Kirkaldy-Willis o.
- Koenig-Wittek o.
- König's o.
- Lange's o.

operation *(continued)*
- L'Episcopo's o.
- Levine's o.
- Littlewood's o.
- Lottes' o.
- Lucas-Cottrell o.
- Luck's o.
- Ludloff's o.
- MacAusland's o.
- Magnuson's o.
- Magnuson-Stack o.
- Mahorner-Mead o.
- Mayo's o.
- Mazur's o.
- McBride's o.
- McCarroll's o.
- McLaughlin's o.
- Mikulicz's o.
- Milch's o.
- Morestin's o.
- Mumford-Gurd o.
- Nélaton's o.
- Nicola's o.
- Ober's o.
- Ogston's o.
- Ollier's o.
- Osborne's o.
- Osgood's o.
- Palmer-Widen o.
- Pauwels' o.
- Pheasant's o.
- Phelps' o.
- Phemister's o.
- Putti-Platt o.
- Reichenheim-King o.
- Ridlon's o.
- Roux-Goldthwait o.
- Schanz's o.

operation *(continued)*
    Schede's o.
    Slocum's o.
    Smith-Petersen o.
    Speed-Boyd o.
    Stamm's o.
    Steindler's o.
    Thomson's o.
    Van Gorder's o.
    Wagoner's o.
    Watson-Jones o.
    Wilson-McKeever o.
    Wladimiroff's o.
    Wyeth's o.
    Yount's o.
    Zahradnicek's o.
os
    o. calcis
Osborne's operation
osfe-. See words beginning
    osphy-.
Osgood's operation
Osgood-Schlatter disease
osphyarthrosis
osphyomyclitis
osseocartilaginous
osseous
ossicle
ossification
ostealgia
ostearthrotomy
ostectomy
osteitis
    o. deformans
    o. fibrosa cystica
    o. ossificans
osteoarthritis
osteoarthropathy

osteoarthrosis
osteoblastoma
osteochondral
osteochondritis
    o. deformans
    o. dissecans
osteochondrodystrophy
osteochondroma
osteochondromatosis
    synovial o.
osteochondrosarcoma
osteochondrosis
osteoclasis
osteoclast
    Collin's o.
    Phelps-Gocht o.
    Rizzoli's o.
osteocystoma
osteodynia
osteodystrophy
osteofibrochondrosarcoma
osteoid
osteoma
    cavalryman's o.
    o. sarcomatosum
    o. spongiosum
osteomalacia
osteominosis
osteomyelitis
    Garré's o.
osteomyelodysplasia
osteopathy
osteoperiosteal
osteoperiostitis
osteopetrosis
osteophyte
osteophytosis
osteoplastica

osteoplasty
osteopoikilosis
osteoporosis
osteoporotic
osteorrhaphy
osteosclerosis
osteostixis
osteosynthesis
osteotome
    Albee's o.
    Alexander's o.
    Blount's o.
    Bowen's o.
    Campbell's o.
    Carroll-Legg o.
    Carroll's o.
    Carroll-Smith-Petersen o.
    Cherry's o.
    Clayton's o.
    Cloward's o.
    Cobb's o.
    Converse's o.
    Cottle's o.
    Crane's o.
    Dingman's o.
    Epstein's o.
    Frazier's o.
    Hibbs' o.
    Hoke's o.
    Howorth's o.
    Kezerian's o.
    Lambotte-Henderson o.
    Lambotte's o.
    Legg's o.
    Leinbach's o.
    Mayfield's o.
    Meyerding's o.
    Miner's o.

osteotome *(continued)*
    Moore's o.
    Rowland's o.
    Sheehan's o.
    Smith-Petersen o.
    Stille's o.
osteotomy
    cup-and-ball o.
    Lorenz's o.
    Macewen's o.
Otto's
    disease
    pelvis
packing
    Gelfoam p.
Paget's
    disease
    quiet necrosis
palm
palma
    p. manus
palmar
palmaris
Palmer-Widen operation
panosteitis
parallagma
paralysis
    Pott's p.
paraplegia
paratarsium
paratenon
paravertebral
paresis
paresthesia
paronychia
    p. tendinosa
parosteitis
parosteosis

patella
patellapexy
patellar
patellectomy
patellofemoral
Patrick's test
Pauwels' operation
Pauzat's disease
pectus
    p. carinatum
    p. excavatum
    p. recurvatum
pedal
pedicle
    p. of vertebral arch
pediculus
    p. arcus vertebrae
Pellegrini-Stieda disease
pelma
pelviotomy
pelvis
    Otto's p.
pelvisacral
pelvisection
pelvitrochanterian
pelvospondylitis
    p. ossificans
periarthritis
perichondritis
perichondrium
pericoxitis
peridesmium
perineum
periosteal
periosteomyelitis
periosteorrhaphy
periosteotome
    Alexander's p.

periosteotome
    Alexander-Farabeuf p.
periosteotomy
periosteum
periostitis
perispondylitis
    Gibney's p.
peritendineum
peritendinitis
    p. calcarea
    p. crepitans
peritenon
peritenoneum
peritenonitis
peroneal
peroneotibial
Perrin-Ferraton disease
Perthes' disease
pes
    p. abductus
    p. adductus
    p. anserinus
    p. cavus
    p. planus
    p. pronatus
    p. supinatus
    p. valgus
phalangeal
phalangectomy
phalanges
phalangette
phalangophalangeal
phalanx
    proximal p.
Pheasant's operation
Phelps-Gocht osteoclast
Phelps' operation
Phemister's operation

physiotherapy
pillion
pin
    Bohlman's p.
    Compere's p.
    Hagie's p.
    Hansen-Street p.
    Hatcher's p.
    Knowles' p.
    Moore's p.
    Rush's p.
    Steinmann's p.
    Street's p.
    Turner's p.
    von Saal's p.
    Zimmer's p.
PIP – proximal interphalan-
    geal
PIPJ – proximal interphalan-
    geal joint
Pirie's bone
Pirogoff's amputation
plantar
plantaris
plate
    Badgley's p.
    Blount's p.
    Deyerle's p.
    Eggers' p.
    Elliott's p.
    Hoen's p.
    Jewett's p.
    Kessel's p.
    Laing's p.
    Lane's p.
    Lawson-Thornton p.
    McLaughlin's p.
    Moe's p.

plate *(continued)*
    Sherman's p.
    Thornton's p.
    Wilson's p.
    Wright's p.
pleurapophysis
plombage
plombierung
poculum
    p. diogenis
pododynia
polyarthritis
polyarticular
polychondritis
polydactylia
polydysspondylism
polymyositis
polytendinitis
polytendinobursitis
poples
popliteal
position
    Bonner's p.
    Brickner p.
    Fowler's p.
    Jones' p.
Pott's
    disease
    fracture
    gangrene
    paralysis
Poulet's disease
Preiser's disease
prehallux
prepatellar
pretarsal
pretibial
probe

probe
    Bunnell's p.
process
    acromion p.
    articular p.
    capitular p.
    condyloid p.
    conoid p.
    intercondylar p.
    odontoid p.
    olecranon p.
    styloid p.
    ungual p.
    xiphoid p.
pronation
pronatoflexor
prosthesis
    Austin-Moore p.
    Bateman's p.
    DePalma's p.
    DePuy's p.
    Eicher's p.
    Judet's p.
    Lippman's p.
    MacIntosh's p.
    Matchett-Brown p.
    McKeever's p.
    Moore's p.
    Neer's p.
    Shier's p.
    Smith-Petersen p.
    Thompson's p.
    Townley's p.
    vitallium p.
    Walldius' p.
    Zimaloy's p.
protractor
    Robinson's p.

protrusion
pseudoluxation
psoas muscle
pubetrotomy
pubic
pubioplasty
pubiotomy
pubis
pubofemoral
pubotibial
Pugh's nail
punch
    Deyerle's p.
Putti-Platt operation
Putti's rasp
pylon
quadratipronator
quadriceps
quadricepsplasty
quadriplegia
Quervain's
    disease
    fracture
rachialgia
rachiocampsis
rachiotomy
rachitis
radial
radicular
radiculectomy
radiculitis
radiculomedullary
radiculomeningomyelitis
radiculomyelopathy
radiculoneuritis
radiobicipital
radiocarpal
radiocarpus

radiohumeral
radiopalmar
radioulnar
radius
rakealjea. See *rachialgia.*
rakeo-. See words beginning *rachio-.*
rakitis. See *rachitis.*
ramus
    r. of pubis
Raney-Crutchfield tong
rasp
    Putti's r.
raspatory
    Kirmission's r.
Rauchfuss' sling
ray
    digital r.
reamer
    Küntscher's r.
    Moore's r.
    Rush's r.
Recklinghausen's disease
recurvation
reduction
    closed r.
reflex
    Bechterew-Mendel r.
    Bechterew's r.
    Mayer's r.
    Stookey r.
    Strümpell's r.
refracture
Reichel's chondromatosis
Reichenheim-King operation
rete
    r. articulare genus
    r. calcaneum

rete
    r. carpi dorsale
retinaculum
retractor
    Beckman-Adson r.
    Blount's r.
    Meyerding's r.
    Rizzo's r.
    Senn's r.
    Sweet's r.
retropatellar
retropulsion
rheumatism
    Besnier's r.
    MacLeod's capsular r.
rhizomelic
rhomboid
    Michaelis's r.
Ricard's amputation
Ridlon's operation
RIF – right iliac fossa
rigidity
    cogwheel r.
rizomelik. See *rhizomelic.*
Rizzo's retractor
Rizzoli's osteoclast
Robinson's protractor
ROM – range of motion
romboid. See *rhomboid.*
roomatizm. See *rheumatism.*
Roux-Goldthwait operation
Rowland's osteotome
Rush's
    mallet
    pin
    reamer
Russell's traction
Ryerson's tenotome

sacral
sacralgia
sacralization
sacrarthrogenic
sacrectomy
sacroanterior
sacrococcygeal
sacrococcyx
sacrocoxalgia
sacrocoxitis
sacrodynia
sacroiliac
sacroiliitis
sacrolisthesis
sacrolumbar
sacroposterior
sacrosciatic
sacrospinal
sacrotomy
sacrovertebral
sacrum
sarcoidosis
    muscular s.
sarcoplasm
sarcoplast
Satterlee's saw
saucerization
saw
    Adams' s.
    Butcher's s.
    Charriere's s.
    Langenbeck's s.
    Satterlee's s.
Sayre's
    apparatus
    bandage
    jacket
    splint

scaphoid
scaphoiditis
    tarsal s.
scaphula
scapula
scapulalgia
scapular
scapulectomy
scapuloclavicular
scapulodynia
scapulohumeral
scapulopexy
scapuloposterior
scapulothoracic
Scarpa's triangle
Schanz's
    disease
    operation
    syndrome
Schede's operation
Scheuermann's
    disease
    kyphosis
Schlatter's disease
Schmorl's
    body
    disease
    nodule
sciatic
sciatica
scissors
    Kreuscher's s.
    Wester's s.
scoliokyphosis
scoliosis
    Brissaud's s.
    cicatricial s.
    coxitic s.

scoliosis *(continued)*
>   empyematic s.
>   ischiatic s.
>   myopathic s.
>   ocular s.
>   ophthalmic s.
>   osteopathic s.
>   paralytic s.
>   rachitic s.
>   rheumatic s.
>   sciatic s.
>   static s.

scoliosometer
scoliotic
scoliotone
scolopsia
screw
>   Basile's s.
>   Bosworth's s.
>   Eggers' s.
>   Kristiansen's s.
>   McLaughlin's s.
>   Sherman's s.
>   Thornton's s.

semilunar
semilunare
Senn's retractor
sequestrectomy
sequestrum
Sever's disease
sfirektome. See *sphyrectomy.*
sfirotome. See *sphyrotomy.*
Sheehan's osteotome
Shepherd's fracture
Sherman's
>   plate
>   screw

Shier's prosthesis

siatik. See *sciatic.*
siatika. See *sciatica.*
sign
>   Allis' s.
>   Coopernail's s.
>   Erichsen's s.
>   Gaenslen's s.
>   Galeazzi's s.
>   Homans' s.
>   Lasègue's s.
>   McMurray's s.
>   Ober's s.
>   Stiller's s.
>   Tinel's s.

simphysis. See *symphysis.*
sin-. See words beginning
>   *syn-.*

sinew
sino-. See words beginning
>   *syno-.*

skeletal
skeleton
skewfoot
Skillern's fracture
sling
>   Glisson's s.
>   Rauchfuss's s.
>   Teare's s.

Slocum's operation
SLR – straight leg raising
Smedberg's drill
Smillie's
>   knife
>   nail

Smith-Petersen
>   nail
>   operation
>   osteotome

Smith-Petersen
    prosthesis
Smith's
    fracture
    dislocation
soas-. See *psoas.*
space
    palmar s.
    thenar s.
    web s's.
Speed-Boyd operation
sphyrectomy
sphyrotomy
spica
    hip s.
spina
    s. bifida occulta
spinal
spinalgia
spine
    cervical s.
spinogalvanization
spinous
splayfoot
splint
    Agnew's s.
    Anderson's s.
    Angle's s.
    Ashhurst's s.
    Balkan s.
    banjo s.
    Baylor's s.
    Böhler-Braun s.
    Böhler's s.
    Bond's s.
    Bowlby's s.
    Brant's s.
    Buck's s.

splint *(continued)*
    Cabot's s.
    Chandler's s.
    cock-up s.
    Colles' s.
    Curry's s.
    Davis' s.
    Denis-Browne club
      foot s.
    DePuy's s.
    drop-foot s.
    Dupuytren's s.
    Eggers' s.
    Engelmann's s.
    Fox's s.
    Gordon's s.
    Hart's s.
    Hodgen's s.
    Jones' s.
    Kanavel's s.
    Keller-Blake s.
    Lewin's s.
    Lewin-Stern s.
    Lytle's s.
    Mason-Allen s.
    protecto s.
    Sayre's s.
    Stader's s.
    Taylor's s.
    Thomas' s.
    Valentine's s.
    Volkmann's s.
    Wertheim's s.
    Zimmer's s.
spondylalgia
spondylarthritis
    s. ankylopoietica
spondylarthrocace

spondylexarthrosis
spondylitis
    s. deformans
    Kümmell's s.
    Marie-Strümpell s.
spondylizema
spondylocace
spondylodesis
spondylodynia
spondylolisthesis
spondylolysis
spondylomalacia
    s. traumatica
spondylopathy
    traumatic s.
spondylopyosis
spondyloschisis
spondylosis
    s. chronica ankylopoi-
      etica
    rhizomelic s.
spondylosyndesis
spondylotomy
spot
    Carleton's s's.
sprain
    riders' s.
Spratt's curet
Sprengel's deformity
spur
    calcaneal s.
    occipital s.
    olecranon s.
Stader's splint
Stamm's operation
Steindler's operation
Steinert's disease

Steinmann's pin
sternoclavicular
sternoscapular
sternotomy
sternovertebral
sternum
Stieda's fracture
Stille's osteotome
Stiller's sign
Stokes' amputation
Stookey reflex
Street's pin
striated
Strümpell's reflex
Stryker's frame
subastragalar
subcapsuloperiosteal
subchondral
subluxation
    Volkmann's s.
subsultus
    s. tendinum
subvertebral
Sudeck's atrophy
sudoluxation. See *pseudo-*
    luxation.
supination
supraclavicular
supracondylar
sura
sural
surgical procedures. See
    operation.
swayback
Swediaur's disease
Sweet's retractor

Syme's amputation
symphysis
synarthrophysis
synarthrosis
synchondrectomy
synchondrosis
synchondrotomy
syndactyly
syndesis
syndesmectomy
syndesmectopia
syndesmitis
    s. metatarsea
syndesmo-odontoid
syndesmopexy
syndesmophyte
syndesmoplasty
syndesmorrhaphy
syndesmosis
syndesmotomy
syndrome
    Albright's s.
    Baastrup's s.
    Bakwin-Eiger s.
    Barré-Liéou s.
    carpal tunnel s.
    Guillain-Barré s.
    Klippel-Feil s.
    Naffziger's s.
    scalenus anticus s.
    Schanz's s.
    Tietze's s.
synosteotomy
synostosis
    radio-ulnar s.
synovectomy
synovia
synovial

synovitis
synovium
syntenosis
synthesis
    s. of continuity
synthetism
syntripsis
tabatière anatomique
taliped
talipes
    t. calcaneovalgus
    t. calcaneovarus
    t. calcaneus
    t. cavovalgus
    t. cavus
    t. equinovalgus
    t. equinovarus
    t. equinus
    t. planovalgus
    t. valgus
    t. varus
talipomanus
Talma's disease
talocalcaneal
talocrural
talofibular
talonavicular
talotibial
talus
tarsal
tarsectomy
tarsectopia
tarsoclasis
tarsomegaly
tarsometatarsal
tarsophalangeal
tarsoptosis
tarsotarsal

tarsotibial
Taylor's
      brace
      splint
Teale's amputation
tear
      bucket-handle t.
Teare's sling
teerfo. See *tirefond.*
template
      Moore's t.
tendinitis
tendinoplasty
tendolysis
tendon
      Achilles' t.
      calcaneal t.
      flexor carpi radialis t.
      flexor digitorum pro-
         fundus t.
      flexor digitorum sub-
         limis t.
      palmaris longus t.
tendoplasty
tenectomy
tenodesis
tenodynia
tenomyotomy
tenonectomy
tenontitis
      t. prolifera calcarea
tenontodynia
tenontophyma
tenontothecitis
tenophyte
tenoplasty
tenorrhaphy
tenositis

tenostosis
tenosuspension
tenosynovectomy
tenosynovitis
tenotome
      Ryerson's t.
tenotomy
tenovaginitis
test
      Finklestein's t.
      McMurray's t.
      Ober's t.
      Patrick's t.
      Trendelenburg's t.
theca
thecitis
thecostegnosis
thenar
Thomas'
      collar
      splint
Thompson's prosthesis
Thomson's operation
thoracicohumeral
thoracispinal
thoracolumbar
Thornton's
      nail
      plate
      screw
thrypsis
thumb
      bifid t.
      tennis t.
tibia
      t. valga
      t. vara
tibial

tibialgia
tibialis
tibiocalcanean
tibiofemoral
tibiofibular
tibionavicular
tibiotarsal
Tietze's syndrome
Tinel's sign
tirefond
tiring
toe
    hammer t.
    Morton's t.
tong
    Barton's t.
    Crutchfield's t.
    Raney-Crutchfield t.
tonus
tophi
tophus
torticollis
tourniquet
    pneumatic t.
Townley's prosthesis
traction
    Buck's t.
    Russell's t.
    skeletal t.
transversectomy
transversotomy
trapeziometacarpal
trapezium
trapezoid
Trendelenburg's test
trephine
    Michele's t.
    Turkel's t.

triangle
    Scarpa's t.
triceps
Tripier's amputation
trochanter
trochanteric
trochanterplasty
trochlea
tubercle
tuberositas
tuberosity
tucker
    Bishop's tendon t.
    Bishop-Black tendon t.
    Bishop-DeWitt tendon t.
    Bishop-Peter tendon t.
    Burch-Greenwood ten-
        don t.
    Fink's tendon t.
tumor
    Ewing's t.
Turkel's
    needle
    trephine
Turner's pin
ulna
Ullmann's line
ulnar
ulnocarpal
ulnoradial
ultrasonics
Valentine's splint
Van Buren's forceps
Van Gorder's operation
vein
    antebrachial cephalic v.
    cephalic v.
    saphenous v.

Velpeau's
  bandage
  deformity
Venable-Stuck nail
vertebra
vertebrae
  cervical v.
  coccygeal v.
  lumbar v.
  sacral v.
  thoracic v.
vertebral
vertebrectomy
vesalianum
volar
volardorsal
volaris
Volkmann's
  contracture
  deformity
  disease
  splint
  subluxation
von Gies' joint
von Recklinghausen's disease
von Saal's pin
Wagoner's operation
Wagstaffe's fracture
Waldenström's disease
Walldius' prosthesis
Watson-Jones operation
Wertheim's splint
Wester's
  clamp
  scissors
Williams'
  clamp
  exercise

Wilman's clamp
Wilson-McKeever operation
Wilson's
  awl
  bolt
  clamp
  plate
  wrench
wire
    Kirschner's w.
Wladimiroff-Mikulicz
    amputation
Wladimiroff's operation
wrench
    Wilson's w.
Wright's plate
wrist
wristdrop
wryneck
Wyeth's operation
xanthoma
    x. disseminatum
xanthomatosis
xanthosarcoma
xiphisternum
xiphocostal
xiphoid
xiphoiditis
xiphopagotomy
Yount's operation
Zahradnicek's operation
zanthoma. See *xanthoma.*
zanthomatosis. See *xanthoma-tosis.*
zanthosarkoma. See *xantho-sarcoma.*
Zenker's
    degeneration

Zenker's
    necrosis
zifisternum. See *xiphisternum.*
zifo-. See words beginning
    xipho-.

zifoid. See *xiphoid.*
Zimaloy's prosthesis
Zimmer's
    pin
    splint

OTORHINOLARYNGOLOGY

Abelson's adenotome
Abraham's cannula
abscess
    Bezold's a.
AC — air conduction
achalasia
acouesthesia
acoumeter
acoumetry
acouometer
acouophone
acouophonia
acoustic
acousticon
acoustics
AD — right ear (auris dextra)
Adams' operation
adaptor
    House's a.
adenocarcinoma
adenofibroma
    a. edematodes
adenoid
adenoidectomy
adenoidism
adenoiditis
adenoma
adenotome
    Abelson's a.
    Kelley's a.

adenotome *(continued)*
    Laforce-Grieshaber a.
    Laforce's a.
    Shambaugh's a.
adenotomy
adenotonsillectomy
adenovirus
aditus
    a. ad antrum
    a. ad antrum mastoid-
        eum
    a. ad antrum tympani-
        cum
    a. laryngis
Adler's punch
Adson's forceps
afagopraksea. See *aphago-*
    praxia.
aftha. See *aphtha.*
aftho-. See words beginning
    aphtho-.
agger
    a. nasi
ala
    a. auris
    a. nasi
Albert-Andrews laryngoscope
Alexander's
    chisel
    gouge

allergy
Allport's
    retractor
    searcher
alveolonasal
ama
ampulla
anastomosis
    Galen's a.
    Jacobson's a.
Andrews'
    applicator
    gouge
Andrews-Hartmann forceps
anesthesia
    endotracheal a.
angina
    Ludwig's a.
    Plaut-Vincent's a.
angle
    Topinard's a.
ankyloglossia
ankylotia
ankylotome
ankylotomy
annulus
    a. tracheae
    tympanic a.
    Vieussens' a.
anosmatic
anosmia
    a. gustatoria
    preferential a.
    a. respiratoria
anosphrasia
anotia
anthelix
Anthony's tube

antihelix
antihistamine
antihistaminic
antitragus
antral
antrectomy
antritis
antroatticotomy
antrocele
antronalgia
antronasal
antroscope
antroscopy
antrostomy
antrotomy
antrotympanic
antrotympanitis
antrum
    attic-aditus a.
    a. auris
    ethmoid a.
    a. ethmoidale
    frontal a.
    a. of Highmore
    a. highmori
    mastoid a.
    a. mastoideum
    a. maxillare
    maxillary a.
    tympanic a.
    a. tympanicum
anvil
apertura
    a. externa aqueductus
      vestibuli
    a. sinus frontalis
    a. sinus sphenoidalis
    a. tympanica canaliculi

apertura
  a. chordae tympani
aperture
  a. of frontal sinus
  a. of sphenoid sinus
  tympanic a. of canalicu-
    lus of chorda tympani
apex
  a. auriculae
aphagopraxia
aphonia
  a. paralytica
  spastic a.
aphtha
aphthosis
aphthous
aponeurosis
applicator
  Andrews' a.
  Brown's a.
  Dean's a.
  Holinger's a.
  Lathbury's a.
  Lejeune's a.
  Pynchon's a.
  Roberts' a.
aqueduct
  a. of cochlea
  a. of Cotunnius
  fallopian a.
  a. of Fallopius
  a. of the vestibule
aqueductus
  a. endolymphaticus
  a. vestibuli
arachnorhinitis
Arbuckle's probe
arch
  a's of Corti

arcus
  a. glossopalatinus
  a. lipoides myringis
  a. palatini
  a. palatoglossus
  a. palatopharyngeus
  a. pharyngopalatinus
area
  Kiesselbach's a.
areepi-. See words beginning
  aryepi-.
aretenoid. See *arytenoid.*
argyria
  a. nasalis
arhinia
ariteno-. See words beginning
  aryteno-.
arjirea. See *argyria.*
Arnold's nerve
artery
  carotid a.
aryepiglottic
aryepiglotticus
aryepiglottidean
arytenoepiglottic
arytenoid
arytenoidectomy
arytenoideus
arytenoiditis
arytenoidopexy
AS – left ear (auris sinistra)
Asch's
  operation
  splint
aspergillosis
aspirator
  Gottschalk's a.
asterion

atelectasis
Atkins-Tucker laryngoscope
atomizer
    Devilbiss' a.
atresia
atrium
    a. glottidis
    a. of glottis
    a. laryngis
    a. of larynx
    a. meatus medii
attic
atticitis
atticoantrotomy
atticomastoid
atticotomy
    transmeatal a.
AU — both ears (aures unitas)
audiogram
audiologist
audiology
audiometer
audiometrician
audiometry
audiosurgery
audiphone
audition
auditive
auditognosis
auditory
    a. canal
Aufricht-Lipsett rasp
Aufricht's
    rasp
    retractor
    speculum
aura
    a. asthmatica

aural
auricle
auricula
auricular
auriculare
auricularis
auriculocranial
auriculotemporal
auriculoventricular
aurilave
aurinarium
aurinasal
auriphone
auripuncture
auris
    a. externa
    a. interna
    a. media
auriscalpium
auriscope
auris dextra
auris sinistra
aurist
auristics
auristillae
auris uterque
aurogauge
aurometer
Avellis' syndrome
Baelz's syndrome
bag
    Politzer's b.
Ballenger's
    curet
    forceps
    knife
Ballenger-Sluder tonsillectome
Bane's forceps

Bárány's
   symptom
   syndrome
   test
Barlow's forceps
Barnhill's curet
BC — bone conduction
Bechterew's nucleus
Beckman-Colver speculum
Beck-Mueller tonsillectome
Beck-Schenck tonsillectome
Beck's knife
Bellocq's cannula
Bell's palsy
Bermingham's nasal douche
Berne's
   forceps
   rasp
Beyer's
   forceps
   rongeur
Bezold's
   abscess
   mastoiditis
Billeau's curet
Billroth's operation
binaural
binauricular
binotic
Bizzarri-Giuffrida laryngo-
   scope
Blakemore's tube
Blake's forceps
Blakesley's forceps
blennorrhea
   Stoerk's b.
Boettcher's
   forceps

Boettcher's *(continued)*
   hook
   scissors
bone
   b. conduction
   hyoid b.
   petrous b.
   squamosal b.
   temporal b.
   tympanic b.
   zygomatic b.
border
   vermilion b.
Bostock's catarrh
Bosworth's snare
Boucheron's speculum
Bouchut's tube
bougie
   Hurst's b.
   Jackson's b.
   Plummer's b.
branchia
branchial
   b. cleft
branchiogenic
branchiogenous
branchioma
branchiomere
branchiomeric
branchiomerism
bronchi
bronchial
bronchiectasis
bronchogram
bronchography
bronchoscope
bronchoscopy
bronchus

Brown's
    applicator
    needle
    retractor
    snare
    tonsillectome
Broyles'
    laryngoscope
    nasopharyngoscope
Bruening's
    forceps
    otoscope
    snare
Brun's curet
Brunton's otoscope
bucca
    b. cavi oris
buccal
buccopharyngeal
Buck's
    curet
    knife
bur
    Diamond b.
    Hall's b.
    Jordan-Day b.
    Lampert's b.
    Wullstein's b.
bursa
    nasopharyngeal b.
    pharyngeal b.
bursitis
    Tornwaldt's b.
calculus
    salivary c.
Caldwell-Luc operation
Caldwell's position

caliculus
    c. gustatorius
canal
    auditory c.
    carotid c.
    c. of Corti
    Huschke's c.
canaliculus
    c. of chorda tympani
    c. chordae tympani
    c. of cochlea
    c. cochleae
    mastoid c.
    c. mastoideus
    tympanic c.
    c. tympanicus
cancrum
    c. nasi
    c. oris
Canfield's knife
cannula
    Abraham's c.
    Bellocq's c.
    Coakley's c.
    Day's c.
    Goodfellow's c.
    Kos' c.
    Krause's c.
    Paterson's c.
    Scott's c.
cannulization
capsule
    articular c.
carcinoma
    schneiderian c.
Carmack's curet
caroticotympanic

carotid
c. artery
Carpenter's knife
Carpue's
operation
rhinoplasty
Carter's
operation
splint
cartilage
arytenoid c.
corniculate c.
cricoid c.
cuneiform c.
epiglottic c.
thyroid c.
cartilaginous
caruncle
sublingual c.
caruncula
c. salivaris
c. sublingualis
Cassel's operation
catarrh
Bostock's c.
catarrhal
catheter
Yankauer's c.
catheterization
laryngeal c.
cauda
c. helicis
cavum
c. conchae
c. infraglotticum
c. laryngis
c. nasi
c. nasi osseum

cavum *(continued)*
c. oris
c. oris externum
c. pharyngis
c. tympani
cecum
cupular c. of cochlear
duct
c. cupulare ductus
cochlearis
vestibular c. of cochlear
duct
c. vestibulare ductus
cochlearis
cellulae
c. ethmoidales osseae
c. mastoideae
c. pneumaticae tubae
auditivae
c. pneumaticae tubariae
c. tympanicae
cephalalgia
histamine c.
pharyngotympanic c.
cephalgia
cerumen
inspissated c.
ceruminal
ceruminolysis
ceruminolytic
ceruminosis
ceruminous
cervical
Cheever's operation
cheilectropion
cheilitis
cheilognathoprosoposchisis
cheilognathoschisis

cheilognathouranoschisis
cheiloplasty
cheiloschisis
cheilosis
chemodectoma
Chevalier-Jackson
    laryngoscope
    operation
    speculum
    tube
chisel
    Alexander's c.
    Converse's c.
    Derlacki's c.
    Derlacki-Shambaugh c.
    Fomon's c.
    Freer's c.
    Hajek's c.
    House's c.
    Killian's c.
    Sewall's c.
    Shambaugh-Derlacki c.
    Sheehan's c.
    Troutman's c.
choana
choanae
    c. osseae
choanal
choanoid
cholesteatoma
    c. tympani
chondroma
chorda
    c. tympani
chordectomy
chorditis
    c. cantorum
    c. fibrinosa

chorditis *(continued)*
    c. nodosa
    c. tuberosa
    c. vocalis
chromorhinorrhea
cicatricial
cicatrix
    manometric c.
Cicherelli's forceps
cilia
Citelli-Meltzer punch
clamp
    Jesberg's c.
Clerf's
    laryngoscope
    saw
Cloquet's ganglion
Coakley's
    cannula
    curet
    forceps
    operation
    speculum
cochlea
cochlear
cochleariform
cochleitis
cochleovestibular
cochlitis
cog-tooth
Cohen's forceps
collum
collunarium
columella
    c. cochleae
    c. nasi
Colver's
    forceps

Colver's
  knife
concha
  c. of auricle
  c. auriculae
  c. bullosa
  ethmoidal c.
  c. nasalis inferior ossea
  c. nasalis media ossea
  c. nasalis superior ossea
  c. nasalis suprema ossea
  nasoturbinal c.
  sphenoidal c.
  c. sphenoidalis
conchae
conchitis
conchoscope
conchotome
conchotomy
conduction
  air c.
  bone c.
conus
  c. elasticus laryngis
Converse's
  chisel
  rongeur
  speculum
cordal
cordectomy
Cordes-New forceps
cordopexy
cordotomy
corniculate
cornu
  ethmoid c.
  c. majus ossis hyoidei
  c. minus ossis hyoidei

corona
coronae
coronal
coronale
coronalis
corone
coronion
coronoid
Corti's
  arch
  canal
  organ
  rod's
  tunnel
Corwin's hemostat
coryza
  allergic c.
  c. oedematosa
Costen's syndrome
Cottle-Arruga forceps
Cottle-Jansen forceps
Cottle-Kazanjian forceps
Cottle-Neivert retractor
Cottle's
  elevator
  forceps
  knife
  osteotome
  rasp
  retractor
  saw
  scissors
  speculum
  tenaculum
Cotunnius
  aqueduct of C.
Craig's forceps
cranioaural

cribriform
cricoarytenoid
cricoid
cricoidectomy
cricoidynia
cricopharyngeal
cricopharyngeus
cricothyreotomy
cricothyroid
cricothyroidotomy
cricotomy
cricotracheotomy
crista
    c. ampullaris
    c. conchalis maxillae
    c. conchalis ossis pala-
      tini
    c. ethmoidalis maxillae
    c. ethmoidalis ossis
      palatini
    c. fenestrae cochleae
    c. frontalis
    c. galli
cristi
    c. nasalis maxillae
    c. tympanica
croup
crura
    c. anthelicis
    c. of anthelix
crus
    anterior c. of stapes
    c. anterius stapedis
    c. breve incudis
    c. helicis
    c. of helix
    posterior c. of stapes
    c. posterius stapedis

cuneiform
cupula
    c. of cochlea
    c. cochleae
curet
    Ballenger's c.
    Barnhill's c.
    Billeau's c.
    Brun's c.
    Buck's c.
    Carmack's c.
    Coakley's c.
    Derlacki's c.
    Faulkner's c.
    Freimuth's c.
    Gross' c.
    Halle's c.
    Hartmann's c.
    Hayden's c.
    Hotz's c.
    House's c.
    Ingersoll's c.
    Jones' c.
    Lempert's c.
    McCaskey's c.
    Middleton's c.
    Mosher's c.
    Myles' c.
    Pratt's c.
    Richards' c.
    Ridpath's c.
    Rosenmueller's c.
    Schaeffer's c.
    Shapleigh's c.
    Spratt's c.
    St. Clair-Thompson's c.
    Stubbs' c.
    Tabb's c.

curet *(continued)*
    Vogel's c.
    Weisman's c.
    Whiting's c.
    Yankauer's c.
Cushing's forceps
cymba
    c. conchae auriculae
Daniels' tonsillectome
Davis' retractor
Davis-Crowe mouth gag
Day's cannula
deafness
    apoplectiform d.
    ceruminous d.
    conduction d.
    labyrinthine d.
    perceptive d.
Dean's
    applicator
    forceps
    knife
    periosteotome
    scissors
decibel
decongestant
Defourmentel's forceps
degeneration
deglutition
Deiters' nucleus
Denhardt-Dingman mouth gag
Denhard's mouth gag
Denonvilliers' operation
Derlacki's
    chisel
    curet
    gouge
    knife

Derlacki's
    mobilizer
Derlacki-Shambaugh chisel
desensitization
Devilbiss' atomizer
Diamond bur
diapason
diastolization
Dingman's
    elevator
    forceps
    osteotome
    retractor
diplacusis
    binaural d.
    d. binauralis dyshar-
      monica
    d. binauralis echoica
    disharmonic d.
    echo d.
    monaural d.
disease
    Hunt's d.
    Legal's d.
    Ménière's d.
    Mikulicz's d.
    Ramsey-Hunt d.
dissector
    Holinger's d.
    Hurd's d.
    McWhinnie's d.
    Pierce's d.
    Rogers' d.
    Walker's d.
diverticula
Donaldson's tube
dorsum
    d. nasi

douche
   Bermingham's nasal d.
Douglas' knife
drugs. See *Medications.*
drumhead
duct
   cochlear d.
   endolymphatic d.
   lacrimal d.
   d's of Rivinus
   Stensen's d.
   Walther's d's.
   Wharton's d.
ductus
   d. cochlearis
   d. endolymphaticus
   d. reuniens
Dufourmental's rongeur
Duplay-Lynch speculum
Duplay's speculum
dysacousia
dysaudia
dysosmia
dysphagia
dysphonia
   d. plicae ventricularis
   d. spastica
dyspnea
EAC — external auditory canal
EAM — external auditory meatus
Eaton's speculum
ecchymosis
edentulous
EENT — eye, ear, nose and throat
electropneumatotherapy

elevator
   Cottle's e.
   Dingman's e.
   Freer's e.
   Hajek-Ballenger e.
   Hamrick's e.
   House's e.
   Killian's e.
   Lamont's e.
   Mackenty's e.
   Pennington's e.
   Proctor's e.
   Ray-Parsons-Sunday e.
   Shambaugh-Derlacki e.
   Shambaugh's e.
   Sunday's e.
eminence
   arytenoid e.
eminentia
   e. articularis ossis temporalis
   e. conchae
   e. fallopii
   e. fossae triangularis auriculae
emissarium
   e. mastoideum
enchondroma
endolaryngeal
endolarynx
endolymph
endolympha
endolymphatic
endomastoiditis
endonasal
English rhinoplasty
ENT — ear, nose and throat
entacoustic

enucleation
eparterial
epiglottectomy
epiglottic
epiglottidean
epiglottidectomy
epiglottiditis
epiglottis
epiglottitis
epiotic
epipharyngeal
epipharyngitis
epipharynx
epistaxis
epiturbinate
epitympanic
epitympanum
Equen-Neuffer knife
equilibrium
Erhardt's speculum
Erich's
    forceps
    splint
errhine
erysipelas
esophagectomy
esophagogram
esophagolaryngectomy
esophagopharynx
esophagoscope
esophagoscopy
esophagostomy
esophagotomy
esophagus
espundia
esthesioneuroblastoma
ethmofrontal
ethmoid

ethmoidal
ethmoidectomy
ethmoiditis
ethmoidotomy
ethmolacrimal
ethmomaxillary
ethmonasal
ethmopalatal
ethmosphenoid
ethmoturbinal
ethmovomerine
ethmyphitis
eustachian
    e. tube
eustachitis
eustachium
Eves' snare
excavator
    Schuknecht's e.
excochleation
exostosis
expectorant
expectoration
explorer
    Rosen's e.
exudate
facial
fahringo-. See words begin-
    ning *pharyngo-*.
Fallopius
    aqueduct of F.
farin-. See words beginning
    pharyn-.
Farrington's forceps
Farrior's speculum
fauces
faucial
faucitis

Faulkner's curet
Fauvel's forceps
fenestra
    f. cochleae
    f. of cochlea
    f. novovalis
    f. ovalis
    f. rotunda
    f. vestibuli
fenestrater
    Rosen's f.
fenestration
Fergusson's
    incision
    operation
Ferris-Robb knife
Ferris-Smith forceps
Ferris-Smith-Kerrison forceps
Ferris-Smith-Sewall retractor
fibers
    Prussak's f's.
fibroangioma
fibroma
Fink's laryngoscope
Fisher's knife
Fish's forceps
fissure
    petrotympanic f.
Flagg's laryngoscope
Flannery's speculum
flebektazea. See *phlebectasia.*
flem. See *phlegm.*
Fletcher's knife
fold
    aryepiglottic f.
    salpingopharyngeal f.
folium
    lingual f.

folliculitis
Fomon's
    chisel
    knife
    periosteotome
    rasp
    scissors
foramen
    Huschke's f.
    f. incisivum
    f. mastoideum
    rivinian f.
    Scarpa's f.
    f. sphenopalatinum
    Stensen's f.
    f. stylomastoideum
forceps
    Adson's f.
    Andrews-Hartmann f.
    Ballenger's f.
    Bane's f.
    Barlow's f.
    Berne's f.
    Beyer's f.
    Blake's f.
    Blakesley's f.
    Boettcher's f.
    Bruening's f.
    Cicherelli's f.
    Coakley's f.
    Cohen's f.
    Colver's f.
    Cordes-New f.
    Cottle-Arruga f.
    Cottle-Jansen f.
    Cottle-Kazanjian f.
    Cottle's f.
    Craig's f.

forceps *(continued)*

- Cushing's f.
- Dean's f.
- Defourmentel's f.
- Dingman's f.
- Erich's f.
- Farrington's f.
- Fauvel's f.
- Ferris-Smith f.
- Ferris-Smith-Kerrison f.
- Fish's f.
- Fraenkel's f.
- Goodhill's f.
- Goldman-Kazanjian f.
- Gruenwald-Bryant f.
- Gruenwald's f.
- Guggenheim's f.
- Hajek-Koffler f.
- Hartmann-Citelli f.
- Hartmann-Gruenwald f.
- Hartmann's f.
- Hoffmann's f.
- House's f.
- Howard's f.
- Hurd's f.
- Imperatori's f.
- Jackson's f.
- Jansen-Middleton f.
- Jansen's f.
- Jansen-Struycken f.
- Juers-Lempert f.
- Jurasz's f.
- Kazanjian's f.
- Knight's f.
- Knight-Sluder f.
- Koffler-Lillie f.
- Koffler's f.
- Krause's f.

forceps *(continued)*

- Lempert's f.
- Lillie's f.
- Littauer's f.
- Lucae's f.
- Luc's f.
- Lutz's f.
- Lynch's f.
- Marshik's f.
- Martin's f.
- McHenry's f.
- McKay's f.
- Metzenbaum's f.
- Moritz-Schmidt f.
- Museholdt's f.
- Myerson's f.
- Myles' f.
- Noyes' f.
- Pang's f.
- Paterson's f.
- Reiner-Knight f.
- Robb's f.
- Robertson's f.
- Rowland's f.
- Ruskin's f.
- Sawtell's f.
- Scheinmann's f.
- Seiffert's f.
- Semken's f.
- Shearer's f.
- Struempel's f.
- Struyken's f.
- Takahashi's f.
- Tivnen's f.
- Tobold's f.
- Tydings' f.
- Tydings-Lakeside f.
- van-Struycken f.

forceps *(continued)*
    Watson-Williams f.
    Weil's f.
    Weingartner's f.
    White-Lillie f.
    White's f.
    Wilde's f.
    Wullstein-House f.
    Wullstein's f.
    Yankauer-Little f.
    Yankauer's f.
Foregger's laryngoscope
formula
    Seiler's f.
fossa
    f. incudis
    f. ovalis
    pharyngomaxillary f.
    Rosenmüller's f.
    triangular f.
Fraenkel's forceps
Frazier's tube
Freer's
    chisel
    elevator
    knife
Freimuth's curet
frenotomy
frenulum
frenum
Friesner's knife
frontomaxillary
frontonasal
fronto-occipital
frontoparietal
frontotemporal
Fröschel's symptom
furcula

furuncular
furunculosis
galea
    g. aponeurotica
    tendinous g.
Galen's anastomosis
Gandhi's knife
ganglion
    Cloquet's g.
    geniculate g.
    g. geniculi nervi facialis
gangosa
geniohyoid
genyantralgia
genyantritis
genyantrum
genycheiloplasty
genyplasty
Gerzog's speculum
Gifford's retractor
Gilles'
    hook
    operation
Gilles-Dingman hook
glabella
glabellad
glabellum
gland
    Rivinus' g.
    salivary g.
glomus
    g. jugulare
glossa
glossal
glossalgia
glossanthrax
glossectomy
glossitis

glossoepiglottidean
glossoncus
glossopharyngeal
glossopharyngeum
glossoplasty
glossoplegia
glossorrhaphy
glossotomy
glottic
glottides
glottis
Goldman-Kazanjian forceps
Goodfellow's cannula
Goodhill's forceps
Good's rasp
Goodyear's knife
Gottschalk's
    aspirator
    saw
gouge
    Alexander's g.
    Andrews' g.
    Derlacki's g.
    Holmes' g.
    Troutman's g.
goundou
groove
    Verga's lacrimal g.
Gross'
    curet
    spoon
    spud
Gruber's speculum
Gruenwald-Bryant forceps
Gruenwald's forceps
Guedel's laryngoscope
Guggenheim's forceps
guillotine

guillotine *(continued)*
    Sluder's g.
    Sluder-Sauer g.
Gundelach's punch
Hajek-Ballenger elevator
Hajek-Koffler forceps
Hajek-Skillern punch
Hajek's
    chisel
    retractor
Halle's
    curet
    speculum
Halle-Tieck speculum
Hall's bur
hammer
    Quisling's h.
Hamrick's elevator
Harrison's knife
Hartmann-Citelli forceps
Hartmann-Dewaxer speculum
Hartmann-Gruenwald forceps
Hartmann-Herzfeld rongeur
Hartmann's
    curet
    forceps
    punch
    rongeur
    speculum
    tuning fork
Haslinger's
    laryngoscope
    retractor
Hayden's curet
HD – hearing distance
HEENT – head, eyes, ears,
   nose and throat
Heerman's incision

Heffernan's speculum
helicotrema
helix
hematoma
    h. auris
hemiglossal
hemiglossectomy
hemiglossitis
hemilaryngectomy
hemostat
    Corwin's h.
Henle's spine
Henner's retractor
herpes
    h. catarrhalis
    h. febrilis
    h. labialis
    h. oticus
    h. simplex
Highmore's antrum
highmoritis
hircus
histamine
hoarseness
Hoffmann's
    forceps
    punch
    rongeur
Holinger's
    applicator
    dissector
    laryngoscope
Holmes'
    gouge
    nasopharyngoscope
hook
    Boettcher's h.
    Gilles' h.

hook *(continued)*
    Gilles-Dingman h.
    House's h.
    Lillie's h.
    Schuknecht's h.
    Shambaugh's h.
Hopmann's polyp
Hotz's curet
Hourin's needle
House-Barbara needle
House-Rosen needle
House's
    adaptor
    chisel
    curet
    elevator
    forceps
    hook
    irrigator
    knife
    needle
    prosthesis
    rod
    scissor
    separator
    tube
House-Urban retractor
Howard's forceps
Huguier's sinus
Hunt's disease
Hurd's
    dissector
    forceps
Hurst's bougie
Huschke's
    canal
    foramen
    valve

Husks' rongeur
hydrocephalus
      otitic h.
hydrorrhea
      nasal h.
hydrotis
hydrotympanum
hypacusis
hyperacusis
hyperemic
hyperkeratosis
      h. lacunaris
hyperptyalism
hyperrhinoplaty
hypoglossal
hypoglottis
hypopharyngoscope
hypopharyngoscopy
hypopharynx
hypotympanotomy
hypotympanum
IA — internal auditory
IAC — internal auditory canal
Imperatori's forceps
incision
      endaural i.
      Fergusson's i.
      Heerman's i.
      Lempert's i.
      meatal i.
      postauricular i.
      retroauricular i.
      Shambaugh's i.
incisura
      i. anterior auris
      i. intertragica
      i. mastoidea ossis
          temporalis

incisura *(continued)*
      i. Rivini
      Santorini's i.
      i. terminalis auris
      i. tympanica
incostapedial
incudal
incudectomy
incudomalleal
incudostapedial
incus
Indian
      operation
      rhinoplasty
infection
      Vincent's i.
Ingals' speculum
Ingersoll's curet
interarytenoid
intramastoiditis
intranarial
intranasal
irrigator
      House's i.
      Shambaugh's i.
Italian
      operation
      rhinoplasty
iter
Ivy's rongeur
Jackson's
      bougie
      forceps
      laryngoscope
      scissors
Jacobsen's nerve
Jacobson's anastomosis
Jansen-Middleton forceps

Jansen-Newhart probe
Jansen-Struycken forceps
Jansen's
    forceps
    operation
    retractor
Jarvis' operation
Jennings' mouth gag
Jesberg's clamp
joint
    incudostapedial j.
Jones'
    curet
    splint
Jordan-Day bur
Joseph-Maltz saw
Joseph's
    knife
    periosteotome
    saw
    scissors
Juers-Lempert forceps
jugomaxillary
jugular
Jurasz's forceps
Kartagener's
    syndrome
    triad
Kazanjian's
    forceps
    splint
Keegan's operation
Kelley's adenotome
keratosis
    k. pharyngeus
Kerrison's rongeur
KHZ – kilohertz

Kiesselbach's
    area
    plexus
Killian's
    chisel
    elevator
    knife
    operation
    speculum
kilo-. See words beginning
    cheilo-.
Knapp's scissors
knife
    Ballenger's k.
    Beck's k.
    Buck's k.
    Canfield's k.
    Carpenter's k.
    Colver's k.
    Cottle's k.
    Dean's k.
    Derlacki's k.
    Douglas' k.
    Equen-Neuffer k.
    Ferris-Robb k.
    Fisher's k.
    Fletcher's k.
    Fomon's k.
    Freer's k.
    Friesner's k.
    Gandhi's k.
    Goodyear's k.
    Harrison's k.
    House's k.
    Joseph's k.
    Killian's k.
    Leland's k.

knife *(continued)*
    Lothrop's k.
    Lynch's k.
    Maltz's k.
    McHugh's k.
    Robertson's k.
    Rosen's k.
    Schuknecht's k.
    Seiler's k.
    Sexton's k.
    Shambaugh-Lempert k.
    Sheehy's k.
    Tobold's k.
    Tydings' k.
    Wullstein's k.
Knight's
    forceps
    scissors
Knight-Sluder forceps
koanah. See *choana.*
Koffler-Lillie forceps
Koffler's forceps
kokle-. See words beginning *cochle-.*
koklea. See *cochlea.*
Kos' cannula
Kramer's speculum
Krause's
    cannula
    forceps
    snare
Kuhnt's operation
Kuster's operation
Kyle's speculum
labial
labium
    anterius ostii pharyngei
        tubae auditivae

labyrinth
    acoustic l.
    ethmoidal l.
    membranous l.
    nonacoustic l.
    osseous l.
labyrinthectomy
labyrinthine
labyrinthitis
labyrinthosis
labyrinthotomy
lacrimation
lacrimonasal
Laforce-Grieshaber adeno-
    tome
Laforce's
    adenotome
    tonsillectome
lahringo-. See words begin-
    ning *laryngo-.*
lamina
    l. spiralis ossea
    l. spiralis secundaria
Lamont's
    elevator
    saw
Lane's mouth gag
LaRocca's tube
laryngalgia
laryngeal
laryngect
laryngectomee
laryngectomy
laryngemphraxis
laryngendoscope
laryngismal
laryngismus
    l. paralyticus

laryngismus
    l. stridulus
laryngitic
laryngitis
    catarrhal l.
    croupous l.
    diphtheritic l.
    phlegmonous l.
    l. sicca
    l. stridulosa
    subglottic l.
    syphilitic l.
    tuberculous l.
laryngocele
laryngocentesis
laryngofission
laryngofissure
laryngogram
laryngograph
laryngography
laryngology
laryngomalacia
laryngometry
laryngoparalysis
laryngopathy
laryngopharyngeal
laryngopharyngectomy
laryngopharyngeus
laryngopharyngitis
laryngopharynx
laryngophony
laryngophthisis
laryngoplasty
laryngoplegia
laryngoptosis
laryngopyocele
laryngorhinology
laryngorrhagia
laryngorrhaphy

laryngorrhea
laryngoscleroma
laryngoscope
    Albert-Andrews l.
    Atkins-Tucker l.
    Bizzarri-Giuffrida l.
    Broyles' l.
    Chevalier-Jackson l.
    Clerf's l.
    Fink's l.
    Flagg's l.
    Foregger's l.
    Guedel's l.
    Haslinger's l.
    Holinger's l.
    Jackson's l.
    Lewy's l.
    Lundy's l.
    Lynch's l.
    MacIntosh's l.
    Roberts' l.
    Rusch's l.
    Sanders' l.
    Siker's l.
    Tucker's l.
    Welch-Allyn l.
    Wis-Foregger's l.
    Wis-Hipple's l.
    Yankauer's l.
laryngoscopic
laryngoscopist
laryngoscopy
laryngospasm
laryngostasis
laryngostat
laryngostenosis
laryngostomy
laryngostroboscope

laryngotome
laryngotomy
    subhyoid l.
    l. thyrohyoid
laryngotracheal
laryngotracheitis
laryngotracheobronchitis
laryngotracheobronchoscopy
laryngotracheoscopy
laryngotracheotomy
laryngotyphoid
laryngovestibulitis
laryngoxerosis
larynx
Lathbury's applicator
Latrobe's retractor
Lauren's operation
Law's position
Legal's disease
Lejeune's
    applicator
    scissors
Leland's knife
Lempert-Colver speculum
Lempert's
    bur
    curet
    elevator
    forceps
    incision
    knife
    operation
    perforator
    retractor
Lermoyez's
    punch
    syndrome
leukoplakia

Lewis'
    rasp
    snare
    tube
Lewy's laryngoscope
ligament
    annular l.
    axis l.
Lillie's
    forceps
    hook
    scissors
    speculum
limen
    l. nasi
Lindeman-Silverstein tube
line
    Topinard's l.
lingua
    l. dissecta
    l. fraenata
    l. geographica
    l. nigra
    l. plicata
    l. villosa nigra
lingual
linguale
lingualis
lingually
lingula
lingulectomy
Littauer's forceps
LM – otitis media
lobule
lobulus
    l. auriculae
Lombard-Boies rongeur
Lombard's test

Lothrop's
    knife
    retractor
loupe
Love's
    retractor
    splint
Lucae's forceps
Luc's forceps
Ludwig's angina
Lundy's laryngoscope
Luongo's retractor
Lutz's forceps
lymphadenectomy
lymphadenitis
lymphadenoid
lymphatic
lymphoblastoma
lymphoepithelioma
lymphosarcoma
lymphotism
lymphotome
Lynch's
    forceps
    knife
    laryngoscope
    scissors
MacIntosh's laryngoscope
Mackenty's
    choanal plug
    elevator
    tube
Mack's tonsillectome
Maclay's scissors
macrocephalia
macrocheilia
macroglossia
macrognathia

macrostomia
macrotia
macula
    m. acustica sacculi
    m. acustica utriculi
    m. sacculi
    m. utriculi
Mahoney's speculum
malar
malleoincudal
malleotomy
malleus
Maltz-Lipsett rasp
Maltz's
    knife
    rasp
    saw
mandible
mandibula
mandibular
mandibulopharyngeal
Mandl's paint
manubria
    m. of malleus
Marshik's forceps
Martin's forceps
mastoid
mastoidal
mastoidale
mastoidalgia
mastoidea
mastoidectomy
mastoideocentesis
mastoideum
mastoiditis
    Bezold's m.
    m. externa
    m. interna

mastoiditis
    sclerosing m.
mastoidotomy
mastoidotympanectomy
Mayer's position
maxilla
maxillary
maxillofacial
Mayer's splint
McCaskey's curet
McCurdy's needle
McHenry's forceps
McHugh's
    knife
    speculum
McIvor's mouth gag
McKay's forceps
McWhinnie's dissector
meatoantrotomy
meatus
    auditory m.
    external acoustic m.
    m. conchae ethmotur-
       binalis minoris
    m. nasi communis osseus
    m. nasopharyngeus
       osseus
Medications
    Achromycin
    Actidil
    Aerosporin
    Alerin
    Allecur
    Ambodryl
    antazoline
    Antistine
    Argyrol
    Aureomycin

Medications *(continued)*
    bacitracin
    Barachlor
    Benadryl
    Bonine
    Boracic acid
    boric acid
    Bradosol
    bromodiphenhydramine
    brompheniramine
    buclizine
    carbinoxamine
    Chestamine
    Chlo-Amine
    Chloramate
    chloramphenicol
    chlorcyclizine
    Chloromycetin
    chlorothen
    chlorpheniramine
    chlortetracycline
    Chlor-Trimeton
    clemizole
    Clistin
    cocaine
    codeine
    Coly-Mycin Otic
    Copavin
    Coricidin
    Cort-Dome
    Cortef
    Cortisol
    Cortril
    Cresatin
    cyclizine
    cyproheptadine
    Decapryn
    dexamethasone

Medications *(continued)*

dexbrompheniramine
dexchlorpheniramine
Diafen
Dimetane
dimethindene
diphenhydramine
diphenylpyraline
Disomer
domiphen
doxylamine
Dramamine
Drize
ephedrine
epinephrine
Erythrocin
erythromycin
Florinef
fludrocortisone
Fludrohydrocortisone
Forhistal
Gantrisin
glycerin
Hispril
Histachlor
Histadur
Histadyl
Histamine
Histaspan
Histionex
Histitrin
Histrey
Hydrillyn
hydrocortisone
Hydrocortone
Ilotycin
isothipendyl
Lullamin

Medications *(continued)*

Marezine
Maxidex
meclizine
Merthiolate
meta-cresylacetate
methapyrilene
methdilazine
methylprednisolone
Neo-Antergan
Neo-Hetramine
neomycin
Orthoboric acid
oxytetracycline
Panmycin
penicillin
Perazil
Periactin
Phenergan
Phenetron
phenindamine
pheniramine
phenol
phenyltoloxamine
Polaramine
Polycycline
polymyxin
prednisolone
promethazine
Pyribenzamine
pyrilamine
Pyronil
pyrrobutamine
Reactrol
rotoxamine
salicylic acid
Semikon
Sodium

Medications *(continued)*
    Ethylmercurithiosali-
      cylate
    Softran
    Stanzamine
    Steclin
    streptomycin
    Suladrin
    sulfadiazine
    sulfisoxazole
    sulfonamide
    sulfur
    Sumadil
    Tacaryl
    Tagathen
    Teldrin
    Temaril
    Terramycin
    tetracycline
    Tetracyn
    Thenfadil
    thenyldiamine
    Thephorin
    Theruhistin
    thimerosal
    thonzylamine
    trimeprazine
    Trimeton
    tripelennamine
    triprolidine
    Twiston
    Tylahist
    xylometazoline
Meltzer's
    nasopharyngoscope
    punch
membrana
    m. basilaris ductus

membrana *(continued)*
      cochlearis
    m. elastica laryngis
    m. fibroelastica laryngis
    m. mucosa nasi
    m. spiralis ductus coch-
      learis
    m. stapedis
    m. tympani secundaria
membrane
    buccopharyngeal m.
    hypoglossal m.
    mucous m.
    Reissner's m.
    Rivinus' m.
    Scarpa's m.
    Shrapnell's m.
    tectorial m.
    tympanic m.
Ménière's disease
meningitis
mesocephalic
mesoturbinal
mesoturbinate
metopantralgia
metopantritis
Metzenbaum-Lipsett scissors
Metzenbaum's
    forceps
    scissors
Meyer's sinus
microglossia
micrognathia
microrhinia
microscope
    Zeiss' m.
microstomia
microtia

Middleton's curet
Mikulicz's
    disease
    syndrome
mobilization
    stapes m.
mobilizer
    Derlacki's m.
modiolus
Moeller's reaction
Moltz-Storz tonsillectome
Morch's tube
Morgagni's
    sinus
    ventricle
Moritz-Schmidt forceps
Mosher's
    curet
    punch
    speculum
mouth gag
    Davis-Crowe m.g.
    Denhardt-Dingman m.g.
    Denhard's m.g.
    Jennings' m.g.
    Lane's m.g.
    McIvor's m.g.
    Roser's m.g.
    Sluder-Jansen m.g.
mucocele
mucoid
mucoperichondrium
mucoperiosteal
mucoperiosteum
mucopurulent
mucosa
mucus
muscle

muscle *(continued)*
    cricoarytenoid m.
    cricopharyngeus m.
    cricothyroid m.
    depressor septi nasi m.
    genioglossus m.
    geniohyoideus m.
    glossopalatinus m.
    glossopharyngeus m.
    helicis m.
    interarytenoid m.
    levator veli palatini m.
    palatoglossus m.
    palatopharyngeus m.
    pharyngeal constrictor
        m.
    pharyngopalatinus m.
    stapedius m.
    stylopharyngeus m.
    tensor veli palatini m.
    thyroarytenoid m.
musculoplasty
Museholdt's forceps
myasthenia
    m. gravis
    m. laryngis
mycosis
    m. leptothrica
Myerson's
    forceps
    saw
Myles'
    curet
    forceps
    punch
    snare
    speculum
    tonsillectome

mylohyoid
myringa
myringectomy
myringitis
    bullous m.
    m. bullosa
myringodectomy
myringodermatitis
myringomycosis
    m. aspergillina
myringoplasty
myringorupture
myringoscope
myringostapediopexy
myringotome
myringotomy
myrinx
nares
naris
nasal
nasalis
nasion
nasitis
nasoantral
nasoantritis
nasobronchial
nasociliary
nasofrontal
nasograph
nasolabial
nasolacrimal
nasomanometer
nasonnement
naso-oral
nasopalatine
nasopharyngeal
nasopharyngitis

nasopharyngoscope
    Broyles' n.
    Holmes' n.
    Meltzer's n.
nasopharynx
nasorostral
nasoscope
nasoseptal
nasoseptitis
nasosinusitis
nasospinale
nasotracheal
nasoturbinal
nasus
    n. externus
Nebinger-Praun operation
needle
    Brown's n.
    Hourin's n.
    House-Barbara n.
    House-Rosen n.
    House's n.
    McCurdy's n.
    Rosen's n.
    Shambaugh's n.
    Updegraff's n.
Neivert's retractor
nerve
    Arnold's n.
    chorda tympani n.
    cochlear n.
    facial n.
    glossopharyngeal n.
    Jacobsen's n.
    petrosal n.
    trigeminal n.
    vestibular n.

neuralgia
- glossopharyngeal n.
- trigeminal n.
- retrobulbar n.

New-Lambotte osteotome
nodular
nodule
noma
nose
- cleft n.
- potato n.
- saddle-back n.
- swayback n.

nostril
notch
- n. of Rivinus
- rivinian n.

Noyes' forceps
Noyes-Shambaugh scissors
NP – nasopharyngeal
- nasopharynx

NT – nasotracheal
nucha
nuchal
nucleus
- Bechterew's n.
- Deiters' n.

numatizashun. See *pneumatization.*

numo-. See words beginning *pneumo-.*

nystagmus
- aural n.
- caloric n.
- labyrinthine n.
- vestibular n.

occipital
occipitofrontal
occipitomastoid
occipitomental
occiput
ogo
Ogston-Luc operation
olfaction
olfactory
operation
- Adams' o.
- Asch's o.
- Billroth's o.
- Caldwell-Luc o.
- Carpue's o.
- Carter's o.
- Cassel's o.
- Cheever's o.
- Chevalier-Jackson o.
- Coakley's o.
- Denonvilliers' o.
- Fergusson's o.
- Gillies' o.
- Indian o.
- Italian o.
- Jansen's o.
- Jarvis' o.
- Keegan's o.
- Killian's o.
- Kuhnt's o.
- Kuster's o.
- Lauren's o.
- Lempert's o.
- Nebinger-Praun o.
- Ogston-Luc o.
- radical antrum o.
- Ridell's o.
- Robert's o.
- Rogue's o.
- Schonbein's o.

operation *(continued)*
    Schwartze's o.
    Sluder's o.
    Sonneberg's o.
    Sourdille's o.
    Stacke's o.
    tagliacotian o.
    Vicq d'Azyr's o.
    Yankauer's o.
opisthogenia
opisthognathism
orbit
orbital
organ
    o. of Corti
organum
    o. spirale
    o. vestibulocochleare
oroantral
oronasal
oropharynx
os
    o. epitympanicum
    o. ethmoidale
    o. frontale
    o. hyoideum
    o. interparietale
    o. lacrimale
    o. mastoideum
    o. nasale
    o. occipitale
    o. orbiculare
    o. palatinum
    o. parietale
    o. sphenoidale
    o. temporale
    o. unguis
    o. zygomaticum

osseosonometry
osseous
ossicle
ossicula
    o. auditus
ossiculectomy
ossiculotomy
ossiculum
osteotome
    Cottle's o.
    Dingman's o.
    New-Lambotte o.
    Rowland's o.
    Silver's o.
otacoustic
otagra
otalgia
    o. dentalis
    o. intermittens
otalgic
otectomy
othelcosis
othematoma
othemorrhea
othygroma
otiatrics
otic
oticodinia
otitic
otitis
    o. crouposa
    o. desquamativa
    o. diphtheritica
    o. externa circumscripta
    o. externa diffusa
    o. externa furunculosa
    o. externa hemorrhagica
    o. externa mycotica

otitis *(continued)*
>   furuncular o.
>   o. haemorrhagica
>   o. labyrinthica
>   o. mastoidea
>   o. media catarrhalis acuta
>   o. media catarrhalis chronica
>   o. media purulenta acuta
>   o. media purulenta chronica
>   o. media sclerotica
>   o. media serosa
>   o. media suppurativa
>   o. media vasomotorica
>   mucosis o.
>   mucosus o.
>   o. mycotica
>   o. sclerotica
otoantritis
otoblennorrhea
otocatarrh
otocephalus
otocerebritis
otocleisis
otoconia
otocranium
otodynia
otoencephalitis
otoganglion
otogenic
otogenous
otography
otohemineurasthenia
otolaryngology
otolith

otolithiasis
otologic
otologist
otology
otomassage
otomastoiditis
otomicroscope
otomicroscopy
otomucormycosis
otomyasthenia
Otomyces
otomycosis
otomyiasis
otoncus
otonecrectomy
otoneuralgia
otoneurasthenia
otopathy
otopharyngeal
otophone
otopiesis
otoplasty
otopolypus
otopyorrhea
otopyosis
otorhinolaryngology
otorhinology
otorrhagia
otorrhea
otosalpinx
otosclerectomy
otoscleronectomy
otosclerosis
otoscope
>   Bruening's o.
>   Brunton's o.
>   Siegle's o.
>   Toynbee's o.

otoscope
Welch-Allyn o.
otoscopy
otosis
otospongiosis
otosteal
otosteon
ototomy
ototoxic
ototoxicity
Owen's position
ozena
o. laryngis
paint
Mandl's p.
palata
palatal
palate
cleft p.
palatine
palatitis
palatoglossal
palatognathous
palatograph
palatography
palatomaxillary
palatomyograph
palatonasal
palatopharyngeal
palatoplasty
palatoplegia
palatoschisis
palatostaphylinus
palatouvularis
palatum
palsy
Bell's p.
Pang's forceps

panotitis
panseptum
pansinuitis
pansinusectomy
pansinusitis
panturbinate
papilla
acoustic p.
p. parotidea
papillae
filiform p.
p. filiformes
p. foliatae
foliate p.
fungiform p.
p. fungiformes
lingual p.
p. linguales
papilloma
paracusia
p. acris
p. duplicata
p. loci
p. willisiana
p. of Willis
paraglossa
paraglossia
paraglossitis
paries
p. externus ductus
cochlearis
p. jugularis cavi
tympani
p. labyrinthicus cavi
tympani
p. mastoideus cavi
tympani
p. medialis orbitae

paries *(continued)*
  p. membranaceus cavi tympani
  p. membranaceus tracheae
  p. tegmentalis cavi tympani
  p. tympanicus ductus cochlearis
  p. vestibularis ductus cochlearis
parietal
parietofrontal
parieto-occipital
parietosphenoid
parietosquamosal
parietotemporal
Parkinson's position
parosmia
parotid
parotidean
parotidectomy
parotitis
pars
  p. flaccida membranae tympani
  p. tensa membranae tympani
patch
  Silastic p.
Paterson's
  cannula
  forceps
peenash
Pennington's elevator
perforator
  Royce's p.
  Thornwald's p.

perforator
  Wellaminski's p.
periauricular
perichondritis
perichondrium
perilymph
perilymphatic
periorbital
periosteotome
  Dean's p.
  Fomon's p.
  Joseph's p.
periosteum
periotic
perirhinal
perisinuitis
perisinuous
perisinusitis
peritonsillar
peritonsillitis
petiolus
  p. epiglottidis
petromastoid
petro-occipital
petropharyngeus
petrosal
petrosectomy
petrositis
petrosphenoid
petrosquamosal
petrous
pharyngalgia
pharyngeal
pharyngectasia
pharyngectomy
pharyngemphraxis
pharyngeus
pharyngism

pharyngismus
pharyngitic
pharyngitid
pharyngitis
    atrophic p.
    catarrhal p.
    croupous p.
    diphtheric p.
    follicular p.
    gangrenous p.
    glandular p.
    granular p.
    p. herpetica
    hypertrophic p.
    p. keratosa
    membranous p.
    phlegmonous p.
    p. sicca
    p. ulcerosa
pharyngoamygdalitis
pharyngocele
pharyngoconjunctivitis
pharyngodynia
pharyngoepiglottic
pharyngoesophageal
pharyngoglossal
pharyngoglossus
pharyngokeratosis
pharyngolaryngeal
pharyngolaryngitis
pharyngolith
pharyngolysis
pharyngomaxillary
pharyngomycosis
pharyngonasal
pharyngo-oral
pharyngopalatine
pharyngoparalysis

pharyngopathy
pharyngoperistole
pharyngoplasty
pharyngoplegia
pharyngorhinitis
pharyngorhinoscopy
pharyngorrhagia
pharyngorrhea
pharyngosalpingitis
pharyngoscleroma
pharyngoscope
pharyngoscopy
pharyngospasm
pharyngostenosis
pharyngostomy
pharyngotherapy
pharyngotome
pharyngotomy
pharyngotonsillitis
pharyngotyphoid
pharynx
phlebectasia
    p. laryngis
phlegm
phonation
photophore
Pierce's
    dissector
    retractor
Pierre Robin syndrome
pillar
pinna
pinnal
piriform
platinectomy
Plaut-Vincent's angina
pledget
plegaphonia

plexus
Kiesselbach's p.
plica
p. stapedis
p. supratonsillaris
p. triangularis
plicotomy
plug
Mackenty's choanal p.
Plummer's bougie
Plummer-Vinson syndrome
PND – postnasal drainage
postnasal drip
pneumatization
pneumothorax
pocket
Rathke's p.
politzerization
Politzer's
bag
speculum
test
treatment
pollinosis
polyp
Hopmann's p.
ponticulus
p. auriculae
p. promontorii
position
Caldwell's p.
Law's p.
Mayer's p.
Owen's p.
Parkinson's p.
Proetz's p.
Rose's p.
Schüller's p.

position *(continued)*
Stenvers' p.
Waters-Waldron p.
postaurale
pouch
Prussak's p.
Rathke's p.
Pratt's curet
preauricular
presbycusis
Prince's scissors
probe
Arbuckle's p.
Jansen-Newhart p.
Rosen's p.
Spencer's p.
Theobald's p.
Welch-Allyn p.
Yankauer's p.
procedure
Valsalva's p.
process
mastoid p.
styloid p.
zygomatic p.
Proctor's
elevator
retractor
Proetz's
position
treatment
prognathism
prognathous
prominentia
p. laryngea
p. styloidea
promontorium
p. faciei

promontorium *(continued)*
   p. tympani
promontory
prosthesis
   House's p.
   Sheehy-House p.
   Teflon p.
Prussak's
   fibers
   pouch
   space
pseudocholesteatoma
Pseudomonas
   P. aeruginosa
pterygomandibular
pterygomaxillary
pterygopalatine
ptyalectasis
ptyalism
ptyalith
ptyalize
ptyalocele
ptyalolithiasis
ptyalorrhea
punch
   Adler's p.
   Citelli-Meltzer p.
   Gundelach's p.
   Hajek-Skillern p.
   Hartmann's p.
   Hoffmann's p.
   Lermoyez's p.
   Meltzer's p.
   Mosher's p.
   Myles' p.
   Schmeden's p.
   Spencer's p.
   Spies' p.

punch *(continued)*
   Takahashi's p.
   Van Struycken's p.
   Wagner's p.
   Watson-Williams p.
   Wilde's p.
   Yankauer's p.
pyemia
   otogenous p.
pyknosis
Pynchon's
   applicator
   speculum
pyothorax
pyramid
   petrous p.
quinsy
   lingual q.
Quisling's hammer
Ramsey-Hunt disease
ranula
raphe
   r. pharyngis
rasp
   Aufricht-Lipsett r.
   Aufricht's r.
   Berne's r.
   Cottle's r.
   Fomon's r.
   Good's r.
   Lewis' r.
   Maltz-Lipsett r.
   Maltz's r.
   Wiener-Pierce r.
Rathke's
   pocket
   pouch
   tumor

Ray-Parsons-Sunday elevator
Ray's speculum
reaction
    Moeller's r.
recess
    Tröltsch's r's.
recessus
    r. cochlearis vestibuli
    r. ellipticus vestibuli
    r. epitympanicus
    r. membranae tympani
        anterior
    r. membranae tympani
        posterior
    r. membranae tympani
        superior
    r. pharyngeus
    r. piriformis
    r. pro utriculo
    r. sphenoethmoidalis
    r. sphenoethmoidalis
        osseus
    r. sphericus vestibuli
Reiner-Beck snare
Reiner-Knight forceps
Reissner's membrane
retractor
    Allport's r.
    Aufricht's r.
    Brown's r.
    Cottle-Neivert r.
    Cottle's r.
    Davis' r.
    Dingman's r.
    Ferris-Smith-Sewall r.
    Gifford's r.
    Hajek's r.
    Haslinger's r.

retractor *(continued)*
    Henner's r.
    House-Urban r.
    Jansen's r.
    Latrobe's r.
    Lothrop's r.
    Love's r.
    Luongo's r.
    Neivert's r.
    Pierce's r.
    Proctor's r.
    Schuknecht's r.
    Senn-Dingman r.
    Shambaugh's r.
    Snitman's r.
    Weitlaner's r.
    White-Proud r.
    Wullstein's r.
retroauricular
retrolabyrinthine
retromandibular
retromastoid
retronasal
retropharyngeal
retropharyngitis
retropharynx
rhinal
rhinalgia
rhinallergosis
rhinedema
rhinenchysis
rhinesthesia
rhineurynter
rhinion
rhinism
rhinitis
    allergic r.
    anaphylactic r.

rhinitis *(continued)*
    atrophic r.
    r. caseosa
    catarrhal r.
    croupous r.
    dyscrinic r.
    fibrinous r.
    gangrenous r.
    hypertrophic r.
    membranous r.
    pseudomembranous r.
    purulent r.
    scrofulous r.
    r. sicca
    syphilitic r.
    tuberculous r.
    vasomotor r.
rhinoanemometer
rhinoantritis
rhinobyon
rhinocephalia
rhinocephalus
rhinocheiloplasty
rhinocleisis
rhinocoele
rhinodacryolith
rhinodynia
rhinogenous
rhinokyphectomy
rhinokyphosis
rhinolalia
    r. aperta
    r. clausa
rhinolaryngitis
rhinolaryngology
rhinolith
rhinolithiasis
rhinologist

rhinology
rhinomanometer
rhinometer
rhinomiosis
rhinomycosis
rhinonecrosis
rhinoneurosis
rhinopathia
    r. vasomotoria
rhinopathy
rhinopharyngeal
rhinopharyngitis
    r. mutilans
rhinopharyngocele
rhinopharyngolith
rhinopharynx
rhinophonia
rhinophore
rhinophyma
rhinoplastic
rhinoplasty
    Carpue's r.
    dactylocostal r.
    English r.
    Indian r.
    Italian r.
    tagliacotian r.
rhinopolypus
rhinoreaction
rhinorrhagia
rhinorrhaphy
rhinorrhea
    cerebrospinal r.
rhinosalpingitis
rhinoscleroma
rhinoscope
rhinoscopic
rhinoscopy

rhinosporidiosis
rhinostegnosis
rhinostenosis
rhinotomy
rhinovaccination
rhinovirus
rhonchal
rhonchial
rhonchus
Richard's curet
Ridell's operation
Ridley's sinus
Ridpath's curet
rima
    r. glottidis
    r. glottidis cartilaginea
    r. glottidis membrana-
      cea
    intercartilaginous r.
    intermembranous r.
    r. oris
    r. vestibuli
    r. vocalis
ring
    Waldeyer's r.
Ringer's solution
Rinne's test
Rivini's incisura
Rivinus'
    ducts
    gland
    membrane
    notch
Robb's forceps
Roberts'
    applicator
    laryngoscope
    operation

Robertson's
    forceps
    knife
rod
    Corti's r's.
    House's r.
Roeder's treatment
Rogers' dissector
rongeur
    Beyer's r.
    Converse's r.
    Dufourmental's r.
    Hartmann-Herz-
      feld r.
    Hartmann's r.
    Hoffmann's r.
    Husks' r.
    Ivy's r.
    Kerrison's r.
    Lombard-Boies r.
    Rowland's r.
    Ruskin's r.
    Tobey's r.
    Whiting's r.
Rosenmueller's
    curet
    fossa
Rosen's
    explorer
    fenestrater
    knife
    needle
    probe
    separator
    tube
Roser's mouth gag
Rose's position
Rouge's operation

Rowland's
    forceps
    osteotome
    rongeur
Royce's perforator
ruga
    r. palatina
Rusch's laryngoscope
Ruskin's
    forceps
    rongeur
saccule
    laryngeal s.
    s. of larynx
sacculus
    s. communis
    s. lacrimalis
    s. laryngis
    s. proprius
    s. rotundus
    s. sphaericus
    s. ventricularis
    s. vestibularis
saliva
salivant
salivary
salivation
salpingitis
    eustachian s.
salpingocatheterism
salpingopharyngeal
salpingoscope
salpingoscopy
salpingostaphyline
Salvatore-Maloney tracheo-
    tome
Sanders' laryngoscope
Santorini's incisura

sarcoma
Sauer's tonsillectome
Sauer-Sluder tonsillectome
saw
    Clerf's s.
    Cottle's s.
    Gottschalk's s.
    Joseph-Maltz s.
    Joseph's s.
    Lamont's s.
    Maltz's s.
    Myerson's s.
    Slaughter's s.
    Woakes' s.
Sawtell's forceps
scala
    s. media
    s. tympani
    s. vestibuli
scapha
Scarpa's
    foramen
    membrane
Schaeffer's curet
Schall's tube
Scheinmann's forceps
Schmeden's punch
Schmincke's tumor
Schonbein's operation
Schuknecht's
    excavator
    hook
    knife
    retractor
Schüller's position
Schwabach's test
Schwartze's
    operation

Schwartze's
  sign
scissors
    Boettcher's s.
    Cottle's s.
    Dean's s.
    Fomon's s.
    House's s.
    Jackson's s.
    Joseph's s.
    Knapp's s.
    Knight's s.
    Lejeune's s.
    Lillie's s.
    Lynch's s.
    Maclay's s.
    Metzenbaum-Lipsett s.
    Metzenbaum's s.
    Noyes-Shambaugh s.
    Prince's s.
    Seiler's s.
Scott's
  cannula
  speculum
scute
  tympanic s.
SD — septal defect
searcher
    Allport's s.
Searcy's tonsillectome
Seiffert's forceps
Seiler's
  formula
  knife
  scissors
sella
  s. turcica
sellar

Semken's forceps
Sengstaken-Blakemore tube
Sengstaken's tube
Senn-Dingman retractor
Senturia's speculum
separator
    House's s.
    Rosen's s.
septal
septectomy
septonasal
septoplasty
septotome
septotomy
septum
    s. cartilagineum nasi
    s. nasi osseum
    s. sinuum frontalium
    s. sinuum sphenoidalium
Sewall's chisel
Sexton's knife
sfeno-. See words beginning
    spheno-.
Shambaugh-Derlacki
  chisel
  elevator
Shambaugh-Lempert knife
Shambaugh's
  adenotome
  elevator
  hook
  incision
  irrigator
  needle
  retractor
Shapleigh's curet
Shearer's forceps
Sheehan's chisel

Sheehy-House prosthesis
Sheehy's
    knife
    tube
Shrapnell's membrane
siagantritis
siagonagra
siagonantritis
sialaden
sialadenitis
sialadenography
sialadenoncus
sialagogic
sialagogue
sialaporia
sialectasia
sialectasis
sialitis
sialoadenectomy
sialoadenitis
sialoadenotomy
sialocele
sialodochiectasis
sialodochitis
sialodochoplasty
sialogram
sialography
sialolith
sialolithiasis
sialolithotomy
sialoma
sialorrhea
sialosis
sialostenosis
sialosyrinx
sialozemia
Siegle's ostoscope
Sierra-Sheldon tracheotome

sign
    Schwartze's s.
    Wreden's s.
    Zaufal's s.
Siker's laryngoscope
Silastic patch
Silver's osteotome
sinobronchitis
sinus
    s. cochleae
    ethmoidal s.
    s. ethmoidalis
    s. frontalis osseus
    Huguier's s.
    laryngeal s.
    mastoid s.
    maxillary s.
    s. maxillaris
    Meyer's s.
    s. of Morgagni
    paranasal s's.
    s. paranasales
    s. posterior cavi tympani
    pyriform s.
    Ridley's s.
    sphenoidal s.
    s. sphenoidalis
    s. tympani
    tympanic s.
sinusitis
sinusotomy
SISI — short increment
    sensitivity index
Sjögren's syndrome
Slaughter's saw
Sluder-Demarest tonsillec-
    tome
Sluder-Jansen mouth gag

Sluder-Sauer
    guillotine
    tonsillectome
Sluder's
    guillotine
    operation
    tonsillectome
SMR — submucous resection
SMR speculum
snare
    Bosworth's s.
    Brown's s.
    Bruening's s.
    Eves' s.
    Krause's s.
    Lewis' s.
    Myles' s.
    Reiner-Beck s.
    Storz-Beck s.
    Stutsman's s.
    Tydings' s.
    Wilde-Bruening s.
    Wright's s.
Snitman's retractor
solution
    Ringer's s.
SOM — secretory otitis media
    serous otitis media
Sonneberg's operation
Sonnenschein's speculum
Sourdille's operation
space
    poststyloid s.
    prestyloid s.
    Prussak's s.
    retropharyngeal s.
speculum
    Aufricht's s.

speculum *(continued)*
    Beckman-Colver s.
    Boucheron's s.
    Chevalier-Jackson s.
    Coakley's s.
    Converse's s.
    Cottle's s.
    Duplay-Lynch s.
    Duplay's s.
    Eaton's s.
    Erhardt's s.
    Farrior's s.
    Flannery's s.
    Gerzog's s.
    Gruber's s.
    Halle's s.
    Halle-Tieck s.
    Hartmann-Dewaxer s.
    Hartmann's s.
    Heffernan's s.
    Ingals' s.
    Killian's s.
    Kramer's s.
    Kyle's s.
    Lempert-Colver s.
    Lillie's s.
    Mahoney's s.
    McHugh's s.
    Mosher's s.
    Myles' s.
    Politzer's s.
    Pynchon's s.
    Ray's s.
    Scott's s.
    Senturia's s.
    SMR s.
    Sonnenschein's s.
    Toynbee's s.

speculum *(continued)*
    Troeltsch's s.
    Vienna's s.
    Welch-Allyn s.
    Yankauer's s.
Spencer's
    probe
    punch
sphenoethmoid
sphenofrontal
sphenoid
sphenoidal
sphenoidectomy
    frontoethmoid s.
sphenoiditis
sphenoidostomy
sphenoidotomy
sphenomaxillary
sphenopalatine
Spies' punch
spine
    s. of Henle
    suprameatal s.
splint
    Asch's s.
    Carter's s.
    Erich's s.
    Jones' s.
    Kazanjian's s.
    Love's s.
    Mayer's s.
spoon
    Gross' s.
Spratt's curet
spud
    Gross' s.
squama
squamomastoid

SRT — speech reception test
    speech reception
       threshold
St. Clair-Thompson's curet
Stacke's operation
stapedectomy
stapedial
stapediolysis
stapedioplasty
stapediotenotomy
stapediovestibular
stapes
staphylagra
staphylectomy
staphyledema
staphylematoma
staphyline
staphylinus
staphylion
staphylitis
staphyloangina
staphyloncus
staphylopharyngorrhaphy
staphyloplasty
staphyloptosia
staphyloptosis
staphylorrhaphy
staphyloschisis
staphylotome
staphylotomy
Stenger's test
Stensen's
    duct
    foramen
stent
Stenvers' position
sternohyoid
sternomastoid

sternothyroid
sternotracheal
Stoerk's blennorrhea
stomatitides
stomatitis
stomatomycosis
stomatoplasty
Storz-Beck snare
Straight's tenaculum
stria
    s. vascularis ductus
      cochlearis
stridor
Struempel's forceps
Struyken's forceps
Stubbs' curet
Stutsman's snare
stylohyal
stylohyoid
styloid
stylomandibular
stylomastoid
subglossitis
subglottic
sublingual
submandibular
submaxillary
submental
sudo-. See words beginning
    pseudo-.
sudokolesteatoma. See
    pseudocholesteatoma.
sulcus
    tympanic s.
summit
    s. of nose
Sunday's elevator
supraclavicular

supraglottic
supramandibular
supramastoid
supramaxillary
supramental
supranasal
supraorbital
suprastapedial
suprasternal
supratemporal
surgical procedures. See
    operations.
suture
    coronal s.
    ethmoideomaxillary s.
    frontal s.
    frontoethmoidal s.
    frontolacrimal s.
    frontomaxillary s.
    frontonasal s.
    frontozygomatic s.
    intermaxillary s.
    internasal s.
    lacrimoconchal s.
    lacrimomaxillary s.
    lambdoid s.
    nasomaxillary s.
    occipitomastoid s.
    palatoethmoidal s.
    parietomastoid s.
    petrosquamous s.
    sagittal s.
    sphenoethmoidal s.
    sphenofrontal s.
    sphenomaxillary s.
    sphenoparietal s.
    sphenosquamous s.
    sphenozygomatic s.

suture *(continued)*
    squamosomastoid s.
    temporozygomatic s.
    zygomaticomaxillary s.
symptom
    Bárány's s.
    Fröschel's s.
synchondrosis
syndrome
    Avellis' s.
    Baelz's s.
    Bárány's s.
    Costen's s.
    Kartagener's s.
    Lermoyez's s.
    Mikulicz's s.
    Pierre Robin s.
    Plummer-Vinson s.
    Sjögren's s.
synechia
Tabb's curet
Takahashi's
    forceps
    punch
tampon
    nasal t.
tantalum
technique
    guillotine t.
Teflon prosthesis
tegmen
    t. antri
    t. mastoideotympanicum
    t. mastoideum
    t. tympani
tegmentum
    t. auris
temple

tempora
temporal
temporalis
temporauricular
temporofacial
temporofrontal
temporohyoid
temporomandibular
temporomaxillary
temporo-occipital
temporoparietal
temporosphenoid
temporozygomatic
tenaculum
    Cottle's t.
    Straight's t.
terigo. See words beginning
    pterygo-.
test
    Bárány's t.
    Lombard's t.
    Politzer's t.
    Rinne's t.
    Schwabach's t.
    Stenger's t.
    watch t.
    Weber's t.
    whisper t.
    whistle t.
Theobald's probe
Thornwald's perforator
thrush
thyrochondrotomy
thyrocricotomy
thyroglossal
thyrohyoid
thyroid
thyromegaly

thyrotomy
tia-. See words beginning
ptya-.
tialektasis. See *ptyalectasis.*
tializm. See *ptyalism.*
tic
    t. doulourex (doo-loo-
      roo)
tinnitus
Tivnen's forceps
TM — tympanic membrane
TMJ — temporomandibular
  joint
Tobey's rongeur
Tobold's
    forceps
    knife
tonguetie
tonsil
tonsilla
    t. lingualis
    t. palatina
    t. pharyngea
    t. tubaria
tonsillar
tonsillectome
    Ballenger-Sluder t.
    Beck-Mueller t.
    Beck-Schenck t.
    Brown's t.
    Daniels' t.
    Laforce's t.
    Mack's t.
    Moltz-Storz t.
    Myles' t.
    Sauer's t.
    Sauer-Sluder t.
    Searcy's t.

tonsillectome *(continued)*
    Sluder-Demarest t.
    Sluder-Sauer t.
    Sluder's t.
    Tydings' t.
    Van Osdel's t.
    Whiting's t.
tonsillectomy
tonsillitis
    caseous t.
    catarrhal t.
    diphtherial t.
    erythematous t.
    follicular t.
    herpetic t.
    lacunar t.
    t. lenta
    lingual t.
    mycotic t.
    parenchymatous t.
    preglottic t.
    pustular t.
    streptococcus t.
    Vincent's t.
tonsilloadenoidectomy
tonsillolith
tonsilloscope
tonsilloscopy
tonsillotome
tonsillotomy
Topinard's
    angle
    line
Tornwaldt's bursitis
torticollis
torus
    t. frontalis
    t. levatorius

torus *(continued)*
    t. occipitalis
    t. palatinus
    t. tubarius
Toynbee's
    otoscope
    speculum
trachea
tracheal
tracheitis
tracheobronchial
tracheobronchitis
tracheobronchoscopy
tracheocele
tracheoesophageal
tracheofissure
tracheofistulization
tracheolaryngeal
tracheolaryngotomy
tracheomalacia
tracheopharyngeal
tracheoplasty
tracheorrhaphy
tracheoscopy
    peroral t.
tracheostenosis
tracheostomy
tracheotome
    Salvatore-Maloney t.
    Sierra-Sheldon t.
tracheotomy
tragus
transillumination
Trautmann's triangle
treatment
    Politzer's t.
    Proetz's t.
    Roeder's t.

trephine
triad
    Kartagener's t.
triangle
    Trautmann's t.
trismus
Troeltsch's speculum
Tröltsch's recesses
Troutman's
    chisel
    gouge
tube
    Anthony's t.
    auditory t.
    Blakemore's t.
    Bouchut's t.
    Chevalier-Jackson t.
    Donaldson's t.
    eustachian t.
    Frazier's t.
    House's t.
    LaRocca's t.
    Lewis' t.
    Lindeman-Silverstein t.
    Mackenty's t.
    Morch's t.
    Rosen's t.
    Schall's t.
    Sengstaken-Blakemore t.
    Sengstaken's t.
    Sheehy's t.
    Voltolini's t.
    Welch-Allyn t.
    Yankauer's t.
tubercle
    darwinian t.
tuborrhea
tubotorsion

tubotympanal
Tucker's laryngoscope
tumefaction
tumor
    Rathke's t.
    Schmincke's t.
tuning fork
    Hartmann's t. f.
tunnel
    t. of Corti
turbinate
    sphenoid t.
turbinectomy
turbinotome
turbinotomy
Tydings'
    forceps
    knife
    snare
    tonsillectome
Tydings-Lakeside forceps
tympanal
tympanectomy
tympanic
tympanichord
tympanichordal
tympanicity
tympanion
tympanitic
tympanitis
tympanoacryloplasty
tympanoeustachian
tympanolabyrinthopexy
tympanomalleal
tympanomandibular
tympanomastoiditis
tympanomeatal
tympanophonia

tympanoplasty
tympanosclerosis
tympanosquamosal
tympanostapedial
tympanosympathectomy
tympanotemporal
tympanotomy
tympanum
tympany
uloglossitis
uloncus
umbo
    u. of tympanic membrane
Updegraff's needle
uraniscochasma
uraniscolalia
uranisconitis
uranoplasty
utricle
uvula
    u. palatina
    palatine u.
uvulectomy
uvulitis
uvuloptosis
uvulotome
uvulotomy
vallecula
    v. epiglottica
Valsalva's procedure
valve
    Huschke's v.
Van Osdel's tonsillectome
Van-Struycken
    forceps
    punch
vas

vasa
  v. auris internae
velum
  v. palatinum
ventricle
  Morgagni's v.
ventricular
ventriculocordectomy
Verga's lacrimal groove
vermilionectomy
vertigo
vestibular
vestibule
vestibulotomy
vestibulum
  v. auris
  v. glottidis
  v. laryngis
  v. nasi
  v. oris
vibrissa
vibrissae
vibromasseur
vibrometer
vicq d' Azyr's operation
Vienna's speculum
Vieussens' annulus
Vincent's
  infection
  tonsillitis
Vogel's curet
Voltolini's tube
vomer
vomeronasal
Wagner's punch
Waldeyer's ring
Walker's dissector
Walther's ducts
Waters-Waldron position

Watson-Williams
  forceps
  punch
Weber's test
Weil's forceps
Weingartner's forceps
Weisman's curet
Weitlaner's retractor
Welch-Allyn
  laryngoscope
  otoscope
  probe
  speculum
  tube
Wellaminski's perforator
Wharton's duct
White-Lillie forceps
White-Proud retractor
White's forceps
Whiting's
  curet
  rongeur
  tonsillectome
Wiener-Pierce rasp
Wilde-Bruening snare
Wilde's
  forceps
  punch
Willis' paracusis
window
  oval w.
  round w.
windowing
Wis-Foregger's laryngoscope
Wis-Hipple's laryngoscope
Woakes' saw
Wreden's sign
Wright's snare

Wullstein-House forceps
Wullstein's
    bur
    forceps
    knife
    retractor
xanthosis
    x. of septum nasi
xeromycteria
xerostomia
Yankauer-Little forceps
Yankauer's
    catheter
    curet
    forceps

Yankauer's *(continued)*
    laryngoscope
    operation
    probe
    punch
    speculum
    tube
Zaufal's sign
Zeiss' microscope
zygoma
zygomatic
zygomaticofacial
zygomaticofrontal
zygomaticomaxillary
zygomaxillary

PEDIATRICS

abetalipoproteinemia
Abderhalden-Fanconi
    syndrome
ABO incompatibility
abscess
    perinephric a.
    retropharyngeal a.
    subphrenic a.
Abt-Letterer-Siwe syndrome
acantholysis
    a. bullosa
achalasia
achondroplasia
acidosis
    diabetic a.
    hyperchloremic renal a.
    metabolic a.
aciduria
    B-aminoisobutyric a.
aclasis
    diaphyseal a.
acne
    a. neonatorum
acrobrachycephaly
acrocephalosyndactylia
acrocyanosis
acrodermatitis
    a. enteropathica
acrodynia
acromegaly
actinomyces

actinomycosis
Addison's disease
adenitis
    cervical a.
    mesenteric a.
adenoiditis
adenoma
    a. sebaceum
adenopathy
    cervical a.
Adie's syndrome
adiponecrosis
    a. subcutanea
        neonatorum
adnexa
adolescence
adrenarche
adrenocortical
aerophore
aftha. See *aphtha.*
agammaglobulinemia
agenesia
    a. corticalis
agglutinin
agranulocytosis
akalazea. See *achalasia.*
akondroplazea. See *achon-
    droplasia.*
akrobrakesefale. See *acro-
    brachycephaly.*

Albers-Schönberg's syndrome
albinism
Albright's snydrome
albuminuria
aldosteronism
    juvenile a.
Aldrich's syndrome
aleukia
    congenital a.
Alexander's disease
alkalosis
allergic
allergy
Alper's disease
Alport's syndrome
alymphocytosis
alymphoplasia
ambient
amebiasis
amenorrhea
aminoacidemia
aminoaciduria
aminoaciduriasis
amnionitis
amyloidosis
amylopectinosis
amyoplasia
    a. congenita
amyotonia
    a. congenita
anaphylaxis
anasarca
ancylostomiasis
Andersen's disease
Andogsky's syndrome
anemia
    aplastic a.
    Cooley's a.

anemia *(continued)*
    Czerny's a.
    erythroblastic a.
    Fanconi's a.
    hemolytic a.
    Jaksch's a.
    Larzel's a.
    Mediterranean a.
    megaloblastic a.
    a. neonatorum
    a. pseudoleukemica in-
        fantum
    sickle cell a.
    von Jaksch's a.
anencephaly
aneurysm
    aortic a.
angiitis
angiocardiography
anorchia
anorchism
anorexia
    a. nervosa
anoxia
ansilostomiasis. See
    ancylostomiasis.
antigen
    Australia a.
anuria
anus
    imperforate a.
aorta
aortitis
Apgar
    rating
    score
aphtha
    Bednar's a.

apnea
    a. neonatorum
appendicitis
arachnidism
arachnodactyly
arachnoiditis
arak-. See words beginning
    arach-.
Aran-Duchenne disease
areflexia
arginosuccinicaciduria
Arnold-Chiari syndrome
arrhythmia
    sinus a.
arteriosclerosis
    infantile a.
arteritis
    a. umbilicalis
arthritis
    rheumatoid a.
arthrogryposis
    a. multiplex congenita
ascariasis
Ascaris
    A. lumbricoides
ascites
    chylous a.
ASD – atrial septal defect
asphyxia
    a. neonatorum
asthma
astigmatism
astrocytoma
ataxia
    cerebellar a.
    Friedreich's a.
atelectasis
athetoid

athetosis
    congenital a.
atopic
atopy
atresia
    biliary a.
    esophageal a.
    tricuspid a.
atrial septal defect
atrophy
    Déjerine-Sottas a.
    Fazio-Londe a.
    Parrot's a. of the
      newborn
Australia antigen
autism
autistic
bacteroidosis
Ballantyne-Runge syndrome
Banti's syndrome
Barlow's disease
Bartter's syndrome
Beckwith's syndrome
Bednar's aphtha
Berger's paresthesia
beriberi
bilirubin
Blalock-Hanlon operation
Blalock-Taussig operation
blefaritis. See *blepharitis*.
blefarospasm. See *blepharo-*
    spasm.
blennorrhea
blepharitis
blepharospasm
Bloch-Sulzberger syndrome
blood
    cord b.

Bloom's syndrome
Bonnevie-Ullrich syndrome
Bornholm's disease
botulism
Bourneville's syndrome
brachycephalic
brachydactyly
bradycardia
Brandt's syndrome
brash
    weaning b.
bronchiectasis
bronchiolitis
bronchitis
bronchopneumonia
brucella
brucellosis
Brudzinski's sign
bruit
    carotid b.
Brushfield's spots
brwe. See *bruit.*
Buhl's disease
Byrd-Dew method
Caffey's disease
Caffey-Silverman syndrome
Caffey-Smyth-Roske
    syndrome
Calvé-Legg-Perthes syndrome
Camurati-Engelmann
    syndrome
Canavan's disease
cancer
cancerous
Candida
    C. albicans
candidiasis
canker

caput
    c. medusae
    c. succedaneum
cardiospasm
cataplexy
cataract
catarrhal
catheter
    arterial c.
    umbilical c.
    venous c.
catheterization
celiaca
cellulitis
cephalhematoma
cerebellar
cerebral
cerebrospinal
cerebrovascular
Chagas' disease
chalasia
chalazion
Chapple's syndrome
Charcot-Marie-Tooth-Hoff-
    mann syndrome
Cheadle's disease
Chédiak-Higashi syndrome
chickenpox
cholangitis
cholera
    c. infantum
chondrodystrophia
    c. calcificans congenita
    c. fetalis calcificans
chondrodystrophy
chorea
    Sydenham's c.
chorioepithelioma

choriomeningitis
  lymphocytic c.
chorioretinitis
chromaffinoma
cirrhonosus
cirrhosis
  biliary c.
citrullinuria
clinodactyly
clonus
  ankle c.
clostridia
clubfoot
CNS – central nervous system
coarctation
  c. of the aorta
coccidiodomycosis
colic
colicky
colitis
  ulcerative c.
coloboma
Colorado tick fever
colostration
colostrum
coma
  diabetic c.
  hyperosmolar c.
Comby's sign
communicable
complex
  Eisenmenger's c.
  Ghon c.
concussion
conjunctivitis
constipation
contusion

conversion
  hysterical c.
convulsion
  febrile c.
Cooley's anemia
Coombs' test
cor
  c. biloculare
  c. triloculare biatriatum
Cori's disease
corpora
  c. quadrigemina
Corrigan's pulse
Corynebacterium
  C. diphtheriae
coryza
coxa
  c. vara
Coxsackie virus
cradle cap
craniopharyngioma
craniostenosis
craniosynostosis
craniotabes
crease
  sole c.
creatinine
crepitation
cretinism
cri-du-chat syndrome
Crigler-Najjar syndrome
crisis
  adrenal c.
croup
Crouzon's disease
crusta
  c. lactea
cryoprecipitate

cryptococcosis
cryptorchidism
Cushing's syndrome
cutis
 c. elastica
 c. hyperelastica
CVP — central venous pressure
cyanosis
cyst
 choledochal c.
 colloid c.
 dermoid c.
 hydatid c.
 omental c.
 porencephalic c's.
 urachal c.
 vitelline duct c.
cystathioninuria
cystinosis
cystinuria
Czerny's anemia
dacryocystostenosis
dance
 St. Vitus' d.
dandruff
Darrow-Gamble syndrome
defect
 atrial septal d.
 ventral septal d.
deficiency
 disaccharidase d.
 erythrocyte glutathione
  peroxidase d.
 Factor VIII d.
 fibrinogen d.
 glucose-6-phosphate de-
  hydrogenase d.
 immunoglobulin d.

deficiency
 riboflavin d.
deformity
 Sprengel's d.
degeneration
 cerebellar d.
 cerebromacular d.
dehydration
Déjerine's disease
Déjerine-Sottas
 atrophy
 disease
deLange's syndrome
delinquency
delirium
dengue
Dennett's diet
Dennie-Marfan syndrome
depigmentation
dermatitis
 atopic d.
 d. excoriativa infantum
 d. exfoliativa infantum
 d. gangrenosa infantum
 Jacquet's d.
 seborrheic d.
 d. venenata
dermatomyositis
dermatophytosis
desensitization
De Toni-Fanconi-Debre
 syndrome
dextrocardia
Dextrostix
diabetes
 d. insipidus
 d. mellitus
diabetic

Diamond-Blackfan syndrome
diarrhea
diastematomyelia
diencephalic syndrome
diet
    Dennett's d.
    Moro-Heisler d.
difenilthiourea. See *diphenyl-thiourea.*
difilobothriasis. See *diphyl-lobothriasis.*
diftherea. See *diphtheria.*
DiGeorge's syndrome
dilatation
    esophageal d.
diphenylthiourea
diphtheria
diphyllobothriasis
diplegia
    atonic-astatic d.
    infantile d.
    spastic d.
Diplococcus
    D. pneumoniae
dis-. See also words beginning *dys-.*
disease
    Addison's d.
    Alexander's d.
    Alper's d.
    Andersen's d.
    Aran-Duchenne d.
    Barlow's d.
    Bornholm's d.
    Buhl's d.
    Caffey's d.
    Canavan's d.
    celiac d.

disease *(continued)*
    central nervous system d.
    Chagas' d.
    Cheadle's d.
    Cori's d.
    Crouzon's d.
    cytomegalic inclusion d. of the newborn
    cytomegalovirus d.
    Déjerine's d.
    Déjerine-Sottas d.
    Factor X deficiency d.
    Feer's d.
    fibrocystic d.
    fifth d.
    Gaucher's d.
    glycogen storage d.
    Hartnup's d.
    hemolytic d. of the newborn
    hemorrhagic d. of newborn
    Henoch's d.
    Hers' d.
    Hirschsprung's d.
    Hodgkin's d.
    Hutinel's d.
    hyaline membrane d.
    Kashin-Bek d.
    Köhler's d.
    Krabbe's d.
    Leber's d.
    Leigh's d.
    Leiner's d.
    Letterer-Siwe d.
    Little's d.
    maple syrup d.
    Marion's d.

disease *(continued)*
    McArdle's d.
    Möller-Barlow d.
    Morquio's d.
    Niemann-Pick d.
    Oppenheim's d.
    Pelizaeus-Merzbacher d.
    Pink d.
    Pompe's d.
    Potter's d.
    Recklinghausen's d.
    Refsum's d.
    Ritter's d.
    Saunders' d.
    Scheuermann's d.
    Schilder's d.
    spinocerebellar degen-
      erative d.
    Sticker's d.
    Still's d.
    Stuart-Prower factor de-
      ficiency d.
    Tay-Sachs d.
    Thomsen's d.
    Underwood's d.
    Unverricht's d.
    von Gierke's d.
    Weil's d.
    Wilkins' d.
    Wilson's d.
    Winckel's d.
disfagia. See *dysphagia.*
disjenisis. See *dysgenesis.*
distaxia
    d. cerebralis infantilis
distress
    idiopathic respiratory d.
     of newborn

diverticulum
    Meckel's d.
Down's syndrome
drooling
drugs. See *Medications.*
Dubin-Johnson syndrome
Dubovitz's syndrome
Duchenne's dystrophy
duct
    Stensen's d.
ductus
    d. arteriosus
dwarfism
    pituitary d.
dysautonomia
    familial d.
dyschondroplasia
dysentery
    amebic d.
    bacillary d.
dysfibrinogenemia
dysfunction
    placental d.
dysgammaglobulinemia
dysgenesis
    gonadal d.
dysgerminoma
dyshepatia
    lipogenic d.
dysmaturity
dysmenorrhea
dysostosis
    cleidocranial d.
    craniofacial d.
    mandibulofacial d.
    d. multiplex
    orodigitofacial d.
dysphagia

dysplasia
 anhidrotic ectodermal d.
 bronchopulmonary d.
 chondroectodermal d.
 diaphysial d.
 ectodermal d.
 polyostotic fibrous d.
 thymic d.
dyspnea
dysrhythmia
dystonia
dystrophy
 Duchenne's d.
 Meesmann's d.
 muscular d.
EBV – Epstein-Barr virus
ecchymosis
Echinococcus
ECHO – enteric cytopatho-
 genic human orphan
 (virus)
ECHO virus
echoencephalography
ecthyma
eczema
 e. herpeticum
 infantile e.
 e. marginatum
 e. neonatorum
efeb-. See words beginning
 epheb-.
efelidez. See *ephelides*.
efelis. See *ephelis*.
effusion
Ehlers-Danlos syndrome
Eisenmenger's complex
ekimosis. See *ecchymosis*.
ekinokokus. See *Echinococcus*.

eksanthem. See *exanthem*.
ekthima. See *ecthyma*.
ekzema. See *eczema*.
electrocardiography
electrodesiccation
electroencephalogram
electrolyte
electrophoresis
elephantiasis
 congenital e.
elliptocytosis
Ellis-Van Creveld syndrome
embolus
embryoma
emesis
emphysema
empyema
emulsion
 Pusey's e.
encephalitis
 viral e.
encephalocele
encephalomyelitis
encephalopathy
 demyelinating e.
enchondroma
encopresis
endocarditis
 subacute bacterial e.
enteritis
 bacterial e.
 regional e.
enterobiasis
Enterobius
 E. vermicularis
enteropathy
enuresis
eosinophilia

ependymoma
ephebiatrics
ephebic
ephebogenesis
ephebogenic
ephebology
ephelides
ephelis
epicanthus
epidermolysis
    e. bullosa
epidermophytosis
epididymis
epifisis. See *epiphysis.*
epilepsy
    abdominal e.
    focal e.
    grand mal e.
    jacksonian e.
    myoclonus e.
    nocturnal e.
    petit mal e.
    psychomotor e.
epileptic
epileptiform
epiloia
epiphysis
epistaxis
epituberculosis
Epstein-Barr virus
Epstein's
    pearls
    symptom
Erb-Duchenne paralysis
erithema. See *erythema.*
erithro-. See words beginning *erythro-.*
Erlacher-Blount syndrome

eruption
    Kaposi's varicelliform e.
Erysipelothrix
erythema
    e. infectiosum
    Jacquet's e.
    e. neonatorum toxicum
    e. streptogenes
erythredema polyneuropathy
erythroblastosis
    e. fetalis
    e. neonatorum
erythroderma
    atopic e.
    e. desquamativum
erythroleukoblastosis
Escherichia
    E. coli
Ewing's
    sarcoma
    tumor
exanthem
exostosis
exstrophy
Factor VIII
    deficiency
    inhibitor
Fallot's tetralogy
Fanconi-Albertini-Zellweger
    syndrome
Fanconi-Petrassi syndrome
Fanconi's
    anemia
    syndrome
Farber's test
farinjitis. See *pharyngitis.*
Fazio-Londe atrophy
feces
Feer's disease

fenilketonurea. See *phenylketonuria.*
feochromocytoma. See *pheochromocytoma.*
fever
    cat scratch f.
    Colorado tick f.
    Haverhill f.
    hay f.
    paratyphoid f.
    Q f.
    relapsing f.
    rheumatic f.
    Rocky Mountain spotted
     f.
    scarlet f.
    South African tick f.
    spotted f.
    Tick f.
    typhoid f.
    undulant f.
    valley f.
    yellow f.
fibrillation
    atrial f.
    ventricular f.
fibroelastosis
    endocardial f.
fibroplasia
    retrolental f.
fibrosis
    cystic f.
fissure
fistula
    tracheoesophageal f.
FJN – familial juvenile
  nephrophthisis
flaccid

flaring
    alar f.
    nasal f.
fobia. See *phobia.*
fokomelea. See *phocomelia.*
folliculitis
fontanelle
fonticulus
foramen
    f. primum
    f. secundum
formiminoglutamicaciduria
fragilitas
    f. ossium
Franceschetti's syndrome
Frei test
Freiberg's infraction
Friedreich's ataxia
fungi
furuncle
furunculosis
galactosemia
gallbladder
gamma globulin
ganglioneuroma
gangrene
gargoylism
gastroenteritis
gastrointestinal
Gaucher's disease
genitalia
German measles
gestation
gestational
Ghon
      complex
      tubercle
gigantism

Gilbert-Dreyfus' syndrome
Gilbert-Lereboullet syndrome
Gilles de la Tourette's
    syndrome
gingivitis
        herpetic g.
gingivostomatitis
        herpetic g.
gland
        parotid g.
        Philip's g's.
        salivary g.
        sublingual g.
        submaxillary g.
Glanzmann's syndrome
glaucoma
glioblastoma
glioma
globulin
glomerulonephritis
glycinuria
glycogen
glycosuria
goiter
gonad
gonorrhea
Goodpasture's syndrome
Gower's sign
G6PD – glucose-6-phosphate
    dehydrogenase
grand mal
granuloma
granulomatosis
Grünfelder's reflex
grunting
Hallermann-Streiff syndrome
Hallervorden-Spatz syndrome
hammer toe

Hand-Schüller-Christian
    syndrome
Hartnup's disease
Hart's syndrome
Haverhill fever
HDN – hemolytic disease of
    the newborn
hebetic
hemangioblastoma
hemangioma
        cavernous h.
hemangiomatosis
hemarthrosis
hematemesis
hematoma
        extradural h.
        subdural h.
        sublingual h.
        submental h.
hematopoiesis
hematuria
hemiatrophy
hemiplegia
hemivertebra
hemochromatosis
hemoglobinopathy
hemolysis
hemolytic
hemophilia
hemophiliac
hemophilus
hemorrhage
        sternocleidomastoid h.
        subarachnoid h.
hemosiderosis
Henoch's disease
hepatic
hepatitis

hepatocellular
hepatolenticular
hepatoma
hepatomegaly
hepatosplenomegaly
heredopathia
    h. atactica polyneuri-
      tiformis
hernia
    diaphragmatic h.
    hiatal h.
    incarcerated h.
    inguinal h.
    umbilical h.
herniorrhaphy
herpangina
herpes
    visceral h. simplex
Hers' disease
hipsarithmea. See *hypsa-*
    rhythmia.
Hirschsprung's disease
histidinemia
histiocytosis
    h. X
histoplasmosis
Hodgkin's disease
homocystinuria
hookworm
hordeolum
Hurler's syndrome
Hutchinson-Gilford syndrome
Hutchinson's syndrome
Hutinel's disease
hydranencephaly
hydroa
    h. puerorum
    h. vacciniforme

hydrocele
hydrocelectomy
hydrocephalic
hydrocephalocele
hydrocephaloid
hydrocephalus
hydrocolpos
hydronephrosis
hydrops
    h. fetalis
hydroxyprolinemia
hygroma
hyperacidity
hyperaldosteronism
hyperbilirubinemia
hyperbilirubinemic
hypercalcemia
    idiopathic h.
hyperemesis
    h. lactentium
hyperglycemia
hyperglycinemia
hyperinsulinism
hyperkalemia
hyperkeratosis
hyperlipidemia
hypernatremia
hyperopia
hyperostosis
    infantile cortical h.
hyperparathyroidism
hyperplasia
hyperprolinemia
hyperpyrexia
hypersensitization
hypersplenism
hypertelorism
hypertension

hyperthyroidism
hypertyrosinemia
hyperuricemia
hypervalinemia
hyperventilation
hypervitaminosis
hypoadrenalism
hypocalcemia
hypocalcemic
hypocapnia
hypochondriasis
hypodermoclysis
hypogammaglobulinemia
hypoglycemia
hypoglycemic
hypokalemia
hypomagnesemia
hyponatremia
hyponatremic
hypoparathyroidism
hypophosphatasia
hypopituitarism
hypopotassemia
hypoproteinemia
hypospadias
hypothermia
hypothyroidism
hypotonia
hypovitaminosis
hypovolemia
hypovolemic
hypoxemic
hypoxia
hypsarhythmia
ichthyosis
icterus
    i. gravis neonatorum
    Liouville's i.

icterus *(continued)*
    i. melas
    i. neonatorum
idiocy
    amaurotic familial i.
    mongolian i.
idiopathic
IDM – infant of diabetic
   mother
iktheosis. See *ichthyosis.*
ileitis
    terminal i.
ileus
    adynamic i.
    meconium i.
imbecile
immunity
immunization
immunoelectrophoresis
impaction
    fecal i.
impetigo
    i. neonatorum
incarceration
incompatibility
    ABO i.
    Rh i.
incontinentia
    i. pigmenti
incubation
incubator
infancy
infant
infantile
infarct
    bilirubin i's.
    uric acid i.
influenza

infraction
    Freiberg's i.
inhibitor
    Factor III i.
insufficiency
    adrenocortical i.
    aortic i.
intertrigo
intussusception
    ileocolic i.
IRDS – idiopathic respiratory
    distress syndrome
iritis
irritability
isohemagglutinin
isoimmunization
isolette
isovalericacidemia
jacksonian epilepsy
Jacquet's
    dermatitis
    erythema
Jaksch's anemia
Jansen's syndrome
jaundice
    physiologic j.
jitteriness
jittery
Joseph's syndrome
kala-azar
kalazea. See *chalasia.*
Kaposi's varicelliform
    eruption
karnikterus. See *kernicterus.*
Kashin-Bek disease
Kaufman's pneumonia
keratitis
    interstitial k.

keratoconjunctivitis
keratolysis
    k. neonatorum
keratopathy
    band k.
keratosis
    k. pilaris
kerion
kernicterus
Kernig's sign
ketoacidosis
    diabetic k.
ketosis
Klebsiella
    K. pneumoniae
Klinefelter's syndrome
Klippel-Feil syndrome
Kloepfer's syndrome
Klumpke's paralysis
Köhler's disease
kolanjitis. See *cholangitis.*
kolera. See *cholera.*
kondro-. See words beginning
    chondro-.
Koplik's spots
korea. See *chorea.*
korio-. See words beginning
    chorio-.
koriza. See *coryza.*
Krabbe's disease
Kussmaul's respiration
kwashiorkor
kyphosis
    k. dorsalis juvenilis
Landau's test
Landry-Guillain-Barre
    syndrome
lanugo

laringoskope. See *laryngo-scope.*
larinks. See *larynx.*
Larsen's syndrome
larva
    l. migrans
laryngoscopy
larynx
Larzel's anemia
Laurence-Moon syndrome
Laurence-Moon-Biedl
  syndrome
lavage
    gastric l.
LE — lupus erythematosus
Leber's disease
Leigh's disease
Leiner's disease
leptomeningitis
Leptospira
    L. icterohaemorrhagiae
leptospirosis
Leptothrix
leptotrichosis
lethargic
Letterer-Siwe disease
leukemia
    aplastic l.
    basophilic l.
    eosinophilic l.
    granulocytic l.
    hemoblastic l.
    leukopenic l.
    lymphocytic l.
    lymphosarcoma cell l.
    mast cell l.
    megakaryocytic l.
    micromyeloblastic l.

leukemia *(continued)*
    myeloblastic l.
    myelogenous l.
leukocytosis
leukodystrophy
    globoid cell l.
    sudanophilic l.
lichen
    l. striatus
Lightwood-Albright syndrome
Liouville's icterus
lipidosis
lipochondrodystrophy
lipogranulomatosis
Little's disease
lupus
    l. erythematosus dissem-
      inatus
Lutembacher's syndrome
luteoma
lymphadenitis
    mesenteric l.
lymphadenopathy
lymphangitis
lymphangioma
    l. circumscriptum
    l. cysticum
lymphocytosis
lymphogranuloma
    l. venereum
lymphoma
lymphoreticulosis
lymphosarcoma
Macewen's sign
macrocephaly
macrogenitosomia
    m. praecox
macroglobulinemia
    Waldenström's m.

Magnus and de Kleijin neck
    reflexes
malaise
malaria
malnutrition
malrotation
marasmus
Marfan's syndrome
Marie's syndrome
Marion's disease
Marmo's method
Maroteaux-Lamy syndrome
mastoiditis
masturbation
McArdle's disease
McCune-Albright syndrome
measles
      German m.
Meckel's diverticulum
meconium
mediastinitis
Medications
    acetaminophen
    acetazolamide
    acetylcysteine
    acetylsalicylic acid
    ACTH
    actinomycin
    adrenalin
    Adroyd
    Aerosporin
    Aldactone
    Aldomet
    Aludrine
    aluminum hydroxide gel
    amantadine
    aminophylline
    aminosalicylic acid

Medications *(continued)*
    ammonium chloride
    amobarbital sodium
    amphetamine sulfate
    amphotericin B.
    ampicillin
    Amytal
    Anadrol
    Ansolysen
    Antepar
    apomorphine
    Apresoline
    Aralen
    Aramine
    Aristocort
    ascorbic acid
    Asdrin
    aspirin
    Atabrine
    Atarax
    atropine
    Avertin
    Azulfidine
    bacitracin
    BAL
    Banthine
    belladonna
    Benadryl
    Benemid
    Benodaine
    Bentyl
    benzathine penicillin G
    Benzedrine
    betamethasone
    Bicillin
    Bisacodyl
    Bonine
    brompheniramine

Medications *(continued)*

busulfan
Cafergot
calcium gluceptate
Caprokol
carbarsone
Carbo-Resin
carisoprodol
cascara sagrada
cedilanid
Celestone
Celontin
cephalothin
chloral hydrate
chlorambucil
chloramphenicol
chlorcyclizine
chlordiazepoxide
Chloromycetin
chloroquine
chlorothiazide
chlorpheniramine
chlorpromazine
Chlor-Trimeton
cholestyramine
codeine
Colace
colistimethate
colistin
Coly-Mycin
Compazine
corticotropin
cortisone
Cosmegen
Cotazym
Cuemid
Cuprimine
curare

Medications *(continued)*

Cyclamycin
cyclophosphamide
cycloserine
cyproheptadine
Cytomel
Cytoxan
Dacapryn
dactinomycin
Daraprim
Darvon
Decadron
Delalutin
Delatestryl
Delestrogen
Deltra
Delvex
Demerol
Dendrid
Depo-Provera
desoxycorticosterone
dexamethasone
Diamox
Dianabol
diazepam
Dicodid
dicyclomine
diethylstilbestrol
Dilantin
dimenhydrinate
Dimercaprol
Dimetane
Dimocillin
dioctyl
Diodoquin
Diodrast
diphenhydramine
diphenoxylate

Medications *(continued)*

- diphenylhydantoin
- dithiazanine
- Diuril
- Doxinate
- doxylamine
- Dramamine
- Dropsprin
- Dulcolax
- Durabolin
- Edecrin
- emetine
- Emivan
- ephedrine
- epinephrine
- Equanil
- ergotamine
- Erythrocin
- erythromycin
- Esidrix
- Estinyl
- estradiol
- Etamon
- ethacrynic acid
- ethamivan
- ethinyl estradiol
- ethosuximide
- ethotoin
- Eumydrin
- fluoxymesterone
- folic acid
- Fulvicin
- Fumagillin
- Fungizone
- furazolidone
- Furoxone
- furtrethonium
- gamma globulin

Medications *(continued)*

- Gantrisin
- Garamycin
- Gemonil
- gentamicin
- gentian violet
- glucagon
- haloperidol
- Halotestin
- heparin
- Herplex
- Hetrazan
- hexylresorcinol
- Histadyl
- Hycodan
- hydralazine
- hydriodic acid
- hydrocortisone
- hydrochlorothiazide
- hydrocodone
- Hydro-Diuril
- hydroxyzine
- Hykinone
- idoxuridine
- Ilosone
- Ilotycin
- Imferon
- imipramine
- insulin
- iodochlorhydroxyquin
- ipecac
- Ismelin
- isoniazid
- isoproterenol
- Isuprel
- kanamycin
- Kantrex
- Kayexalate

Medications *(continued)*

Keflin
Kenacort
Konakion
Lasix
Lastrogen
Lentopen
Leukeran
levallorphan
Levophed
Librium
lidocaine
Lincocin
lincomycin
Liquiprin
Lomotil
Lorfan
Lugol's solution
lypressin
magnesium sulfate
Mandelamine
mannitol
Mebral
mechlorethamine
Mecholyl
meclizine
Medrol
medroxyprogesterone
Mellaril
menadione
mepacrine
meperidine
mephenesin
mephenytoin
mephobarbital
meprobamate
meralluride
Mesantoin

Medications *(continued)*

Mestinon
metaraminol
methacholine
methacycline
methantheline
methapyrilene
metharbital
methdilazine
methenamine
methicillin
methoxamine
methsuximide
methylcellulose
methyldopa
methylphenylethyl-
   hydantoin
methylprednisolone
methylrosaniline
methyltestosterone
Meticorten
Milontin
Miltown
morphine sulfate
Mucomyst
Mustargen
Mycifradin
Mycostatin
Myleran
Mysoline
nalidixic acid
Nalline
nalorphine
nandrolone
NegGram
Nembutal
Neo-Calglucon
Neo-cultol

Medications *(continued)*
- Neolin
- neomycin
- neostigmine
- Neo-Synephrine
- niacinamide
- nicotinamide
- nitrogen mustard
- Noctec
- norepinephrine
- Norisodrine
- nystatin
- Omnipen
- Oncovin
- Oreton
- Osmitrol
- Oxacillin
- oxymetholone
- papaverine
- Paradione
- paraldehyde
- paramethadione
- paregoric
- PAS
- Pediamycin
- Penbritin
- penicillamine
- penicillin
- pentobarbital
- pentolinium
- Pentothal
- Perazil
- Periactin
- Permapen
- Phenergan
- phenobarbital
- phensuximide
- phentolamine

Medications *(continued)*
- phenylephrine
- pilocarpine
- piperazine
- piperoxan
- Polycillin
- polymyxin B
- potassium chloride
- potassium iodide
- prednisolone
- prednisone
- primidone
- Priscoline
- Pro-Banthine
- probenecid
- procainamide
- prochlorperazine
- progesterone
- Progestoral
- promethazine
- Pronestyl
- propantheline
- propoxyphene
- propranolol
- Prostigmin
- pseudoephedrine
- Pyribenzamine
- pyridostigmin
- Questran
- quinacrine
- quinidine
- quinine
- Regitine
- reserpine
- Restophen
- RhoGAM
- Ritalin
- Robaxin

Medications *(continued)*

Romilar
Rondomycin
salicylazosulfapyridine
Salrin
Sansert
scopolamine
secobarbital
Seconal
Seromycin
Serpasil
sodium bicarbonate
sodium salicylate
Soma
spironolactone
Staphcillin
Stoxil
Sudafed
sulfisoxazole
sulfonamide
Sus-Phrine
Symmetrel
TAO — triacetyloleando-
    mycin
Tapazole
Teldrin
Tempra
testosterone
tetrachloroethylene
tetracycline
thioridazine
Thorazine
Tigan
Tofranil
tolazoline
Tolserol
triacetyloleandomycin
triamcinolone

Medications *(continued)*

tribromoethanol
triethylenemelamine
    (TEM)
trimethobenzamide
tripelennamine
Tri-Vi-Sol
tubocurarine
Tylenol
Unipen
Valium
vasopressin
Vasoxyl
Velban
vincristine
Vioform
Viokase
Winstrol
Wyamine
Wydase
Xylocaine
Zarontin
Mediterranean anemia
medulloblastoma
Meesmann's dystrophy
megacolon
    congential m.
megalencephaly
melena
    m. neonatorum
menarche
meningioma
meningismus
meningitis
    aseptic m.
    tuberculous m.
meningocele
meningococcemia

meningococcus
meningomyelocele
menstruation
mesenteric
metastasis
metatarsus
    m. varus
methemoglobinemia
methemoglobinuria
method
    Byrd-Dew m.
    Marmo's m.
Metopirone test
micrencephaly
microangiopathy
    thrombotic m.
microcephaly
microcytosis
Microsporum
    M. audouini
    M. furfur
    M. lanosum
mielitis. See *myelitis.*
mielo. See words beginning
    myelo-.
migraine
miksedema. See *myxedema.*
milium
mio-. See words beginning
    myo-.
Möbius' syndrome
Möller-Barlow disease
molluscum
mongolian
mongolism
    double-trisomy m.
mongoloid
moniliasis

mononucleosis
    infectious m.
monosomy
morbilliform
Moro-Heisler diet
Moro reflex
Morquio's disease
mucoviscidosis
mumps
murmur
    diastolic m.
    holosystolic m.
    pansystolic m.
    systolic ejection m.
myalgia
myasthenia
    m. gravis
Mycobacterium
    M. leprae
    M. tuberculosis
Mycoplasma
mycosis
myelitis
    transverse m.
myelodysplasia
myelofibrosis
myelomeningocele
myelophthisis
myeloproliferative
myocardial
myocarditis
myocardium
myoclonic
myoclonus
myopia
myotonia
    m. congenita
    m. neonatorum

myxedema
    infantile m.
narcolepsy
nares
naris
nasopharyngeal
nausea
nefritis. See *nephritis.*
nefrosis. See *nephrosis.*
neonatal
neonate
neoplasm
nephritis
nephrosis
Nettleship's syndrome
neuritis
neuroblastoma
neurofibromatosis
neutropenia
nevi
nevoxanthoendothelioma
nevus
    n. flammeus
    n. pilosus
    n. spilus
    n. verrucosus
Niemann-Pick disease
Nocardia
noma
    n. pudendi
    n. vulvae
normocephalic
numo-. See words beginning
    pneumo-.
obesity
ofthalmea. See *ophthalmia.*
oksesefale. See *oxycephaly.*
okseuriasis. See *oxyuriasis.*

oliguria
Ollier's syndrome
omphalocele
operation
    Blalock-Hanlon o.
    Blalock-Taussig o.
ophthalmia
    o. neonatorum
opisthotonos
    o. fetalis
Oppenheim's disease
orchitis
organomegaly
orkitis. See *orchitis.*
oropharynx
Ortolani's test
Osgood-Schlatter syndrome
osteitis
    o. condensans
        generalisata
osteochondritis
    o. deformans juvenilis
    o. dissecans
    o. ischiopubica
osteochondrodystrophy
osteochondroma
osteochondrosis
    o. deformans tibiae
osteodystrophia
    o. juvenilis
osteogenesis
    o. imperfecta
    o. imperfecta cystica
osteoma
    osteoid o.
osteomalacia
    juvenile o.
osteomyelitis

osteopetrosis
osteoporosis
osteopsathyrosis
osteotabes
otitis
    o. media
oxycephaly
oxygen
oxyuriasis
palsy
    brachial plexus p.
    cerebral p.
pancreas
pancreatitis
panencephalitis
papilledema
papilloma
paracentesis
parainfluenza
paralysis
    Erb-Duchenne p.
    Klumpke's p.
    spastic p.
    Werdnig-Hoffmann p.
parapertussis
paraplegia
parathyroid
paresthesia
    Berger's p.
paroksizmal. See *paroxysmal.*
paronychia
parotitis
paroxysmal
Parrot's atrophy of the
    newborn
Pastia's sign
Patau's syndrome
patent ductus arteriosus

pavor
    p. diurnus
    p. nocturnus
PDA – patent ductus
    arteriosus
pearl
    Epstein's p's.
pedarthrocace
pediatric
pediatrician
pedicterus
pediculosis
pedobaromacrometer
pedobarometer
pedologist
pedometer
Pelizaeus-Merzbacher disease
pellagra
Pellizzi's syndrome
Pendred's syndrome
Perez's sign
periarteritis
    p. nodosa
pericarditis
perinephritis
peritonitis
pertussis
petechia
petit mal
pharyngitis
    lymphonodular p.
    purulent p.
    streptococcal p.
    viral p.
Pehistix
phenomenon
    Rumpel-Leede p.
phenylketonuria

pheochromocytoma
Philip's glands
phobia
phocomelia
phonocardiography
pica
Pierre Robin syndrome
pigeon toe
piknocytosis. See
pyknocytosis.
pilitis. See *pyelitis.*
pilonephritis. See
pyelonephritis.
pinealoma
Pink disease
pink-eye
pinna
pinworm
pityriasis
PKU – phenylketonuria
placentitis
plague
pleurisy
pleurodynia
pneumococcus
pneumomediastinum
pneumonia
    aspiration p.
    Kaufman's p.
    lobar p.
pneumonitis
pneumopericardium
pneumoperitoneum
pneumothorax
poisoning
    barbiturate p.
    lead p.
    petroleum distillate p.

poisoning *(continued)*
    phenothiazine p.
    salicylate p.
    scopolamine p.
    strychnine p.
    thallium p.
polioencephalitis
    bulbar p.
poliomyelitis
polyarteritis
polyarthritis
polycythemia
    p. vera
polydactylia
polydactyly
polydipsia
polydysplasia
    hereditary ectodermal p.
polyneuropathy
polyp
    intestinal p.
polyserositis
    idiopathic p.
Pompe's disease
porencephalia
porphyria
port wine mark
Potter's disease
precocity
premature
prematurity
prepubertal
progeria
projectile
pronate
prostration
proteinuria
    orthostatic p.

proteinuria
    postural p.
prurigo
pruritus
    p. ani
pseudohermaphroditism
pseudohypoparathyroidism
pseudoleukemia
    p. infantile
pseudomenstruation
Pseudomonas
    P. aeruginosa
pseudoparalysis
pseudotumor
    p. cerebri
psittacosis
psoriasis
psychosis
    symbiotic p.
PTA – plasma thromboplastin
    antecedent
pterygium
    p. colli
ptosis
pubarche
pubertas
    p. praecox
puberty
pubescent
Pudenz'
    reservoir
    shunt
pulse
    Corrigan's p.
puncture
    bone marrow p.
    cisternal p.
    lumbar p.

puncture *(continued)*
    pericardial p.
    subdural p.
purpura
    anaphylactoid p.
    p. fulminans
    p. hemorrhagica
    Schönlein-Henoch p.
    thrombocytopenic p.
    thrombotic p.
Pusey's emulsion
pustulosis
    p. vacciniformis acuta
pyelitis
pyelonephritis
pyknocytosis
pyuria
Q fever
quarantine
rabies
ragadez. See *rhagades.*
rales
rating
    Apgar r.
Recklinghausen's disease –
    von Recklinghausen's
    disease
reflex
    Grünfelder's r.
    Magnus and de Kleijn
      neck r's.
    Moro r.
    sucking r.
Refsum's disease
reservoir
    Pudenz' r.
respiration
    Kussmaul's r.

respiratory
resuscitation
retardation
    mental r.
reticuloendotheliosis
retinitis
    r. pigmentosa
Reye's syndrome
rhagades
Rh incompatibility
rheumatic fever
rheumaticosis
rhinitis
Rhus
    R. diversiloba
    R. toxicodendron
    R. venenata
rickets
rickettsiae
rickettsial
rickettsialpox
Riley-Day syndrome
Riley-Shwachman syndrome
ringworm
Ritter's disease
Rocky Mountain spotted
    fever
Romaña's sign
roomatikosis. See
    rheumaticosis.
roseola
    r. infantum
Rothmund's syndrome
roundworm
Roussy-Lévy syndrome
RS virus
rubella
    r. scarlatinosa

rubeola
    r. scarlatinosa
Rubinstein-Taybi syndrome
Rumpel-Leede phenomenon
rus. See *Rhus.*
salicylism
salmonella
salmonellosis
sarcoidosis
sarcoma
sarcosinemia
Saunders' disease
scabies
scaphocephaly
scarlatina
Scheuermann's disease
Scheuthauer-Marie-Sainton
    syndrome
Schick test
Schilder's disease
schizophrenia
Schönlein-Henoch purpura
scissoring
scleredema
    s. neonatorum
sclerema
    s. neonatorum
scleroderma
sclerosis
    tuberous s.
scoliosis
score
    Apgar s.
    Silverman's s.
scrofula
scurvy
    hemorrhagic s.
    infantile s.

seborrhea
sefalhematoma. See
   cephalhematoma.
seizure
seminoma
sepsis
septal
septicemia
sferositosis. See *spherocytosis.*
shigella
shigellosis
shock
   anaphylactic s.
   bacteremic s.
   cardiogenic s.
   endotoxic s.
   hypovolemic s.
shunt
   parietal s.
   Pudenz' s.
   ventricular atrial s.
   ventriculoperitoneal s.
SID – sudden infant death
SIDS – sudden infant death
   syndrome
sifilis. See *syphilis.*
sign
   Brudzinski's s.
   Comby's s.
   Gowers' s.
   Kernig's s.
   Macewen's s.
   Pastia's s.
   Perez's s.
   Romaña's s.
   Wreden's s.
sikosis. See *psychosis.*
silicosis

Silverman's score
Silver's syndrome
Similac
sinobronchitis
sinus
   pilonidal s.
sinusitis
sirronosus. See *cirrhonosus.*
sirrosis. See *cirrhosis.*
sitakosis. See *psittacosis.*
skafosefale. See *scaphocephaly.*
skizofrenea. See
   schizophrenia.
SLE – systemic lupus
   erythematosus
smallpox
soriasis. See *psoriasis.*
South African tick fever
spasm
spastic
spaticity
spherocytosis
spina
   s. bifida
spirillum
spirochetal
spirochete
splenomegaly
spondylitis
   ankylosing s.
spongioblastoma
spot
      Brushfield's s's.
      Koplik's s's.
Sprengel's deformity
sprue
squint
St. Vitus' dance

stafilokokkis. See
  staphylococcus.
stammering
staphylococcus
starvation
status
    s. asthmaticus
    s. dysmyelinatus
    s. dysmyelinisatus
    s. epilepticus
steatorrhea
    idiopathic s.
stenosis
    aortic s.
    esophageal s.
    mitral s.
    pulmonic s.
    pyloric s.
    valvular pulmonic s.
Stensen's duct
Stevens-Johnson syndrome
Sticker's disease
Stilling-Türk-Duane syndrome
Still's disease
Stock-Spielmeyer-Vogt
    syndrome
stomatitis
    herpetic s.
strabismus
strawberry mark
streptococci
streptococcus
    beta hemolytic s.
Streptothrix
stricture
    esophageal s.
stridor
strophulus

Stuart-Prower factor
    deficiency disease
Sturge-Weber syndrome
stuttering
sty
sucking
sudo-. See words beginning
    pseudo-.
surgical procedures. See
    operation.
suture
    sagittal s.
Sydenham's chorea
symptom
    Epstein's s.
syncope
syndactyly
syndrome
    Abderhalden-Fanconi s.
    Abt-Letterer-Siwe s.
    Adie's s.
    adrenogenital s.
    Albers-Schönberg's s.
    Albright's s.
    Aldrich's s.
    Alport's s.
    Andogsky's s.
    Arnold-Chiari s.
    Ballantyne-Runge s.
    Banti's s.
    Bartter's s.
    battered child s.
    Beckwith's s.
    Bloch-Sulzberger s.
    Bloom's s.
    Bonnevie-Ullrich s.
    Bourneville's s.
    Brandt's s.

syndrome *(continued)*
- Caffey-Silverman s.
- Caffey-Smyth-Roske s.
- Calvé-Legg-Perthes s.
- Camurati-Englemann s.
- Chapple's s.
- Charcot-Marie-Tooth-Hoffmann s.
- Chédiak-Higashi s.
- cri-du-chat s.
- Crigler-Najjar s.
- Cushing's s.
- Darrow-Gamble s.
- de Lange's s.
- Dennie-Marfan s.
- DeToni-Fanconi-Debre s.
- Diamond-Blackfan s.
- diencephalic s.
- DiGeorge's s.
- Down's s.
- Dubin-Johnson s.
- Dubovitz's s.
- Ehlers-Danlos s.
- Ellis-Van Creveld s.
- Erlacher-Blount s.
- Fanconi's s.
- Fanconi-Albertini-Zellweger s.
- Fanconi-Petrassi s.
- Franceschetti's s.
- Gilbert-Dreyfus s.
- Gilbert-Lereboullet s.
- Gilles de la Tourette's s.
- Glanzmann's s.
- Goodpasture's s.
- Hallermann-Streiff s.
- Hallervordan-Spatz s.
- Hand-Schüller-Christian s.

syndrome *(continued)*
- Hart's s.
- Hurler's s.
- Hutchinson-Gilford s.
- Hutchinson's s.
- idiopathic respiratory distress s.
- Jansen's s.
- Joseph's s.
- Klinefelter's s.
- Klippel-Feil s.
- Kloepfer's s.
- Landry-Guillain-Barré s.
- Larsen's s.
- Laurence-Moon s.
- Laurence-Moon-Biedl s.
- Lightwood-Albright s.
- Lutembacher's s.
- malabsorption s.
- Marfan's s.
- Marie's s.
- Maroteaux-Lamy s.
- McCune-Albright s.
- methionine malabsorption s.
- Möbius' s.
- nephrotic s.
- Nettleship's s.
- Ollier's s.
- Osgood-Schlatter s.
- Patau's s.
- Pellizzi's s.
- Pendred's s.
- Pierre Robin s.
- placental dysfunction s.
- postperfusion s.
- Reye's s.
- Riley-Day s.

syndrome *(continued)*
    Riley-Shwachman s.
    Rothmund's s.
    Roussy-Lévy s.
    Rubinstein-Taybi s.
    Scheuthauer-Marie-
      Sainton s.
    Silver's s.
    Stevens-Johnson s.
    Stilling-Türk-Duane s.
    Stock-Spielmeyer-Vogt s.
    Sturge-Weber s.
    testicular feminizing s.
    Treacher Collins' s.
    triplo-X s.
    trisomy 13-15 s.
    trisomy 18 s.
    Turner's s
    Werdnig-Hoffmann s.
    Wiedemann's s.
    Willebrand-Jürgens s.
    Wilson-Mikity s.
    Wiskott-Aldrich s.
    Wolff-Parkinson-White s.
synostosis
    tribasilar s.
synovitis
syphilis
tabes
    hereditary t.
    t. infantum
    t. mesaraica
    t. mesenterica
tachycardia
    paroxysmal t.
tachypnea
taeniasis
takekardea. See *tachycardia.*

takipnea. See *tachypnea.*
talipes
    t. calcaneovalgus
    t. cavus
    t. equinovarus
tamponade
    cardiac t.
tapeworm
Tay-Sachs disease
telangiectasia
teratoma
terijeum. See *pterygium.*
test. See also *Laboratory*
    terminology.
    Coombs' t.
    Farber's t.
    Frei t.
    Landau's t.
    Metopirone t.
    Ortolani's t.
    Schick t.
    Tine t.
testes
    undescended t.
testicle
testicular
tetanus
tetany
tetralogy
    t. of Fallot
thalassemia
thelarche
therapy
    aerosol t.
    hyperbaric oxygen t.
Thomsen's disease
thoracentesis
thorax

thrombasthenia
thrombin
thrombocytopenia
    idiopathic t.
thrombosis
thrombus
thrush
thumbsucking
thyroid
thyroiditis
thyrotoxicosis
tic
Tick fever
Tine test
tinea
    t. capitis
    t. corporis
    t. cruris
    t. versicolor
titer
    antistreptolysin t.
tonsillitis
    white t.
torticollis
torulosis
tosis. See *ptosis.*
Toxocara
toxocariasis
toxoid
Toxoplasma
toxoplasmosis
trachea
tracheostomy
tracheotomy
trachoma
transfusion
    exchange t.
transillumination

transposition
    t. of great vessels
Treacher Collins' syndrome
tremulous
trichinosis
trismus
    t. nascentium
    t. neonatorum
trisomy
tryptophanuria
tubercle
    Ghon t.
tuberculoma
tuberculosis
    t. papulonecrotica
tularemia
tumor
    Ewing's t.
    granulosa cell t.
    pineal t.
    pontine t.
    theca cell t.
    Wilms' t.
Turner's syndrome
tympanites
typhoid
typhus
tyrosinosis
ulcer
    duodenal u.
    peptic u.
umbilical
umbilicus
Underwood's disease
Unverricht's disease
urachus
    patent u.
uremia

URI — upper respiratory infection
urinalysis
urticaria
    u. pigmentosa
uveitis
vaccine
Valley fever
valve
    mitral v.
valvotomy
varicella
    v. gangrenosa
    v. inoculata
    pustular v.
    v. pustulosa
    vaccination v.
varicelliform
variola
varioliform
varix
vasospasm
venipuncture
ventricular septal defect
ventriculogram
ventriculography
vernix
    v. caseosa
verruca
    v. plana juvenilis
vertebra
    v. plana
virus
    Coxsackie v.
    ECHO v.
    Epstein-Barr v.
    herpes simplex v.
    RS v.

visceromegaly
vitiligo
VMA — vanillylmandelic acid
volvulus
    v. neonatorum
vomiting
    projectile v.
von Gierke's disease
von Jaksch's anemia
VSD — ventricular septal defect
vulvovaginitis
Waldenström's macroglobulinemia
weaning
Weil's disease
Werdnig-Hoffmann
    paralysis
    syndrome
whooping cough
Wiedemann's syndrome
Wilkins' disease
Willebrand-Jürgens syndrome
Wilms' tumor
Wilson-Mikity syndrome
Wilson's disease
Winckel's disease
Wiskott-Aldrich syndrome
Wolff-Parkinson-White syndrome
Wreden's sign
wryneck
xanthomatosis
xerophthalmia
zanthomatosis. See *xanthomatosis.*
zerofthalmea. See *xerophthalmia.*
zygodactyly

PLASTIC SURGERY

Abbe's operation
Adams' operation
akinesia
    O'Brien a.
    Van Lint a.
ala
    a. nasi
alar
Alexander's operation
allograft
alloplasty
allotransplantation
allotriodontia
Allport's operation
Alsus-Knapp operation
alveolar
alveolus
Alvis' operation
anaplasty
anaplerosis
anesthesia
    endotracheal a.
Angelucci's operation
angkilo-. See words beginning
    ankylo-.
ankyloblepharon
ankylochilia
anthelix
antitragus
aponeurosis

arch
    zygomatic a.
area
    Kiesselbach's a.
areolar
Arlt's operation
Asch's forceps
atrium
auricle
auricula
auricular
Austin's knife
autocystoplasty
autograft
autografting
Baker's velum
bandage
    Kerlix b.
    Thillaye's b.
bar
    Erich's arch b.
    Passavant's b.
Bard-Parker blade
Barsky's
    elevator
    operation
Beard-Cutler operation
Becker's operation
Bell's operation
Berke-Motais operation

Berke's operation
Binnie's operation
bistoury
    Brophy's b.
blade
    Bard-Parker b.
Blair-Brown
    knife
    operation
Blair's
    knife
    operation
    serrefine
Blaskovics' operation
blef-. See words beginning
   bleph-.
blepharophryplasty
blepharoplasty
blepharoptosis
blepharorrhaphy
blepharostat
bone
    malar b.
    maxillary b.
    sesamoid b's.
border
    vermilion b.
bow
    Logan's b.
Brauer's operation
Braun's operation
Braun-Wangensteen operation
Brophy's
    bistoury
    knife
    operation
Brown-Blair operation
Browne's needle

Brown's
    dermatome
    knife
    operation
    splint
buccal
bulla
    ethmoid b.
Burow's operation
caliper
    Ladd's c.
Caltagirone's knife
canthus
cartilage
    septal c.
cartilaginous
caruncula
cauda
    c. helicis
cavum
    c. conchae
cephaloauricular
cephalocaudad
cervicoplasty
chalinoplasty
cheilectomy
cheilectropion
cheilitis
cheilognathoprosoposchisis
cheilognathoschisis
cheilognathouranoschisis
cheiloplasty
cheilorrhaphy
cheiloschisis
cheilostomatoplasty
cheiroplasty
choana
ciliary

clamp
    Hunt's c.
clinoid
columella
    c. nasi
columna
concha
    c. auriculae
    c. sphenoidalis
conchae
conjunctiva
conjunctivoplasty
contracture
Crawford's operation
cribriform
Crile's knife
crista
    c. galli
    c. nasalis maxillae
    c. nasalis ossis palatini
Cronin's operation
crura
    c. anthelicis
crus
Cutler's operation
cymba
    c. conchae auriculae
Davis and Kitlowski operation
Davis' graft
debridement
Demel and Ruttin operation
Denhardt-Dingman mouth gag
Denis-Browne needle
Derby's operation
dermabraded
dermabrader
    Iverson's d.
dermabrasion

dermanaplasty
dermatochalasis
dermatome
    Brown's d.
    Padgett's d.
dermatoplasty
Dieffenbach's operation
Dieffenbach-Warren operation
Dingman's
    elevator
    forceps
    osteotome
    retractor
Dorrance's operation
Dott's mouth gag
Douglas' operation
Dragstedt's operation
drain
    Penrose d.
dressing
    Telfa d.
drugs. See *Medications.*
duct
    lacrimal d.
Duke-Elder operation
Dupuy-Dutemps operation
Eckstein-Kleinschmidt
  operation
ectropion
Eitner's operation
electrocoagulation
elevator
    Barsky's e.
    Dingman's e.
    Freer's e.
    McIndoe's e.
    Veau's e.
ellipse

elliptical
Elschnig's operation
eminence
 malar e.
eminentia
 e. conchae
 e. triangularis
entropion
epidermatoplasty
Erich's
 arch bar
 operation
Esmarch's operation
Esser's operation
ethmofrontal
ethmoid
Everbusch's operation
facioplasty
faringoplasty. See
 pharyngoplasty.
farinjeal. See *pharyngeal.*
fascia
 f. lata femoris
fasciaplasty
fascioplasty
fauces
Fergus' operation
Fergusson's incision
filtrum. See *philtrum.*
fissura
 f. antitragohelicina
 antitragohelicine f.
fixation
 intermaxillary f.
flap
 skin f.
fold
 semilunar f.

Fomon's operation
foramen
 greater palatine f.
 Scarpa's f.
foramina
 lesser palatine f.
forceps
 Asch's f.
 Dingman's f.
 Walsham's f.
fornix
 f. conjunctivae
fossa
 hypophyseal f.
 Rosenmüller's f.
 scaphoid f.
 f. triangularis auriculae
Fox's operation
fracture
 blow-out f.
 comminuted f.
 nasomaxillary f.
 zygomaticomaxillary f.
Freer's elevator
French method
frenulum
Fricke's operation
Friedenwald-Guyton operation
Gabarro's operation
Gaillard's operation
Gavello's operation
Gayet's operation
genioplasty
genitoplasty
genycheiloplasty
genyplasty
Gifford's operation
Gigli's saw

Gilles-Dingman hook
Gilles' hook
Gillies'
    graft
    operation
Gillies-Fry operation
Giralde's operation
gland
    meibomian g.
glossoplasty
gnathodynia
gnathoplasty
gnathoschisis
graft
    chessboard g.
    Davis' g.
    fascia lata g.
    free g.
    full thickness skin g.
    Gillies' g.
    Ollier-Thiersch g.
    Padgett's g.
    pedicle g.
    Reverdin's g.
    split thickness skin g.
    stent g.
    Wolfe-Krause g.
Grimsdale's operation
Guyton's operation
Hagedorn-LeMesurier
  operation
Hagedorn's operation
Hagerty's operation
hamular
hamulus
harelip
Harman's operation
helix

hemisection
Hess' operation
heterograft
hiatus
    h. semilunaris
Holmes' operation
homeotransplant
homograft
homoplastic
homoplasty
hook
    Gilles-Dingman h.
    Gilles' h.
Hotz' operation
Hughes' operation
Hunt's clamp
hypognathous
Iliff's operation
implant
    silastic i.
incision
    Fergusson's i.
    z-i.
incisura
    i. intertragica
Indian method
infraorbital
infundibulum
    ethmoidal i.
injection
    silastic i.
intercartilaginous
isograft
isthmus
    i. faucium
Italian method
Iverson's dermabrader
Jaesche's operation

jenekiloplaste. See
   genycheiloplasty.
jeneplaste. See *genyplasty.*
Johnson's operation
Jones' operation
Joseph's operation
Keith's needle
keloplasty
Kerlix bandage
Kiesselbach's area
Kilner's operation
kilo-. See words beginning
   cheilo-.
kiroplaste. See *cheiroplasty.*
Kirschner's wire
Kitlowski's operation
knife
     Austin's k.
     Blair-Brown k.
     Blair's k.
     Brophy's k.
     Brown's k.
     Caltagirone's k.
     Crile's k.
     MacKenty's k.
     Virchow's k.
koana-. See *choana.*
Kolle-Lexer operation
Konig's operation
Kowalzig's operation
Krause-Wolfe operation
Krönlein's operation
Kuhnt-Szymanowski operation
labial
lacus
     l. lacrimalis
Ladd's caliper
Lagleyze's operation

lamina
Lancaster's operation
Langenbeck's operation
Latrobe's retractor
Leahey's operation
LeMesurier's operation
leukoplakia
Lexer's operation
ligament
     medial palpebral l.
lip
     cleft l.
lobule
lobulus
     l. auriculae
Logan's bow
Luckett's operation
Machek's operation
MacKenty's knife
macrocheilia
macrostomia
macrotia
Magnus' operation
Malbec's operation
Malbran's operation
maloplasty
mammoplasty
     augmentation m.
mandible
Marcks' operation
Martin's retractor
mastoid
maxilla
maxillary
maxillectomy
McCash-Randall operation
McDowell's operation
McIndoe's elevator

meatus
    acoustic m.
Medications
    Achromycin
    adrenalin
    Bacitracin
    carbocaine
    cocaine hydrochloride
    Demerol
    gentian violet
    Hyper-Tet
    Lidocaine
    Mepivacaine
    pHisoHex
    Pontocaine
    procaine
    streptomycin
    Tetracaine
    xeroform
    Xylocaine
    Zephiran
meloncus
meloplasty
mental
mentalis
mentolabial
method
    French m.
    Indian m.
    Italian m.
metopoplasty
micrognathia
micrognathism
microstomia
Millard's operation
Minsky's operation
Mirault-Brown-Blair operation
Mirault's operation

Monks' operation
Motais' operation
mouth gag
    Denhardt-Dingman m. g.
    Dott's m. g.
mucomembranous
mucoperichondrium
mucoperiosteal
mucoperiosteum
Mueller's operation
Mules' operation
Müller's muscle
muscle
    m. adductor pollicis
    m. extensor pollicis
      brevis
    m. extensor pollicis
      longus
    m. flexor pollicis brevis
    m. flexor pollicis longus
    frontalis m.
    glossopalatine m.
    levator m. of palatine
      velum
    m. levator palpebrae
      superioris
    m. orbicularis oculi
    Müller's m.
    pharyngopalatine m.
    platysma m.
    Riolan's m.
    temporalis m.
musculi
    m. levator veli palatini
    m. temporoparietalis
    m. tensor veli palatini
musculus
    m. pectoralis major

musculus *(continued)*
    m. pectoralis minor
    m. salpingopharyngeus
myoplasty
nares
naris
nasion
nasofrontal
nasolabial
nasolacrimal
nasopalatine
nasopharyngeal
nasoseptal
nasoturbinal
nasus
    n. externus
natho-. See words beginning
    gnatho-.
needle
    Browne's n.
    Denis-Browne n.
    Keith's n.
    Reverdin's n.
neoplasty
nostril
notch
    intertragic n.
O'Brien akinesia
oculi
    orbicularis o.
Ollier-Thiersch
    graft
    operation
operation
    Abbe's o.
    Adams' o.
    Alexander's o.
    Allport's o.

operation *(continued)*
    Alsus-Knapp o.
    Alvis' o.
    Angelucci's o.
    Arlt's o.
    Barsky's o.
    Beard-Cutler o.
    Becker's o.
    Bell's o.
    Berke-Motais o.
    Berke's o.
    Binnie's o.
    Blair-Brown o.
    Blair's o.
    Blaskovics' o.
    Brauer's o.
    Braun's o.
    Braun-Wangensteen o.
    Brophy's o.
    Brown-Blair o.
    Brown's o.
    Burow's o.
    Crawford's o.
    Cronin's o.
    Cutler's o.
    Davis and Kitlowski o.
    Demel and Ruttin o.
    Derby's o.
    Dieffenbach's o.
    Dieffenbach-Warren o.
    Dorrance's o.
    Douglas' o.
    Dragstedt's o.
    Duke-Elder o.
    Dupuy-Dutemps o.
    Eckstein-Kleinschmidt o.
    Eitner's o.
    Elschnig's o.

operation *(continued)*
- Erich's o.
- Esmarch's o.
- Esser's o.
- Everbusch's o.
- Fergus' o.
- Fomon's o.
- Fox's o.
- Fricke's o.
- Friedenwald-Guyton o.
- Gabarro's o.
- Gaillard's o.
- Gavello's o.
- Gayet's o.
- Gifford's o.
- Gillies' o.
- Gillies-Fry o.
- Giralde's o.
- Grimsdale's o.
- Guyton's o.
- Hagedorn-LeMesurier o.
- Hagedorn's o.
- Hagerty's o.
- Harman's o.
- Hess' o.
- Holmes' o.
- Hotz' o.
- Hughes' o.
- Illiff's o.
- Jaesche's o.
- Johnson's o.
- Jones' o.
- Joseph's o.
- Kilner's o.
- Kitlowski's o.
- Kolle-Lexer o.
- Konig's o.
- Kowalzig's o.

operation *(continued)*
- Krause-Wolfe o.
- Krönlein's o.
- Kuhnt-Szymanowski o.
- Lagleyze's o.
- Lancaster's o.
- Langenbeck's o.
- Leahey's o.
- LeMesurier's o.
- Lexer's o.
- Luckett's o.
- Machek's o.
- Magnus' o.
- Malbec's o.
- Malbran's o.
- Marcks' o.
- McCash-Randall o.
- McDowell's o.
- Millard's o.
- Minsky's o.
- Mirault-Brown-Blair o.
- Mirault's o.
- Monks' o.
- Motais' o.
- Mueller's o.
- Mules' o.
- Ollier-Thiersch o.
- Owens' o.
- Pagenstecher's o.
- Panas' o.
- Parkhill's o.
- Pfeifer's o.
- Pierce-O'Connor o.
- Randall's o.
- Reese's o.
- Reverdin's o.
- Rose's o.
- Rosenburg's o.

operation *(continued)*
    Savin's o.
    Sayoc's o.
    Schimek's o.
    Schuchardt-Pfeifer o.
    Simon's o.
    Snellen's o.
    Sourdille's o.
    Spaeth's o.
    Stallard's o.
    Straith's o.
    Swenson's o.
    Szymanowski's o.
    tagliacotian o.
    Tansley's o.
    Teale's o.
    Tennison's o.
    Thiersch's o.
    Thompson's o.
    Trainor-Nida o.
    Tripier's o.
    Truc's o.
    Ulloa's o.
    Van Millingen's o.
    Veau-Axhausen o.
    Veau's o.
    Verhoeff's o.
    Verweys' o.
    Vogel's o.
    von Blaskovics-Doyen o.
    von Langenbeck's o.
    V-Y o.
    Wardill-Kilner o.
    Webster's o.
    Wheeler's o.
    Wicherkiewicz' o.
    Wiener's o.
    Wolfe's o.

operation *(continued)*
    Wolff's o.
    Worth's o.
    Wright's o.
    W-Y o.
    Young's o.
orbicular
orbital
osteoplastic
osteoplasty
osteoseptum
osteotome
    Dingman's o.
osteotomy
ostium
otoplasty
Owens' operation
Padgett's
    dermatome
    graft
Pagenstecher's operation
palatal
palate
    cleft p.
palatine
palatognathous
palatomaxillary
palatonasal
palatoplasty
palatum
    p. durum
    p. durum osseum
    p. fissum
    p. molle
    p. ogivale
    p. osseum
palpebra
palpebral

Panas' operation
Parkhill's operation
Passavant's bar
pedicle
pedunculated
Penrose drain
periosteum
Pfeifer's operation
pharyngeal
pharyngoplasty
philtrum
Pierce-O'Connor operation
pillar
piriform
plica
    p. semilunaris
ponticulus
    p. auriculae
preauricular
process
    mastoid p.
prognathism
prognathous
pterygium
    p. colli
pterygoid
pterygomandibular
pterygomaxillary
pterygopalatine
ptosis
rafe. See *raphe.*
Randall's operation
raphe
    palatine r.
reaction
    antigen-antibody r.
    immunity r.
Reese's operation

repair
    Rose-Thompson r.
resection
    submucous r.
retractor
    Dingman's r.
    Latrobe's r.
    Martin's r.
    Senn-Dingman r.
    Sluder's r.
retrenchment
retroauricular
Reverdin's
    graft
    needle
    operation
rhinocheiloplasty
rhinokyphectomy
rhinokyphosis
rhinoplasty
rhytidectomy
rhytidoplasty
rhytidosis
rino-. See words beginning
    rhino-.
Riolan's muscle
Ritchie's tenaculum
ritidektome. See *rhytidectomy.*
ritido-. See words beginning
    rhytido-.
Rosenburg's operation
Rosenmüller's fossa
Rose's operation
Rose-Thompson repair
ruga
    r. palatina
rugae
salpingopharyngeal

Savin's operation
saw
      Gigli's s.
Sayoc's operation
scapha
scarification
Scarpa's foramen
Schimek's operation
Schuchardt-Pfeifer operation
sefalo-. See words beginning
    cephalo-.
Senn-Dingman retractor
septum
    deviated nasal s.
    nasal s.
serrefine
    Blair's s.
sfeno-. See words beginning
    spheno-.
sfenoid. See *sphenoid*.
sfenoidal. See *sphenoidal*.
silastic
Simon's operation
sinus
    paranasal s.
skafa. See *scapha*.
Sluder's retractor
Snellen's operation
Sourdille's operation
Spaeth's operation
sphenoethmoid
sphenofrontal
sphenoid
sphenoidal
sphenopalatine
splint
    Brown's s.
    volar s.

Stallard's operation
staphylectomy
staphyloplasty
staphylorrhaphy
staphylotomy
stomatoplasty
Straith's operation
submental
sulcus
    s. anthelicis transversus
    s. nasolabialis
    retroauricular s.
    tympanic s.
supra-auricular
surgical procedures. See
    operation.
suture
    Zytor's s.
Swenson's operation
syndrome
    Treacher-Collins s.
Szymanowski's operation
tagliacotian operation
Tansley's operation
tarsal
tarsoplasty
tarsorrhaphy
tarsus
    t. inferior palpebrae
    t. superior palpebrae
Teale's operation
tectonic
Telfa dressing
temporal
temporomandibular
tenaculum
    Ritchie's t.
Tennison's operation

tenomyoplasty
tenoplastic
tenoplasty
terigo-. See words beginning
   pterygo-.
terigoid. See *pterygoid.*
terijeum. See *pterygium.*
Thiersch's operation
Thillaye's bandage
Thompson's operation
torus
    t. frontalis
    t. levatorius
    t. mandibularis
    t. palatinus
tosis. See *ptosis.*
tracheostomy
tragus
Trainor-Nida operation
transplantation
Treacher-Collins syndrome
Tripier's operation
Truc's operation
tube
    orotracheal t.
tunica
    t. conjunctiva
     palpebrarum
turbinate
Ulloa's operation
unciform
uncinate
uranoplasty
uranoschisis
uranoschism
uranostaphyloplasty
uranostaphylorrhaphy
uranostaphyloschisis

uvula
    u. palatina
Van Lint akinesia
Van Millingen's operation
Veau-Axhausen operation
Veau's
    elevator
    operation
velopharyngeal
velum
    Baker's v.
Verhoeff's operation
vermilion
vermilionectomy
Verweys' operation
vestibule
Virchow's knife
Vogel's operation
vomer
vomeronasal
von Blaskovics-Doyen
   operation
von Langenbeck's operation
V-Y operation
Walsham's forceps
Wardill-Kilner operation
Webster's operation
Wheeler's operation
Wicherkiewicz' operation
Wiener's operation
wire
    interdental w.
    Kirschner's w.
Wolfe-Krause graft
Wolfe's operation
Wolff's operation
Worth's operation
Wright's operation

W-Y operation
xenotransplantation
Young's operation
zeno-. See also words
beginning *xeno-*.
zenograft
Z incision

zoografting
Z-plasty
zygomatic
zygomaticofrontal
zygomaticomaxillary
zygomaticotemporal
Zytor's suture

PSYCHIATRY AND NEUROLOGY

AA — achievement age
    Alcoholics Anonymous
abalienated
abalienatio
    a. mentis
abalienation
abasia
    a. atactica
    choreic a.
    paralytic a.
    paroxysmal trepidant a.
    spastic a.
    trembling a.
    a. trepidans
abasic
abducens
abducent
aberration
ablutomania
abreaction
abscess
    Dubois' a.
absentia
    a. epileptica
abstinence
abulia
    cyclic a.
abulic
abulomania
acalculia
acarophobia
acatamathesia
acataphasia

accident prone
acervulus
Achilles tendon reflex
acousma
acousmatagnosis
acousmatamnesia
acrobrachycephaly
acrocephalosyndactylia
acrodynia
acromania
acroneuropathy
acroneurosis
acroparalysis
acroparesthesia
acrophobia
acting out
adaptation
addict
addiction
    polysurgical a.
addictologist
addictology
adhesio
    a. interthalamica
adiadochokinesia
adiadochokinesis
Adie's syndrome
adiposis
    a. cerebralis
    a. dolorosa
    a. orchalis
    a. orchica
    a. tuberosa simplex

adipositas
    a. cerebralis
adiposity
    cerebral a.
Adler's theory
adolescence
adoyomanea. See *aidoiomania.*
adrenergic
Adson's
    bur
    cannula
    chisel
    clip
    conductor
    drill
    elevator
    forceps
    hook
    knife
    needle
    retractor
    scissors
    suction tube
adventitial
adventitious
adynamia
    a. episodica hereditaria
aero-asthenia
aerodromophobia
aeroneurosis
aerophagia
aerophagy
aerophobia
afazea. See *aphasia.*
afefobea. See *aphephobia.*
afemea. See *aphemia.*
affect

affection
affective
affectivity
affectomotor
affektepilepsie
afonea. See *aphonia.*
African meningitis
agenesia
    a. corticalis
agenesis
    callosal a.
aggression
agitated
agitation
agitographia
agitolalia
agitophasia
agnosia
agoraphobia
agrammatica
agrammatism
agrammatologia
agraphia
    absolute a.
    acoustic a.
    a. amnemonica
    a. atactica
    cerebral a.
    jargon a.
    literal a.
    mental a.
    motor a.
    optic a.
    verbal a.
agraphic
agromania
agyria

ahmiel-. See words beginning
   amyel-.
ahmio-. See words beginning
   amyo-.
ahservulus. See *acervulus*.
aichmophobia
aidoiomania
ailurophilia
ailurophobia
AJ — ankle jerk
akatamathesia
akatanoesis
akathisia
akinesia
akinesis
akinesthesia
akinetic
akmofobea. See *aichmophobia*.
ala
   a. cerebelli
   a. cinerea
alalia
   a. cophica
   a. organica
   a. physiologica
   a. prolongata
alalic
alcoholic
alcoholism
alcoholomania
alcoholophilia
alexanderism
Alexander's operation
alexia
alexic
algophilia
algophily
algophobia

algopsychalia
alienation
alienism
alienist
allochiria
alteregoism
alurofilea. See *ailurophilia*.
alurofobea. See *ailurophobia*.
Alzheimer's
   dementia
   disease
   sclerosis
   syndrome
amathophobia
amaurosis
   a. centralis
   a. cerebral
amaxophobia
ambivalence
ambivalent
ambiversion
ambivert
amenomania
ament
amentia
   a. agitata
   a. attonita
   nevoid a.
   a. occulta
   a. paranoides
   phenylpyruvic a.
   Stearn's alcoholic a.
amential
amerisia
ametamorphosis
amimia
   amnesic a.
   ataxic a.

amine
Ammon's horn
amnemonic
amnesia
    anterograde a.
    auditory a.
    Broca's a.
    infantile a.
    lacunar a.
    localized a.
    olfactory a.
    patchy a.
    posthypnotic a.
    retroactive a.
    retrograde a.
    tactile a.
amnesiac
amnesic
amnestic
amok
amoral
amoralia
amoralis
amphetamine
amychophobia
amyelia
amyelineuria
amyelotrophy
amyostasia
amyostatic
amyosthenia
amyosthenic
amyotonia
    a. congenita
amyotrophia
    neuralgic a.
    a. spinalis progressiva
amyotrophic

amyotrophy
    diabetic a.
    neuralgic a.
anaclitic
analgesia
analysand
analysis
analysor
analytic
anamnesis
anamnestic
anancastic
anarithmia
anarthria
    a. literalis
Anders' disease
anencephalia
anencephalic
anencephalohemia
anencephalous
anesthesia
    Corning's a.
    endotracheal a.
aneurysm
    berry a.
    cirsoid a.
    innominate a.
    intracranial a.
    miliary a.
    mycotic a.
    racemose a.
aneurysmal
aneurysmectomy
angioblastoma
angioma
    a. arteriale racemosum
    a. cavernosum
    cavernous a.

angioma *(continued)*
    encephalic a.
        a. venosum racemosum
angioneurosis
angiospasm
angophrasia
angzietas. See *anxietas.*
anhedonia
anima
animus
anisocoria
anomia
anorexia
    a. nervosa
anosmic
ansa
    a. cervicalis
    a. hypoglossi
    a. of lenticular nucleus
    a. lenticularis
    a. subclavia
    a. of Vieussens
ansae
ansae nervorum spinalium
ansotomy
anticonvulsant
anticonvulsive
antidepressant
antihallucinatory
antisocial
antisocialism
anurizm. See *aneurysm.*
anxietas
    a. presenilis
    a. tibiarum
anxiety
    free floating a.
apandria

apanthropia
apanthropy
apastia
apastic
apathetic
apathic
apathism
apathy
Apert's syndrome
aphasia
    ageusic a.
    amnemonic a.
    amnesic a.
    amnestic a.
    anosmic a.
    associative a.
    Broca's a.
aphemia
aphephobia
aphonia
    hysteric a.
    a. paranoica
apicotomy
aplasia
    a. axialis extracorticalis
        congenita
apnea
apocarteresis
apophyseal
apophysis
    cerebral a.
    a. cerebri
    genial a.
apoplexy
    Broadbent's a.
    cerebellar a.
    cerebral a.
    fulminating a.

apoplexy *(continued)*
    ingravescent a.
    meningeal a.
    pontile a.
    Raymond's a.
    thrombotic a.
apperception
apperceptive
appersonification
apractic
apraxia
    akinetic a.
    a. algera
    amnestic a.
    cortical a.
    ideational a.
    ideokinetic a.
    ideomotor a.
    innervation a.
    limb-kinetic a.
    motor a.
    sensory a.
    transcortical a.
apraxic
aprophoria
aprosexia
apselaphesia
apsithyria
apsychia
apyschosis
aqueduct
    cerebral a.
    a. of midbrain
    a. of Sylvius
    a. of vestibule
aqueductus
    a. cerebri
arachnitis

arachnoid
arachnoidea
    a. encephali
    a. spinalis
arachnoideae
arachnoiditis
arachnophobia
Aran-Duchenne muscular
    disease
Arantius
    ventricle of A.
archipallial
archipallium
area
    Broca's a.
    Obsteiner-Redlich a.
areflexia
arhinencephalia
arithmomania
Arnold-Chiari
    deformity
    syndrome
arteriogram
arteriosclerosis
asaphia
asemasia
asemia
    a. graphica
    a. mimica
    a. verbalis
association
astasia
    a. abasia
astatic
astereocognosy
astereognosis
asterixis

asthenia
asthenic
asthenophobia
astrapophobia
astrocytoma
asynchronism
asynergia
asynergy
    appendicular a.
    axial a.
    axioappendicular a.
    trunkal a.
ataractic
ataraxia
ataraxic
ataraxy
ataxia
    autonomic a.
    Briquet's a.
    Broca's a.
    central a.
    cerebellar a.
    cerebral a.
    Fergusson and
      Critchley's a.
    Friedreich's a.
    frontal a.
    hereditary cerebellar a.
    hysteric a.
    intrapsychic a.
    kinetic a.
    labyrinthic a.
    Leyden's a.
    Marie's a.
    motor a.
    noothymopsychic a.
    Sanger-Brown's a.
    spinal a.

ataxia *(continued)*
    spinocerebellar a.
    static a.
    a. telangiectasia
    thermal a.
    vasomotor a.
ataxiagram
ataxiamnesic
ataxiaphasia
athetoid
athetosis
atonia
atremia
atrophy
    Aran-Duchenne
      muscular a.
    Charcot-Marie-Tooth a.
    circumscribed a. of brain
    convolutional a.
    Cruveilhier's a.
    degenerative a.
    Dejerine-Sottas a.
    denervated muscle a.
    Duchenne-Aran
      muscular a.
    Erb's a.
    facioscapulohumeral a.
    Fazio-Londe a.
    Hoffmann's a.
    Hunt's a.
    idiopathic muscular a.
    Landouzy-Dejerine a.
    lobar a.
    myelopathic muscular a.
    neural a.
    neuritic muscular a.
    neuropathic a.
    neurotic a.

atrophy *(continued)*
 neurotrophic a.
 olivopontocerebellar a.
 Parrot's a. of the
  newborn
 peroneal a.
 Pick's convolutional a.
 pseudohypertrophic
  muscular a.
 spinoneural a.
 trophoneurotic a.
 Vulpian's a.
 Werdnig-Hoffmann a.
ATS — anxiety tension state
atypical
aula
aulatela
aulic
auliplexus
aura
autism
autistic
autocerebrospinal
autoerotic
autoeroticism
autoerotism
autognosis
autognostic
autokinesis
autokinetic
automatism
autonomic
autopunition
aversive
awla. See *aula.*
awlatela. See *aulatela.*
awlepleksus. See *auliplexus.*
awlik. See *aulic.*

Aztec idiocy
Baastrup's syndrome
Babcock's needle
Babinski-Nageotte syndrome
Babinski's
 law
 phenomenon
 reflex
 sign
 syndrome
Bacon's forceps
Bailey's
 conductor
 leukotome
Balint's syndrome
Ballet's
 disease
 sign
ballismus
band
 Meckel's b.
Bane's forceps
Bárány's
 pointing test
 syndrome
Barré-Liéou syndrome
Barrett-Adson retractor
Barton-Cone tongs
Bärtschi-Rochain's syndrome
basicranial
basilar
basilaris
 b. cranii
basioccipital
basion
basophobia
basophobiac
Beard's syndrome

Beckman-Adson retractor
Beckman-Eaton retractor
Beckman's retractor
Beck's syndrome
behavior
behaviorism
Bell-Magendie law
Bell's
    law
    mania
    nerve
    palsy
    phenomenon
Bender-Gestalt test
Berger rhythm
Bergeron's chorea
bestiality
bifrontal
Binswanger's
    dementia
    disease
biodynamics
Biot's respiration
bisexual
bisexuality
bitemporal
biventer
    b. cervicis
block
    spinal subarachnoid b.
    stellate b.
    sympathetic b.
    ventricular b.
body
    pacchionian b's.
    pineal b.
    Schmorl's b.
Bonhoeffer's symptom

Bonnet's syndrome
boopia
Bourneville's disease
brace
    Hudson's b.
brachium
    b. cerebelli
    b. cerebri
    b. of colliculus
    b. conjunctivum
    b. copulativum
    b. of mesencephalon
    b. opticum
    b. pontis
    b. quadrigeminum
bradwemaw. See
    bredouillement.
bradyphasia
bradyphrasia
bradyphrenia
bradypsychia
Bragard's sign
Brain's reflex
Bravais-jacksonian epilepsy
bredouillement
bregma
Briquet's
    ataxia
    syndrome
Brissaud's reflex
Brissaud-Sicard syndrome
Bristowe's syndrome
Broadbent's apoplexy
Broca's
    amnesia
    aphasia
    area
    ataxia

Broca's *(continued)*
    center
    convolution
    fissure
    gyrus
    space
Brown-Séquard syndrome
Brudzinski's sign
Bruns' syndrome
Brushfield-Wyatt disease
Bucy-Frazier cannula
Bucy's
    knife
    retractor
bulbonuclear
bulbopontine
bulimia
bundle
    Helweg's b.
bur
    Adson's b.
    D'Errico's b.
    Hudson's b.
    McKenzie's b.
Burdach's tract
CA – chronological age
cacergasia
cacesthenic
cacesthesia
cachinnation
cacodemonomania
cafard
Cairns' forceps
callomania
callosal
calvaria
Campbell's elevator
camptocormia

camptocormy
canalicular
canaliculus
canalization
cannula
    Adson's c.
    Bucy-Frazier c.
    Cone's c.
    Cooper's c.
    Frazier's c.
    Haynes' c.
    Kanavel's c.
    Scott's c.
    Seletz's c.
cannulation
Capgras's syndrome
captation
carcinophobia
carfol-. See words beginning
    carphol-.
carnal
carnophobia
carotid
carphologia
carphology
castration
catalepsy
cataleptic
cataleptiform
cataleptoid
cataphasia
cataphora
cataphoric
cataphrenia
cataplectic
cataplexie
    c. du reveil
cataplexis

cataplexy
catapophysis
catathymic
catatonia
catatonic
catatony
catecholamine
catharsis
cathectic
cathexis
cathisophobia
cauda
    c. cerebelli
    c. equina
causalgia
cavity
    Meckel's c.
cavum
    c. epidurale
    c. septi pellucidi
    c. subarachnoideale
    c. subdurale
    c. vergae
cella
    c. lateralis ventriculi
      lateralis
    c. media ventriculi
      lateralis
censor
    freudian c.
    psychic c.
center
    Broca's c.
    Setchenow's c's.
centripetal
cephalalgia
cephalhematocele
    Stromeyer's c.

cephalhematoma
    c. deformans
cephalhydrocele
cephalic
cephalocentesis
cephalogyric
cephalomeningitis
cephalometry
cephalomotor
cephaloplegia
cephalorhachidian
cerebellar
cerebellifugal
cerebellipetal
cerebellitis
cerebellofugal
cerebello-olivary
cerebellopontile
cerebellopontine
cerebellorubral
cerebellorubrospinal
cerebellospinal
cerebellum
cerebral
cerebralgia
cerebrasthenia
cerebration
    unconscious c.
cerebriform
cerebrifugal
cerebripetal
cerebritis
    saturnine c.
cerebrocardiac
cerebrocentric
cerebrogalactose
cerebrohyphoid
cerebroid

cerebrol
cerebrolein
cerebroma
cerebromalacia
cerebromedullary
cerebromeningeal
cerebromeningitis
cerebrometer
cerebron
cerebro-ocular
cerebropathia
    c. psychica toxemica
cerebropathy
cerebrophysiology
cerebropontile
cerebropsychosis
cerebrorachidian
cerebrosclerosis
cerebroscope
cerebroscopy
cerebrosis
cerebrospinal
cerebrospinant
cerebrospinase
cerebrostimulin
cerebrotonia
cerebrovascular
cerebrum
Céstan-Chenais syndrome
Chaddock's
    reflex
    sign
Chandler's
    forceps
    retractor
Charcot-Marie-Tooth atrophy
Charcot's
    disease

Charcot's
    gait
chemopallidectomy
chemopallidothalamectomy
cheromania
Cherry-Kerrison forceps
Cherry's
    osteotome
    retractor
    tongs
Cheyne-Stokes psychosis
chisel
    Adson's c.
cholesteatoma
cholinergic
chordotomy
chorea
    automatic c.
    Bergeron's c.
    button-makers' c.
    chronic c.
    c. cordis
    dancing c.
    diaphragmatic c.
    c. dimidiata
    Dubini's c.
    electric c.
    epidemic c.
    c. festinans
    fibrillary c.
    c. gravidarum
    habit c.
    hemilateral c.
    Henoch's c.
    hereditary c.
    Huntington's c.
    hyoscine c.
    hysterical c.

chorea *(continued)*
    imitative c.
    c. insaniens
    juvenile c.
    laryngeal c.
    limp c.
    local c.
    c. major
    malleatory c.
    maniacal c.
    methodic c.
    mimetic c.
    c. minor
    c. mollis
    Morvan's c.
    c. nocturna
    c. nutans
    one-sided c.
    paralytic c.
    posthemiplegic c.
    prehemiplegic c.
    procursive c.
    rhythmic c.
    rotary c.
    saltatory c.
    school-made c.
    Schrötter's c.
    c. scriptorum
    senile c.
    simple c.
    Sydenham's c.
    tetanoid c.
    tic c.
choreal
choreiform
choreoathetoid
choreoathetosis
choreoid

choreomania
choreophrasia
choriomeningitis
    lymphocytic c.
    pseudolymphocytic c.
choroidectomy
chromosomes
Chvostek's sign
cinerea
cingulum
cingulumotomy
circle
    c. of Willis
circumstantiality
cistern
    cerebellomedullary c.
    c. of fossa of Sylvius
    c. of lateral fossa of
      cerebrum
    c. of Pecquet
    subarachnoidal c's.
    c. of Sylvius
cisterna
    c. ambiens
    c. basalis
    c. cerebellomedullaris
    c. chiasmatica
    c. chiasmatis
    c. fossae lateralis cerebri
    c. fossae Sylvii
    c. intercruralis profunda
    c. interpeduncularis
    c. magna
    c. sulci lateralis
    c. Sylvii
    c. venae magnae cerebri
cisternae
    c. subarachnoidales

cisternae
    c. subarachnoideales
cisternal
clairaudience
clairsentience
clairvoyance
clamp
    bulldog c.
    Crutchfield's c.
    Gandy's c.
    Salibi's c.
classification
    Kraepelin's c.
Claude's
    hyperkinesis sign
    syndrome
claudication
    intermittent c.
    venous c.
claustra
claustrophilia
claustrophobia
claustrum
clava
climacteric
clip
    Adson's c.
    McKenzie's c.
    Olivecrona's c.
    Raney's c.
    Schutz's c.
    Sugar's c.
clivus
clonic
clonism
clonus
    ankle c.
Cloward-Hoen retractor

CNS – central nervous system
coconscious
coconsciousness
cognition
cognitive
coma
comatose
commissura
    c. alba medulae spinalis
    c. anterior cerebri
    c. cerebelli
    c. habenularum
commissure
    Meynert's c.
commitment
commotio
    c. cerebri
    c. spinalis
compensation
complex
    castration c.
    Electra c.
    inferiority c.
    Oedipus c.
compression
compulsion
compulsive
conamen
conarium
conation
conative
concept
conception
conconscious
concretism
concussion
condensation
conditioning

conduction
    bone c.
conductor
    Adson's c.
    Bailey's c.
    Davis' c.
    Kanavel's c.
Cone's
    cannula
    needle
    retractor
confabulation
confidentiality
configuration
conflict
confluens
    c. sinuum
confusion
congenital
connector
    Rochester's c.
Conolly's system
conscience
conscious
consciousness
constellation
constitution
    ideo-obsessional c.
    psychopathic c.
content
    latent c.
Contour's retractor
conus
    c. medullaris
conversion
convexobasia
convolution
    Broca's c.

convolution *(continued)*
    c's of cerebrum
    Heschl's c.
    occipitotemporal c.
    Zuckerkandl's c.
convulsant
convulsibility
convulsion
    choreic c.
    clonic c.
    coordinate c.
    epileptiform c.
    hysteroid c.
    mimetic c.
    mimic c.
    puerperal c.
    salaam c.
    static c.
    tetanic c.
    tonic c.
    uremic c.
convulsive
Cooper's cannula
coprolagnia
coprolalomania
coprophagia
coprophagy
coprophilia
coprophiliac
coprophobia
Corning's
    anesthesia
    puncture
cornu
    c. anterius ventriculi
      lateralis
    c. inferius ventriculi
      lateralis

cornu
    c. medulae spinalis
corona
    c. radiata
corpora
    c. amylacea
    c. arenacea
    c. bigemina
    c. flava
    c. quadrigemina
    c. restiformia
corpus
    c. amygdaloideum
    c. callosum
    c. fornicis
    c. medullare cerebelli
    c. medullare vermis
    c. nuclei caudati
    c. ossis sphenoidalis
    c. pineale
    c. pyramidale medulae
    c. rhomboidale
    c. striatum
    c. trapezoideum
correlation
cortex
cortical
corticectomy
corticoautonomic
corticobulbar
corticocerebral
corticodiencephalic
corticomesencephalic
corticopeduncular
corticopontine
corticospinal
Cotard's syndrome
counterphobia
countertransference
Craig's scissors
Crane's mallet
cranial
cranialis
craniamphitomy
craniectomy
cranioacromial
cranioaural
craniocele
craniocerebral
craniomalacia
craniomeningocele
craniopharyngioma
cranioplasty
craniopuncture
craniorachischisis
cranioschisis
craniosclerosis
cranioscopy
craniospinal
craniostenosis
craniostosis
craniosynostosis
craniotabes
craniotome
craniotomy
craniotonoscopy
craniotopography
craniotympanic
cranitis
cranium
crescent
crescentic
cretin
cretinism
cretinistic
cretinoid
cretinous

cribriform
Crile's knife
criminaloid
criminosis
crisis
    Lundvall's blood c.
Crouzon's disease
crura
crus
    c. cerebelli ad pontem
    c. cerebri
Crutchfield-Raney tongs
Crutchfield's
    clamp
    drill
    tongs
Cruveilhier's atrophy
cryptomnesia
cryptomnesic
cryptoneurous
cryptopsychic
cryptopsychism
CSF – cerebrospinal fluid
CSM – cerebrospinal
   meningitis
CST – convulsive shock
   therapy
culmen monticuli
cuneate
cuneus
cunnilingus
curet
    Govons' c.
    Hibbs' c.
    Pratt's c.
    Raney's c.
Cushing's
    depressor

Cushing's *(continued)*
    disease
    drill
    forceps
    law
    medulloblastoma
    reaction
    retractor
    spatula
    spoon
    syndrome
    tumor
cushinoid
CVA – cerebrovascular
   accident
cybernetics
cyclothymia
cyclothymiac
cyclothymic
cyclothymosis
daler. See *délire.*
Dandy's
    hook
    scissors
Dandy-Walker syndrome
Darkschewitsch's
    fibers
    nucleus
Davidoff's retractor
Davidson's retractor
Davis'
    conductor
    forceps
    retractor
    spatula
dazhah aproova. See *déjà
   éprouvé.*
dazhah fa. See *déjà fait.*

dazhah ontondoo. See *déjà entendu.*
dazhah ponsa. See *déjà pensé.*
dazhah rakonta. See *déjà raconté.*
dazhah vakoo. See *déjà vécu.*
dazhah voo. See *déjà vu.*
dazhah vooloo. See *déjà voulu.*
dazhanara. See *degéneré.*
decerebellation
decerebrate
decerebration
decerebrize
decision
 Durham's d.
declinator
declive
 d. monticuli cerebelli
decompression
 cerebral d.
decortication
decursus
 d. fibrarum cerebralium
decussation
 Forel's d.
 fountain d. of Meynert
defecalgesiophobia
deflection
deformity
 Arnold-Chiari d.
degeneration
 wallerian d.
degéneré
degenitalize
dehumanization
déjà entendu
déjà éprouvé
déjà fait

déjà pensé
déjà raconté
déjà vécu
déjà voulu
déjà vu
dejection
Dejerine-Roussy syndrome
Dejerine-Sottas atrophy
Dejerine's
 sign
 syndrome
delinquent
deliquium
 d. animi
délire
 d. de toucher
deliria
deliriant
delirifacient
delirious
delirium
 d. mussitans
 d. schizophrenoides
 d. sine delirio
 d. tremens
de lunatico inquirendo
delusion
delusional
dement
demented
dementia
 Alzheimer's d.
 Binswanger's d.
 epileptic d.
 d. myoclonica
 paralytic d.
 d. paralytica
 d. paranoides

dementia *(continued)*
    paretic d.
    d. praecox
    d. praesenilis
    d. pugilistica
    semantic d.
    senile d.
    terminal d.
    toxic d.
demonomania
demyelinate
dependence
dependency
depersonalization
depraved
deprementia
depressant
depressed
depression
    pacchionian d's.
depressive
depressor
    Cushing's d.
deprivation
deranencephalia
Dercum's disease
dereism
dereistic
derencephalocele
D'Errico-Adson retractor
D'Errico's
    bur
    forceps
    retractor
desensitization
deterioration
determinism
    psychic d.

Devic's syndrome
DeVilbiss'
        forceps
        trephine
diachesis
diadochokinesia
diadochokinesis
diadochokinetic
diakesis. See *diachesis.*
diaphragma
        d. sellae
diastematocrania
diastematomyelia
diatela
diaterma
diencephalic
diencephalohypophysial
diencephalon
Dimitri's disease
dinomania
diocoele
diplegia
diploë
diplopia
diplopiaphobia
dipsomania
dipsopathy
dipsosis
dis-. See also words beginning
    dys-.
disease
        Alzheimer's d.
        Anders' d.
        Aran-Duchenne d.
        Ballet's d.
        Binswanger's d.
        Bourneville's d.
        Brushfield-Wyatt d.

disease *(continued)*
    Charcot's d.
    Crouzon's d.
    Cushing's d.
    Dercum's d.
    Dimitri's d.
    Down's d.
    Dubini's d.
    Dubois' d.
    Duchenne's d.
    Duchenne-Aran d.
    Economo's d.
    Erb-Charcot d.
    Erb-Goldflam d.
    Erb-Landouzy d.
    Erb's d.
    Frankl-Hochwart's d.
    Friedreich's d.
    Fürstner's d.
    Gerlier's d.
    Gilles de la Tourette's d.
    Goldflam's d.
    Hunt's d.
    Janet's d.
    Kalischer's d.
    Koshevnikoff's d.
    Krabbe's d.
    Lasègue's d.
    Little's d.
    Merzbacher-Pelizaeus d.
    Mills's d.
    Morel-Kraepelin d.
    Niemann-Pick d.
    Parkinson's d.
    Pick's d.
    Rendu-Osler-Weber d.
    Romberg's d.
    Roth-Bernhardt d.

disease *(continued)*
    Roth's d.
    Schilder's d.
    Schmorl's d.
    Simmonds' d.
    Steiner's d.
    Sturge-Weber d.
    Tay-Sachs d.
    Thomsen's d.
    Tourette's d.
    Unverricht's d.
    Vogt's d.
    von Hippel-Lindau d.
    von Recklinghausen's d.
    Weber's d.
    Wernicke's d.
    Winkelman's d.
    Ziehen-Oppenheim d.
disfajea. See *dysphagia.*
disfazea. See *dysphasia.*
disfemia. See *dysphemia.*
disfonia. See *dysphonia.*
disfor-. See words beginning
    dysphor-.
disfrasia. See *dysphrasia.*
disfrenia. See *dysphrenia.*
disk
    intervertebral d.
diskectomy
diskogram
disorientation
displacement
dissector
    Oldberg's d.
dissociation
distaxia
    cerebral d.
distortion

distractibility
disvolution
divagation
DNA — deoxyribonucleic acid
dolichocephalic
dolichocephalism
domatophobia
dominance
Down's
    disease
    syndrome
dramatism
dramatization
drapetomania
dream
    clairvoyant d.
    veridical d.
drill
    Adson's d.
    Crutchfield's d.
    Cushing's d.
    McKenzie's d.
    Raney's d.
    Stille's d.
dromomania
dromophobia
drugs. See *Medications.*
DTP — distal tingling on
    percussion
DTR — deep tendon reflex
DT's — delirium tremens
Dubini's
    chorea
    disease
Dubois'
    abscess
    disease
    method

Duchenne-Aran
    disease
    muscular atrophy
Duchenne-Erb paralysis
Duchenne's disease
ductus
    d. perilymphatici
Duncan's ventricle
dura
dural
dura mater
    d. m. of brain
    d. m. encephali
    d. m. of spinal cord
    d. m. spinalis
duramatral
duraplasty
durematoma
Durham's decision
duroarachnitis
durosarcoma
dysarthria
    d. literalis
    d. syllabaris spasmodica
dysarthric
dysautonomia
dysbasia
    d. angiosclerotica
    d. angiospastica
    d. intermittens
        angiosclerotica
    d. lordotica progressiva
    d. neurasthenica
        intermittens
dysbulia
dysbulic
dyscephaly
dyschiria

dysergasia
dysergastic
dysergia
dysesthesia
dysgraphia
dyskinesia
    d. algera
dyskinetic
dyslalia
dyslexia
dyslogia
dysmetria
dysnomia
dyspareunia
dysphagia
dysphasia
dysphemia
dysphonia
dysphoretic
dysphoria
dysphoriant
dysphoric
dysphrasia
dysphrenia
dyspraxia
dysrhythmia
dyssocial
dyssymbolia
dyssymboly
dyssynergia
    d. cerebellaris
      myoclonica
    d. cerebellaris
      progressiva
dystaxia
    d. agitans
dystectia
dysthymia

dystonia
    d. musculorum
      deformans
dystrophoneurosis
dystrophy
    Erb's d.
    Landouzy-Déjérine d.
    muscular d.
    thyroneural d.
dystropic
dystropy
Ebbinghaus' test
eccentric
ecchordosis physaliphora
ecdemomania
echogram
echographia
echokinesis
echolalia
echolalus
echomimia
echomotism
echopathy
echophrasia
echopraxia
echopraxis
eclampsia
eclysis
ecmnesia
ecomania
Economo's disease
ecophobia
ecphoria
ecphorize
ecphory
ECT — electric convulsive
    therapy
ectocinerea

edema
>Huguenin's e.
edipism
edipus. See *Oedipus.*
EEE – eastern equine encephalomyelitis
EEG – electroencephalogram
ego
egocentric
egodystonic
egomania
egosyntonic
egotistical
egotropic
eidetic
eko-. See words begining *echo-.*
elaboration
elation
Electra complex
electrocorticography
electroencephalogram
electroencephalograph
electroencephalography
electromyography
electronarcosis
electroplexy
electroshock
electrospectrography
electrospinogram
electrostimulation
elevator
>Adson's e.
>Campbell's e.
>Frazier's e.
>Freer's e.
>Hajek-Ballenger e.
>Hibbs' e.
>Killian's e.

elevator *(continued)*
>Love-Adson e.
>Rochester's e.
ellipsis
emasculate
emasculation
embolism
>cerebral e.
embololalia
embolus
emotion
emotional
empathize
empathy
emprosthotonos
encephalalgia
encephalatrophy
encephalemia
encephalic
encephalitis
encephaloarteriography
encephalocele
encephalocoele
encephalocystocele
encephalogram
encephalolith
encephaloma
encephalomalacia
encephalomeningitis
encephalomeningocele
encephalomeningopathy
encephalomyelitis
encephalomyelocele
encephalomyeloneuropathy
encephalomyelopathy
encephalomyeloradiculitis
encephalomyeloradiculo-
>neuritis

encephalomyeloradiculopathy
encephalomyocarditis
encephalon
encephalonarcosis
encephalopathia
    e. alcoholica
encephalopathy
      Wernicke's e.
encephalophyma
encephalopsychosis
encephalopuncture
encephalopyosis
encephalorrhagia
encephalosclerosis
encephaloscope
encephaloscopy
encephalosepsis
encephalosis
encephalothlipsis
encephalotome
encephalotomy
encopresis
endocrinasthenia
endomorph
endomorphic
endomorphy
endothelioma
    dural e.
engram
enomania
enosimania
ensef-. See words beginning
    enceph-.
entropy
enuresis
environment
EOM — extraocular
   movements

epencephalic
epencephalon
ependopathy
ependyma
ependymal
ependymitis
ependymoblast
ependymoblastoma
ependymocyte
ependymocytoma
ependymoma
ependymopathy
epicoele
epidemiology
epidermoid
epidermoidoma
epidural
epilepsia
    e. gravior
    e. major
    e. minor
    e. mitior
    e. nutans
    e. partialis continua
    e. procursiva
    e. rotatoria
    e. tarda
epilepsy
    abdominal e.
    Bravais-jacksonian e.
    cortical e.
    cryptogenic e.
    diurnal e.
    focal e.
    grand mal e.
    hysterical e.
    idiopathic e.
    jacksonian e.

epilepsy *(continued)*
    larval e.
    latent e.
    matutinal e.
    menstrual e.
    musicogenic e.
    myoclonus e.
    nocturnal e.
    petit mal e.
    physiologic e.
    procursive e.
    psychic e.
    psychomotor e.
    reflex e.
    rolandic e.
    sensory e.
    serial e.
    symptomatic e.
    tardy e.
    tonic e.
    traumatic e.
    uncinate e.
epileptic
    e. equivalent
    e. seizure
epileptiform
epileptogenic
epileptogenous
epileptoid
epileptologist
epileptology
epileptosis
epiloia
episode
    psycholeptic e.
epithalamus
epithelioma

epithelioma
    e. myxomatodes
        psammosum
epithelium
    mesenchymal e.
Erb-Charcot disease
Erb-Goldflam disease
Erb-Landouzy disease
Erb's
    atrophy
    disease
    dystrophy
    sclerosis
    syndrome
eremophobia
erethism
erethisophrenia
erethistic
erethitic
ergasia
ergasiatrics
ergasiatry
ergasiology
ergasiomania
ergasiophobia
ergasthenia
ergomania
ergomaniac
erithredema. See
    erythredema.
erithro-. See words beginning
    erythro-.
erogenous
erotic
eroticism
erotism
    anal e.
    muscle e.

erotism
    oral e.
eroticomania
erotogenesis
erotogenic
erotographomania
erotomania
erotomaniac
erotopath
erotopathy
erotophobia
erotopsychic
erotosexual
erratic
erythredema polyneuropathy
erythromelalgia
erythrophobia
eschar
    neuropathic e.
ESP — extrasensory
   perception
EST — electroshock therapy
estheticokinetic
eunoia
euphoretic
euphoria
euphoriant
euphoric
euphorigenic
excitability
excitable
excitation
excitomotor
exencephalia
exhibitionism
exhilarant
existential
existentialism

exteroceptive
exterofection
exterofective
extradural
extrapsychic
extrapyramidal
extraversion
extrovert
facetectomy
facies
    Parkinson's f.
factitious
falik. See *phallic.*
falx
    f. cerebelli
    f. cerebri
fan-. See words beginning
   phan-.
Fañana
    glia of F.
fantasy. See *phantasy.*
fasciculation
fasciculus
    f. aberrans of Monokow
    f. of Foville
    f. of Gowers
fastigium
Fazio-Londe atrophy
feeblemindedness
fellatio
felo-de-se
fenil-. See words beginning
   phenyl-.
fenomenon. See *phenomenon.*
fenotype. See *phenotype.*
Fergusson and Critchley's
    ataxia
Ferris-Smith forceps

fetish
fetishism
fiber
    Darkschewitsch's f's.
fibroblastoma
    meningeal f.
figure
    fortification f's.
fila
    f. olfactoria
    f. radicularia nervorum
      spinalium
filum
    f. durae matris spinalis
    f. of spinal dura mater
    f. terminale
fissure
    Broca's f.
    Pansch's f.
    f. of Sylvius
fixation
    freudian f.
fizeo-. See words beginning
    physio-.
flagellantism
Flatau's law
flegmatik. See *phlegmatic*.
flexibilitas
    f. cerea
flight
    f. of ideas
floccilation
flocculus
fluid
    xanthochromic f.
fobia. See *phobia*.
fobic. See *phobic*.
fobofobia. See *phobophobia*.

Foix-Alajouanine syndrome
fold
    Veraguth's f.
folee. See *folie*.
folia cerebelli
folie
    f. à deux
    f. circulaire
    f. du doute
    f. du pourquoi
    f. gemellaire
    f. musculaire
    f. raisonnante
folium
    f. cacuminis
    f. vermis
fontanelle
foramen
    f. caecum medullae
      oblongatae
    Luschka's f.
    Magendie's f.
    f. magnum
    f. of Monro
    f. occipitale magnum
foramina
foraminotomy
forceps
    Adson's f.
    Bacon's f.
    Bane's f.
    Cairns' f.
    Chandler's f.
    Cherry-Kerrison f.
    Cushing's f.
    Davis' f.
    D'Errico's f.
    DeVilbiss' f.

forceps *(continued)*
    Ferris-Smith f.
    Gerald's f.
    Gruenwald's f.
    Hudson's f.
    Hurd's f.
    Leksell's f.
    Lewin's f.
    Love-Gruenwald f.
    Love-Kerrison f.
    Luer's f.
    McKenzie's f.
    Oldberg's f.
    Raney's f.
    Ruskin's f.
    Schlesinger's f.
    Schutz's f.
    Scoville's f.
    Sewall's f.
    Spence-Adson f.
    Spence's f.
    Spurling's f.
    Stevenson's f.
    Stille-Luer f.
    Wilde's f.
foreconscious
Forel's decussation
formication
fornix
    f. cerebri
Förster-Penfield operation
fossa
    cerebellar f.
    cerebral f.
    cranial f.
    f. cranii anterior
    f. cranii media
    f. cranii posterior

fossa
    posterior f.
fovea
Foville's
    fasciculus
    syndrome
    tract
frame
    Stryker's f.
Francke's striae
Frankl-Hochwart's disease
Frazier's
    cannula
    elevator
    hook
    retractor
    suction tube
Freer's elevator
fren-. See words beginning
    phren-.
French s-shaped retractor
frenetic
freno-. See words beginning
    phreno-.
frenzy
Freud's
    cathartic method
    theory
freudian
Friedmann's vasomotor
    syndrome
Friedreich's
    ataxia
    disease
    tabes
frigidity
Fröhlich's syndrome
Froin's syndrome

frons
    f. cranii
frustration
fugue
    epileptic f.
functional
fundus
funduscope
funicular
funiculitis
funiculus
    f. cuneatus
    f. gracilis medullae
      oblongatae
    f. medullae spinalis
    f. solitarius
    f. teres
    f. ventralis
furibund
furor
    f. epilepticus
Fürstner's disease
gait
    ataxic g.
    cerebellar g.
    Charcot's g.
    Oppenheim's g.
    scissor g.
    steppage g.
galea
    g. aponeurotica
    tendinous g.
Galt's trephine
galvanism
galvanopalpation
Gandy's clamp
ganglion
    gasserian g.

ganglion *(continued)*
    Meckel's g.
    trigeminal g.
ganglionectomy
gangliosympathectomy
Ganser's
    symptom
    syndrome
Garcin's syndrome
Gardner's needle
gargoylism
gelasmus
Gélineau's syndrome
gene
genetic
geniculum
genotype
genu
    g. corporis callosi
    g. nervi facialis
geophagia
gephyrophobia
Gerald's forceps
geriatric
geriatrics
geriopsychosis
Gerlier's disease
Gerstmann's syndrome
Gestalt theory
gestaltism
Gifford's retractor
Gigli's saw
Gilles de la Tourette's
    disease
    syndrome
glabella
glia
    cytoplasmic g.

glia
>g. of Fañana

glioblast

glioblastoma
>g. multiforme

gliocytoma

gliogenous

glioma
>ependymal g.
>ganglionic g.
>g. multiforme
>g. sarcomatosum

gliomatosis

gliomatous

gliomyoma

gliomyxoma

glioneuroma

gliophagia

gliopil

gliosa

gliosarcoma

gliosis
>basilar g.
>cerebellar g.
>diffuse g.
>hemispheric g.
>hypertrophic nodular g.
>lobar g.
>perivascular g.
>spinal g.
>unilateral g.

gliosome

globus
>g. hystericus

glossolalia

glycorrhachia

Goldflam's disease

Goll's tract

gouge
>Hibbs' g.

Govons' curet

Gowers
>fasciculus of G.

Gradenigo's syndrome

Graham's hook

grandiosity

gratification

Gruenwald's forceps

GSR – galvanic skin response

guard
>Sachs' g.

Guillain-Barré syndrome

gumma

gustatory

gyri
>g. annectentes
>g. breves insulae
>g. cerebri
>g. insulae
>g. occipitales
>g. operti
>g. orbitales
>g. profundi cerebri
>g. transitivi cerebri

gyrus
>g. angularis
>Broca's g.
>g. callosus
>g. cinguli
>g. dentatus
>g. fasciolaris
>g. fornicatus
>g. fusiformis
>g. hippocampi
>g. infracalcarinus
>g. limbicus

gyrus *(continued)*
    g. lingualis
    g. marginalis
    g. olfactorius
    g. parahippocampalis
    g. paraterminalis
    g. precentralis
    g. rectus
    g. temporalis
    g. uncinatus
habenula
habitual
habituation
habromania
Haenel's symptom
Hajek-Ballenger elevator
Hallervorden-Spatz syndrome
Hall's neurotome
hallucination
    auditory h.
    depressive h.
    gustatory h.
    haptic h.
    hypnagogic h.
    lilliputian h.
    olfactory h.
    reflex h.
    stump h.
    tactile h.
    visual h.
hallucinative
hallucinatory
hallucinogen
hallucinogenesis
hallucinogenetic
hallucinogenic
hallucinosis
hallucinotic

Hamby's retractor
haut-mal
Haynes'
    cannula
    operation
hebephrenia
hebephreniac
hebetude
heboid
heboidophrenia
hedonia
hedonic
hedonism
hedonophobia
Helweg's
    bundle
    tract
hemangioblastoma
hematoma
    subdural h.
hematomyelia
hemianesthesia
hemianopia
hemiballismus
hemicraniectomy
hemihypesthesia
hemilaminectomy
hemiparesis
hemiplegia
hemisphere
    cerebellar h.
    cerebral h.
hemispherectomy
hemispherium
    h. cerebelli
Henoch's chorea
hereditary
heredity

heredoataxia
hermaphrodite
Heschl's convolution
heteroerotism
heterosexual
heterosexuality
heterosuggestion
heterotonic
heterotopia
Hibbs'
    curet
    elevator
    gouge
hipnagojik. See *hypnagogic.*
hipno-. See words beginning
    hypno-.
hipo-. See words beginning
    hypo-.
hippocampus
    h. leonis
    h. nudus
Hirschberg's reflex
hodology
Hoen's skull plate
Hoffmann's
    atrophy
    sign
holergasia
holergastic
holism
holistic
holorachischisis
Homén's syndrome
homicidomania
homilophobia
homosexual
homosexuality
homunculus

hook
    Adson's h.
    Dandy's h.
    Frazier's h.
    Graham's h.
horn
    Ammon's h.
Horsley's separator
hostility
Hudson's
    brace
    bur
    forceps
Huguenin's edema
Huntington's chorea
Hunt's
    atrophy
    disease
    neuralgia
    paradoxical phenomenon
    striatal syndrome
    tremor
Hurd's forceps
Hurler's syndrome
hydranencephaly
hydrencephalocele
hydrencephalomeningocele
hydrocephalic
hydrocephalocele
hydrocephaloid
hydrocephalus
    communicating h.
    noncommunicating h.
    obstructive h.
    otitic h.
hydromeningocele
hydromyelia
hydromyelomeningocele

hygroma
    subdural h.
hyla
hypalgesia
hypencephalon
hyperalgesia
hyperesthesia
hyperkinesia
hyperkinesis
hyperkinetic
hypernea
hypernoia
hyperostosis
    h. cranii
    h. frontalis interna
    Morgagni's h.
hyperphrenia
hyperreflexia
hypertarachia
hyperthymergasia
hyperthymia
hyperventilation
hypnagogic
hypnoanalysis
hypnoanesthesia
hypnobatia
hypnogenic
hypnolepsy
hypnonarcoanalysis
hypnonarcosis
hypnopompic
hypnosia
hypnosis
hypnotherapy
hypnotic
hypnotism
hypnotize
hypoactive

hypochondria
hypochondriac
hypochondriacal
hypochondriasis
hypoesthesia
hypoglycorrhachia
hypokinesia
hypomania
hypomaniac
hypomanic
hypophrenosis
hypophyseal
hypophysectomy
hypophysis
    h. cerebri
hypophysitis
hypophysoma
hyporeflexia
hypotelorism
    orbital h.
hypothalamotomy
hypothalamus
hypothermia
hypotonic
hysteria
    anxiety h.
    canine h.
    conversion h.
    fixation h.
    h. libidinosa
    monosymptomatic h.
hysteric
hysterical
hystericism
hystericoneuralgic
hysteriform
hysteroepilepsy
hysteroepileptogenic

hysteroerotic
hysterogenic
hysteroid
hysteromania
hysteronarcolepsy
hysteroneurasthenia
hysteroneurosis
hysteropia
hysteropsychosis
iatrogenic
ICT – insulin coma therapy
ictal
ictus
    i. epilepticus
    i. paralyticus
    i. sanguinis
id
ideal
    ego i.
idealization
ideation
    incoherent i.
ideational
idée
    i. fixe
identification
ideodynamism
ideogenetic
idetik. See *eidetic.*
idiocy
    absolute i.
    amaurotic familial i.
    athetosic i.
    Aztec i.
    cretinoid i.
    developmental i.
    diplegic i.
    eclamptic i.

idiocy *(continued)*
    epileptic i.
    genetous i.
    hemiplegic i.
    hydrocephalic i.
    intrasocial i.
    Kulmuk i.
    microcephalic i.
    Mongolian i.
    paralytic i.
    paraplegic i.
    plagiocephalic i.
    scaphocephalic i.
    sensorial i.
    traumatic i.
idioglossia
idioglottic
idioimbecile
idioneural
idioneurosis
idiopathic
idiophrenic
idiopsychologic
idiosyncrasy
idiosyncratic
idiot
    erethistic i.
    Mongolian i.
    pithecoid i.
    profound i.
    i. -savant
    superficial i.
    torpid i.
idiotropic
illusion
illusional
image
imagines

imago
imbecile
imbecility
immature
impotence
imprinting
impulse
    irresistible i.
impulsion
    wandering i.
inadequate
inadequacy
incallosal
incest
incision
    coronal i.
    suboccipital i.
    vermis i.
incoherent
incompetent
incoordination
incubus
indifference
    belle i.
indifferent
Indoklon therapy
indusium griseum
ineon. See *inion.*
infantile
infantilism
infarction
    cerebral i.
infundibulum
    i. hypothalami
inhibition
iniencephaly
inion

insane
insanity
    adolescent i.
    affective i.
    alcoholic i.
    alternating i.
    anticipatory i.
    choreic i.
    circular i.
    climacteric i.
    communicated i.
    compound i.
    compulsive i.
    consecutive i.
    cyclic i.
    doubting i.
    emotional i.
    hereditary i.
    homicidal i.
    homochronous i.
    hysteric i.
    idiophrenic i.
    impulsive i.
    manic-depressive i.
    moral i.
    perceptional i.
    periodic i.
    polyneuritic i.
    primary i.
    puerperal i.
    recurrent i.
    senile i.
    simultaneous i.
    toxic i.
insanoid
insensible
insight

insolation
      hyperpyrexial i.
insomnia
insomniac
insomnic
inspectionism
instinct
      death i.
      ego i.
      herd i.
instinctive
insula
insultus
      i. hystericus
integration
intellect
intellection
intellectualization
intelligence
interneuron
interpretation
intervertebral
intracephalic
intracerebellar
intracerebral
intracisternal
intracranial
intralobar
intramedullary
intrapsychic
intraspinal
intraventricular
introjection
introspection
introversion
introvert
inversion
      sexual i.

invert
involuntary
involutional
iodoventriculography
IQ – intelligence quotient
irascibility
irreversible
irritability
irritation
      cerebral i.
      spinal i.
ischogyria
ismus. See *isthmus.*
isolation
IST – insulin shock therapy
isthmus
      i. of cingulate gyrus
jacksonian epilepsy
Jackson's
      law
      rule
      syndrome
Jakob-Creutzfeld syndrome
Janet's
      disease
      test
Jansen's retractor
jefirofobea. See *gephyrophobia.*
Joffroy's reflex
Jolly's reaction
Jung's method
juvenile
kakergasea. See *cacergasia.*
kakesthenik. See *cacesthenic.*
kakesthezea. See *cacesthesia.*
kakinashun. See *cachinnation.*
kakodemonomanea. See
      cacodemonomania.

Kalischer's disease
Kanavel's
    cannula
    conductor
Kanner's syndrome
karnshvoont. See
    kernschwund.
kemo-. See words beginning
    chemo-.
kenophobia
kernicterus
Kernig's sign
kernschwund
keromanea. See *cheromania*.
Killian's elevator
Kiloh-Nevin syndrome
kinanesthesia
kinesioneurosis
kinesodic
kinesthesia
kinesthetic
KJ – knee jerk
KK – knee kicks
kleptolagnia
kleptomania
kleptomaniac
kleptophobia
Klippel-Feil syndrome
Klippel-Feldstein syndrome
Klüver-Bucy syndrome
knife
    Adson's k.
    Bucy's k.
    Crile's k.
kolesteatoma. See
    cholesteatoma
kolinerjik. See *cholinergic*.
kooroo. See *kuru*.

kor-. See words beginning
    chor-.
koro
Korsakoff's
    psychosis
    syndrome
Koshevnikoff's disease
Krabbe's
    disease
    sclerosis
Kraepelin's classification
Krause's ventricle
Kretschmer types
Kulmuk idiocy
kuru
labile
lability
labiochorea
Lafora's sign
laliophobia
laloneurosis
lalophobia
lambda
Lambotte's osteotome
lamella
lamina
    inferior l. of sphenoid
      bone
    l. medullaris lateralis
      corporis striati
    l. medullaris medialis
      corporis striati
    l. ossium cranii
laminae
    l. albae cerebelli
    l. medullares cerebelli
    l. medullares thalami
laminectomy

laminotomy
Landouzy-Déjérine
    atrophy
    dystrophy
Landry's paralysis
lapsus
    l. linguae
    l. memoriae
Lasègue's
    disease
    sign
latah
latency
latent
laterality
lateropulsion
law
    Babinski's l.
    Bell-Magendie l.
    Bell's l.
    Cushing's l.
    Flatau's l.
    Jackson's l.
    Magendie's l.
    wallerian l.
Leichtenstern's sign
Leksell's forceps
lemniscus
lenticular
lenticulo-optic
leptocephalia
leptomeninges
leptomeningioma
leptomeningitis
leptomeninx
Leri's sign
lesbian
lesbianism

lethargy
    hysteric l.
    induced l.
    lucid l.
lethe
letheomania
lethologica
leukodystrophy
leukoencephalitis
leukomyelitis
leukomyelopathy
leukotome
    Bailey's l.
    Love's l.
leukotomy
Lewin's forceps
Leyden's ataxia
Lhermitte's sign
libidinal
libidinous
libido
    bisexual l.
    ego l.
Lichtheim's
    plaques
    sign
ligamentum
    l. denticulatum
    l. flavum
likenshadel. See *lückenschädel.*
lingula
    l. cerebelli
Lissauer's tract
Little's disease
lobectomy
lobotomy
    frontal l.
    prefrontal l.

lobotomy
    transorbital l.
lobus
    l. frontalis
    l. occipitalis
    l. olfactorius
    l. parietalis
    l. temporalis
lobulus
    l. centralis cerebelli
    l. paracentralis
    l. parietalis
    l. quadrangularis
      cerebelli
    l. semilunaris
logagnosia
logagraphia
logamnesia
logaphasia
logasthenia
logoklony
logokophosis
logomania
logoneurosis
logopathy
logoplegia
logorrhea
logospasm
lordosis
Love-Adson elevator
Love-Gruenwald forceps
Love-Kerrison forceps
Love's
    leukotome
    retractor
LSD – lysergic acid
    diethylamide
Lucae's mallet

lucid
lückenschädel
Luer's forceps
luko-. See words beginning
    leuko-.
lumbosacral
lunacy
lunatic
lunatism
Lundvall's blood crisis
lura
lural
Luschka's foramen
Lust's reflex
MA – mental age
macrencephalia
macrocrania
macrogyria
macromania
macromelia
    m. paraesthetica
maculocerebral
Magendie's
    foramen
    law
    spaces
maladjustment
malingerer
malingering
malleation
mallet
    Crane's m.
    Lucae's m.
    Meyerding's m.
maneuver
    Valsalva's m.
mania
    acute hallucinatory m.

mania *(continued)*
    akinetic m.
    m. à potu
    Bell's m.
    dancing m.
    doubting m.
    epileptic m.
    hysterical m.
    m. mitis
    periodical m.
    puerperal m.
    Ray's m.
    reasoning m.
    religious m.
    m. secandi
    transitory m.
    unproductive m.
maniac
maniaphobia
manic
manifest
mannerism
MAOI – monoamine oxidase
    inhibitor
Marchiafava-Bignami
    syndrome
Marie's
    ataxia
    sclerosis
marital
marrowbrain
masochism
masochist
McCarthy's reflex
McKenzie's
    bur
    clip
    drill

McKenzie's
    forceps
MD – muscular dystrophy
mechanism
    defense m.
    neutralizing m.
Meckel's
    band
    cavity
    ganglion
Medications
    acetophenazine
    Amfedsul
    amitriptyline
    Amphedroxyn
    amphetamine
    Amsustain
    Atarax
    Aventyl
    benactyzine
    Benzedrine
    benzphetamine
    buclizine
    butabarbital
    butaperazine
    Butisol
    caffeine
    captodiame
    carphenazine
    Celontin
    Cendex
    chloral hydrate
    chlordiazepoxide
    chlormezanone
    chlorpromazine
    chlorprothixene
    Compazine

Medications *(continued)*
- Coramine
- Dalmane
- Daro-Tab
- Dartal
- Deaner
- deanol acetamidobenzoate
- desipramine
- Desoxyn
- Dexedrine
- dextroamphetamine
- diazepam
- Didrex
- Dilantin
- diphenylhydantoin
- Doriden
- doxepin
- Drinalfa
- droperidol
- Efroxine
- Elavil
- Enanthate
- Equanil
- Eskalith
- ethchlorvynol
- ethosuximide
- ethotoin
- fluphenazine
- flurazepam
- flurothyl
- Gemonil
- glutethimide
- Haldol
- haloperidol
- hydroxyzine
- imipramine
- Inapsine

Medications *(continued)*
- Indoklon
- isocarboxazid
- Libritabs
- Librium
- Lithane
- lithium
- Lithonate
- Luminal
- Marplan
- Mebaral
- Mellaril
- mephenytoin
- mephobarbital
- meprobamate
- Meratran
- Mesantoin
- mesoridazine
- methamphetamine
- methaqualone
- metharbital
- Methedrine
- methsuximide
- methylphenidate
- Methylphenylsuccini-mide
- methyprylon
- Metrazol
- Milontin
- Miltown
- Mysoline
- Nardil
- Navane
- Nembutal
- nialamide
- Niamid
- nikethamide
- Noctec

Medications *(continued)*

- Noludar
- Norodin
- Norpramin
- nortriptyline
- oxazepam
- Oxydess
- Paracetaldehyde
- Paradione
- paraldehyde
- paramethadione
- Parnate
- Peganone
- pentobarbital
- pentylenetetrazol
- Perke-One
- Permitil
- perphenazine
- Pertofrane
- Phedrisox
- phenacemide
- phenaglycodol
- phenelzine
- phenobarbital
- phenothiazine
- phensuximide
- Phenurone
- picrotoxin
- piperacetazine
- pipradrol
- Placidyl
- primidone
- prochlorperazine
- Proketazine
- Prolixin
- promazine
- protriptyline
- Quaalude

Medications *(continued)*

- Quide
- Raphetamine
- Repoise
- Ritalin
- secobarbital
- Seconal
- Semoxydrine
- Serax
- Serentil
- Sinequan
- Softran
- Solacen
- Somnafac
- Somnos
- Sparine
- Stelazine
- Suavitil
- Suvren
- Synatan
- Syndrox
- Taractan
- thiopropazate
- thioridazine
- thiothixene
- Thorazine
- Tindal
- Tofranil
- Trancopal
- tranylcypromine
- Tridione
- trifluoperazine
- triflupromazine
- Trilafon
- trimethadione
- tybamate
- Ultran
- Valium

Medications *(continued)*
    Vesprin
    Vistaril
    Vivactil
    Zamitam
    Zarontin
medicerebellar
medicerebral
medulla
    m. oblongata
    m. spinalis
medullary
medullispinal
medullitis
medulloblast
medulloblastoma
    Cushing's m.
medulloencephalic
medulloepithelioma
megalomania
megalomaniac
melancholia
    affective m.
    m. agitata
    agitated m.
    m. attonita
    m. with delirium
    flatuous m.
    m. hypochondriaca
    involution m.
    m. religiosa
    stuporous m.
melancholiac
melomania
memory
    affect m.
    anterograde m.
menarche

Mendel-Bechterew reflex
Ménière's syndrome
meningeal
meningematoma
meningeocortical
meningeoma
meningeorrhaphy
meninges
meninghematoma
meningina
meninginitis
meningioma
    angioblastic m.
    olfactory groove m.
meningiomatosis
meningism
meningismus
meningitic
meningitides
meningitis
    acute aseptic m.
    African m.
    aseptic m.
    benign lymphocytic m.
    cerebral m.
    cerebrospinal m.
    gummatous m.
    lymphocytic m.
    meningococcic m.
    metastatic m.
    m. necrotoxica reactiva
    occlusive m.
    m. ossificans
    otitic m.
    parameningococcus m.
    purulent m.
    Quincke's m.
    septicemic m.

meningitis *(continued)*
    m. serosa
    m. serosa circumscripta
    m. serosa circumscripta
      cystica
    serous m.
    m. sympathica
    torula m.
    torular m.
    tubercular m.
    tuberculous m.
meningitophobia
meningoarteritis
meningoblastoma
meningocele
meningocephalitis
meningocerebritis
meningococcemia
    acute fulminating m.
meningococci
meningococcidal
meningococcin
meningococcosis
meningococcus
meningocortical
meningoencephalitis
meningoencephalocele
meningoencephalomyelitis
meningoencephalopathy
meningoexothelioma
meningofibroblastoma
meningoma
meningomalacia
meningomyelitis
meningomyelocele
meningomyeloradiculitis
meningomyelorrhaphy
meningo-osteophlebitis

meningopathy
meningopneumonitis
meningorachidian
meningoradicular
meningoradiculitis
meningorecurrence
meningorrhagia
meningorrhea
meningothelioma
meningotyphoid
meningovascular
meninguria
meninx
    m. fibrosa
    m. serosa
    m. tenuis
    m. vasculosa
mentalia
meralgia
    m. paresthetica
merergastic
merorachischisis
Merzbacher-Pelizaeus disease
mesencephalon
mesencephalotomy
mesmerism
metacoele
metaphrenia
metaplexus
metapsyche
metapsychics
metapsychology
metatela
metathalamus
metencephal
metencephalic
metencephalon
metencephalospinal

method
    Dubois' m.
    Freud's cathartic m.
    Jung's m.
    Pavlov's m.
methomania
metonymy
Meyerding's
    curet
    gouge
    mallet
    osteotome
Meyer's theory
Meynert's
    commissure
    decussation
microcephaly
microcrania
micromania
microneurosurgery
microsurgery
miel-. See words beginning
    myel-.
mielo-. See words beginning
    myelo-.
migraine
    fulgurating m.
    ophthalmic m.
    ophthalmoplegic m.
migrateur
milieu
Millard-Gubler syndrome
Mills's disease
Minnesota Multiphasic
    Personality Inventory test
mio-. See words beginning
    myo-.
misaction

misandria
misanthropia
miso-. See also words
    beginning *myso-*.
misocainia
misogamy
misogyn
misogyny
misologia
misoneism
misopedia
mitho-. See words beginning
    mytho-.
MMPI — Minnesota Multi-
    phasic Personality
    Inventory
M'Naghten rule
Monckeberg's sclerosis
Mongolian idiot
mongolism
mongoloid
Monokow
    fasciculus aberrans of M.
monomania
monomoria
monoplegia
monorecidive
Monro
    foramen of M.
monticulus
    m. cerebelli
Morel-Kraepelin disease
Morgagni's hyperostosis
moria
moron
moronity
morphinomania
Morvan's chorea

motorium
    m. commune
MS – multiple sclerosis
Munchausen's syndrome
mutation
mute
mutism
    akinetic m.
    hysterical m.
myalgia
myasthenia
    m. gravis pseudo-
       paralytica
myatonia
mydriasis
    spinal m.
myelalgia
myelanalosis
myelapoplexy
myelasthenia
myelatelia
myelatrophy
myelauxe
myelencephalitis
myelencephalon
myelencephalospinal
myelencephalous
myeleterosis
myelic
myelin
myelinopathy
myelinosis
myelitis
myelobrachium
myelocele
myelocoele
myelocystocele
myelocystomeningocele

myelodysplasia
myeloencephalic
myeloencephalitis
myelofibrosis
myelogram
myelography
myeloid
myeloma
myelomalacia
myelomeningitis
myelomeningocele
myeloneuritis
myeloparalysis
myelopathy
myelophthisis
myeloradiculitis
myeloradiculodysplasia
myeloradiculopathy
myelorrhagia
myelorrhaphy
myelosarcoma
myeloschisis
myelosclerosis
myelosis
myelospasm
myelosyphilis
myelotome
myelotomy
    commissural m.
myoclonia
    m. epileptica
myoclonic
myoclonus
myohypertrophia
    m. kymoparalytica
myokymia
myoneural
mysophilia

mysophobia
mythomania
mythophobia
mythoplasty
Naffziger's syndrome
napex
narcism
narcissism
narcissistic
narcoanalysis
narcodiagnosis
narcohypnosis
narcolepsy
narcoleptic
narcolysis
narcomania
narcosis
narcosomania
narcosynthesis
narcotic
nasion
necrencephalus
necromania
necrophilia
necrophilism
necrophobia
necrosadism
needle
 Adson's n.
 Babcock's n.
 Cone's n.
 Gardner's n.
 New's n.
 Sachs' n.
 Ward-French n.
neencephalon
negativism
neocerebellum

neokinetic
neolallia
neolallism
neologism
neopallium
neophilism
neophobia
neophrenia
neoplasm
neostriatum
neothalamus
nerve
 Bell's n.
 trochlear n.
neural
neuralgia
 Hunt's n.
 trigeminal n.
neurapraxia
neurarchy
neurasthenia
neurastheniac
neurasthenic
neurataxia
neurataxy
neuratrophia
neuratrophic
neuratrophy
neuraxis
neuraxitis
neurectasia
neurectomy
 presacral n.
neurexeresis
neurilemoma
neurinoma
neuritis
neuroanastomosis

neuroanatomy
neuroblast
neuroblastoma
neurobrucellosis
neuroclonic
neurocytoma
neuroencephalomyelopathy
neuroepithelium
neurofibroma
neurofibromatosis
neuroglia
neurogliocytoma
neuroglioma
neurogliosis
neurohypophysis
neurolemma
neuroleptic
neurologia
neurological
neurologist
neurology
neurolysis
neuroma
neuromalacia
neuromatosis
neuromere
neuromyelitis
neuron
neuroparalysis
neuroparalytic
neuropath
neuropathic
neuropathogenesis
neuropathology
neuropathy
neurophonia
neuroplasty
neuropsychiatrist

neuropsychiatry
neuropsychic
neuropsychopathy
neuropsychosis
neuropyra
neuropyretic
neuroradiology
neurorecidive
neurorecurrence
neuroregulation
neurorelapse
neuroretinopathy
    hypertensive n.
neurorrhaphy
neurorrheuma
neurosarcokleisis
neurosarcoma
neurosclerosis
neurosecretion
neurosensory
neuroses
neurosis
    anxiety n.
    association n.
    cardiac n.
    compensation n.
    compulsion n.
    conversion n.
    depersonalization n.
    depressive n.
    expectation n.
    fatigue n.
    fixation n.
    gastric n.
    homosexual n.
    hypochondriacal n.
    hysterical n.
    intestinal n.

neurosis *(continued)*
    obsessional n.
    obsessive-compulsive n.
    occupation n.
    pension n.
    phobic n.
    professional n.
    rectal n.
    regression n.
    sexual n.
    torsion n.
    transference n.
    traumatic n.
    vegetative n.
    war n.
neurosism
neuroskeletal
neuroskeleton
neurosome
neurospasm
neurosplanchnic
neurospongioma
neurospongium
neurostatus
neurosthenia
neurosurgeon
neurosurgery
neurosyphilis
    ectodermogenic n.
    meningeal n.
    meningovascular n.
    mesodermogenic n.
    paretic n.
    tabetic n.
neurosystemitis
    n. epidemica
neurotabes
    n. diabetica

neurotherapy
neurothlipsis
neurotic
neurotica
neuroticism
neurotome
    Hall's n.
neurotomy
    retrogasserian n.
neurotripsy
neurotrophasthenia
New's needle
Niemann-Pick disease
nihilism
nimfo-. See words beginning
    nympho-.
nistagmus. See *nystagmus.*
noctiphobia
nodule
    Schmorl's n.
non compos mentis
notencephalocele
Nothnagel's
    sign
    syndrome
notomyelitis
nuclei
    n. arcuati
nucleus
    n. ambiguus
    cuneate n.
    Darkschewitsch's n.
    n. gracilis
    n. lateralis medullae
        oblongatae
    n. pulposus
numo-. See words beginning
    pneumo-.

nura-. See words beginning
    neura-.
nuro-. See words beginning
    neuro-.
nympholepsy
nymphomania
nymphomaniac
nystagmus
nystagmus-myoclonus
Obersteiner-Redlich area
obex
obliteration
    cortical o.
obnubilation
OBS — organic brain
    syndrome
obsession
obsessive
obsessive-compulsive
obtund
occipital
occipitalis
occipitalization
occipito-atloid
occipito-axoid
occipitobasilar
occipitobregmatic
occipitocervical
occipitofacial
occipitofrontal
occipitomastoid
occipitomental
occipitoparietal
occipitotemporal
occipitothalamic
occiput
oedipism
Oedipus complex

Oehler's symptom
ofthal-. See words beginning
    ophthal-.
oksesefale. See *oxycephaly*.
Oldberg's
    dissector
    forceps
    retractor
olfactory
oligergasia
oligergastic
oligodendroglia
oligodendroglioma
oligomania
oligophrenia
    phenylpyruvic o.
    o. phenylpyruvica
oligopsychia
oligoria
oliva
olivary
olivipetal
Olivecrona's clip
olivopontocerebellar
omahl. See *haut-mal*.
onanism
oneiric
oneirism
oneiroanalysis
oneirodynia
oneirogenic
oneirophrenia
oneiroscopy
onikotilomanea. See
    onychotillomania.
oniomania
onirik. See *oneiric*.
onirizm. See *oneirism*.

oniro-. See words beginning
   oneiro-.
onomatomania
onomatopoiesis
onychotillomania
operation
   Alexander's o.
   Förster-Penfield o.
   Haynes's o.
   Puusepp's o.
opercula
operculum
ophthalmencephalon
ophthalmoplegia
opisthion
opisthotonos
Oppenheim's
   gait
   sign
orientation
oriented
orthopsychiatry
oscillopsia
osteogenic
osteoma
osteoplastic
osteoplasty
osteotome
   Cherry's o.
   Lambotte's o.
osteotomy
otohemineurasthenia
overcompensation
overdetermination
overlay
   emotional o.
   psychogenic o.
overt

overtone
   psychic o.
oxycephaly
pachycephalia
pachyleptomeningitis
pachymeningitis
pakeonean. See *pacchionian*.
paleencephalon
paleocerebellar
paleocerebellum
paleocortex
paleophrenia
paleothalamus
palikinesia
palilalia
palinphrasia
pallidal
pallidectomy
pallidofugal
pallidotomy
pallidum
pallium
palsy
   Bell's p.
Pandy's test
panic
panophobia
Pansch's fissure
pantaphobia
pantophobia
pantophobic
papilledema
papilloma
   p. neuroticum
paracoele
paraganglioma
paraganglion
paragrammatism

paragraphia
paralexia
paralogia
    thematic p.
paralogism
paralysis
    Duchenne-Erb p.
    Landry's p.
    Werdnig-Hoffmann p.
paramyoclonus
paramyotonia
paranoia
    p. hallucinatoria
    heboid p.
    litigious p.
    p. originaria
    querulous p.
    p. simplex
paranoiac
paranoic
paranoid
paranoidism
paranomia
paranormal
paranosic
paranosis
paraparesis
parapathia
paraphasia
paraphasic
paraphasis
paraphemia
paraphia
paraphilia
paraphiliac
paraphobia
paraphora
paraphrasia

paraphrenia
    p. confabulans
    p. expansiva
    p. phantastica
    p. systematica
paraphrenic
paraphronia
paraplegia
paraplegic
parapraxia
parapsychology
parapsychosis
parareaction
parataxic
    p. distortion
paratrophy
parergasia
parergastic
paresis
paresthesia
parietal
parietofrontal
parieto-occipital
parietotemporal
Parinaud's syndrome
Parkinson's
    disease
    facies
    syndrome
parkinsonian
parkinsonism
    postencephalitis p.
paroksizmal. See *paroxysmal.*
parorexia
paroxysmal
Parrot's
    atrophy of the newborn
    sign

pars
- p. centralis ventriculi lateralis cerebri
- p. cervicalis medullae spinalis
- p. frontalis radiationis corporis callosi
- p. inferior fossae rhomboideae
- p. inferior gyri frontalis medii
- p. intermedia fossae rhomboideae
- p. lumbalis medullae spinalis
- p. marginalis sulci cinguli
- p. occipitalis radiationis corporis callosi
- p. opercularis gyri frontalis inferioris
- p. orbitalis gyri frontalis inferioris
- p. parasympathica systematis nervosi autonomici
- p. parietalis operculi
- p. parietalis radiationis corporis callosi
- p. petrosa ossis temporalis
- p. posterior commissurae anterioris cerebri
- p. posterior rhinencephali
- p. subfrontalis sulci cinguli
- p. superior fossae

pars *(continued)*
- rhomboideae
- p. superior gyri frontalis medii
- p. sympathica systematis nervosi autonomici

pathergasia
pathognomonic
pathognomy
pathophobia
Pavlov's method
pavor
- p. diurnus
- p. nocturnus

Pecquet's cistern
pederasty
pederosis
pedophilia
pedophilic
pedophobia
peduncle
- cerebellar p.
- cerebral p.
- p. of flocculus
- p. of hypophysis
- olfactory p.
- olivary p. of Schwalbe
- pineal p.
- p. of pineal body
- p. of thalamus, inferior

pedunculotomy
pedunculus
- p. cerebellaris, inferior, medius, superior
- p. cerebri
- p. corporis callosi
- p. corporis pinealis
- p. flocculi

pedunculus
    p. thalami inferior
PEG – pneumoencephalog-
   raphy
pellagra
perception
    extrasensory p.
perceptorium
pericranitis
pericranium
periosteal
periosteum
pero
perseveration
persona
personality
    alternating p.
    anancastic p.
    antisocial p.
    asthenic p.
    cyclothymic p.
    disordered p.
    double p.
    dual p.
    explosive p.
    hysterical p.
    inadequate p.
    multiple p.
    obsessive compulsive p.
    paranoid p.
    passive-aggressive p.
    psychopathic p.
    schizoid p.
    seclusive p.
    shut-in p.
perversion
pervert
pessimism

petit mal
petrosal
pfropfhebephrenia
pfropfschizophrenia
phallic
phaneromania
phantasm
phantasmatomoria
phantasmoscopia
phantasy
pharmacomania
pharmacophilia
pharmacophobia
pharmacopsychosis
phenomenology
phenomenon
    Babinski's p.
    Bell's p.
    Hunt's paradoxical p.
    Trousseau's p.
phenotype
phenylketonuria
phenylpyruvic
    p. oligophrenia
phlegmatic
phobia
phobic
phobophobia
phrenemphraxis
phrenic
phrenicectomy
phreniclasia
phreniconeurectomy
phrenicotomy
phrenicotripsy
phrenology
phrenopathic
phrenopathy

phrenoplegia
phthisiomania
phthisiophobia
physiopathic
physiopsychic
pia
    p. mater
pia-arachnitis
pia-arachnoid
piaglia
pial
pia mater
    p. m. encephali
    p. m. spinalis
piamatral
piarachnitis
piarachnoid
pica
Pick's
    convolutional atrophy
    disease
piknic. See *pyknic.*
pikno-. See words beginning
    pykno-.
pileum
pileus
pineal
pinealectomy
pinealoma
Pinel's system
pira-. See words beginning
    pyra-.
piro-. See words beginning
    pyro-.
pituitary
pituitectomy
PKU – phenylketonuria
plagiocephaly

plaque
    Lichtheim's p's.
    Redlich-Fisher miliary
        p's.
    senile p's.
plate
    Hoen's skull p.
platybasia
pleocytosis
plexus
    brachial p.
    carotid p.
    cervical p.
    p. cervicobrachialis
    choroid p.
    p. choroideus ventriculi
        lateralis
    p. choroideus ventriculi
        quarti
    p. choroideus ventriculi
        tertii
    p. vertebralis
pneumocephalon
    p. artificiale
pneumocephalus
pneumoencephalogram
pneumoencephalography
pneumoencephalomyelogram
pneumoencephalomyelog-
    raphy
pneumoencephalos
pneumomyelography
poliencephalomyelitis
polioclastic
polioencephalitis
polioencephalomeningo-
    myelitis
polioencephalopathy

poliomyelencephalitis
poliomyelitis
    bulbar p.
poliomyelopathy
polioneuromere
polyclonia
polyparesis
polyphagia
pons
    p. cerebelli
    p. varolii
pons-oblongata
pontibrachium
ponticulus
pontile
pontine
pontobulbia
pontocerebellar
porencephalia
porencephalic
porencephalitis
poriomania
pornographomania
pornolagnia
porphyria
postictal
potency
pouch
    Rathke's p.
Pratt's curet
precocious
precocity
precognition
preconscious
preconvulsant
preconvulsive
precuneus
predisposition

prefrontal
pregenital
preoblongata
priapism
projection
pronation
propons
prosencephalon
protuberance
    occipital p.
psalis
psalterium
pseudocoele
pseudologia
    p. fantastica
pseudosclerosis
    p. spastica
pseudotabes
psychalgalia
psychalgia
psychalgic
psychalia
psychanalysis
psychanopsia
psychasthene
psychasthenia
psychasthenic
psychataxia
psyche
psycheclampsia
psychedelic
psychiater
psychiatric
psychiatrics
psychiatrist
psychiatry
psychic
psychics

psychinosis
psychlampsia
psychoalgalia
psychoallergy
psychoanaleptic
psychoanalysis
psychoanalyst
psychoanalytic
psychoanalyze
psychoasthenics
psychoauditory
psychobacillosis
psychobiological
psychobiology
psychocatharsis
psychocentric
psychochemistry
psychochrome
psychochromesthesia
psychocoma
psychocortical
psychodelic
psychodiagnosis
psychodiagnostics
psychodometer
psychodometry
psychodrama
psychodynamics
psychodysleptic
psychoepilepsy
psychogalvanometer
psychogenesis
psychogenia
psychogenic
psychogenous
psychogeriatrics
psychognosis
psychognostic

psychogogic
psychogram
psychograph
psychokinesia
psychokinesis
psychokym
psycholagny
psycholepsy
psycholeptic
psycholinguistics
psychologic
psychological
psychologist
psychology
psychomathematics
psychometer
psychometrics
psychometry
psychomotor
psychoneuroses
psychoneurosis
    p. maidica
    paranoid p.
psychonomy
psychonosema
psychonosis
psychoparesis
psychopath
psychopathia
    p. martialis
    p. sexualis
psycopathic
psychopathist
psychopathology
psychopathosis
psychopathy
psychopharmacology
psychophonasthenia

psychophylaxis
psychophysical
psychophysics
psychophysiology
psychoplegia
psychoplegic
psychopneumatology
psychoprophylactic
psychoprophylaxis
psychoreaction
psychorhythmia
psychorrhagia
psychorrhea
psychorrhexis
psychosensorial
psychosensory
psychoses
psychosexual
psychosis
    Cheyne-Stokes p.
    gestational p.
    idiophrenic p.
    Korsakoff's p.
    manic p.
    manic-depressive p.
    paranoiac p.
    paranoid p.
    polyneuritic p.
    p. polyneuritica
    postpartum p.
    puerperal p.
    schizoaffective p.
    senile p.
    situational p.
    toxic p.
    zoophil p.
psychosolytic
psychosomatic

psychosomaticist
psychosomimetic
psychosurgery
psychotechnics
psychotherapeutics
psychotherapy
psychotic
psychotogenic
psychotomimetic
psychotonic
psychotropic
psychrophobia
ptosis
Pudenz'
    shunt
    tube
    valve
puerile
puerilism
pulvinar
puncture
    cisternal p.
    Corning's p.
    lumbar p.
    thecal p.
    ventricular p.
putamen
Puusepp's
    operation
    reflex
pyknic
pyknoepilepsy
pyknophrasia
pyramid
pyramidal
pyramidotomy
pyramis
pyrolagnia

pyromania
quadrantanopia
quadriplegia
Queckenstedt's sign
querulous
Quincke's meningitis
Quinquaud's sign
rachialbuminimetry
rachialgia
rachicentesis
rachidial
rachidian
rachilysis
rachiocampsis
rachiochysis
rachiodynia
rachiomyelitis
rachiotomy
rachischisis
rachitis
rachitome
rachitomy
radicular
radiculectomy
radiculitis
radiculoganglionitis
radiculomedullary
radiculomeningomyelitis
radiculomyelopathy
radiculoneuritis
radiculopathy
radioencephalogram
radioencephalography
Raeder's syndrome
rafe. See *raphe.*
rahpor. See *rapport.*
rake-. See words beginning
    rachi-.

rakeal-. See words beginning
    rachial-.
rakeo-. See words beginning
    rachio-.
rakiskisis. See *rachischisis.*
rakitis. See *rachitis.*
ramisection
ramitis
ramus
Raney's
        clip
        curet
        drill
        forceps
raphe
rapport
Rathke's
        pouch
        tumor
rational
rationalization
Raymond's apoplexy
Ray's mania
reaction formation
reaction
        Cushing's r.
        Jolly's r.
receptor
recessus
        r. infundibuli
        r. lateralis fossae
            rhomboidei
        r. lateralis ventriculi
            quarti
        r. pinealis
        r. suprapinealis
        r. triangularis
recidivism
recidivist

Redlich-Fisher miliary plaques
reflex
    Achilles tendon r.
    Babinski's r.
    Brain's r.
    Brissaud's r.
    carotid sinus r.
    cerebral cortex r.
    Chaddock's r.
    Hirschberg's r.
    Joffroy's r.
    Lust's r.
    McCarthy's r.
    Mendel-Bechterew r.
    Puusepp's r.
    quadrupedal extensor r.
    Remak's r.
    Riddoch's mass r.
    Rossolimo's r.
    Schaefer's r.
    tarsophalangeal r.
    Throckmorton's r.
    wrist clonus r.
regression
    atavistic r.
reinnervation
REM – rapid eye movement
Remak's reflex
Rendu-Osler-Weber disease
Rendu's tremor
repression
resistance
respiration
    Biot's r.
restibrachium
retardate
retardation
    psychomotor r.

rete
    r. canalis hypoglossi
retractor
    Adson's r.
    Barrett-Adson r.
    Beckman-Adson r.
    Beckman-Eaton r.
    Beckman's r.
    Bucy's r.
    Chandler's r.
    Cherry's r.
    Cloward-Hoen r.
    Cone's r.
    Contour's r.
    Cushing's r.
    Davidoff's r.
    Davidson's r.
    Davis' r.
    D'Errico-Adson r.
    D'Errico's r.
    Frazier's r.
    French s-shaped r.
    Gifford's r.
    Hamby's r.
    Jansen's r.
    Love's r.
    Meyerding's r.
    Oldberg's r.
    Sachs' r.
    Scoville's r.
    Sheldon's r.
    Snitman's r.
    Taylor's r.
    Tower's r.
    Tuffier-Raney r.
    Tuffier's r.
    Ullrich's r.
    Weitlaner's r.

retrobulbar
retrogasserian
retropulsion
rhinencephalon
rhinorrhea
    cerebrospinal r.
rhizotomy
rhombencephalon
rhombocoele
rhythm
    alpha r.
    Berger r.
    beta r.
    gamma r.
Riddoch's mass reflex
rigidity
    cerebellar r.
    hemiplegic r.
    lead-pipe r.
    nuchal r.
rigor
    r. nervorum
    r. tremens
Rimbaud-Passouant-Vallat
  syndrome
rimula
rinensefalon. See
  rhinencephalon.
rinorea. See *rhinorrhea.*
risus
    r. caninus
    r. sardonicus
rizotomee. See *rhizotomy.*
RNA – Ribonucleic acid
Rochester's
    connector
    elevator
rolandometer

rombensefalon. See
  rhombencephalon.
rombergism
Romberg's
    disease
    sign
rombosel. See *rhombocoele.*
Rorschach test
Rossolimo's reflex
rostrum
    r. corporis callosi
Roth-Bernhardt disease
Roth's disease
Roussy-Cornil syndrome
rule
    Jackson's r.
    M'Naghten r.
rumination
    obsessive r.
Rumpf's sign
Ruskin's forceps
Sachs'
    guard
    needle
    retractor
    spatula
    suction tube
sacroiliac
sacrospinal
sacrovertebral
sadism
sadist
sadistic
sadomasochistic
Saenger's sign
sagittal
sal-. See words beginning *psal-.*
Salibi's clamp

saltation
saltereum. See *psalterium.*
Sanger-Brown's ataxia
Sarbó's sign
satellitosis
satyriasis
satyromania
saw
      Gigli's s.
scaphocephalia
Schaefer's reflex
Schilder's disease
schizocephalia
schizogyria
schizoid
schizoidism
schizophasia
schizophrenia
schizophreniac
schizophrenic
schizophreniform
schizophrenosis
Schlesinger's forceps
Schmorl's
      body
      disease
      nodule
Schrötter's chorea
Schutz's
      clip
      forceps
Schwalbe
      olivary peduncle of S.
schwannoma
Schwann's
      sheath
      white substance
sciatica

scissors
      Adson's s.
      Craig's s.
      craniotomy s.
      Dandy's s.
      Smellie's s.
      Stevenson's s.
      Strully's s.
      Taylor's s.
scleromeninx
sclerosis
      Alzheimer's s.
      amyotrophic lateral s.
      annular s.
      anterolateral s.
      arterial s.
      arteriolar s.
      arteriopapillary s.
      benign s.
      bone s.
      bulbar s.
      cerebellar s.
      cerebral s.
      cerebrospinal s.
      cervical s.
      s. circumscripta
        pericardii
      disseminated s.
      Erb's s.
      familial centrolobar s.
      hyperplastic s.
      insular s.
      Krabbe's s.
      Marie's s.
      miliary s.
      Mönckeberg's s.
      multiple s.
      nodular s.

sclerosis *(continued)*
    posterolateral s.
    presenile s.
    s. redux
    renal arteriolar s.
    s. tuberosa
    tuberous s.
    unicellular s.
    vascular s.
    venous s.
    ventrolateral s.
scoliosis
scotoma
scotomization
scotophobia
Scott's cannula
Scoville's
    forceps
    retractor
sefal-. See words beginning
    cephal-.
Seguin's signal symptom
seizure
    audiogenic s.
    cerebral s.
    photogenic s.
    psychic s.
    psychomotor s.
sejunction
selenoplegia
selenoplexia
Seletz's cannula
self-suspension
sella
    s. turcica
semicoma
semicomatose
semicretinism

seminarcosis
sensorial
sensorium
sensory
separator
    Horsley's s.
septum
    s. pellucidum
    s. pontis
serotonin
Setchenow's centers
Sewall's forceps
sfeno-. See words beginning
    spheno-.
sfenoid. See *sphenoid.*
sheath
    Schwann's s.
Sheldon's retractor
shunt
    Pudenz' s.
    Silastic ventricular-
        peritoneal s.
shwonnoma. See *schwannoma.*
siatika. See *sciatica.*
sibling
sifilis. See *syphilis.*
sifilo-. See words beginning
    syphilo-.
sign
    Babinski's s.
    Ballet's s.
    Bragard's s.
    Brudzinski's s.
    Chaddock's s.
    Chvostek's s.
    Claude's hyperkinesis s.
    Déjerine's s.
    Hoffmann's s.

sign *(continued)*
  Kernig's s.
  Lafora's s.
  Laségue's s.
  Leichtenstern's s.
  Leri's s.
  Lhermitte's s.
  Lichtheim's s.
  Nothnagel's s.
  Oppenheim's s.
  Parrot's s.
  Queckenstedt's s.
  Quinquaud's s.
  Romberg's s.
  Rumpf's s.
  Saenger's s.
  Sarbo's s.
  Tinel's s.
  Trousseau's s.
  Wartenberg's s.
  Weber's s.
  Westphal's s.
sika-. See words beginning
 psycha-.
sikal-. See words beginning
 psychal-.
sikan-. See words beginning
 psychan-.
sikas-. See words beginning
 psychas-.
sike-. See words beginning
 psyche-.
siki-. See words beginning
 psychi-.
siko-. See words beginning
 psycho-.
Silastic ventricular-
 peritoneal shunt

siliqua
 s. olivae
Simmonds' disease
sin-. See also words beginning
 cin-, and words beginning
 syn-.
sinciput
sinerea. See *cinerea.*
singulum. See *cingulum.*
singulumotome. See
 cingulumotomy.
sinistrocerebral
sinistrosis
siringo-. See words beginning
 syringo-.
skafosefalea. See
 scaphocephalia.
skizo-. See words beginning
 schizo-.
sklero-. See words beginning
 sclero-.
skull
SLR – straight leg raising
Smellie's scissors
Snitman's retractor
sociology
sociopath
sodomy
soma
somatic
somatization
somatophrenia
somatopsychic
somatopsychosis
somnambulism
somniloquism
somnipathy
somnolence

somnolentia
somnolism
somopsychosis
space
    Broca's s.
    Magendie's s's.
spasm
spastic
spatula
    Cushing's s.
    Davis' s.
    Sachs' s.
Spence-Adson forceps
Spence's forceps
sphenoethmoid
sphenofrontal
sphenoid
sphenoidal
spina
    s. bifida
    s. bifida occulta
spine
spinobulbar
spinocerebellar
spinogalvanization
spinous
splanchnicectomy
splanchnicotomy
splanknekotome. See
    splanchnicotomy.
splanknesektome. See
    splanchnicectomy.
splenium
    s. corporis callosi
spondylitis
spondylodesis
spondylolisthesis
spondylolysis

spondylomalacia
spondylopathy
spondylopyosis
spondyloschisis
spondylosis
    s. chronica ankylopoi-
        etica
    rhizomelic s.
spondylosyndesis
spondylotomy
spongioblast
spongioblastoma
spongiocyte
spoon
    Cushing's s.
spot
    Trousseau's s.
spreader
    Turek's s.
    Wiltberger's s.
Spurling's forceps
stability
stammering
Stanford-Binet test
stasiphobia
status
    s. choreicus
    s. convulsivus
    s. cribalis
    s. cribrosus
    s. dysgraphicus
    s. dysmyelinatus
    s. dysmyelinisatus
    s. dysraphicus
    s. epilepticus
    s. hemicranicus
    s. lacunaris
    s. lacunosus

status *(continued)*
    s. marmoratus
    petit mal s.
    s. spongiosus
    s. verrucosus
    s. vertiginosus
Stearn's alcoholic amentia
stefaneon. See *stephanion.*
Steiner's disease
stellate
stellectomy
stenion
stephanion
stereoencephalotomy
stereognosis
stereotypy
Stevenson's
    forceps
    scissors
Stille-Luer forceps
Stille's drill
stimulate
stimulus
stratum
    s. album profundum
      corporis quadrigemini
    s. gangliosum cerebelli
    s. gelatinosum
    s. granulosum cerebelli
    s. griseum centrale
      cerebri
    s. griseum colliculi
      superioris
    s. interolivare lemnisci
    s. moleculare cerebelli
    s. nucleare medullae
      oblongatae
    s. olfactorium

stratum *(continued)*
    s. opticum
    s. pyramidale
    s. reticulatum
    s. zonale corporis
      quadrigemini
    s. zonale thalami
strephosymbolia
stria
    s. fornicis
    habenular s.
    s. lancisii
    s. medullaris thalami
    meningitic s.
    olfactory s.
    s. pinealis
    s. terminalis
striae
    Francke's s.
    s. medullares acusticae
    s. medullares fossae
      rhomboideae
    s. medullares ventriculi
      quarti
strikninomanea. See
    strychninomania.
Stromeyer's cephalhematocele
Strully's scissors
strychninomania
Stryker's frame
stupor
    anergic s.
    delusion s.
    epileptic s.
    lethargic s.
    postconvulsive s.
stuporous
Sturge's disease

Sturge-Weber
    disease
    syndrome
stuttering
    labiochoreic s.
subarachnoid
subarachnoiditis
subconscious
subconsciousness
subcortical
subdural
subgaleal
subjective
sublimate
sublimation
subpial
subpontine
substance
    white s. of Schwann
substantia
    s. alba
    c. cinerea
    s. corticalis cerebelli
    s. gelatinosa
    s. grisea
    s. innominata
    s. nigra
    s. perforata
    s. reticularis alba gyri
      fornicati
substitution
subthalamus
suction tube
    Adson's s. t.
    Frazier's s. t.
    Sachs' s. t.
sudo-. See words beginning
    pseudo-.

Sugar's clip
suicide
sulcus
    s. basilaris pontis
    calcarine s.
    callosal s.
    cingulate s.
    s. collateralis
    s. corporis callosi
    s. hippocampi
    s. hypothalamicus
    s. limitans
    s. lunatus
    paramedial s.
superdural
superego
supination
suppression
surgical procedures. See
    operation.
surrogate
Sydenham's chorea
Sylvii
    cisterna S.
    cisterna fossae S.
Sylvius
    aqueduct of S.
    cistern of fossa of S.
    cistern of S.
    fissure of S.
    ventricle of S.
symbiosis
symbol
    phallic s.
symbolism
symbolization
symbolophobia
sympathectomy

sympathicotripsy
sympathomimetic
symptom
 Bonhoeffer's s.
 Ganser's s.
 Haenel's s.
 Oehler's s.
 Seguin's signal s.
 Trendelenburg's s.
synclonus
syncopal
syncope
syndrome
 Adie's s.
 Alzheimer's s.
 Apert's s.
 Arnold-Chiari s.
 Baastrup's s.
 Babinski-Nageotte s.
 Babinski's s.
 Balint's s.
 Bárány's s.
 Barré-Liéou s.
 Bärtschi-Rochain's s.
 Beard's s.
 Beck's s.
 Bonnet's s.
 Briquet's s.
 Brissaud-Sicard s.
 Bristowe's s.
 Brown-Séquard s.
 Bruns' s.
 callosal s.
 Capgras's s.
 capsular thrombosis s.
 capsulothalamic s.
 Céstan-Chenais s.
 Claude's s.

syndrome *(continued)*
 Cotard's s.
 Cushing's s.
 Dandy-Walker s.
 Déjerine-Roussy s.
 Déjerine's s.
 Devic's s.
 Down's s.
 Erb's s.
 Foix-Alajouanine s.
 Foville's s.
 Friderichsen-Waterhouse s.
 Friedmann's vasomotor s.
 Fröhlich's s.
 Froin's s.
 Ganser's s.
 Garcin's s.
 Gélineau's s.
 Gerstmann's s.
 Gilles de la Tourette's s.
 Gradenigo's s.
 Guillain-Barré s.
 Hallervorden-Spatz s.
 Homén's s.
 Hunt's striatal s.
 Hurler's s.
 Jackson's s.
 Jakob-Creutzfeld s.
 Kanner's s.
 Kiloh-Nevin s.
 Klippel-Feil s.
 Klippel-Feldstein s.
 Klüver-Bucy s.
 Korsakoff's s.
 Marchiafava-Bignami s.
 Ménière's s.

syndrome *(continued)*
  Millard-Gubler s.
  Munchausen's s.
  Naffziger's s.
  Nothnagel's s.
  Parinaud's s.
  Parkinson's s.
  Raeder's s.
  Rimbaud-Passouant-
   Vallat s.
  Roussy-Cornil s.
  scalenus anticus s.
  Sturge-Weber s.
  Vogt-Koyanagi-Harada's
   s.
  Vogt's s.
  Wallenberg's s.
  Waterhouse-Friderich-
   sen s.
  Wernicke-Korsakoff s.
synesthesia
synesthesialgia
synkinesis
synthesis
syntonic
syphilis
syphilophobia
syphilopsychosis
syringobulbia
syringocele
syringocoele
syringoencephalia
syringoencephalomyelia
syringomeningocele
syringomyelia
  s. atrophica
syringomyelitis
syringomyelocele

syringomyelus
syringopontia
system
  Conolly's s.
  Pinel's s.
tabes
  cerebral t.
  diabetic t.
  t. dorsalis
  t. ergotica
  Friedreich's t.
  t. spinalis
tabetic
taboparesis
tache
  t. cerebrale
  t. meningeale
  t. spinale
tachyphrasia
tachyphrenia
taedium
  t. vitae
taenia
  t. chorioidea
  t. cinerea
  t. fimbriae
  t. fornicis
  t. hippocampi
  t. medullaris thalami
   optici
  t. pontis
  t. semicircularis
   corporis striati
  t. tectae
  t. thalami
  t. violacea
taeniae
  t. acusticae

taeniae
> t. telarum

tahsh. See *tache.*

tantalum sheet

tapeinocephaly

tapetum
> t. corporis callosi
> t. ventriculi

tasikinesia

TAT — thematic apperception test

Taylor's
> retractor
> scissors

Tay-Sachs disease

tedeum. See *taedium.*

tegmentum
> hypothalamic t.
> t. rhombencephali
> subthalamic t.

telencephalon

telepathy

temp. dext. — to the right temple

tempora

temporal

temporalis

temporoauricular

temporofacial

temporofrontal

temporohyoid

temporomalar

temporomandibular

temporomaxillary

temporo-occipital

temporoparietal

temporopontile

temporosphenoid

temporozygomatic

temp. sinist. — to the left temple

tenia
> t. choroidea
> t. telae

teniola

tentorium
> t. cerebelli
> t. of hypophysis

tephromalacia

tephromyelitis

test
> Barany's pointing t.
> Bender-Gestalt t.
> Ebbinghaus' t.
> finger-nose t.
> finger-to-finger t.
> heel-knee t.
> Janet's t.
> Minnesota Multiphasic Personality Inventory t.
> Pandy's t.
> Rorschach t.
> Stanford-Binet t.
> thematic apperception t.
> Tobey-Ayer t.
> Walter's bromide t.
> Wechsler's Adult Intelligence Scale t.
> Weschler's Intelligence Scale for Children t.
> Wittenborn Psychiatric Rating Scale t.
> Yerkes-Bridges t.
> Ziehen's t.

tetraplegia

thalamencephalon
thalamotomy
thalamus
theory
    Adler's t.
    Freud's t.
    Gestalt t.
    Meyer's t.
therapy
    carbon dioxide t.
    convulsive shock t.
    electric convulsive t.
    electroshock t.
    group t.
    Indoklon t.
    lithium t.
    milieu t.
    shock t.
Thomsen's disease
Throckmorton's reflex
thrombosis
thymergastic
thymopathy
tic
    t. de pensée
    t. de sommeil
    t. douloureux
    t. nondouloureux
Tinel's sign
titubation
    lingual t.
tizeo-. See words beginning
   phthisio-.
Tobey-Ayer test
tongs
    Barton-Cone t.'s.
    Cherry's t.'s.
    Crutchfield-Raney t.'s.

tongs
    Crutchfield's t.'s.
tonsil
    t. of cerebellum
tonsilla
    t. cerebelli
    t. of cerebellum
tonus
    neurogenic t.
topagnosis
topectomy
torticollis
tosis. See *ptosis.*
Tourette's disease
Tower's retractor
toxiphrenia
trabecula
    t. cerebri
    t. cinerea
    t. cranii
trabs
    t. cerebri
trachelism
trachelismus
tract
    Burdach's t.
    Foville's t.
    Goll's t.
    Helweg's t.
    Lissauer's t.
tractotomy
    mesencephalic t.
trait
trance
tranquilizer
transference
transorbital
transvestism

trauma
    psychic t.
traumasthenia
treatment
    Weir Mitchell t.
tremor
    epileptoid t.
    flapping t.
    Hunt's t.
    intention t.
    intermittent t.
    kinetic t.
    t. linguae
    motofacient t.
    t. potatorum
    Rendu's t.
    striocerebellar t.
    volitional t.
tremulous
Trendelenburg's symptom
trephination
trephine
    DeVilbiss' t.
    Galt's t.
trichologia
trichotillomania
trigone
trigonocephaly
trigonum
    t. acustici
    t. cerebrale
    t. collaterale
    t. habenulae
    t. lemnisci
    t. nervi hypoglossi
    t. olfactorium
triplegia
trismus

trisomy 13, 18, 21
Trousseau's
    phenomenon
    sign
    spot
    twitching
truncal
truncus
    t. corporis callosi
    t. lumbosacralis
    t. sympathicus
tube
    Pudenz' t.
tuber
    t. annulare
    t. anterius hypothalami
    t. cinereum
    t. vermis
tuberculoma
    t. en plaque
tuberculum
Tuffier-Raney retractor
Tuffier's retractor
tumor
    Cushing's t.
    Rathke's t.
Turek's spreader
twitch
twitching
    fascicular t.
    fibrillar t.
    Trousseau's t.
type
    Kretschmer t's.
ufor-. See words beginning
    euphor-.
ulegyria
Ullrich's retractor

unconscious
uncus
underhorn
unoia. See *eunoia.*
Unverricht's disease
urolagnia
urophobia
vadum
vagabondage
vagal
vagotomy
vagotonia
vallecula
    v. cerebelli
    v. sylvii
Valsalva's maneuver
valve
    Pudenz' v.
varolian
velamenta cerebri
velum
    medullary v.
ventricle
    v. of Arantius
    v's of the brain
    v. of cerebrum
    v. of cord
    Duncan's v.
    Krause's v.
    v. of myelon
    v. of Sylvius
    terminal v. of spinal cord
    Verga's v.
    Vieussen's v.
ventricornu
ventricornual
ventricose
ventricular

ventriculitis
ventriculoatriostomy
ventriculocisternostomy
ventriculogram
ventriculography
ventriculometry
ventriculopuncture
ventriculoscope
ventriculoscopy
ventriculostium
ventriculostomy
ventriculosubarachnoid
ventriculus
    v. dexter cerebri
    v. lateralis cerebri
    v. quartus cerebri
    v. sinister cerebri
    v. terminalis medullae
      spinalis
    v. tertius cerebri
Veraguth's fold
verbigeration
verbomania
Verga's ventricle
vermis
    v. cerebelli
vertebra
vertebrae
vertebral
vertex
    v. cranii
    v. cranii ossei
vertigo
    encephalic v.
    hysterical v.
    neurasthenic v.
    paralyzing v.
vesania

vibratory
vicious
Vieussens'
    ansa
    ventricle
visuopsychic
vitselzookt. See *witzelsucht.*
Vogt-Koyanagi-Harada's
    syndrome
Vogt's
    disease
    syndrome
volition
volitional
von Hippel-Lindau disease
von Recklinghausen's disease
voyeurism
Vulpian's atrophy
WAIS — Wechsler's Adult
    Intelligence Scale
Wallenberg's syndrome
wallerian
    degeneration
    law
Walter's bromide test
Ward-French needle
Wartenberg's sign
Waterhouse-Friderichsen
    syndrome
wave
    alpha w's.
    beta w's.
    brain w's.
    delta w's.
    random w's.
    theta w's.
Weber's
    disease

Weber's
    sign
Wechsler's Adult Intelligence
    Scale test
Wechsler's Intelligence Scale
    for Children test
WEE — western equine
    encephalomyelitis
Weir Mitchell treatment
Weitlaner's retractor
Werdnig-Hoffman
    atrophy
    paralysis
Wernicke-Korsakoff syndrome
Wernicke's
    disease
    encephalopathy
Westphal's sign
Wilde's forceps
Willis' circle
Wiltberger's spreader
wing
    sphenoid w.
Winkelman's disease
WISC — Wechsler's
    Intelligence Scale for
    Children
Wittenborn Psychiatric Rating
    Scale test
witzelsucht
WPRS — Wittenborn
    Psychiatric Rating Scale
xanthochromia
xanthochromic
xanthocyanopsia
xanthogranulomatosis
xenophobia
Yerkes-Bridges test

zan-. See words beginning *xan-*.
zelotypia
zenophobia. See *xenophobia*.
Ziehen-Oppenheim disease
Ziehen's test
zona
      a. rolandica
      z. spongiosa
zoophobia
Zuckerkandl's convolution

zygion
zygoma
zygomatic
zygomaticofacial
zygomaticofrontal
zygomaticomaxillary
zygomatico-orbital
zygomaticosphenoid
zygomaticotemporal
zygomaxillary

RESPIRATORY SYSTEM

aasmus
Abelson's cannula
Abraham's
    cannula
    sign
Actinomyces
    A. bovis
actinomycosis
    pulmonary a.
Adair's forceps
adenocarcinoma
adenoma
    bronchial a.
adenomatosis
    pulmonary a.
adenovirus
aeration
aerodermectasia
aeroemphysema
aeroionotherapy
aeroporotomy
aerosol
agenesis
agent
    Eaton a.
airway
    a. resistance
Albert's bronchoscope
Allis' forceps
alveobronchiolitis
alveolar

alveoli
    a. pulmonis
alveolitis
    diffuse sclerosing a.
amebiasis
    pulmonary a.
amyloidosis
anapnoic
anapnotherapy
Andrews' retractor
Andrews-Pynchon tube
anesthesia
    cocaine a.
    endotracheal a.
    intravenous a.
aneurysm
angiogram
angiography
    pulmonary a.
anomaly
    Freund's a.
anthracosis
anthropotoxin
aorta
    retroesophageal a.
apicolysis
apneumatosis
apneumia
apneusis
apparatus
    Fell-O'Dwyer a.

applicator
  Plummer-Vinson
    radium a.
arch
  aortic a.
arcus
  a. costarum
ARD – acute respiratory
  disease
area
  Krönig's a.
Arneth's syndrome
artery
  pulmonary a.
  subclavian a.
arytenoid
asbestosis
aspergillosis
  pulmonary a.
asphyxia
aspirator
  Broyles' a.
Assmann's
  focus
  infiltrate
asthma
  bronchial a.
atelectasis
  compression a.
atelectatic
Atkins-Cannard tube
Atlee's clamp
atmograph
atmotherapy
atresia
atrium
  pulmonary a.
auscultation

Ayerza's
  disease
  syndrome
azygography
azygos
Babcock's forceps
Bacteroides
bagassosis
Bailey's catheter
Balme's cough
Bard's syndrome
baritosis
Bársony-Polgár syndrome
Beatty-Bright friction
  sound
Belsey's repair
Benedict's gastroscope
Bernay's retractor
berylliosis
Bethune's tourniquet
Biermer's change
bifurcatio
  b. trachea
bifurcation
bilharziasis
biopsy
  scalene lymph node b.
bistoury
  Jackson's b.
Blakemore's tube
Blalock-Taussig operation
blastomycosis
bleb
blennothorax
Boies' forceps
bolus
Bornholm's disease
Boros' esophagoscope

bougie
 Hurst's b.
 Jackson's b.
 Trousseau's b.
BP – bronchopleural
Bragg-Paul pulsator
Brewster's retractor
Brock's syndrome
bronchadenitis
bronchi
 hyparterial b.
 lobar b.
 b. lobares
 segmental b.
 b. segmentales
bronchia
bronchial
bronchiectasis
 capillary b.
 pseudocylindrical b.
 saccular b.
bronchiectatic
bronchiloquy
bronchiocele
bronchiocrisis
bronchiole
 alveolar b's.
 respiratory b's.
 terminal b's.
bronchiolectasis
bronchioli respiratorii
bronchiolitis
 acute obliterating b.
 b. exudativa
 b. fibrosa obliterans
 vesicular b.
bronchiolus
bronchiospasm

bronchitic
bronchitis
 arachidic b.
 Castellani's b.
 catarrhal b.
 croupous b.
 exudative b.
 fibrinous b.
 hemorrhagic b.
 membranous b.
 b. obliterans
 phthinoid b.
 plastic b.
 polypoid b.
 productive b.
 pseudomembranous b.
 putrid b.
 staphylococcus b.
 streptococcus b.
 suffocative b.
 verminous b.
 vesicular b.
bronchium
bronchoalveolar
bronchoaspergillosis
bronchobiliary
bronchoblastomycosis
bronchoblennorrhea
bronchocandidiasis
bronchocavernous
bronchocele
bronchocephalitis
bronchoclysis
bronchoconstrictor
bronchodilatation
bronchodilation
bronchodilator
bronchoesophageal

bronchoesophagology
bronchoesophagoscopy
bronchogenic
bronchogram
bronchography
broncholith
broncholithiasis
bronchomalacia
bronchomycosis
bronchonocardiosis
broncho-oidiosis
bronchopathy
bronchophony
bronchoplasty
bronchoplegia
bronchopleural
bronchopleuropneumonia
bronchopneumonia
bronchopneumonitis
bronchopneumopathy
bronchopulmonary
bronchoradiography
bronchorrhagia
bronchorrhaphy
bronchorrhea
bronchoscope
 Albert's b.
 Broyles' b.
 Bruening's b.
 Chevalier-Jackson b.
 Davis' b.
 Emerson's b.
 Foregger's b.
 Haslinger's b.
 Holinger-Jackson b.
 Holinger's b.
 Jackson's b.
 Jesberg's b.

bronchoscope *(continued)*
 Kernan-Jackson b.
 Michelson's b.
 Moersch's b.
 Negus' b.
 Overholt-Jackson b.
 Pilling's b.
 Riecker's b.
 Safar's b.
 Staple's b.
 Tucker's b.
 Waterman's b.
 Yankauer's b.
bronchoscopic
bronchoscopy
bronchosinusitis
bronchospasm
bronchospirochetosis
bronchospirography
bronchospirometer
bronchospirometry
bronchostaxis
bronchostenosis
bronchostomy
bronchotetany
bronchotome
bronchotomy
bronchotracheal
bronchovesicular
bronchus
 apical b.
 cardiac b.
 eparterial b.
 main stem b.
 b. principalis dexter
 b. principalis sinister
 stem b.
 tracheal b.

brong-. See words beginning
   bronch-.
Broyles'
   aspirator
   bronchoscope
   dilator
   esophagoscope
   forceps
   telescope
   tube
Bruening's
   bronchoscope
   esophagoscope
   forceps
bruit
   b. dairain (brwe da ra)
   b. de bois (brwe duh
     bwah)
   b. de craquement (brwe
     duh krak maw)
   b. de cuir neuf (brwe
     duh kwer nuf)
   b. de frolement (brwe
     duh frol maw)
   b. de grelot (brwe duh
     gruh lo)
   b. de pôt felé (brwe duh
     po fe la)
brwe. See *bruit*.
Buhl's desquamative
   pneumonia
Burghart's symptom
button
   Moore's tracheostomy
     b's.
byssinosis
calcicosilicosis
calcicosis

calcification
cancrocirrhosis
Candida
   C. albicans
candidiasis
cannula
   Abelson's c.
   Abraham's c.
   Pritchard's c.
   Rockey's c.
cannulation
Caplan's syndrome
Carabelli's tube
carcinoma
   anaplastic c.
   bronchiolar c.
   bronchogenic c.
   squamous cell c.
cardia
   incompetent c.
cardiopulmonary
carina
   c. of trachea
Carlens' catheter
Carswell's grapes
caseation
Castellani's bronchitis
catheter
   Bailey's c.
   Carlens' c.
   Lloyd's c.
   Metras' c.
   Thompson's c.
   Zavod's c.
caval
cavernoscopy
cavernostomy
cavernous

cavitary
cavitation
cavum
Celestin's tube
cell
  Langhans' c.'s.
chalicosis
change
  Biermer's c.
  Gerhardt's c. of sound
Chaussier's tube
chemotherapy
Chevalier-Jackson
  bronchoscope
  esophagoscope
  tube
cholesterohydrothorax
chondroadenoma
chondroma
chylomediastinum
chylopleura
chylopneumothorax
chylorrhea
chylothorax
cinebronchogram
cineradiography
circumscribed
clamp
  Atlee's c.
  Davidson's c.
  Hudson's c.
  Kantrowicz's c.
  Kapp-Beck c.
  Kinsella-Buie c.
  Lees' c.
  Mueller's c.
  Price-Thomas c.
  Ralks' c.

clamp *(continued)*
  Rockey's c.
  Rubin's c.
  Sarot's c.
  Thomson's c.
clavicle
clavicular
clavipectoral
coalescence
coarctation
Coccidioides
  C. immitis
coccidioidomycosis
collapse
  c. of the lung
collapsotherapy
congestion
  pleuropulmonary c.
coniosporosis
coniotoxicosis
COPD – chronic obstructive
  pulmonary disease
cor
  c. pulmonale
Cordes' forceps
costa
costal
costophrenic
costopleural
costopneumopexy
costovertebral
cough
  Balme's c.
  compression c.
  extrapulmonary c.
  Morton's c.
  productive c.
  Sydenham's c.

cough
    whooping c.
    winter c.
Crafoord's
    forceps
    scissors
crepitant
cricoid
cricopharyngeus
cricotracheotomy
croup
croupette
croupy
crura
crus
cryptococcosis
Cryptococcus
    C. neoformans
cupula
    c. of pleura
CVA – costovertebral angle
cyanosis
    pulmonary c.
cyst
    bronchogenic c.
    dermoid c.
    enteric c.
    neurenteric c.
    pericardial c.
    thymic c.
Daniel's operation
Darling's disease
Davidson's clamp
Davis' bronchoscope
Debove's membrane
decannulation
decarbonization
décollement

decortication
    d. of lung
degeneration
    trabecular d.
Délorme's operation
Depaul's tube
Desnos'
    disease
    pneumonia
desquamative
diaphragm
diaphragmatic
dilator
    Broyles' d.
    Einhorn's d.
    Jackson's d.
    Jackson-Trousseau d.
    Laborde's d.
    Patton's d.
    Plummer's d.
    Plummer-Vinson d.
    Sippy's d.
    Steele's d.
    Trousseau-Jackson d.
    Trousseau's d.
diminution
DIP – desquamative
    interstitial pneumonitis
Diplococcus
    D. pneumoniae
discission
    d. of pleura
disease
    Ayerza's d.
    Bornholm's d.
    Darling's d.
    Desnos' d.
    Hamman's d.

disease *(continued)*
    Hodgkin's d.
    hyaline membrane d.
    Kartagener's d.
    Löffler's d.
    Lucas-Championnière's d.
    Shaver's d.
    Woillez' d.
dissector
    Lynch's d.
diverticulum
    pharyngoesophageal d.
    Rokitansky's d.
    supradiaphragmatic c.
    Zenker's d.
drainage
    Monaldi's d.
    postural d.
    underwater seal d.
    waterseal d.
drugs. See *Medications.*
Duguet's siphon
Durham's tube
Duval-Crile forceps
dysphagia
dyspnea
    expiratory d.
    inspiratory d.
    nonexpansional d.
    Traube's d.
Eaton agent
edema
    pulmonary e.
    vernal e.
Eder-Hufford esophagoscope
effusion
    pleural e.

EGL – eosinophilic granuloma of the lung
egophony
Einhorn's dilator
electrocardiogram
elevator
    Jackson's e.
embolism
    pulmonary e.
Emerson's bronchoscope
emphysema
    alveolar e.
    bullous e.
    centrilobular e.
    compensatory e.
    gangrenous e.
    hypertrophic e.
    interlobular e.
    interstitial e.
    Jenner's e.
    mediastinal e.
    obstructive e.
    pulmonary e.
    subcutaneous e.
    subfascial e.
    vesicular e.
emphysematous
empyema
    interlobar e.
    metapneumonic e.
    synpneumonic e.
    thoracic e.
endobronchial
endobronchitis
endoscopy
endotracheal
endotracheitis
eparterial

epicardia
epiglottis
Equen's magnet
Erich's forceps
Escherichia
    E. coli
esofa-. See words beginning
  esopha-.
esophagalgia
esophageal
esophagectasia
esophagectomy
esophagism
   hiatal e.
esophagitis
   reflux e.
esophagocele
esophagocologastrostomy
esophagoduodenostomy
esophagodynia
esophagoenterostomy
esophagofundopexy
esophagogastrectomy
esophagogastroanastomosis
esophagogastroplasty
esophagogastroscopy
esophagogastrostomy
esophagogram
esophagography
esophagojejunogastrostomosis
esophagojejunostomy
esophagolaryngectomy
esophagomalacia
esophagometer
esophagomycosis
esophagomyotomy
esophagopharynx
esophagoplasty

esophagoplication
esophagoptosis
esophagosalivation
esophagoscope
   Boros' e.
   Broyles' e.
   Bruening's e.
   Chevalier-Jackson e.
   Eder-Hufford e.
   Haslinger's tracheo-
     broncho- e.
   Holinger's e.
   Jackson's e.
   Jesberg's e.
   Lell's e.
   Moersch's e.
   Mosher's e.
   Moure's e.
   Roberts' e.
   Schindler's e.
   Tucker's e.
   Yankauer's e.
esophagoscopy
esophagospasm
esophagostenosis
esophagostoma
esophagostomy
esophagotome
esophagotomy
esophagus
Estlander's operation
evagination
eventration
    diaphragmatic e.
Ewart's sign
expansion
expectorant
expectoration

expiration
expiratory
exsufflation
exsufflator
extratracheal
faringo-. See words beginning
    pharyngo-.
farinjeal. See *pharyngeal.*
farinks. See *pharynx.*
Fauvel's granules
FEF – forced expiratory flow
Fell-O'Dwyer apparatus
fever
    Q. f. (Q. for query)
fiberscope
    Hirschowitz's gastro-
        duodenal f.
fibrogastroscopy
fibrosis
    diffuse interstitial pul-
        monary f.
    mediastinal f.
    pulmonary f.
fibrothorax
fibrotic
fibrous
field
    Krönig's f.
FIF – forced inspiratory flow
Finochietto's forceps
Fischer's needle
fissure
    f. of lung
fistula
    bronchopleural f.
    esophagobronchial f.
    pulmonary arterioven-
        ous f.

fistula
    tracheal f.
flem. See *phlegm.*
Floyd's needle
fluoroscopy
flutter
    mediastinal f.
focus
    Assmann's f.
foramen
    f. ovale basis cranii
    f. ovale ossis sphenoi-
        dalis
forceps
    Adair's f.
    Allis' f.
    Babcock's f.
    Boies' f.
    Broyles' f.
    Bruening's f.
    Cordes' f.
    Crafoord's f.
    Duval-Crile f.
    Erich's f.
    Finochietto's f.
    Fraenkel's f.
    Harrington-Mayo f.
    Holinger's f.
    Jackson's f.
    Johnson's f.
    Julian's f.
    Kahler's f.
    Killian's f.
    Kocher's f.
    Kolb's f.
    Krause's f.
    Leyro-Diaz f.
    Lovelace's f.

forceps *(continued)*
    Lynch's f.
    Mayo-Russian f.
    Moersch's f.
    Myerson's f.
    Nelson's f.
    New's f.
    Patterson's f.
    Pennington's f.
    Price-Thomas f.
    Roberts' f.
    Rockey's f.
    Russian f.
    Sam Roberts f.
    Sarot's f.
    Scheinmann's f.
    Seiffert's f.
    Tobold-Fauvel f.
    Tuttle's f.
    Yankauer-Little f.
Foregger's bronchoscope
Forlanini's treatment
fossa
    supraclavicular f.
Fowler's operation
Fraenkel's forceps
Frederick's needle
fremitus
    bronchial f.
    pleural f.
    rhonchal f.
    tactile f.
    tussive f.
fren-. See words beginning
    phren-.
Freund's anomaly
Friedländer's
    bacillus pneumonia

Friedländer's
    pneumobacillus
Friedrich's operation
furrow
    Schmorl's f.
Gabriel-Tucker tube
gastrocamera
    Olympus model GTF-A g.
gastroscope
    Benedict's g.
geotrichosis
Gerhardt's change of sound
Ghon tubercle
Gibson's rule
Goodpasture's syndrome
granule
    Fauvel's g's.
granuloma
granulomatosis
    Wegener's g.
granulomatous
grape
    Carswell's g's.
Guisez's tube
Haight's retractor
hamartoma
Hamman-Rich syndrome
Hamman's
    disease
    sign
Harrington-Mayo forceps
Haslinger's
    bronchoscope
    tracheo-broncho-
        esophagoscope
Heaf test
heaves
hemangioendothelioma

hemangioma
hemidiaphragm
hemithorax
Hemophilus
    H. influenzae
    H. pertussis
hemopneumothorax
hemoptysis
    Manson's h.
    parasitic h.
hemosiderosis
    idiopathic pulmonary h.
hemothorax
hernia
    diaphragmatic h.
    hiatal h.
    hiatus h.
hernial
hiatus
    esophageal h.
hibernoma
hiccup
hilar
hilum
hilus
    h. pulmonis
Himmelstein's valvulotome
Hirschowitz's gastroduodenal
    fiberscope
Hirtz's rale
histiocytosis
    h. X.
Histoplasma
    H. capsulatum
histoplasmosis
Hodgkin's disease
Holinger-Jackson
    bronchoscope

Holinger's
    bronchoscope
    esophagoscope
    forceps
    laryngoscope
    telescope
    tube
hook
    New's h.
Hopp's laryngoscope
Horner's syndrome
Hudson's clamp
Hurst's bougie
Hurwitz's trocar
hyalinization
hydropneumothorax
hydrothorax
    chylous h.
hygroma
hyparterial
hypercapnia
hyperlucency
hyperresonance
hyperventilation
hypoxemia
hypoxia
IC – inspiratory capacity
I/E – inspiratory-expiratory
    ratio
impaction
    mucoid i.
impressio
    i. cardiaca pulmonis
incarcerated
incision
    periscapular i.
infarction
    pulmonary i.

infiltrate
    Assmann's tuberculous i.
infiltration
inflation
influenza
inhalant
    antifoaming i.
inhalation
inhaler
inspiration
inspiratory
inspissated
insufficiency
    pulmonary i.
insufflation
    endotracheal i.
interlobar
interstitial
intrabronchial
intracavitary
intractable
intrapleural
intrathoracic
intratracheal
IPPB — intermittent positive
    pressure breathing
isotope
    radioactive i.
isthmus
    Krönig's i.
IT — inhalation test
    inhalation therapy
    intratracheal tube
Jackson's
    bistoury
    bougie
    bronchoscope
    dilator

Jackson's *(continued)*
    elevator
    esophagoscope
    forceps
    laryngoscope
    retractor
    scalpel
    scissors
    tenaculum
    tube
Jackson-Trousseau dilator
Jenner's emphysema
Jesberg's
    bronchoscope
    esophagoscope
Johnson's forceps
Julian's forceps
Kahler's forceps
Kantrowicz's clamp
Kaplan's needle
Kapp-Beck clamp
Kartagener's
    disease
    syndrome
    triad
Kaufman's pneumonia
kemotherapy. See *chemo-*
    therapy.
Kernan-Jackson bronchoscope
Killian's
    forceps
    tubes
kilo-. See words beginning
    chylo-.
Kinsella-Buie clamp
Kistner's tube
Klebsiella
    K. pneumoniae

knife
    Lynch's k.
Kocher's forceps
Kolb's forceps
kondro-. See words beginning
    chondro-.
Krause's forceps
krico-. See words beginning
    crico-.
Krönig's
    area
    field
    isthmus
    percussion
Kveim test
Laborde's dilator
Laennec's pearls
Langhans' cells
laparothoracoscopy
laringo-. See words beginning
    laryngo-.
larinjeal. See *laryngeal*.
larinks. See *larynx*.
laryngeal
laryngitis
laryngopharyngitis
laryngopharynx
laryngoscope
    Holinger's l.
    Hopp's l.
    Jackson's l.
    Lewy's l.
    Welch-Allyn l.
laryngoscopy
laryngospasm
laryngotomy
laryngotracheal
laryngotracheitis

laryngotracheobronchitis
laryngotracheobronchoscopy
laryngotracheoscopy
laryngotracheotomy
larynx
lavage
Lees' clamp
Legroux's remission
leiomyoma
Leitner's syndrome
Lell's esophagoscope
Lennarson's tube
Lepley-Ernst tube
leptospirosis
lesion
    coin l.
Lewis' tube
Lewy-Rubin needle
Lewy's laryngoscope
Leyro-Diaz forceps
Linguatula
lingula
    l. pulmonis sinistri
lingulectomy
Linton's tube
lipoma
LL – left lung
LLL – left lower lobe
Lloyd's catheter
lobar
lobectomy
lobitis
lobostomy
Löffler's
    disease
    pneumonia
    syndrome
Lore-Lawrence tube

Lovelace's forceps
Lowenstein's medium
LTB − laryngotracheobron-
    chitis
Lucas-Championnière's
    disease
Luer's tube
Lukens' retractor
LUL − left upper lobe
lung
    hyperlucent l.
lymphadenitis
lymphoblastoma
lymphoma
Lynch's
    dissector
    forceps
    knife
    scissors
magnet
    Equen's m.
Malm-Himmelstein valvulo-
    tome
maneuver
    Müller's m.
    Valsalva's m.
Manson's hemoptysis
Mantoux test
manubrium
Martin's tube
Maugeri's syndrome
Mayo-Russian forceps
Mayo's scissors
mediastinal
mediastinitis
mediastinography
mediastinopericarditis
mediastinoscopy

mediastinotomy
mediastinum
Medications
    acetazolamide
    acetylcysteine
    ACTH
    Adrenalin
    amantadine hydro-
        chloride
    aminophylline
    aminosalicylic acid
    ammonium carbonate
    ammonium chloride
    ampicillin
    Atabrine
    benzonatate
    calcium iodide
    Capastat
    capreomycin sulfate
    Capromycin
    carbetapentane citrate
    carbon dioxide with
        oxygen
    cephalothin
    chlophedianol hydro-
        chloride
    chloral hydrate
    chloramphenicol
    codeine
    corticotropin
    cycloserine
    Demerol
    dextromethorphan
        hydrobromide
    Dicodid
    dihydrocodeinone
        bitartrate
    Dionosil (contrast medium)

Medications *(continued)*

Dopram
doxapram hydrochloride
Emivan
ephedrine
epinephrine
erythromycin
ethambutol hydrochloride
ethamivan
ethionamide
glyceryl guaiacolate
α-Glyceryl Guaiacol Ether
Guaianesin
Hycodan
hydriodic acid
INH – isonicotinic acid hydrazide
iodinated glycerol
Iprenol
isoniazid
Isonicotinic acid hydrazide
Isopropylarterenol solution
isoproterenol
Isuprel
kanamycin
levopropoxyphene napsylate
lidocaine
lincomycin
lobeline
Medihaler-Iso
meperidine

Medications *(continued)*

Mercodinone
methicillin
Methorate
Mucomyst
Myambutal
Narcotine
Nectadon
Nembutal
Niconyl
Norisodrine
noscapine
Novrad
Nydrazid
Organidin
Oxycel gauze
Pamisyl
Para-Aminosalicylic acid
Parapas
Parasal
PAS – para-aminosalicylic acid
penicillin G
penicillin V.
pentobarbital sodium
pipazethate hydrochloride
potassium iodide
propyliodone (contrast medium)
pyrazinamide
Pyribenzamine
Quibron
quinacrine
Respaire
Rifadin
Rifaldazine

Medications *(continued)*
    Rifampicin
    rifampin
    Rifamycin
    Rimactane
    Rimifon
    Robitussin
    Romilar
    Seromycin
    streptomycin
    Superinone
    Symmetrel
    terpin hydrate
    Tessalon
    theophylline ethylene-
      diamine
    Theratuss
    Thioamide
    thio-tepa
    Toclase
    Trecator
    tripelennamine citrate
    Triton WR-1339
    tyloxapol
    Tyvid
    Ulo
    Valium
    vanillic diethylamide
    Vapo-N-Iso
    Vinactane
    Viocin
    viomycin sulfate
    Xylocaine
medicolegal
medicothorax
medium
    Lowenstein's m.
Meigs' syndrome

melioidosis
    pulmonary m.
membrane
    Debove's m.
Mendelson's syndrome
mesothelioma
metastases
    pleural m.
Metras' catheter
Metzenbaum's scissors
Michelson's bronchoscope
microlithiasis
    pulmonary alveolar m.
mist
    ultrasonic m.
Moersch's
    bronchoscope
    esophagoscope
    forceps
Monaldi's drainage
Monilia
    M. albicans
Moore's tracheostomy
    buttons
Morch's tube
Morton's cough
Mosher's
    esophagoscope
    tube
Moure's esophagoscope
mucoid
mucopurulent
Mucor
mucormycosis
mucoviscidosis
mucus
Mueller's clamp
Müller's maneuver

murmur
    cardiopulmonary m.
    cardiorespiratory m.
    respiratory m.
muscle
    scalenus m.
    serratus m.
Mycobacterium
    M. tuberculosis
Mycoplasm
    M. pneumoniae
Myerson's
    forceps
    saw
Nachlas' tube
Naffziger's syndrome
nebulizer
needle
    Fischer's n.
    Floyd's n.
    Frederick's n.
    Kaplan's n.
    Lewy-Rubin n.
Negus' bronchoscope
Nelson's
    forceps
    scissors
neurofibroma
New's
    forceps
    hook
    tube
Nocardia
    N. asteroides
nocardial
nocardiosis
numektome. See
    pneumectomy.

numo-. See words beginning
    pneumo-.
obturator
Octomyces
    O. etiennei
oleothorax
Olympus model GTF-A
    gastrocamera
operation
    Blalock-Taussig o.
    Daniel's o.
    Delorme's o.
    Estlander's o.
    Fowler's o.
    Friedrich's o.
    Overholt's o.
    Ransohoff's o.
    Schede's o.
    Sembs's o.
    Wilms' o.
ornithosis
orthopnea
orthopneic
Overholt-Jackson
    bronchoscope
Overholt's operation
oxyetherotherapy
P & A – percussion and
    auscultation
Pancoast's
    syndrome
    tumor
PAP – primary atypical
    pneumonia
paracentesis
    p. pulmonis
    p. thoracis
paragonimiasis

Paragonimus
    P. westermani
para-influenzal
parenchyma
paries
    p. membranaceus
      bronchi
    p. membranaceus
      tracheae
parietal
paroxysm
paroxysmal
pars
    p. thoracalis esophagi
Patterson's
    forceps
    trocar
Patton's dilator
patulous
PE – pharyngoesophageal
    pleural effusion
    pulmonary edema
    pulmonary embolism
pearl
    Laennec's p's.
pectoral
pectoralis
pectoriloquy
pectorophony
pectus
    p. carinatum
    p. excavatum
    p. gallinatum
    p. recurvatum
pedunculated
penicilliosis
Penicillium
Pennington's forceps

percussion
    Krönig's p.
peribronchial
peribronchiolar
peribronchiolitis
peribronchitis
pericarditis
    tuberculous p.
periesophageal
periesophagitis
perihilar
peripneumonia
    p. notha
pertussis
Peyrot's thorax
PFT – pulmonary function
    test
pharyngeal
pharyngitis
pharyngoesophageal
pharyngospasm
pharyngostenosis
pharyngotomy
pharynx
phlegm
phonation
photofluorogram
photofluorography
phrenic
phrenicectomy
phrenicoexeresis
phrenicotomy
phrenicotripsy
phrenitis
phthisis
    pulmonary p.
PI – pulmonary incompetence
    pulmonary infarction

PIE – pulmonary infiltration and eosinophilia
pulmonary interstitial emphysema
Pilling's
    bronchoscope
    tube
piriform
plaque
plasmocytoma
platysma
pleura
    costal p.
    diaphragmatic p.
    mediastinal p.
    parietal p.
    pericardiac p.
    pulmonary p.
    visceral p.
pleuracotomy
pleural
pleurectomy
pleurisy
pleuritic
pleurobronchitis
pleurocele
pleuroclysis
pleurodynia
pleurography
pleurolith
pleuroparietopexy
pleuropericardial
pleuropericarditis
pleuroperitoneal
pleuroperitoneum
pleuropneumonia
pleuropneumonia-like
pleuropneumonolysis

pleuropulmonary
pleuroscopy
pleurothoracopleurectomy
pleurotome
pleurotomy
plexus
    p. aorticus thoracicus
    brachial p.
    esophageal p.
    mediastinal p.
    p. pulmonalis
    subpleural mediastinal p.
plication
    fundal p.
plombage
    extraperiosteal p.
Plummer's dilator
Plummer-Vinson
    dilator
    radium applicator
PND – paroxysmal nocturnal dyspnea
pneumal
pneumatic
pneumatocele
pneumatodyspnea
pneumatometer
pneumatosis
    p. pulmonum
pneumectomy
pneumoalveolography
pneumoangiography
pneumobacillus
    Friedländer's p.
pneumobronchotomy
pneumobulbar
pneumocardial
pneumocentesis

pneumochirurgia
pneumocholecystitis
pneumochysis
pneumococcal
pneumococcic
pneumococcus
pneumoconiosis
    mica p.
    p. siderotica
    talc p.
pneumoenteritis
pneumoerysipelas
pneumogastric
pneumogram
pneumography
pneumohemothorax
pneumohydrothorax
pneumolithiasis
pneumomalacia
pneumomediastinography
pneumomediastinum
pneumomycosis
pneumonectasis
pneumonectomy
pneumonedema
pneumonemia
pneumonere
pneumonia
    abortive p.
    anthrax p.
    p. apostematosa
    aspiration p.
    atypical p.
    bronchial p.
    Buhl's desquamative p.
    catarrhal p.
    deglutition p.
    Desnos' p.

pneumonia *(continued)*
    p. dissecans
    ephemeral p.
    Friedländer's bacillus p.
    Kaufman's p.
    Klebsiella p.
    lingular p.
    lobar p.
    Löffler's p.
    migratory p.
    parenchymatous p.
    pleurogenetic p.
    pneumococcal p.
    pneumocystis carinii p.
    Riesman's p.
    staphylococcus p.
    Stoll's p.
    streptococcus p.
    suppurative p.
    tuberculous p.
    tularemic p.
    unresolved p.
    varicella p.
pneumonic
pneumonitis
    cholesterol p.
    desquamative inter-
      stitial p.
pneumonocentesis
pneumonochirurgia
pneumonocirrhosis
pneumonography
pneumonolysis
pneumonomelanosis
pneumonomoniliasis
pneumonopathy
    eosinophilic p.
pneumonophthisis

pneumonorrhaphy
pneumonosis
pneumonotomy
pneumoparesis
pneumopericardium
pneumoperitoneum
pneumopexy
pneumopleuritis
pneumopleuroparietopexy
pneumopyothorax
pneumoresection
pneumorrhagia
pneumosepticemia
pneumoserothorax
pneumosilicosis
pneumothorax
    artificial p.
    clicking p.
    extrapleural p.
    spontaneous p.
    valvular p.
pneumotoxin
Polisar-Lyons tube
polycythemia
posttussis
poudrage
    pleural p.
PP − pink puffers (emphysema)
PPB − positive pressure breathing
PPD − purified protein derivative
PPLO − pleuropneumonia-like organism
Price-Thomas
    clamp
    forceps

Pritchard's cannula
proteinosis
    pulmonary alveolar p.
Proteus
pseudobronchiectasis
pseudocoarctation
Pseudomonas
    P. aeruginosa
psittacosis
pulmogram
pulmolith
pulmometer
pulmometry
pulmonary
pulmonic
pulmonitis
pulmonohepatic
pulmonology
pulmonoperitoneal
pulmotor
pulsator
    Bragg-Paul p.
purulent
PX − pneumothorax
pyopneumothorax
pyothorax
Q fever (Q for query)
radiogram
radiography
radioisotope
radiolucent
radiopaque
rale
    amphoric r.
    atelectatic r.
    bubbling r.
    cavernous r.
    clicking r.

rale *(continued)*
    collapse r.
    consonating r.
    crackling r.
    crepitant r.
    r. de retour
    extrathoracic r.
    gurgling r.
    Hirtz's r.
    r. indux
    r. muqueux
    pleural r.
    r. redux
    sibilant r.
    Skoda's r.
    sonorous r.
    subcrepitant r.
    tracheal r.
    vesicular r.
    whistling r.
Ralks' clamp
Ransohoff's operation
RDS — respiratory distress
   syndrome
reflux
regurgitation
    esophageal r.
remission
    Legroux's r's.
repair
    Belsey's r.
resonance
    bankbox r.
    bell-metal r.
    cracked-pot r.
    shoulder-strap r.
    skodaic r.
resonant

respiration
respirator
respiratory
retractor
    Andrews' r.
    Bernay's r.
    Brewster's r.
    Haight's r.
    Jackson's r.
    Lukens' r.
    Robinson's r.
    Shurly's r.
retrosternal
rhonchal
rhonchial
rhonchus
RI — respiratory illness
rickettsial
Riecker's bronchoscope
Riesman's pneumonia
ring
    Schatzki's r.
RL — right lung
RLC — residual lung capacity
RLL — right lower lobe
RM — respiratory movement
RML — right middle lobe
Roberts'
    esophagoscope
    forceps
Robinson's retractor
Rockey's
    cannula
    clamp
    forceps
    scope
roentgenography
Rokitansky's diverticulum

rong-. See words beginning
 rhonc-.
RS – respiratory syncytial
RTF – respiratory tract fluid
Rubin's clamp
RUL – right upper lobe
rule
 Gibson's r.
Russian forceps
RV – respiratory volume
Safar's bronchoscope
Salvatore-Maloney tracheo-
 tome
Sam Roberts forceps
sarcoid
sarcoidosis
sarcoma
Sarot's
 clamp
 forceps
saw
 Myerson's s.
scalene
scalenectomy
scalenotomy
scalpel
 Jackson's s.
Schatzki's ring
Schede's operation
Scheinmann's forceps
Schindler's esophagoscope
schistosomiasis
 pulmonary s.
Schmorl's furrow
scissors
 Crafoord's s.
 Jackson's s.
 Lynch's s.

scissors *(continued)*
 Mayo's s.
 Metzenbaum's s.
 Nelson's s.
 Sweet's s.
scleroderma
 pulmonary s.
scope
 Rockey's s.
segment
 bronchopulmonary s.
segmenta
 s. bronchopulmonalia
segmental
Seiffert's forceps
Semb's operation
Sengstaken-Blakemore tube
septum
 s. bronchiale
sequestration
 pulmonary s.
sequoiosis
serpiginous
Shaver's disease
shunt
 portacaval s.
Shurly's retractor
siderosilicosis
siderosis
Sierra-Sheldon tracheotome
sign
 Abrahams' s.
 Ewart's s.
 Hamman's s.
 Skoda's s.
silicatosis
silicosiderosis
silicosis

silicotuberculosis
singultus
sinobronchitis
sinus
    s. trunci pulmonalis
siphon
    Duguet's s.
Sippy's dilator
sitakosis. See *psittacosis*.
situs
    s. inversus viscerum
Skoda's
    rale
    sign
    tympany
sound
    Beatty-Bright friction s.
    cracked-pot s.
    esophageal s.
    hipprocratic s.
    respiratory s.
    to-and-fro s.
Souttar's tube
space
    Traube's s.
spirochetosis
    bronchopulmonary s.
spirogram
spirograph
spirography
spirometer
spirometry
    bronchoscopic s.
spirophore
splenization
    hypostatic s.
splenopneumonia
sputum

sputum *(continued)*
    s. aeroginosum
    albuminoid s.
    s. coctum
    s. crudum
    s. cruentum
    egg yolk s.
    globular s.
    icteric s.
    moss-agate s.
    nummular s.
    prune juice s.
    rusty s.
stannosis
Staphylococcus
    S. aureus
Staple's bronchoscope
status
    s. asthmaticus
Steele's dilator
stenosis
stereoscopy
sternal
sternoclavicular
sternocostal
sternotomy
sternotracheal
sternum
stethoscope
Stoll's pneumonia
stricture
stridor
    s. serraticus
study
    cytological s.
    enzyme s.
subpleural
substernal

succussion
> hippocratic s.

suctioning
> endotracheal-bronchial
> s.

sudo-. See words beginning
> *pseudo-*.

suffocation

sulcate

sulcus
> s. pulmonalis thoracis
> subclavian s. of lung
> s. subclavius pulmonis

surgical procedures. See
> *operation.*

Sweet's scissors

Sydenham's cough

symptom
> Burghart's s.

syndrome
> Arneth's s.
> Ayerza's s.
> Bard's s.
> Bársony-Polgár s.
> Brock's s.
> Caplan's s.
> Goodpasture's s.
> Hamman-Rich s.
> Horner's s.
> Kartagener's s.
> Leitner's s.
> Löffler's s.
> Maugeri's s.
> Meigs' s.
> Mendelson's s.
> Naffziger's s.
> Pancoast's s.
> Wilson-Mikity s.

telescope
> Broyles' t.
> Holinger's t.
> right-angle t.

tenaculum
> Jackson's t.

teratoma

test
> coccidioidin t.
> Heaf t.
> histoplasmin skin t.
> Kveim t.
> Mantoux t.
> patch t.
> Tine t.
> Vollmer's t.

Thompson's catheter

Thomson's clamp

thoracentesis

thoracic

thoracicoabdominal

thoracobronchotomy

thoracocautery

thoracocentesis

thoracocyllosis

thoracocyrtosis

thoracogastroschisis

thoracograph

thoracolaparotomy

thoracolysis
> t. praecordiaca

thoracoplasty
> costoversion t.

thoracopneumograph

thoracopneumoplasty

thoracoschisis

thoracoscope

thoracoscopy

thoracostenosis
thoracostomy
thoracotomy
thorax
    barrel-shaped t.
    Peyrot's t.
    pyriform t.
thrombosis
thymectomy
thymoma
thymus
thymusectomy
Tine test
tisis. See *phthisis*.
TLC − total lung capacity
    total lung compliance
Tobold-Fauvel forceps
tomography
torulosis
tourniquet
    Bethune's t.
toxoplasmosis
trachea
tracheal
tracheitis
tracheobronchial
tracheobronchitis
tracheobronchoscopy
tracheocele
tracheoesophageal
tracheofissure
tracheophony
tracheoplasty
tracheorrhaphy
tracheoscopy
tracheostenosis
tracheostoma
tracheostomy

tracheotome
    Salvatore-Maloney t.
    Sierra-Sheldon t.
tracheotomy
transillumination
transthoracic
transthoracotomy
transtracheal
Traube's
    dyspnea
    space
treatment
    Forlanini's t.
tree
    bronchial t.
    tracheobronchial t.
triad
    Kartagener's t.
Trichomonas
    T. pulmonalis
trocar
    Hurwitz's t.
    Patterson's t.
Trousseau-Jackson dilator
Trousseau's
    bougie
    dilator
truncus
    t. bronchomediastinalis
      dexter
    t. pulmonalis
tube
    Andrews-Pynchon t.
    Atkins-Cannard t.
    Blakemore's t.
    Broyles' t.
    Carabelli's t.
    Celestin's t.

tube *(continued)*
  Chaussier's t.
  Chevalier-Jackson t.
  Depaul's t.
  Durham's t.
  Gabriel-Tucker t.
  Guisez's t.
  Holinger's t.
  intubation t.
  Jackson's t.
  Killian's t's.
  Kistner's t.
  Lennarson's t.
  Lepley-Ernst t.
  Lewis' t.
  Linton's t.
  Lore-Lawrence t.
  Luer's t.
  Martin's t.
  Morch's t.
  Mosher's t.
  Nachlas' t.
  New's t.
  Pilling's t.
  Polisar-Lyons t.
  Sengstaken-Blakemore t.
  Souttar's t.
  thoracostomy t.
  tracheostomy t.
  Tucker's t.
tubercle
  Ghon t.
  scalene t.
tubercular
tuberculin
tuberculoid
tuberculoma
tuberculosilicosis

tuberculosis
  exudative t.
  hilus t.
  miliary t.
  pulmonary t.
  tracheobronchial t.
tuberculous
Tucker's
  bronchoscope
  esophagoscope
  tube
tumor
  alveolar cell t.
  amyloid t.
  Pancoast's t.
  teratoid t.
  thymic t.
tunica
  t. adventitia esophagi
  t. mucosa bronchiorum
  t. mucosa esophagi
  t. mucosa laryngis
  t. mucosa tracheae
  t. muscularis esophagi
  t. muscularis tracheae
Tuttle's forceps
tympanic
tympany
  bell t.
  skodaic t.
  Skoda's t.
underwater seal drainage
URI – upper respiratory
  infection
Valsalva's maneuver
valvulotome
  Himmelstein's v.
  Malm-Himmelstein v.

varix
vein
    azygos v.
    brachial v.
    cephalic v.
    innominate v.
    thymic v.
vena
    v. cava
venesection
venogram
virus
    Coxsackie v.
    ECHO v. — enteric cyto-
      pathogenic human
      orphan v.
    parainfluenza v.
    respiratory syncytial v.
visceropleural
visualization
    laryngoscopic v.

Vollmer's test
Waterman's bronchoscope
Wegener's granulomatosis
Welch-Allyn laryngoscope
wheeze
whooping cough
Wilms' operation
Wilson-Mikity syndrome
Woillez' disease
xiphocostal
xiphoid
Yankauer-Little forceps
Yankauer's
    bronchoscope
    esophagoscope
Zavod's catheter
Zenker's diverticulum
zifo-. See words beginning
    xipho-.

UROLOGY

aberrant
acetonuria
achromaturia
Acmi-Valentine tube
aconuresis
acraturesis
actinomycosis
acuminata
    condylomata a.
    verruca a.
adapter
    Ralks' a.
Addison's disease
Addis's method
adenitis
adenoacanthoma
adenocarcinoma
adenoma
    cortical a's.
adenomyosarcoma
adenosarcoma
    embryonal a.
adiposis
    a. orchalis
    a. orchica
adrenal
    Marchand's a's.
adrenalectomy
adrenalinuria
adrenalism
adrenalitis
adrenalopathy
adrenic
adrenin

adrenitis
adrenocortical
adrenogenous
adrenokinetic
adrenomedullotropic
adrenomegaly
adrenopathy
adrenopause
adrenoprival
adrenostatic
adrenotoxin
adrenotropic
adrenotropin
adrenotropism
adventitia
aerocystography
aerocystoscope
aerocystoscopy
afferent
agenesis
agenitalism
agenosomia
aglomerular
aidoiitis
Albarran's
    gland
    test
    tubules
albiduria
albuginea
    a. penis
albugineotomy
albumin
albuminaturia

albuminuria
  adventitious a.
  globular a.
  nephrogenous a.
  postrenal a.
  renal a.
  residual a.
albuminuric
Alcock's catheter
Alcock-Timberlake obturator
alcoholuria
alginuresis
Allemann's syndrome
Allis' forceps
Alyea's clamp
amebiasis
  a. of bladder
ampulla
  a. ductus deferentis
  Henle's a.
  a. of vas deferens
amyloidosis
anastomosis
  pyeloileocutaneous a.
  transuretero-ureteral a.
Andrews' operation
anesthesia
  fluothane a.
  pentothal a.
aneurysm
aneurysmal
aneurysmatic
angiography
angle
  costovertebral a.
angulation
anischuria
ankylurethria

annulus
  a. urethralis
anorchia
anorchid
anorchidic
anorchidism
anorchis
anorchism
anovesical
anuresis
anuretic
anuria
  angioneurotic a.
  calculous a.
  postrenal a.
  prerenal a.
  renal a.
anuric
aorta
aorticorenal
apex
  a. of bladder
  a. prostatae
  a. vesicae urinariae
aponeurosis
  Denonvilliers' a.
arcuate
ardor
  a. urinae
areolar
Arnold and Gunning's
  method
arteriole
  glomerular a.
  glomerular a., afferent
  glomerular a., efferent
  Isaacs-Ludwig a.
  postglomerular a.

arteriole
    preglomerular a.
arteriorenal
arteriosclerotic
arteriovenous
ascites
aspermatism
aspermatogenesis
aspermia
asthenospermia
atonic
atony
atresia
atrophic
atrophy
azoospermatism
azoospermia
azotemia
    extrarenal a.
    prerenal a.
azoturia
azoturic
Babcock's clamp
backflow
    pyelovenous b.
bah-fon. See *bas-fond.*
balanic
balanitis
    b. circinata
    b. diabetica
    Follmann's b.
    b. gangraenosa
    gangrenous b.
    b. xerotica obliterans
balanoblennorrhea
balanocele
balanoplasty
balanoposthitis

balanoposthomycosis
balanopreputial
balanorrhagia
balanus
bar
    Mercier's b.
Bardenheuer's incision
Bardex's catheter
Bard's catheter
Bartter's syndrome
bas-fond
basket
    Browne's b.
    Councill's b.
    Dormia's b.
    Ferguson's b.
    Howard's b.
    Johnson's b.
    Mitchell's b.
Bates' operation
Baumrucker's resectoscope
Belfield's operation
Bellini's
    ducts
    tubules
Bell's muscle
Bence-Jones
    cylinders
    method
    proteinuria
    urine
Benedict and Franke's
    method
Benedict and Osterberg's
    method
Bengt-Johanson repair
benign
Bennett's operation

Bergenhem's operation
Bergman-Israel incision
Bergmann's incision
Bertin's column
Bertrand's method
Bethune's rib cutter
Bevan-Rochet operation
Bevan's operation
bifid
bifurcation
Bigelow's
    lithotrite
    operation
bilabe
Bittorf's reaction
bladder
    atonic b.
    autonomic b.
    dome of b.
    fasciculated b.
    irritable b.
    nervous b.
    neurogenic b.
    sacculated b.
    stammering b.
    urinary b.
Blakes' forceps
Blasucci's catheter
blennorrhagia
blennorrhea
blennuria
Boari's operation
body
    b. of Highmore
    wolffian b.
boggy
boo-zhe. See *bougie.*
Bottini's operation

bougie
    b. à boule
    acorn-tipped b.
    Coude's b.
    LeFort's b.
    olive tip b.
    Otis' b.
    Philips' b.
    Ruschelit's b.
boutonniére
Bowman's capsule
Bozeman's forceps
BPH – benign prostatic
    hypertrophy
Braasch's
    catheter
    cystoscope
    forceps
Brewer's infarcts
Bricker's operation
brightism
Bright's disease
Brodny's clamp
Broedel's line
Brown-Buerger cystoscope
Browne's basket
bubo
    chancroidal b.
    gonorrheal b.
    venereal b.
bubonulus
Buck's fascia
Buerger-McCarthy forceps
Bugbee's electrode
bulbitis
bulbocavernosus
bulbourethral
bulbous

bulbus
    b. penis
    b. urethrae
bullous
Bumpus'
    forceps
    resectoscope
Bunim's forceps
Buschke-Loewenstein tumor
Butterfield's cystoscope
Bywaters' syndrome
Cacchi-Ricci syndrome
cachexia
    urinary c.
calcification
calculi
calculus
    alternating c.
    coral c.
    cystine c.
    decubitus c.
    dendritic c.
    encysted c.
    fibrin c.
    indigo c.
    nephritic c.
    prostatic c.
    renal c.
    spermatic c.
    stag-horn c.
    urinary c.
    urostealith c.
    vesical c.
    vesicoprostatic c.
caliber
calibrated
calibration
calibrator

caliceal
calicectasis
calicectomy
calices
calices renales
calices renales majores
calices renales minores
calicine
caliectasis
caliectomy
calix
calyceal
calycectasis
calycectomy
calyces
calyces renales
calyces renales majores
calyces renales minores
calyx
Campbell's
    catheter
    forceps
    retractor
    sound
    trocar
capistration
capsula
    c. adiposa renis
    c. fibrosa renis
    c. glomeruli
capsulae renis
capsular
capsule
    Bowman's c.
    fibrous c. of corpora
      cavernosa penis
    Gerota's c.
    glomerular c.

capsule *(continued)*
>
> c. of glomerulus
> müllerian c.
> pelvioprostatic c.
> perinephric c.
> suprarenal c.

capsulectomy

capsuloma

capsuloplasty

capsulorrhaphy

capsulotomy

caput
>
> c. gallinaginis

carcinoma
>
> epibulbar c.
> c. scroti
> squamous cell c.

Carson's catheter

caruncle
>
> morgagnian c.

castrate

castration

C & S – culture and
sensitivity

Cathelin's segregator

catheter
>
> acmistat c.
> acorn tip c.
> Alcock's c.
> Bard's c.
> Bardex's c.
> Blasucci's c.
> Braasch's c.
> Campbell's c.
> Carson's c.
> cathematic c.
> Coude's c.
> Councill's c.

catheter *(continued)*
>
> Coxeter's c.
> de Pezzer's c.
> Emmett-Foley c.
> filiform c.
> Foley c.
> Foley-Alcock c.
> French-Robinson c.
> Furniss' c.
> indwelling c.
> latex c.
> LeFort's c.
> Malecot's c.
> McIver's c.
> Nelaton's c.
> olive tip c.
> Owens' c.
> Pezzer's c.
> Philips' c.
> polyethylene c.
> red Robinson c.
> retention c.
> return flow hemostatic c.
> silastic mushroom c.
> spiral tip c.
> Tiemann's c.
> ureteral c.
> whistle tip c.
> Winer's c.
> Wishard's c.

catheterization
>
> retrourethral c.

catheterize

cauda
>
> c. epididymidis

cavernous

cavum
>
> c. retzii

C-clamp
Cecil's repair
cell
    Leydig's c's.
    Sertoli's c.
cellule
chancre
    Nisbet's c.
chancroid
chemolysis
chorda
    c. gubernaculum
    c. spermatica
chordae
chordee
chorditis
choriocarcinoma
chorioepithelioma
Churny's incision
chylocele
    parasitic c.
chyloderma
chyluria
circumcise
circumcision
circumferential
Civiale's operation
clamp
    Alyea's c.
    Babcock's c.
    Brodny's c.
    C-c.
    Cunningham's c.
    Goldblatt's c.
    Gomco's c.
    Guyon-Pean c.
    Guyon's c.
    Halsted's c.

clamp *(continued)*
    Herrick's c.
    Hyams' c.
    Kantor's c.
    Mayo's c.
    Ockerblad's c.
    pedicle c.
    penile c.
    rubber-shod c.
    Stille's c.
    Stockman's c.
    Tatum's c.
    Walther-Crenshaw c.
    Walther's c.
    Wertheim-Cullen c.
    Wertheim-Reverdin c.
    Wertheim's c.
    Young's c.
    Zipser's c.
Clark's operation
cloaca
    congenital c.
    persistent c.
Cock's operation
collecting system
Colles' fascia
colliculectomy
colliculi
colliculitis
colliculus
    bulbar c.
    seminal c.
    c. seminalis
Collings' electrode
colloid
collum
    c. glandis penis
colony count

column
> Bertin's c.
> c. of Sertoli

concentric

concrement

concretion

condyloma
> c. acuminatum
> c. latum

continence

continent

contracture

convoluted

Cooke-Apert-Gallais
syndrome

cooler
> Eissner's prostatic c.

Cooper's irritable testis

Coppridge's forceps

copulation

copulatory

Corbus' disease

cord
> genital c.
> gubernacular c.
> nephrogenic c.
> spermatic c.

corditis

corona
> c. glandis penis
> c. of glans penis

coronal

corpora

corpus
> c. cavernosum penis
> c. cavernosum urethrae
>   virilis
> c. epididymidis

corpus *(continued)*
> c. glandulae
>   bulbourethralis
> c. glandulare prostatae
> c. Highmori
> c. highmorianum
> c. penis
> c. spongiosum penis
> c. vesicae urinariae
> c. vesiculae seminalis
> c. Wolffi

cortex
> adrenal c.
> c. glandulae suprarenalis
> renal c.
> c. renis

cortiadrenal

cortical

Coude's
> bougie
> catheter

Councill's
> basket
> catheter
> stone dislodger

Cowper's gland

Coxeter's catheter

creatinine

Creevy's evacuator

cremaster
> internal c. of Henle

cremasteric

Crenshaw's forceps

crisis
> Dietl's c.

crista
> c. urethralis masculinae
> c. urethralis virilis

crura
crus
    c. penis
cryptorchid
cryptorchidectomy
cryptorchidism
cryptorchidopexy
cryptorchidy
cryptorchism
crystalloid
crystalluria
crystalluridrosis
cuneiform
Cunningham's clamp
CVA – costovertebral angle
cylinders
    Bence Jones c's.
cylindruria
cyst
    wolffian c.
cystalgia
cystathioninuria
cystatrophia
cystauchenitis
cystauchenotomy
cystauxe
cystectasia
cystectasy
cystectomy
cysteine
cystelcosis
cystendesis
cysterethism
cysthypersarcosis
cystic
cystidolaparotomy
cystidotrachelotomy
cystine

cystinosis
cystinuria
cystistaxis
cystitis
    allergic c.
    amicrobic c.
    bacterial c.
    catarrhal c.
    chemical c.
    c. colli
    croupous c.
    cystic c.
    c. cystica
    diphtheritic c.
    c. emphysematosa
    eosinophilic c.
    exfoliative c.
    c. follicularis
    gangrenous c.
    c. glandularis
    hemorrhagic c.
    incrusted c.
    interstitial c.
    mechanical c.
    panmural c.
    c. papillomatosa
    c. senilis feminarum
    subacute c.
    submucous c.
cystocele
cystochrome
cystochromoscopy
cystocolostomy
cystodynia
cystoenterocele
cystoepiplocele
cystogram
    air c.

cystogram *(continued)*
    excretory c.
    gravity c.
    postvoiding c.
cystography
cystolith
cystolithectomy
cystolithiasis
cystolithic
cystolithotomy
cystometer
    Lewis' c.
cystometrogram
cystometrography
cystometry
cystonephrosis
cystoneuralgia
cystoparalysis
cystopexy
cystophotography
cystophthisis
cystoplasty
cystoplegia
cystoproctostomy
cystoptosis
cystopyelitis
cystopyelogram
cystopyelography
cystopyelonephritis
cystoradiography
cystorectostomy
cystorrhagia
cystorrhaphy
cystorrhea
cystoschisis
cystoscirrhus
cystoscope
    Braasch's c.

cystoscope *(continued)*
    Brown-Buerger c.
    Butterfield's c.
    fiberoptic c.
    Kelly's c.
    Lowsley-Peterson c.
    McCarthy-Campbell c.
    McCarthy-Peterson c.
    McCarthy's c.
    National c.
    Nesbit's c.
    Ravich's c.
    Wappler's c.
cystoscopic
cystoscopy
cystospasm
cystospermitis
cystostaxis
cystostomy
cystotome
cystotomy
    suprapubic c.
cystotrachelotomy
cystoureteritis
cystoureterogram
cystoureteropyelitis
cystoureteropyelonephritis
cystourethritis
cystourethrocele
cystourethrogram
cystourethropexy
cystourethroscope
cystous
dartoic
dartoid
dartos
dartrous
Davat's operation

Davis'
> sound
> stone dislodger

Deaver's retractor
decapsulation
decortication
> renal d.

Dees' needle
Defer's method
Del Castillo's syndrome
demasculinization
Deming's operation
Demme's method
Dennis-Brown technique
Denonvilliers'
> aponeurosis
> fascia
> operation

de Pezzer's catheter
descending
descensus
> d. testis

Desjardin's forceps
detrusor
> d. urinae

dialysance
dialysate
dialysis
> renal d.

dialyzer
diaphragm
> urogenital d.

Dietl's crisis
diffusion
dilatation
dilator
> French's d. Nos. 8 to 36
> Guyon's d.

dilator *(continued)*
> Kollmann's d.
> Leader-Kollmann d.
> Van Buren's d.
> Walther's d.

disease
> Addison's d.
> Bright's d.
> Corbus' d.
> Ducrey's d.
> Durand-Nicolas-Favre d.
> Ebstein's d.
> Kleb's d.
> Lindau's d.
> Peyronie's d.
> Reiter's d.
> Stuhmer's d.

Dittel's
> operation
> sound

diureses
diuresis
> tubular d.

diuretic
> hydragogue d.
> refrigerant d.

diuria
diverticula
> d. ampullae ductus
>   deferentis

diverticulectomy
diverticuleve
diverticulitis
diverticulum
> calyceal d.
> vesical d.

Doppler's operation
Dorian's rib stripper

Dormia's
> basket
> stone dislodger

Douglas' pouch

Doyen's operation

drain
> Malecot's d.
> Penrose d.
> Pezzer's d.
> sump d.

dribbling

drugs. See *Medications.*

Ducrey's disease

duct
> Bellini's d's.
> ejaculatory d.
> Leydig's d.
> mesonephric d.
> d. of Wolff
> wolffian d.

ductuli

ductuli aberrantes

ductuli prostatica

ductulus
> d. aberrans superior

ductus
> d. aberrans
> d. deferens
> d. ejaculatorius
> d. epididymidis
> d. excretorius glandulae bulbourethrales
> d. excretorius vesiculae seminalis
> d. glandulae bulbourethralis
> d. mesonephricus
> d. Muelleri

ductus *(continued)*
> d. paraurethrales
> d. prostatica
> d. spermaticus
> d. wolffi

Duplay's operation

Dupuytren's hydrocele

Durand-Nicolas-Favre disease

dynamoscope

dynamoscopy

dysgenesis
> gonadal d.

dysgenitalism

dysgerminoma

dysgonesis

dysuresia

dysuria
> psychic d.
> spastic d.

dysuriac

dysuric

dyszoospermia

echinococcosis

ectopia
> e. testis
> e. vesicae

Edebohls' operation

efferent

efflux

Eissner's prostatic cooler

ejaculate

ejaculatio
> e. deficiens
> e. praecox
> e. retardata

ejaculation

ejaculatory

ejaculum

electrocystography
electrode
    ball tip e.
    bayonet tip e.
    Bugbee's e.
    Collings' e.
    conical tip e.
    Hamm's e.
    McCarthy's e.
    Neil-Moore e.
    ureteral meatotomy e.
electromyography
    ureteral e.
electrotome
    Stern-McCarthy e.
elephantiasis
    e. scroti
Ellik's evacuator
embolism
embryonal
emission
Emmett-Foley catheter
endometriosis
    e. vesicae
endoscope
    Kelly's e.
endoscopic
endoscopy
endourethral
enorchia
enucleation
enucleator
    Young's e.
enuresis
    diurnal e.
    nocturnal e.
enuretic
epicystitis

epicystotomy
epidermoid
epididymal
epididymectomy
epididymis
epididymitis
epididymodeferentectomy
epididymodeferential
epididymo-orchitis
epididymotomy
epididymovasectomy
epididymovasostomy
epinephrectomy
epinephritis
epinephroma
epinephros
epispadia
epispadiac
epispadial
epispadias
epistaxis
    Gull's renal e.
epithelial
Epstein's
    nephrosis
    syndrome
erectile
erection
erythroplasia
    e. of Queyrat
    Zoon's e.
Esbach's method
evacuator
    Creevy's e.
    Ellik's e.
    McCarthy's e.
    Toomey's e.
Everett-TeLinde operation

exophytic
exsanguinate
exstrophy
    e. of the bladder
extravasation
exudate
exudative
fal-. See words beginning
    phal-.
Fanconi's syndrome
fascia
    Buck's f.
    Colles' f.
    cremasteric f.
    f. cremasterica
    dartos f. of scrotum
    Denonvilliers' f.
    Gerota's f.
    f. penis profunda
    f. penis superficialis
    f. propria cooperi
    f. of prostate
    Scarpa's f.
    spermatic f., external
    spermatic f., internal
    f. spermatica externa
    f. spermatica interna
    f. of urogenital trigone
Feleki's instrument
feminization
    testicular f.
feo-. See words beginning
    pheo-.
Ferguson's basket
fi-. See words beginning *phi-.*
filariasis
filiform
Fishberg's method

fistula
flebo-. See words beginning
    phlebo-.
fluid
    straw colored f.
fluoresceinuria
Foley-Alcock catheter
Foley
    catheter
    forceps
Folin's gravimetric method
Folin's method
Folin and Bell's method
Folin and Berglund's method
Folin and Denis' method
Folin and Farmer's method
Folin and Flander's method
Folin and Hart's method
Folin and Macallum's method
Folin and Wright's method
Folin and Youngburg's method
Folin-Benedict and Myers'
    method
Folin, McEllroy and Peck's
    method
Follmann's balanitis
follower
forceps
    Allis' f.
    Blakes' f.
    Bozeman's f.
    Braasch's f.
    Buerger-McCarthy f.
    Bumpus' f.
    Bunim's f.
    Campbell's f.
    Coppridge's f.
    Crenshaw's f.

forceps *(continued)*
>Desjardin's f.
>Foley's f.
>Harris' f.
>Kelly's f.
>Lewis' f.
>Lewkowitz's f.
>Lowsley's f.
>Mathieu's f.
>McCarthy-Alcock f.
>McCarthy's f.
>McNealy-Glassman-Babcock f.
>Millin's f.
>Pitha's f.
>Poutasse's f.
>Randall's f.
>Ratliff-Blake f.
>Ray's f.
>Rochester-Pean f.
>Skillern's f.
>White-Oslay f.
>Young's f.

foreskin
Formad's kidney
foroblique
fossa
>f. of Morgagni
>navicular f. of male urethra
>f. navicularis urethrae
>f. ovalis

Fowler's sound
Franco's operation
Franklin-Silverman needle
French-McCarthy panendo-scope
French-Robinson catheter

French's dilator
frenulum
>f. of prepuce of penis
>f. preputii penis

frenum
frequency
Freyer's operation
friable
fulguration
fundic
fundiform
fundus
>f. of bladder
>f. of urinary bladder
>f. vesicae urinariae

funiculitis
funiculopexy
funiculus
>f. spermaticus

Furniss' catheter
galactosuria
galacturia
GC – gonococcus
genital
genitalia
genitocrural
genitofemoral
genitoinfectious
genitoplasty
genitourinary
Gerota's
>capsule
>fascia

Gibbon's hydrocele
Gibson's incision
Gilbert-Dreyfus syndrome
Gilbert's syndrome
Giraldes' organ

gland
    Albarran's g.
    Cowper's g.
    Littre's g's.
    Skene's g.
glans
    g. penis
gleet
glischruria
globulinuria
globus
    g. major epididymidis
    g. minor epididymidis
glomerular
glomeruli
    g. renis
    Ruysch's g.
glomerulitis
glomerulonephritis
glomerulopathy
glomerulosclerosis
glomerulose
glomerulus
glycosuria
Goldblatt's
    clamp
    hypertension
Gomco's clamp
gonad
gonadal
gonadectomize
gonadectomy
gonadial
gonadopathy
gonadotherapy
gonadotropin
    chorionic g.
gonadotropism

gonaduct
gonangiectomy
gonecyst
gonecystis
gonecystitis
gonecystolith
gonecystopyosis
gonocele
gonococcal
gonococci
gonococcus
gonophore
gonorrhea
gonorrheal
gorget
    Teale's g.
graft
    Thiersch's g.
granuloma
    g. inguinale
gravity
    specific g.
Grawitz's tumor
groin
GU — genitourinary
gubernaculum
    chorda g.
    Hunter's g.
    g. testis
Gull's renal epistaxis
gumma
Guyon-Pean clamp
Guyon's
    clamp
    dilator
    sound
Hagner's operation
Halsted's clamp

Hamm's electrode
Harrington's retractor
Harris'
      forceps
      segregator
Heintz's method
Heller-Nelson syndrome
hemangioma
hemangiosarcoma
hematocele
      scrotal h.
hematoma
hematoscheocele
hematospermatocele
hematospermia
hematuria
      angioneurotic h.
      endemic h.
      essential h.
      microscopic h.
      renal h.
      urethral h.
      vesical h.
hemaurochrome
hemodialysis
hemospermia
hemostatic bag
      Pilcher's h.b.
Hendrickson's lithotrite
Henle's
      ampulla
      internal cremaster of H.
      loop
      sphincter
      tubules
hermaphrodism
hermaphrodite
hermaphroditism

herpes
      h. praeputialis
      h. progenitalis
      h. simplex
      h. zoster
Herrick's clamp
Hesselbach's triangle
Heyd's syndrome
Highmore's body
Highmori
      corpus of H.
hilar
hili
hilum
hilus
      h. glandulae supra-
         renalis
      h. of kidney
      h. renalis
      h. of suprarenal gland
hind-kidney
Hinman's reflux
Hippel-Lindau syndrome
hook
      Kimball's h.
Howard's basket
Huggins' operation
Hunner's stricture
Hunter's gubernaculum
Hurwitz's trocar
Hutchins' needle
hyaline
Hyams' clamp
hydatid
      h. of Morgagni
      sessile h.
hydatidocele
hydatiduria

hydrocele
    chylous h.
    h. colli
    communicating h.
    Dupuytren's h.
    encysted h.
    funicular h.
    Gibbon's h.
    Maunoir's h.
    noncommunicating h.
    scrotal h.
hydrocelectomy
hydronephrosis
hydronephrotic
hydroperinephrosis
hydropyonephrosis
hydrosarcocele
hydroscheocele
hydroureter
hydroureterosis
hydrouria
hyperemia
hypernephritis
hypernephroid
hypernephroma
hyperorchidism
hyperoxaluria
hyperplasia
hypertension
    adrenal h.
    Goldblatt's h.
    renal h.
hypertonic
hypertrophy
hypogastric
hypogonadism
hypoplasia
hypospadiac

hypospadias
hypotonia
hypotonic
Iglesias' resectoscope
iliac
iliocostal
iliohypogastric
ilioinguinal
Immergut's tube
implant
    silastic i.
impotence
impotentia
    i. coeundi
    i. erigendi
incision
    Bardenheuer's i.
    Bergman-Israel i.
    Bergmann's i.
    Churny's i.
    dorsolateral i.
    flank i.
    Gibson's i.
    Langenbeck's i.
    lateral flank i.
    midline i.
    paramedian i.
    parerectus i.
    Pean's i.
    Pfannenstiel's i.
    pyelotomy i.
    rectus i.
    Simon's i.
    stabwound i.
    subcostal i.
    suprapubic i.
    transverse i.
    vertical i.

incontinence
  paradoxical i.
  paralytic i.
  stress i.
  urinary i.
  i. of urine
incontinent
incontinentia
  i. urinae
indoluria
indoxyl
indoxyluria
induration
  penile i.
indwelling
infarct
  bilirubin i's.
  Brewer's i's.
  uric acid i.
inflammatory
infundibula
  i. of kidney
infundibular
infundibuliform
infundibulopelvic
infundibulum
  i. of urinary bladder
inguinal
inguinocrural
inguinoscrotal
insertion
  cystoradium i.
instrument
  Feleki's i.
integument
intercostal
intercourse
interlobar

interlobular
interstitial
interureteral
interureteric
intrarenal
intratesticular
intraureteral
intraurethral
intravesical
intussusception
Isaacs-Ludwig arteriole
ischiopubic
ischiorectal
Israel's operation
isthmus
  i. prostatae
  i. urethrae
isuria
IVP – intravenous pyelogram
Jacobson's retractor
Jewett's sound
Johnson's
  basket
  needle holder
  stone dislodger
Judd-Masson retractor
junction
  ureteropelvic j.
  ureterovesical j.
Kantor's clamp
Keitzer's urethrotome
Kelly-Deming operation
Kelly's
  cystoscope
  endoscope
  forceps
  operation
Kelly-Stoeckel operation

kidney
- amyloid k.
- arteriosclerotic k.
- artificial k.
- atrophic k.
- cake k.
- cicatricial k.
- cirrhotic k.
- clump k.
- contracted k.
- cyanotic k.
- cystic k.
- disk k.
- doughnut k.
- floating k.
- Formad's k.
- fused k.
- granular k.
- hind k.
- horseshoe k.
- lardaceous k.
- lump k.
- mortar k.
- mural k.
- myelin k.
- pelvic k.
- polycystic k.
- primordial k.
- putty k.
- Rokitansky's k.
- Rose-Bradford k.
- sacciform k.
- sclerotic k.
- sigmoid k.
- soapy k.
- sponge k.
- supernumerary k.
- wandering k.

kidney *(continued)*
- waxy k.

kilo-. See words beginning *chylo-.*
Kimball's hook
Kimmelstiel-Wilson syndrome
Kleb's disease
Klinefelter's syndrome
Kocher's retractor
Kollmann's dilator
kor-. See words beginning *chor-.*
kraurosis
- k. penis

KUB – kidney, ureter and bladder
Labbé's syndrome
lactosuria
lacuna
- great l. of urethra
- l. magna

lacunae
lacunae of Morgagni
lacunae Morgagnii urethrae mulliebris
lacunae of urethra
lacunae urethrales
lamella
lamina
- l. visceralis tunicae vaginalis propriae testis
- l. visceralis tunicae vaginalis testis

Lancereaux's nephritis
Langenbeck's incision
laparonephrectomy
Lapides' needle holder
Lashmet and Newburgh method

Leader-Kollmann dilator
LeFort's
    bougie
    catheter
    sound
Legueu's retractor
leiomyoma
leiomyosarcoma
Leriche's syndrome
leukoplakia
    l. penis
Levant's stone dislodger
Lewis'
    cystometer
    forceps
Lewkowitz's forceps
leydigarche
Leydig's
    cells
    duct
libidogen
lichen
    l. planus
lienorenal
Lindau's disease
line
    Broedel's l.
linea
    l. alba
lipoma
liposarcoma
liquor
    l. prostaticus
    l. seminis
lithangiuria
lithectasy
lithocenosis
lithoclysmia

lithocystotomy
lithodialysis
lithokonion
litholabe
litholapaxy
litholysis
litholyte
lithometer
lithomyl
lithonephria
lithonephritis
lithonephrotomy
lithophone
lithoscope
lithotripsy
lithotriptic
lithotriptor
lithotriptoscope
lithotriptoscopy
lithotrite
    Bigelow's l.
    Hendrickson's l.
    Reliquet's l.
lithotrity
lithous
lithoxiduria
lithuresis
lithureteria
lithuria
Littre's glands
lobule
    cortical l's. of kidney
    l's. of testis
lobuli corticales renis
lobuli epididymidis
lobuli testis
lobulus
Löhlein's nephritis

Longuet's operation
loop
    Henle's l.
Lowsley-Peterson cystoscope
Lowsley's
    forceps
    operation
    tractor
Luder-Sheldon syndrome
lumen
lumbosacral
luxation
Luy's segregator
lymphangiogram
lymphangioma
lymphangiosarcoma
lymphogranuloma
    l. inguinale
    venereal l.
    l. venereum
lymphopathia
    l. venereum
Maisonneuve's urethrotome
Makka's operation
malacoplakia
    m. vesicae
Malecot's
    catheter
    drain
Marañon's syndrome
Marchand's adrenals
Marian's operation
Marshall-Marchetti operation
Marshall-Marchetti-Krantz
   operation
Marshall's
    surgical sucker
Martin's operation

Martius' operation
Martius-Harris operation
Masson-Judd retractor
Mathieu's forceps
Maunoir's hydrocele
Mayo's clamp
Mays' operation
McCarthy-Alcock forceps
McCarthy-Campbell
   cystoscope
McCarthy-Peterson
   cystoscope
McCarthy's
    cystoscope
    electrode
    evacuator
    forceps
    foroblique panendoscope
    resectoscope
    telescope
McCrea's sound
McGill's operation
McIver's catheter
McNealy-Glassman-Babcock
   forceps
meatal
meatome
meatometer
meatorrhaphy
meatoscope
meatoscopy
meatotome
meatotomy
meatus
    m. urinarius
median-bar
mediastinum
    m. testis

Medications

- adrenalin
- Aerosporin
- Almetropin
- ammonium chloride
- ammonium mandelate
- Amnestrogen
- ampicillin
- Anestacon
- Antuitrin
- Anturane
- atropine
- Azo Gantanol
- Azo-Gantrisin
- Azo-Mandelamine
- B & O suppositories
- bromophenol blue
- chlormerodrin
- Chloromycetin
- Chorex
- chorionic gonadotropin
- Chymoral
- Clinistix
- colistin
- Coly-Mycin
- Conestron
- cranberry juice
- cupric sulfate
- Daricon
- Delatestryl
- Delestrogen
- Depo-Testosterone
- Dicorvin
- diethylstilbestrol
- Diuril
- Donnasep
- Dyclone
- dyphylline

Medications *(continued)*

- Elase
- Enarax
- Estinyl
- estradiol
- Estradurin
- ethoxazene hydrochloride
- Flagyl
- fluoxymesterone
- Furacin
- Furadantin
- Gantrisin
- Glucose oxidase reagent
- Halotestin
- Hema-Combistix
- Hexalet
- Hiprex
- hydrochloric acid
- Hypaque
- Indigo Carmine
- kanamycin
- Kantrex
- Keflin
- Labstix
- Lugol's solution
- Macrodantin
- Mandacon
- Mandalay
- Mandelamine
- mandelic acid
- mannitol
- meralluride
- mercaptomerin
- Mesulfin
- Metandren
- methenamine
- methotrexate
- methylene blue

Medications *(continued)*

Methyl Red-Bromothymol blue reagent
methyltestosterone
Methylthionine Chloride
Mycifradin
nalidixic acid
NegGram
neomycin
Neo-Polycin
Neosporin
Neothylline
Nitranitol
Nitrazine
nitrofurantoin
Ora-Testryl
Oreton
Ovocyclin
Penbritin
penicillin
Perandren
pH
phenaphthazine
phenazopyridine
Phenol red
phenolsulfonphthalein
pHisoHex
Polycillin
polymyxin B
potassium chloride
Pregnyl
Premarin
Profenil
Proklar
Prostaphlin
Pyridium
Renelate

Medications *(continued)*

Retropaque (contrast media)
Serenium
Skiodan (contrast media)
sodium biphosphate
sodium indigotindisulfonate
sodium para-aminohippurate
Sonilyn
Staphcillin
Stemutrolin
Stilbestrol
Stilbetin
Stilphostrol
streptomycin
sulfinpyrazone
sulfonamide
sulfosalicylic acid
Syncillin
TACE
Talwin
Tes-Tape
testosterone
testryl
tetracycline
theophylline
Thiosulfil
Trasentine
Trocinate
Ultandren
Urecholine
Urised
Urisedamine
Uristix
Uritone
Urolitia

Medications *(continued)*
    Uro-Phosphate
    Urostat-2X
    Usanol
    Utrasul
    Xylocaine
    Zephiran
medorrhea
medulla
    adrenal m.
    m. glandulae suprarenalis
    m. of kidney
    m. nephrica
    m. renis
    m. of suprarenal gland
    suprarenal m.
medullae
medullary
medullectomy
medulliadrenal
medulloadrenal
medulloid
medullosuprarenoma
megabladder
megalopenis
megaloureter
melasma
    m. addisonii
    m. suprarenale
Mercier's
    bar
    operation
mesenchymal
mesonephric
mesonephroma
mesonephron
mesonephros
mesothelioma

metanephroi
metanephros
method
    acid hematin m.
    Addis's m.
    Arnold and Gunning's m.
    Bence Jones protein m.
    Benedict and Franke's m.
    Benedict and
      Osterberg's m.
    Bertrand's m.
    Defer's m.
    Demme's m.
    Esbach's m.
    Fishberg's m.
    Folin's m.
    Folin's gravimetric m.
    Folin and Bell's m.
    Folin-Benedict and
      Myers' m.
    Folin and Berglund's m.
    Folin and Denis' m.
    Folin and Farmer's m.
    Folin and Flander's m.
    Folin and Hart's m.
    Folin and Macallum's m.
    Folin, McEllroy and
      Peck's m.
    Folin and Wright's m.
    Folin and Youngburg's
      m.
    Heintz's m.
    Lashmet and Newburgh
      m.
    Naunyn-Minkowski m.
    Osborne and Folin's m.
    permutit m.
    Power and Wilder's m.

method *(continued)*
    Shohl and Pedley's m.
    Sjöqvist's m.
    Sumner's m.
    Volhard and Fahr m.
Metzenbaum's scissors
microrchidia
miction
micturate
micturition
Miller's syndrome
Millin-Bacon
    retractor
    spreader
Millin's
    forceps
    tube
Mitchell's basket
mononephrous
morcellement
Morgagni
    fossa of M.
    hydatid of M.
    lacunae of M.
Mosher's speculum
Moynihan's
    probe
    scoop
Muelleri
    ductus M.
muscle
    Bell's m.
    bulbocavernous m.
    cremaster m.
    ischiocavernous m.
    psoas m.
musculus levator prostate
musculus obturatorius externus

musculus obturatorius internus
musculus pubovaginalis
musculus pubovesicalis
musculus quadratus lumborum
musculus rectourethralis
musculus rectovesicalis
musculus sphincter urethrae
musculus sphincter vesicae
    urinariae
musculus transversus
    abdominis
musculus transversus perinei
    superficialis
myoma
myxocystitis
myxoma
myxosarcoma
Narath's operation
National cystoscope
Naunyn-Minkowski method
needle
    Dees' n.
    Franklin-Siverman n.
    Hutchins' n.
    Turkel's n.
    Veenema-Gusberg n.
    Vim-Silverman n.
needle holder
    Johnson's n.h.
    Lapides' n. h.
    Stratte's n. h.
    Young-Millin n. h.
    Young's n. h.
Neil-Moore electrode
Nelaton's
    catheter
    spincter
neoplastic

nephradenoma
nephralgia
    idiopathic n.
nephralgic
nephrapostasis
nephrasthenia
nephratonia
nephratony
nephrauxe
nephrectasia
nephrectasis
nephrectasy
nephrectomize
nephrectomy
nephredema
nephrelcosis
nephremia
nephremphraxis
nephria
nephric
nephridium
nephrism
nephritic
nephritides
nephritis
    albuminous n.
    arteriosclerotic n.
    azotemic n.
    bacterial n.
    capsular n.
    n. caseosa
    catarrhal n.
    cheesy n.
    chloroazotemic n.
    clostridial n.
    congenital n.
    croupous n.
    degenerative n.

nephritis *(continued)*
    desquamative n.
    diffuse n.
    n. dolorosa
    dropsical n.
    exudative n.
    fibrolipomatous n.
    fibrous n.
    focal n.
    glomerular n.
    glomerulocapsular n.
    n. gravidarum
    hemorrhagic n.
    hydremic n.
    hydropigenous n.
    hypogenetic n.
    idiopathic n.
    indurative n.
    interstitial n.
    Lancereaux's n.
    lipomatous n.
    Löhlein's n.
    n. mitis
    parenchymatous n.
    pneumococcus n.
    n. of pregnancy
    productive n.
    n. repens
    saturnine n.
    scarlatinal n.
    subacute n.
    suppurative n.
    syphilitic n.
    tartrate n.
    transfusion n.
    trench n.
    tubal n.
    tuberculous n.

nephritis *(continued)*
  vascular n.
  Volhard's n.
  war n.
nephritogenic
nephroabdominal
nephroangiosclerosis
nephroblastoma
nephrocalcinosis
nephrocapsectomy
nephrocardiac
nephrocele
nephrocirrhosis
nephrocolic
nephrocolopexy
nephrocoloptosis
nephrocystanastomosis
nephrocystitis
nephrocystosis
nephroerysipelas
nephrogastric
nephrogenic
nephrogenous
nephrogram
nephrography
nephrohemia
nephrohydrosis
nephrohypertrophy
nephroid
nephrolith
nephrolithiasis
nephrolithotomy
nephrologist
nephrology
nephrolysis
nephroma
nephromalacia
nephromegaly

nephron
nephroncus
nephro-omentopexy
nephroparalysis
nephropathic
nephropathy
  dropsical n.
  hypazoturic n.
  hypochloruric n.
nephropexy
nephrophagiasis
nephropoietic
nephropoietin
nephroptosia
nephroptosis
nephropyelitis
nephropyelolithotomy
nephropyeloplasty
nephropyosis
nephrorosein
nephrorrhagia
nephrorrhaphy
nephroscleria
nephrosclerosis
  arteriolar n.
  benign n.
  intercapillary n.
  malignant n.
  senile n.
nephroses
nephrosis
  amyloid n.
  Epstein's n.
  larval n.
  lipid n.
  lipoid n.
  lower nephron n.
  necrotizing n.

nephrosis
  toxic n.
nephrospasis
nephrosplenopexy
nephrostomy
nephrotic
nephrotome
nephrotomography
nephrotomy
  abdominal n.
  lumbar n.
nephrotoxic
nephrotoxicity
nephrotoxin
nephrotresis
nephrotropic
nephrotuberculosis
nephrotyphoid
nephrotyphus
nephroureterectomy
nephroureterocystectomy
nephrozymase
nephrozymosis
Nesbit's
  cystoscope
  resectoscope
Nisbet's chancre
nocturia
Nonnenbruch's syndrome
Nourse's syringe
NSU – nonspecific urethritis
obturator
  Alcock-Timberlake o.
  Timberlake's o.
Ochsner's
  probe
  trocar
Ockerblad's clamp

O'Conor's operation
oligohydruria
oligonecrospermia
oligophosphaturia
oligospermatism
oligospermia
oliguria
Ombrédanne's operation
opacity
operation
  Andrews' o.
  Bates' o.
  Belfield's o.
  Bennett's o.
  Bergenhem's o.
  Bevan-Rochet o.
  Bevan's o.
  Bigelow's o.
  Boari's o.
  Bottini's o.
  Bricker's o.
  Civiale's o.
  Clark's o.
  Cock's o.
  Davat's o.
  Deming's o.
  Denonvilliers' o.
  Dittel's o.
  Doppler's o.
  Doyen's o.
  Duplay's o.
  Edebohls' o.
  Everett-TeLinde o.
  Franco's o.
  Freyer's o.
  Hagner's o.
  Huggins' o.
  Israel's o.

operation *(continued)*
   Kelly's o.
   Kelly-Deming o.
   Kelly-Stoeckel o.
   Longuet's o.
   Lowsley's o.
   Makka's o.
   Marian's o.
   Marshall-Marchetti o.
   Marshall-Marchetti-
     Krantz o.
   Martin's o.
   Martius' o.
   Martius-Harris o.
   Mays' o.
   McGill's o.
   Mercier's o.
   Narath's o.
   O'Conor's o.
   Ombrédanne's o.
   Petersen's o.
   Poncet's o.
   Rigaud's o.
   Stanischeff's o.
   Steinach's o.
   Torek's o.
   Tuffier's o.
   van Hook's o.
   Vidal's o.
   Vogel's o.
   Volkmann's o.
   von Bergmann's o.
   von Hacker's o.
   Voronoff's o.
   Wheelhouse's o.
   White's o.
   Wood's o.
   Young's o.

orchialgia
orchichorea
orchidalgia
orchidectomy
orchidic
orchiditis
orchidocelioplasty
orchidoepididymectomy
orchidoncus
orchidopathy
orchidopexy
orchidoplasty
orchidoptosis
orchidorrhaphy
orchidotherapy
orchidotomy
orchiectomy
orchiencephaloma
orchiepididymitis
orchilytic
orchiocatabasis
orchiocele
orchiococcus
orchiodynia
orchiomyeloma
orchioncus
orchioneuralgia
orchiopathy
orchiopexy
orchioplasty
orchiorrhaphy
orchioscheocele
orchioscirrhus
orchiotomy
orchis
orchitic
orchitis
   metastatic o.

orchitis *(continued)*
    o. parotidea
    o. variolosa
orchitolytic
orchotomy
organ
    o. of Giraldes
orgasm
orifice
    o. of male urethra
    o. of ureter
    o. of urethra
    vesicourethral o.
os
    o. penis
    o. pubis
Osborne and Folin's method
osteoma
Otis'
    bougie
    sound
    urethrotome
Owens' catheter
pampiniform
panendoscope
    French-McCarthy p.
    McCarthy's foroblique p.
panendoscopy
papilla
papillary
paradidymal
paradidymis
paragenitalis
paraglobulinuria
paranephric
paranephritis
    lipomatous p.
paranephroma

paranephros
paraphimosis
pararenal
paraurethra
paraurethral
paraurethritis
paravesical
parenchyma
    p. testis
    p. of testis
parenchymal
parietal
pars
    p. abdominalis ureteris
    p. cavernosa urethrae virilis
    p. convoluta lobuli corticalis renis
    p. membranacea urethrae masculinae
    p. membranacea urethrae virilis
    p. pelvina ureteris
    p. prostatica urethrae masculinae
    p. prostatica urethrae virilis
    p. radiata lobuli corticalis renis
    p. spongiosa urethrae masculinae
partes genitales externae viriles
partes genitales masculinae externae
Pean's incision
pedicle
pelves

pelvilithotomy
pelvioileoneocystostomy
pelviolithotomy
pelvioneostomy
pelvioperitonitis
pelvioplasty
pelvioradiography
pelvioscopy
pelviostomy
pelviotomy
pelviradiography
pelvirectal
pelviroentgenography
pelvis
penial
penile
penis
    clubbed p.
    p. plastica
penischisis
penitis
penoscrotal
Penrose drain
periarteritis
    p. gummosa
    p. nodosa
pericystitis
perineal
perineoscrotal
perineostomy
perinephric
perinephritic
perinephritis
perinephrium
perineum
periorchitis
    p. adhaesiva
    p. purulenta

periorchium
peripenial
periprostatic
periprostatis
perirenal
perispermatitis
    p. serosa
peritoneal
peritoneum
periureteric
periureteritis
periurethral
periurethritis
perivesical
perivesicular
perivesiculitis
permutit method
Petersen's operation
Peyronie's disease
Pezzer's
    catheter
    drain
Pfannenstiel's incision
phallalgia
phallanastrophe
phallaneurysm
phallectomy
phallic
phallitis
phallocampsis
phallocrypsis
phallodynia
phalloncus
phalloplasty
phallorrhagia
phallorrhea
phallotomy
phallus

phenolsulfonphthalein
pheochromocytoma
Phiefer-Young retractor
Philips'
    bougie
    catheter
phimosiectomy
phimosis
phimotic
phlebolith
photoscan
pielo-. See words beginning
    pyelo-.
Pilcher's hemostatic bag
pio-. See words beginning
    pyo-.
Pitha's forceps
plexus
    p. cavernosus penis
    cavernous p. of penis
    pampiniform p.
    p. pampiniformis
    prostatic p.
    prostaticovesical p.
    p. prostaticus
    renal p.
    p. renalis
    Santorini's p.
    spermatic p.
    p. spermaticus
    suprarenal p.
    p. suprarenalis
    testicular p.
    p. testicularis
    ureteric p.
    p. uretericus
    p. venosus prostaticus
    vesical p.

plexus *(continued)*
    p. vesicale
    p. vesicalis
    vesicoprostatic p.
plica
    p. pubovesicalis
    p. vesicalis transversa
pneumaturia
polycystic
polyorchidism
polyorchis
polyspermia
polyspermism
polyspermy
polyuria
Poncet's operation
porphyria
porphyrinuria
porphyruria
position
    dorsal lithotomy p.
    lithotomy p.
    supine p.
posthetomy
posthioplasty
posthitis
postholith
Potain's trocar
pouch
    p. of Douglas
Poutasse's forceps
Power and Wilder's method
Pratt's sound
preperitoneal
prepuce
    p. of penis
preputial
preputiotomy

preputium
    p. penis
preurethritis
prevesical
priapism
priapitis
priapus
probe
    Moynihan's p.
    Ochsner's p.
progenital
pronephros
properitoneal
prostata
prostatalgia
prostatauxe
prostate
prostatectomy
    perineal p.
    retropubic prevesical p.
    suprapubic transvesical
      p.
    transurethral p.
prostatelcosis
prostateria
prostatic
prostaticovesical
prostaticovesiculectomy
prostatism
    vesical p.
prostatisme
    p. sans prostate
prostatitic
prostatitis
    granulomatous p.
    tuberculous p.
prostatocystitis
prostatocystotomy

prostatodynia
prostatography
prostatolith
prostatolithotomy
prostatomegaly
prostatometer
prostatomy
prostatomyomectomy
prostatorrhea
prostatotomy
prostatotoxin
prostatovesiculectomy
prostatovesiculitis
prosthesis
    silastic testicular p.
proteinuria
    Bence-Jones p.
proteinuric
pseudohermaphrodism
pseudohermaphrodite
pseudohermaphroditism
psoas muscle
PSP — phenolsulfonphthalein
ptosis
    p. of kidney
pubes
pubetrotomy
pubic
pubioplasty
pubiotomy
pubis
puboprostatic
pubovesical
pudendal
PVC — postvoiding cystogram
pyelectasia
pyelectasis
pyelic

pyelitic
pyelitis
    calculous p.
    p. cystica
    defloration p.
    encrusted p.
    p. glandularis
    p. granulosa
    p. gravidarum
    hematogenous p.
    hemorrhagic p.
    suppurative p.
    urogenous p.
pyelocaliectasis
pyelocystanastomosis
pyelocystitis
pyelocystostomosis
pyelofluoroscopy
pyelogram
    intravenous p.
pyelograph
pyelography
    air p.
    ascending p.
    drip p.
    excretion p.
    infusion p.
    intravenous p.
    respiration p.
    retrograde p.
pyeloileocutaneous
pyelointerstitial
pyelolithotomy
pyelometer
pyelometry
pyelonephritis
    xanthogranulomatous p.
pyelonephrosis

pyelopathy
pyelophlebitis
pyeloplasty
pyeloplication
pyeloscopy
pyelostomy
pyelotomy
pyelotubular
pyeloureterectasis
pyeloureterogram
pyeloureterography
pyeloureterolysis
pyeloureteroplasty
pyelovenous
pyocalix
pyocele
pyogenic
pyonephritis
pyonephrolithiasis
pyonephrosis
pyonephrotic
pyospermia
pyoureter
pyovesiculosis
pyramid
    p's. of kidney
    renal p's.
pyuria
Queyrat's erythroplasia
rabdo-. See words beginning
    rhabdo-.
radiolucent
rafe. See *raphe.*
Ralks' adapter
Randall's forceps
Rankin's retractor
raphe
    r. penis

raphe *(continued)*
    r. of perineum
    r. scroti
    r. of scrotum
Ratliff-Blake forceps
Ravich's cystoscope
Ray's forceps
reaction
    Bittorf's r.
recessus
    r. hepatorenalis
rectourethral
rectovesical
rectovestibular
red Robinson catheter
reflux
    Hinman's r.
    urethrovesiculodifferential r.
Reifenstein's syndrome
Reiter's disease
Reliquet's lithotrite
renal
renculi
renicapsule
renicardiac
reniculi
reniculus
renin
renipelvic
reniportal
renipuncture
renocortical
renocutaneous
renogastric
renogram
renography
renointestinal

renoprival
renopulmonary
renotrophic
renotropic
repair
    Bengt-Johanson r.
    Cecil's r.
resectoscope
    Baumrucker's r.
    Bumpus' r.
    cold punch r.
    Iglesias' r.
    McCarthy's r.
    Nesbit's r.
    Stern-McCarthy r.
    Thompson's r.
residual
rete
    r. testis
retractor
    Campbell's r.
    Deaver's r.
    Harrington's r.
    Jacobson's r.
    Judd-Masson r.
    Kocher's r.
    Legueu's r.
    Masson-Judd r.
    Millin-Bacon r.
    Phiefer-Young r.
    Rankin's r.
    self retaining r.
    Veenema's r.
    Young's r.
retrograde
retroperitoneal
Retzius' space
rhabdomyoma

rhabdosarcoma
    renal r.
rib cutter
    Bethune's r. c.
rib stripper
    Dorian's r. s.
Rigaud's operation
Robinson's stone dislodger
Roche's sign
Rochester-Pean forceps
Rokitansky's kidney
Rose-Bradford kidney
Rosenthal's speculum
ruga
rugae
Ruschelit's bougie
Ruysch's glomeruli
sacculation
sacculus
sacral
Santorini's plexus
sarcocele
sarcoma
scapus
    s. penis
Scarpa's fascia
schistosomiasis
    urinary s.
    vesical s.
Schmidt's syndrome
scissors
    Metzenbaum's s.
sclerosis
    renal arteriolar s.
scoop
    Moynihan's s.
scrotal
scrotectomy

scrotitis
scrotocele
scrotoplasty
scrotum
    s. lapillosum
    lymph s.
    watering-can s.
segregator
    Cathelin's s.
    Harris' s.
    Luy's s.
semen
semenuria
seminal
semination
seminiferous
seminologist
seminology
seminoma
seminuria
septa of testis
septum
    s. bulbi urethrae
    s. glandis penis
    s. of glans penis
    s. pectiniforme
    s. penis
    rectovesical s.
    s. rectovesicale
    s. renis
    s. scroti
    s. of scrotum
serosa
Sertoli's
    cell
    column
shangker. See *chancre.*
Shohl and Pedley's method

sign
   Gilbert's s.
   Roche's s.
Simon's incision
sinus
   s. epididymidis
   s. of epididymis
   prostatic s.
   s. prostaticus
   renal s.
   s. renalis
Sjöqvist's method
Skene's gland
Skillern's forceps
skis-. See words beginning
   schis-.
smegma
   s. praeputii
sois. See *psoas.*
sound
   Campbell's s.
   Davis' s.
   Dittel's s.
   Fowler's s.
   Guyon's s.
   Jewett's s.
   LeFort's s.
   McCrea's s.
   Otis' s.
   Pratt's s.
   Van Buren's s.
   Walther's s.
space
   Retzius' s.
specific gravity
speculum
   Mosher's s.
   Rosenthal's s.

sperm
   muzzled s.
spermacrasia
spermagglutination
spermalist
spermatemphraxis
spermatic
spermaticide
spermatid
spermatin
spermatism
spermatitis
spermatoblast
spermatocele
spermatocelectomy
spermatocidal
spermatocyst
spermatocystectomy
spermatocystitis
spermatocystotomy
spermatocytal
spermatocyte
spermatocytogenesis
spermatogenesis
spermatogenic
spermatogenous
spermatogeny
spermatogone
spermatogonium
spermatoid
spermatology
spermatolysin
spermatolysis
spermatolytic
spermatomere
spermatometrite
spermatopathia
spermatopoietic

spermatorrhea
spermatoschesis
spermatovum
spermatozoa
spermatozoal
spermatozoon
spermaturia
spermectomy
spermia
spermiation
spermicidal
spermicide
spermiduct
spermiocyte
spermiogenesis
spermioteleosis
spermioteleotic
spermium
spermoblast
spermoculture
spermolith
spermoloropexy
spermoneuralgia
spermophlebectasia
spermoplasm
spermosphere
spermotoxic
spermotoxin
sphincter
    Henle's s.
    Nélaton's s.
    s. urethrae
    s. vesicae
spreader
    Millin-Bacon s.
stain
    Ziehl-Neelsen s.
Stanischeff's operation

stasis
    urinary s.
Steinach's operation
stellate
stenosis
stenotic
sterile
sterility
Stern-McCarthy
    electrotome
    resectoscope
Stille's clamp
Stockman's clamp
stone dislodger
    Councill's s. d.
    Davis' s. d.
    Dormia's s. d.
    Johnson's s. d.
    Levant's s. d.
    Robinson's s. d.
    woven loop s. d.
stranguria
strangury
Stratte's needle holder
stricture
    Hunner's s.
stroma
Stühmer's disease
stuttering
    urinary s.
stylet
sucker
    Marshall's surgical s.
sulcus
Sulkowitch's test
summit
    s. of bladder
Sumner's method

suprapubic
suprarenal
suprarenalectomy
suprarenalism
suprarenalopathy
suprarene
suprarenoma
surgical procedures. See
   operation.
suspensory
symphysis
   s. pubica
   s. pubis
syndrome
   adrenogenital s.
   Allemann's s.
   Bartter's s.
   Bywaters' s.
   Cacchi-Ricci s.
   Cooke-Apert-Gallais s.
   Del Castillo's s.
   Epstein's s.
   Fanconi's s.
   Gilbert-Dreyfus s.
   Gilbert's s.
   Heller-Nelson s.
   Heyd's s.
   Hippel-Lindau s.
   Kimmelstiel-Wilson s.
   Klinefelter's s.
   Labbé's s.
   Leriche's s.
   Luder-Sheldon s.
   Marañon's s.
   Miller's s.
   Nonnenbruch's s.
   Reifenstein's s.
   Schmidt's s.

syndrome *(continued)*
   suprarenogenic s.
   Thorn's s.
   Turner's s.
   Waterhouse-
      Friderichsen s.
synorchidism
synorchism
synoscheos
syphilis
syphilitic
syringe
   Nourse's s.
   Toomey's s.
Tatum's clamp
Teale's gorget
technique
   Dennis-Brown t.
telescope
   McCarthy's t.
   Vest's t.
tenesmus
   vesical t.
teratocarcinoma
teratoma
test
   Albarran's t.
   creatinine clearance t.
   nitrogen retention t.
   proteinuria t.
   radioisotope renogram t.
   serum creatinine t.
   specific gravity t.
   Sulkowitch's t.
   urine chloride t.
   Watson-Schwartz t.
testes
testicle

testicular
testiculoma
testiculus
testis
> Cooper's irritable t.
> inverted t.
> obstructed t.
> pulpy t.
> t. redux
> retained t.
> undescended t.

testitis
testitoxicosis
testoid
testopathy
Thiersch's graft
Thompson's resectoscope
Thorn's syndrome
Tiemann's catheter
Timberlake's obturator
Toomey's
> evacuator
> syringe

Torek's operation
torsion
torus
> t. uretericus

tosis. See *ptosis.*
tour
> t. de maitre

trabecula
trabeculae
trabeculae corporis spongiosi
> penis

trabeculae corporum caverno-
> sorum penis

trabecular
trabeculation

tractor
> Lowsley's t.
> Young's t.

transillumination
transitional
transplant
transureteroureterostomy
transurethral
transversalis
transverse
transversourethralis
transversus
transvesical
transvestism
transvestite
triangle
> Hesselbach's t.

trichiasis
Trichomonas
> T. urethritis

trichomoniasis
trigone
> urogenital t.

trigonectomy
trigonitis
trigonotome
trigonum
> t. urogenitale
> t. vesicae

trocar
> Campbell's t.
> Hurwitz's t.
> Ochsner's t.
> Potain's t.

tube
> Acmi-Valentine t.
> Immergut's t.
> Millin's t.

tube
- Valentine's t.

tuberculosis
- adrenal t.
- t. of kidney and bladder

tubule
- Albarran's t's.
- Bellini's t's.
- Henle's t's.
- mesonephric t's.
- metanephric t's.
- renal t's.
- seminiferous t's.
- uriniferous t's.
- uriniparous t's.

Tuffier's operation

tumor
- Buschke-Loewenstein t.
- Grawitz's t.
- Wilms' t.

tunica
- t. adnata testis
- t. adventitia
- t. adventitia ductus deferentis
- t. adventitia ureteris
- t. adventitia vesiculae seminalis
- t. albuginea
- t. albuginea corporis spongiosi
- t. albuginea corporum cavernosorum
- t. albuginea testis
- t. dartos
- t. mucosa ductus deferentis
- t. mucosa ureteris

tunica *(continued)*
- t. mucosa vesicae urinariae
- t. mucosa vesiculae seminalis
- t. muscularis ductus deferentis
- t. muscularis renis
- t. muscularis ureteris
- t. muscularis vesicae urinariae
- t. muscularis vesiculae seminalis
- t. propria tubuli testis
- t. serosa testis
- t. serosa vesicae urinariae
- t. vaginalis communis testis et funiculi spermatica
- t. vaginalis propria testis
- t. vaginalis testis
- t. vasculosa

tunicae funiculi spermatici

tunicae funiculi spermatici et testis

TUR — transurethral resection

Turkel's needle

Turner's syndrome

ulceration

ulcus
- u. syphiliticum

UPJ — ureteropelvic junction

urachal

urachovesical

urachus

uracrasia

uracratia

uragogue
uremia
    azotemic u.
    extrarenal u.
    prerenal u.
    retention u.
uremic
ureter
    ectopic u.
ureteral
ureteralgia
ureterectasia
ureterectasis
ureterectomy
ureteric
    u. ridge
ureteritis
    u. cystica
    u. glandularis
ureterocele
ureterocervical
ureterocolostomy
ureterocutaneostomy
ureterocutaneous
ureterocystanastomosis
ureterocystoneostomy
ureterocystoscope
ureterocystostomy
ureterodialysis
ureteroduodenal
ureteroenteric
ureteroenteroanastomosis
ureteroenterostomy
ureterogram
ureterography
ureteroileostomy
ureterointestinal
ureterolith

ureterolithiasis
ureterolithotomy
ureterolysis
ureteroneocystostomy
ureteroneopyelostomy
ureteronephrectomy
ureteropathy
ureteropelvic
ureteropelvioneostomy
ureterophlegma
ureteroplasty
ureteroproctostomy
ureteropyelitis
ureteropyelography
ureteropyeloneostomy
ureteropyelonephritis
ureteropyelonephrostomy
ureteropyeloplasty
ureteropyelostomy
ureteropyosis
ureterorectal
ureterorectoneostomy
ureterorectostomy
ureterorrhagia
ureterorrhaphy
ureterosigmoid
ureterosigmoidostomy
ureterostegnosis
ureterostenoma
ureterostenosis
ureterostoma
ureterostomosis
ureterostomy
    cutaneous u.
ureterotomy
ureterotrigonoenterostomy
ureterotrigonosigmoidostomy
ureteroureteral

ureteroureterostomy
ureterouterine
ureterovaginal
ureterovesical
ureterovesicoplasty
ureterovesicostomy
urethra
    u. masculina
    u. virilis
urethral
urethralgia
urethratresia
urethrectomy
urethremphraxis
urethreurynter
urethrism
urethritis
    u. cystica
    u. glandularis
    gonorrheal u.
    gouty u.
    u. granulosa
    nonspecific u.
    u. orificii externi
    u. petrificans
    polypoid u.
    prophylactic u.
    specific u.
    u. venerea
urethroblennorrhea
urethrobulbar
urethrocele
urethrocystitis
urethrocystogram
urethrocystography
urethrocystopexy
urethrodynia
urethrogram

urethrograph
urethrography
urethrometer
urethrometry
urethropenile
urethroperineal
urethroperineoscrotal
urethropexy
urethrophraxis
urethrophyma
urethroplasty
urethroprostatic
urethrorectal
urethrorrhagia
urethrorrhaphy
urethrorrhea
urethroscope
urethroscopic
urethroscopy
urethroscrotal
urethrospasm
urethrostaxis
urethrostenosis
urethrostomy
urethrotome
    Keitzer's u.
    Maisonneuve's u.
    Otis' u.
urethrotomy
urethrovaginal
urethrovesical
uretic
urhidrosis
uric
uricaciduria
urina
    u. chyli
    u. cibi

urina *(continued)*
    u. cruenta
    u. galactodes
    u. hysterica
    u. jumentosa
    u. potus
    u. sanguinis
    u. spastica
urinable
urinal
urinalysis
urinary
    u. frequency
    u. retention
    u. sphincter
    u. tract
urinate
urination
    precipitant u.
    stuttering u.
urine
    anemic u.
    Bence-Jones u.
    black u.
    chylous u.
    clean catch u. culture
    crude u.
    diabetic u.
    dyspeptic u.
    febrile u.
    gouty u.
    hysterical u.
    milky u.
    nebulous u.
    nervous u.
    residual u.
    straw colored u.
    voided u.

urinemia
urinemucoid
uriniferous
uriniparous
urinocryoscopy
urinogenital
urinogenous
urinologist
urinology
urinoma
urinometer
urinometry
urinosexual
urinous
urobilinogenuria
urobilinuria
urocele
urochezia
urochrome
urochromogen
uroclepsia
urocrisia
urocrisis
urocriterion
urocyst
urocystic
urocystis
urocystitis
urodeum
urodialysis
urodochium
urodynia
uroerythrin
urofuscin
urofuscohematin
urogenital
urogenous
uroglaucin

urogram
    excretory u.
urography
    ascending u.
    cystoscopic u.
    descending u.
    excretion u.
    excretory u.
    intravenous u.
    oral u.
    retrograde u.
urohematin
urohematonephrosis
urohematoporphyrin
urohypertensin
urokinase
urokinetic
urokymography
urolith
urolithiasis
urolithic
urolithology
urologic
urological
urologist
urology
urolutein
uromancy
uromantia
uromelanin
urometer
uroncus
uronephrosis
uronology
urononcometry
uronophile
uronoscopy
uropathogen

uropathy
    obstructive u.
uropenia
uropepsin
urophanic
urophein
urophobia
uroplania
uropoiesis
uropoietic
uroporphyrin
uropsammus
uropterin
uropyonephrosis
uropyoureter
uroreaction
urorhythmography
urorrhagia
urorrhea
urorrhodin
urorrhodinogen
urorubin
urorubinogen
urorubrohematin
urosaccharometry
uroscheocele
uroschesis
uroscopic
uroscopy
urosemiology
urosepsin
urosepsis
uroseptic
urosis
urospectrin
urostalagmometry
urostealith
urotherapy

urotoxia
urotoxic
urotoxicity
urotoxin
uroureter
uroxanthin
utricle
    prostatic u.
    urethral u.
utricular
utriculi
utriculitis
utriculosaccular
utriculus
    u. masculinus
    u. prostaticus
    u. vestibuli
UVJ – ureterovesical junction
uvula
    u. of bladder
    u. vesicae
Valentine's tube
Van Buren's
    dilator
    sound
van Hook's operation
varicocele
varicocelectomy
varix
vas
    v. aberrans
    v. afferens glomeruli
    v. deferens
    v. efferens glomeruli
    v. epididymidis
vasectomized
vasectomy
vasitis

vasoepididymostomy
vasoligation
vaso-orthidostomy
vasopuncture
vasoresection
vasorrhaphy
vasosection
vasostomy
vasotomy
vasovasotomy
vasovesiculectomy
vasovesiculitis
Veenema-Gusberg needle
Veenema's retractor
venae cavernosae penis
venereal
ventral
venulae rectae renis
venulae stellatae renis
venule
    stellate v's. of kidney
    straight v's. of kidney
verruca
    v. acuminata
vertex
    v. of urinary bladder
    v. vesicae urinariae
verumontanitis
verumontanum
Ves. – vesica – the bladder
vesica
    v. prostatica
    v. urinaria
vesicae
vesical
vesicle
    prostatic v.
    spermatic v.

vesicoabdominal
vesicocele
vesicocervical
vesicoclysis
vesicocolonic
vesicoenteric
vesicofixation
vesicointestinal
vesicoperineal
vesicoprostatic
vesicopubic
vesicorectal
vesicorenal
vesicosigmoid
vesicosigmoidostomy
vesicospinal
vesicotomy
vesicoumbilical
vesicourachal
vesicoureteral
vesicourethral
vesicouterine
vesicouterovaginal
vesicovaginal
vesicovaginorectal
vesicula
    v. prostatica
    v. seminalis
vesiculase
vesiculectomy
vesiculitis
vesiculogram
vesiculography
vesiculotomy
Vest's telescope
Vidal's operation
Vim-Silverman needle
viscus

Vogel's operation
void
Volhard and Fahr method
Volhard's nephritis
Volkmann's operation
von Bergmann's operation
von Hacker's operation
Voronoff's operation
Walther-Crenshaw clamp
Walther's
    clamp
    dilator
    sound
Wappler's cystoscope
Waterhouse-Friderichsen
    syndrome
Watson-Schwartz test
Wertheim-Cullen clamp
Wertheim-Reverdin clamp
Wertheim's clamp
Wheelhouse's operation
White-Oslay forceps
White's operation
Wilms' tumor
Winer's catheter
Wishard's catheter
Wolff
    duct of W.
Wolffi
    corpus W.
wolffian
    body
    cyst
    duct
Wood's operation
XC – excretory cystogram
XU – excretory urogram
Young-Millin needle holder

Young's
  clamp
  enucleator
  forceps
  needle holder
  operation
  retractor

Young's
  tractor
Ziehl-Neelsen stain
Zipser's clamp
Zoon's erythroplasia
zoospermia

ABBREVIATIONS AND SYMBOLS

A . . . . absolute temperature
absorbance
accommodation
acetum
Actinomyces
age
allergy
ampere
Angstrom unit
anode
Anopheles
anterior
artery
atropine
axial
before (ante)
mass number
start of anesthesia
total acidity
water (aqua)
A_2 . . . . second aortic sound
AA . . . . acetic acid
achievement age
alveolar-arterial
aminoacetone
arteries
ascending aorta
of each (ana)
A&A . . . . aid and attendance
AAA . . . . abdominal aortic aneurysm
amalgam
androgenic anabolic agent

AAL. . . . . anterior axillary line
AAR . . . . antigen-antiglobulin reaction
AAS . . . . aortic arch syndrome
AAT. . . . . alpha-antitrypsin
AB . . . . abnormal
                    abortion
                    alcian blue
                    asbestos body
                    asthmatic bronchitis
                    axiobuccal
A/B . . . . acid-base ratio
ABA. . . . . antibacterial activity
ABC . . . . absolute basophil count
                    axiobuccocervical
ABD. . . . . abdomen
                    abdominal
ABD HYST . . . . . . abdominal hysterectomy
ABDOM . . . . abdomen
                    abdominal
ABE . . . . acute bacterial endocarditis
ABG. . . . . axiobuccogingival
ABL . . . . a-beta-lipoproteinemia
                    axiobuccolingual
ABLB. . . . . alternate binaural loudness balance
ABN. . . . . abnormal
ABNORM . . . . abnormal
ABO. . . . . absent bed occupancy
                    blood groups (named for agglutinogens)
ABP . . . . arterial blood pressure
ABS FEB . . . . while the fever is absent (absente febre)
abst., abstr. . . . . . . abstract
AC . . . . acromioclavicular
                    acute
                    adrenal cortex
                    air conduction
                    alternating current
                    anodal closure
                    anticoagulant

AC *(continued)* ... anticomplementary
anti-inflammatory corticoid
aortic closure
atriocarotid
auriculocarotid
axiocervical
before meals (ante cibum)
ACA............. adenocarcinoma
ACAD .... academy
ACC............ adenoid cystic carcinoma
anodal closure contraction
Acc.............. accommodation
ACCL........... anodal closure clonus
ACD............ absolute cardiac dullness
acid, citrate, dextrose
anterior chest diameter
ACE............. adrenocortical extract
ACG............ apexcardiogram
Ac-G............ accelerator globulin
ACH............ adrenal cortical hormone
ACh............. acetylcholine
ACHE .... acetylcholinesterase
ACl .... aspiryl chloride
ACM .... albumin-calcium-magnesium
ACO............ anodal closing odor
ACP .... acid phosphatase
acyl-carrier protein
anodal closing picture
aspirin, caffeine, phenacetin
ACS .... anodal closing sound
antireticular cytotoxic serum
ACT............ activated coagulation time
anticoagulant therapy
ACTe .... anodal closure tetanus
ACTH .... adrenocorticotropic hormone
ACTP........... adrenocorticotropin polypeptide
ACVD .... acute cardiovascular disease
AD .... admitting diagnosis

AD *(continued)* . . . Aleutian disease
anodal duration
average deviation
axiodistal
axis deviation
right ear (auris dextra)
A&D. . . . . ascending and descending
ad . . . . adde (add)
addetur (let there be added)
Ad def. an   to the point of fainting
(ad defectionem animi)
Ad deliq. . . . . ad deliquium (to fainting)
Ad grat. Acid . . . . . to an agreeable sourness
(ad gratum acid-itatem)
Ad lib. . . . . as desired (ad libitum)
Ad pond. om . . . . . to the weight of the whole
(ad pondus omnium)
Ad 2 vic. . . . . for two doses (ad duas vices)
ADA. . . . . adenosine deaminase
anterior descending artery
ADA# . . . . American Diabetes Association diet number
ADC. . . . . anodal duration contraction
average daily census
axiodistocervical
ADEM . . . . acute disseminated encephalomyelitis
ADG. . . . . axiodistogingival
ADH. . . . . alcohol dehydrogenase
antidiuretic hormone
Adhib. . . . . to be administered (adhibendus)
ADI . . . . axiodistoincisal
ADL . . . . activities of daily living
ADM . . . . administrative medicine
administrator
admission
admit
Admov. . . . . let there be added (admove)
ADO . . . . axiodisto-occlusal
ADP. . . . . adenosine diphosphate
automatic data processing

ADPL .... average daily patient load
ADS............ antibody deficiency syndrome
　　　　　　　　　 antidiuretic substance
Adst. feb. .... while fever is present (adstante febre)
ADT............ adenosine triphosphate
　　　　　　　　　 anything desired
Adv .... against (adversum)
AE .... antitoxineinheit (antitoxin unit)
AEG .... air encephalogram
Aeg .... the patient (aeger)
AEP .... average evoked potential
AEq .... age equivalent
AER　　　　　　　 aldosterone excretion rate
　　　　　　　　　 auditory evoked response
　　　　　　　　　 average evoked response
AET............ absorption-equivalent thickness
Aet .... age (aetas)
　　　　　　　　　 aged (aetatis)
AF .... acid-fast
　　　　　　　　　 aldehyde fuchsin
　　　　　　　　　 amniotic fluid
　　　　　　　　　 antibody-forming
　　　　　　　　　 aortic flow
　　　　　　　　　 atrial fibrillation
　　　　　　　　　 atrial flutter
AFB............ acid fast bacilli
AFC............ antibody-forming cells
AFI .... amaurotic familial idiocy
AFIB .... atrial fibrillation
AFL............ atrial flutter
AFP .... anterior faucial pillar
AG .... antiglobulin
　　　　　　　　　 atrial gallop
　　　　　　　　　 axiogingival
A/G .... albumin-globulin ratio
AGA .... appropriate for gestational age
AGG .... agammaglobulinemia
　　　　　　　　　 aggravated
Aggred. feb ...... while the fever is coming on

Aggred. feb *(continued)*

(aggrediente febre)

Agit	shake
Agit. vas	the vial being shaken (agitato vase)
AGL	acute granulocytic leukemia
	aminoglutethimide
AGMK	African green monkey kidney
AGN	acute glomerulonephritis
AGS	adrenogenital syndrome
AGT	antiglobulin test
AGTT	abnormal glucose tolerance test
AGV	aniline gentian violet
AH	abdominal hysterectomy
	acetohexamide
	amenorrhea and hirsutism
	aminohippurate
	antihyaluronidase
	arterial hypertension
	hypermetropic astigmatism
AHA	acquired hemolytic anemia
	autoimmune hemolytic anemia
AHD	atherosclerotic heart disease
	arteriosclerotic heart disease
AHF	antihemophilic factor
AHG	antihemophilic globulin
	antihuman globulin
AHH	alpha-hydrazine analogue of histidine
	arylhydrocarbon hydroxylase
AHLE	acute hemorrhagic leukoencephalitis
AHLS	antihuman-lymphocyte serum
AHP	air at high pressure
AHT	augmented histamine test
AI	accidentally incurred
	aortic incompetence
	aortic insufficiency
	apical impulse
	axioincisal
AIB	aminoisobutyric acid

AIC . . . . aminoimidazole carboxamide
AID . . . . acute infectious disease
　　　　　　　　　　　artificial insemination donor
AIEP . . . . amount of insulin extractable from the
　　　　　　　　　　　　　　pancreas
AIH . . . . artificial insemination, homologous
AIHA . . . . autoimmune hemolytic anemia
AIP. . . . . acute intermittent porphyria
　　　　　　　　　　　average intravascular pressure
AIU . . . . absolute iodine uptake
AJ . . . . ankle jerk
AK . . . . above knee
AKA . . . . above knee amputation
AL . . . . albumin
　　　　　　　　　　　axiolingual
ALA . . . . aminolevulinic acid
　　　　　　　　　　　axiolabial
ALAD . . . . abnormal left axis deviation
　　　　　　　　　　　aminolevulinic acid dehydrase
ALAG . . . . axiolabiogingival
A.La.L. . . . . axiolabiolingual
Alb. . . . . albumin
　　　　　　　　　　　white
ALC . . . . approximate lethal concentration
　　　　　　　　　　　axiolinguocervical
Ald. . . . . aldolase
ALG . . . . antilymphocyte globulin
　　　　　　　　　　　axiolinguogingival
ALH . . . . anterior lobe hormone
　　　　　　　　　　　anterior lobe of the hypophysis
Alk. . . . . alkaline
Alk phos . . . . alkaline phosphatase
ALL . . . . acute lymphoblastic leukemia
　　　　　　　　　　　acute lymphocytic leukemia
All. . . . . allergies
ALME . . . . acetyl-lysine methyl ester
ALMI . . . . anterior lateral myocardial infarct
ALN . . . . anterior lymph node
ALO . . . . axiolinguo-occlusal

ALP . . . . alkaline phosphatase
                                antilymphocyte plasma
ALS . . . . amyotrophic lateral sclerosis
                                antilymphatic serum
                                antilymphocyte serum
Alt. dieb. . . . . every other day (alternis diebus)
Alt. hor. . . . . every other hour (alternis horis)
Alt. noc. . . . . every other night (alternis nocte)
ALTEE . . . . acetyl-L-tyrosine ethyl ester
Alv. adst. . . . . when the bowels are constipated
                                (alvo adstricta)
Alv. deject . . . . alvine dejections
ALW . . . . arch-loop-whorl
AM . . . . alveolar macrophage
                                ametropia
                                amperemeter
                                anovular menstruation
                                arithmetic mean
                                aviation medicine
                                axiomesial
                                morning
                                myopic astigmatism
Am . . . . meter-angle
AMA . . . . against medical advice
                                American Medical Association
AMB . . . . ambulatory
AMC . . . . axiomesiocervical
AMD . . . . alpha-methyldopa
                                axiomesiodistal
AMG . . . . antimacrophage globulin
                                axiomesiogingival
AMH . . . . automated medical history
                                mixed astigmatism with myopia
                                  predominating
AMI . . . . acute myocardial infarction
                                amitriptyline
                                axiomesioincisal
AML . . . . acute monocytic leukemia

AML *(continued)*. . acute myelocytic leukemia
AMLS . . . . antimouse lymphocyte serum
AMM . . . . agnogenic myeloid metaplasia
      ammonia
AMML . . . . acute myelomonocytic leukemia
AMO . . . . axiomesio-occlusal
AMOL . . . . acute monocytic leukemia
AMP . . . . acid mucopolysaccharide
      adenosine monophosphate
      ampicillin
      amputation
      average mean pressure
Amp. . . . . ampere
AMPS . . . . abnormal mucopolysacchariduria
      acid mucopolysaccharides
AMS . . . . aggravated in military service
      antimacrophage serum
      automated multiphasic screening
AMT . . . . alpha-methyltyrosine
      amethopterin
      amount
Amy. . . . . amylase
An. . . . . anisometropia
      anodal
      anode
      anterior
ANA . . . . acetylneuraminic acid
      antinuclear antibodies
      aspartyl naphthylamide
Anal. . . . . analysis
      analyst
Anat. . . . . anatomical
      anatomy
ANCC . . . . anodal closure contraction
AnDTe. . . . . anodal duration tetanus
Anes . . . . anesthesia
      anesthesiology
Anesth. . . . . anesthesia

Anesth. *(continued)*

	anesthesiology
ANF	alpha-naphthoflavone
	antinuclear factor
Ang.	angiogram
Ank.	ankle
ANOC	anodal opening contraction
ANOV	analysis of variance
ANS	antineutrophilic serum
	arteriolonephrosclerosis
	autonomic nervous system
Ant.	anterior
Ant. ax. line	anterior axillary line
Ante	before
Ante cibum	before meals (ante sibum)
ANTR	apparent net transfer rate
ANTU	alpha-naphthylthiourea
AO	anodal opening
	anterior oblique
	aorta
	aortic opening
	axio-occlusal
	opening of the atrioventricular valves
AOB	alcohol on breath
AOC	anodal opening contraction
AOCL	anodal opening clonus
AOD	arterial occlusive disease
AOO	anodal opening odor
AOP	anodal opening picture
Aort. regurg.	aortic regurgitation
Aort. sten.	aortic stenosis
AOS	anodal opening sound
AOTe.	anodal opening tetanus
AP	acid phosphatase
	action potential
	acute proliferative
	alkaline phosphatase
	aminopeptidase

AP *(continued)* ... angina pectoris
antepartum
anterior pituitary
anteroposterior
appendix
arterial pressure
association period
axiopulpal
A & P .... anterior and posterior
auscultation and percussion
APA .... aldosterone-producing adenoma
aminopenicillanic acid
antipernicious anemia factor
APB .... atrial premature beat
auricular premature beat
APC .... acetylsalicylic acid, phenacetin, caffeine
adenoidal-pharyngeal-conjunctival
aspirin, phenacetin, caffeine
atrial premature contraction
APC-C .... aspirin, phenacetin, caffeine;
with codeine
APD .... action potential duration
APE .... adapted physical educator
aminophylline, phenobarbital, ephedrine
anterior pituitary extract
APF .... animal protein factor
APGL .... alkaline phosphatase activity of the
granular leukocytes
APH .... antepartum hemorrhage
APHP.......... antipseudomonas human plasma
AP & Lat. .... anteroposterior and lateral
APL .... accelerated painless labor
anterior pituitary-like
APN .... average peak noise
APP .... alum-precipitated pyridine
App .... appendix
Appy. .... appendectomy
APR .... amebic prevalence rate

APT . . . . alum precipitated toxoid
APTT . . . . activated partial thromboplastin time
AQ . . . . achievement quotient
Aq. . . . . water (aqua)
Aq. bull . . . . boiling water (aqua bulliens)
Aq. dest. . . . . distilled water (aqua destillata)
Aq. ferv. . . . . hot water (aqua fervens)
Aq. frig. . . . . cold water (aqua frigida)
Aq. pur. . . . . pure water (aqua pura)
Aq. tep. . . . . tepid water (aqua tepida)
AQS . . . . additional qualifying symptoms
AR . . . . alarm reaction
                        aortic regurgitation
                        Argyll Robertson (pupil)
                        artificial respiration
                        at risk
ARD . . . . acute respiratory disease
                        anorectal dressing
ARF . . . . acute respiratory failure
Arg. . . . . silver (argentum)
ARL . . . . average remaining lifetime
ARM . . . . artificial rupture of the membranes
ARP . . . . at risk period
ARS . . . . antirabies serum
Art. . . . . artery
AS . . . . acetylstrophanthidin
                        Adams-Stokes (disease)
                        androsterone sulfate
                        antistreptolysin
                        aortic stenosis
                        arteriosclerosis
                        astigmatism
                        left ear (aúris sinístra)
ASA . . . . acetylsalicylic acid
                        Adams-Stokes attack
                        arylsulfatase-A
ASCVD . . . . arteriosclerotic cardiovascular disease
                        atherosclerotic cardiovascular disease

ASD . . . . aldosterone secretion defect
atrial septal defect
ASF . . . . aniline, formaldehyde, and sulfur
ASH . . . . hypermetropic astigmatism
ASHD . . . . arteriosclerotic heart disease
ASIS . . . . anterior superior iliac spine
ASK . . . . antistreptokinase
ASL . . . . antistreptolysin
ASLO . . . . antistreptolysin-O
ASM . . . . myopic astigmatism
ASMI . . . . anteroseptal myocardial infarct
ASN . . . . alkali-soluble nitrogen
ASO . . . . antistreptolysin-O
arteriosclerosis obliterans
ASP . . . . area systolic pressure
ASR . . . . aldosterone secretion rate
aldosterone secretory rate
ASS . . . . anterior superior spine
Asst. . . . . assistant
Ast. . . . . astigmatism
Asth. . . . . asthenopia
ASTO . . . . antistreptolysin-O
ASV . . . . antisnake venom
A.T. . . . . old tuberculin (Alt Tuberculin)
AT . . . . antitrypsin
At. wt. . . . . atomic weight
AT-10 . . . . Dihydrotachysterol
ATA . . . . anti-Toxoplasma antibodies
atmosphere absolute
autintricarboxylic acid
ATB . . . . at the time of the bombing
ATD . . . . asphyxiating thoracic dystrophy
ATE . . . . adipose tissue extract
ATEE . . . . acetyltyrosine ethyl ester
ATG . . . . antithyroglobulin
ATN . . . . acute tubular necrosis
ATP . . . . adenosine triphosphate

ATPS . . . . ambient temperature and pressure,
                       saturated with water vapor
ATR . . . . Achilles tendon reflex
Atr. fib. . . . . atrial fibrillation
ATS . . . . antitetanic serum
                       antithymocyte serum
                       anxiety tension state
                       arteriosclerosis
ATT . . . . aspirin tolerance time
Att. . . . . attending
AU . . . . Angstrom unit
                       antitoxin unit
                       arbitrary units
                       Australia (antigen)
                       azauridine
                       both ears (aures unitas)
                       each ear (auris uterque)
AUL . . . . acute undifferentiated leukemia
Aur. fib. . . . . auricular fibrillation
Ausc. . . . . auscultation
AV . . . . arteriovenous
                       atrioventricular
                       average
                       avoirdupois
AV/AF . . . . anteverted, anteflexed
AVCS . . . . atrioventricular conduction system
AVF . . . . arteriovenous fistula
AVH . . . . acute viral hepatitis
AVI . . . . air velocity index
AVN . . . . atrioventricular node
AVR . . . . aortic valve replacement
AVRP . . . . atrioventricular refractory period
AVT . . . . Allen vision test
AW . . . . anterior wall
A & W . . . . alive and well
AWI . . . . anterior wall infarction
AWMI . . . . anterior wall myocardial infarction
Ax. . . . . axis

Az. . . . . azote
                  nitrogen
AZ test . . . . Aschheim-Zondek test
Azg. . . . . azaguanine
AZO . . . . (indicates presence of the group) —N:N—
AZT . . . . Aschheim-Zondek test
AZUR . . . . azauridine
B . . . . bacillus
                  base
                  bath (balneum)
                  Baume's scale
                  behavior
                  Benoist's scale
                  bicuspid
                  born
                  Brucella
                  buccal
                  sand bath (balneum arenae)
                  symbol of gauss
B4 . . . . before
BA . . . . bacterial agglutination
                  betamethasone acetate
                  blocking antibody
                  bone age
                  bovine albumin
                  branchial artery
                  bronchial asthma
                  buccoaxial
BAC . . . . blood alcohol concentration
                  buccoaxiocervical
Bact. . . . . bacterium
BAEE . . . . benzoyl arginine ethyl ester
                  benzylarginine ethyl ester
BAG . . . . buccoaxiogingival
BAIB . . . . beta-aminoisobutyric acid
BAL . . . . bath
                  British Anti-Lewisite
Bals. . . . . balsam

BAME . . . . benzoylarginine methyl ester
BAO . . . . basal acid output
BAP . . . . blood agar plate
BASH . . . . body acceleration given synchronously
                             with the heartbeat
Baso. . . . . basophile
BB . . . . blood bank
                         blood buffer base
                         blue bloaters (emphysema)
                         both bones
                         breakthrough bleeding
                         breast biopsy
                         buffer base
BBA . . . . born before arrival
BBB . . . . blood-brain barrier
                         bundle branch block
BBT . . . . basal body temperature
BC . . . . bactericidal concentration
                         battle casualty
                         bone conduction
                         buccocervical
BCB . . . . brilliant cresyl blue
BCE . . . . basal cell epithelioma
BCG . . . . bacille Calmette Guerin (vaccine)
                         ballistocardiogram
                         bicolor guaiac (test)
BCNU. . . . . bischloroethyl-nitrosourea
                         bischloronitrosourea
BCW . . . . biological and chemical warfare
BD . . . . base deficit
                         base of prism down
                         bile duct
                         buccodistal
                         twice a day (bis die)
BDE . . . . bile duct exploration
BE . . . . Bacillen emulsion (tuberculin)
                         bacterial endocarditis
                         barium enema

BE *(continued)* . . . base excess
bovine enteritis
BEI . . . . butanol-extractable iodine
BEV . . . . billion electron volts
BF . . . . blood flow
bouillon filtrate (tuberculin)
B/F . . . . bound-free ratio
BFC . . . . benign febrile convulsion
BFP . . . . biologic false-positive
BFR . . . . biologic false-positive reactor
blood flow rate
bone formation rate
BFT . . . . bentonite flocculation test
BG . . . . blood glucose
bone graft
buccogingival
BGH . . . . bovine growth hormone
BGP . . . . beta-glycerophosphatase
BGSA . . . . blood granulocyte-specific activity
BGTT . . . . . . : . . . borderline glucose tolerance test
BH . . . . benzalkonium and heparin
BHA . . . . butylated hydroxyanisole
BHC . . . . benzene hexachloride
BHI . . . . brain-heart infusion
BHS . . . . beta-hemolytic streptococcus
BHT . . . . butylated hydroxytoluene
BH/VH . . . . body hematocrit-venous hematocrit ratio
BI . . . . bacteriological index
base of prism in
burn index
Bib. . . . . drink (bibe)
BID . . . . twice a day (bis in die)
BIDLB . . . . block in the postero-inferior division
of the left branch
BIH . . . . benign intracranial hypertension
BIL . . . . bilateral
bilirubin
BILAT . . . . bilateral

BIN . . . . twice a night (bis in nocte)
BIP. . . . . bismuth iodoform paraffin
Bis. . . . . twice
BJ . . . . Bence Jones
BJP . . . . Bence Jones protein
BK . . . . below knee
BKA . . . . below-knee amputation
Bkfst. . . . . breakfast
BL . . . . baseline
                          Bessey-Lowry (units)
                          bleeding
                          blood loss
                          buccolingual
                          Burkitt's lymphoma
Bl. cult. . . . . blood culture
Bl. Pr. . . . . blood pressure
BLB . . . . Boothby, Lovelace, Bulbulian (mask)
BLG. . . . . beta-lactoglobulin
BLN. . . . . bronchial lymph nodes
BLT . . . . blood-clot lysis time
BLU . . . . Bessey-Lowry units
BM . . . . basement membrane
                          body mass
                          bone marrow
                          bowel movement
                          buccomesial
                          sea-water bath (balneum maris)
Bmk. . . . . birthmark
BMR . . . . basal metabolic rate
BN . . . . branchial neuritis
BNO . . . . bladder neck obstruction
BNPA . . . . binasal pharyngeal airway
BO . . . . base of prism out
                          bowel obstruction
                          bucco-occlusal
B & O . . . . belladonna and opium
BOEA . . . . Ethyl biscoumacetate
Bol. . . . . pill (bolus)

BOM . . . . bilateral otitis media
BP . . . . back pressure
                         bathroom privileges
                         behavior pattern
                         benzopyrene
                         birthplace
                         blood pressure
                         boiling point
                         bronchopleural
                         buccopulpal
BPH . . . . benign prostatic hypertrophy
BPL . . . . beta-propiolactone
BPO . . . . benzylpenicilloyl
BPRS . . . . brief psychiatric rating scale
                         brief psychiatric reacting scale
BR . . . . bathroom
                         bed rest
                         bilirubin
                         Brucella
BRBC . . . . bovine red blood cells
Brkf . . . . breakfast
Brkt. . . . . breakfast
BRM . . . . biuret reactive material
BRP . . . . bathroom privileges
                         bilirubin production
Brth. . . . . breath
BS . . . . blood sugar
                         bowel sounds
                         breaking strength
                         breath sounds
BSA . . . . bismuth-sulphite agar
                         body surface area
                         bovine serum albumin
BSB . . . . body surface burned
BSDLB . . . . block in the anterosuperior division of
                         the left branch
BSF . . . . back scatter factor
BSI . . . . bound serum iron

BSO . . . . bilateral salpingo-oophorectomy
BSP . . . . Bromsulphalein
BSR . . . . basal skin resistance
BSS . . . . balanced salt solution
                       black silk suture
                       buffered saline solution
BT . . . . bladder tumor
                       brain tumor
BTB . . . . breakthrough bleeding
BTPS . . . . body temperature, ambient pressure,
                       saturated with water
BTR . . . . Bezold-type reflex
BTU . . . . British thermal unit
BU . . . . base of prism up
                       Bodansky units
                       burn unit
BUDR . . . . bromodeoxyuracil
                       bromodeoxyuridine
Bull . . . . let it boil (bulliat)
BUN . . . . blood urea nitrogen
BUS glands . . . . . . Bartholin's, urethral, Skene's glands
But . . . . butter (butyrum)
BV . . . . biologic value
                       blood vessel
                       blood volume
                       bronchovesicular
                       vapor bath (valneum vaporis)
BVH . . . . biventricular hypertrophy
BVI . . . . blood vessel invasion
BVV . . . . bovine vaginitis virus
BW . . . . biological warfare
                       birth weight
                       body water
                       body weight
BX . . . . biopsy
C . . . . calculus
                       calorie (large)
                       canine

C *(continued)* .... carbohydrate
cathode
Caucasian
Celsius
centigrade
certified
cervical
chest
clearance rate
clonus
Clostridium
closure
color sense
compound
contracture
correct
Cryptococcus
cup
cylinder
gallon
hundred
velocity of light
C_{alb} .... albumin clearance
C_{am} .... amylase clearance
C_{cr} .... creatinine clearance
C_{in} .... insulin clearance
C_{PAH} .... para-aminohippurate clearance
C_u .... urea clearance
C' .... complement
c .... calorie (small)
curie
with (cum)
CA .... cancer
carcinoma
cardiac arrest
cathode
cervicoaxial
chronological age

CA *(continued)* . . . cold agglutinin
common antigen
coronary artery
corpora amylacea
croup associated (virus)
Ca . . . . calcium
about (circa)
CACC . . . . cathodal closure contraction
CAD . . . . coronary artery disease
CADTe. . . . . cathodal duration tetanus
CAG. . . . . chronic atrophic gastritis
CAH. . . . . chronic active hepatitis
congenital adrenal hyperplasia
CAHD . . . . coronary atherosclerotic heart disease
CAI . . . . computer-assisted instruction
CAL. . . . . computer-assisted learning
Cal . . . . large calorie
cal . . . . small calorie
Calef. . . . . warmed (calefactus)
CAM . . . . chorioallantoic membrane
contralateral axillary metastasis
CAMP. . . . . computer-assisted menu planning
cyclic adenosine monophosphate
CAO. . . . . chronic airway obstruction
CAP . . . . capsule
cellulose acetate phthalate
chloramphenicol
cystine aminopeptidase
let him take (capiat)
Card. . . . . cardiology
Cardiol. . . . . cardiology
CAT. . . . . Children's Apperception Test
Computer of Average Transients
Cath. . . . . cathartic
catheter
catheterize
CAV. . . . . congenital absence of vagina
congenital adrenal virilism

CB . . . . chronic bronchitis
CBA . . . . chronic bronchitis with asthma
CBC . . . . complete blood count
CBD . . . . common bile duct
CBF . . . . cerebral blood flow
                    coronary blood flow
CBG . . . . corticosteroid-binding globulin
                    cortisol-binding globulin
CBOC . . . . completion bed occupancy care
CBS . . . . chronic brain syndrome
CBV . . . . central blood volume
                    circulating blood volume
                    corrected blood volume
CBW . . . . chemical and biological warfare
CC . . . . cardiac cycle
                    chief complaint
                    clinical course
                    commission certified
                    compound cathartic
                    cord compression
                    costochondral
                    creatinine clearance
cc. . . . . cubic centimeter
CCA . . . . chick-cell agglutination
                    chimpanzee coryza agent
                    common carotid artery
CCAT . . . . conglutinating complement absorption test
CCC . . . . cathodal closing contraction
                    chronic calculous cholecystitis
                    consecutive case conference
CCCL . . . . cathodal closure clonus
CCF . . . . cephalin-cholesterol flocculation
                    compound comminuted fracture
                    congestive cardiac failure
CCK . . . . cholecystokinin
CCK-PZ . . . . cholecystokinin pancreozymin
CCN . . . . coronary care nursing
CCP . . . . ciliocytophthoria

CCS	casualty clearing station
CCT	composite cyclic therapy
CCTe	cathodal closure tetanus
CCU	Cherry-Crandall units
	community care unit
	coronary care unit
CCW.	counterclockwise
CD	cadaver donor
	cardiac disease
	cardiac dullness
	cardiovascular disease
	caudal
	common duct
	conjugata diagonalis
	consanguineous donor
	curative dose
	cystic duct
C/D	cigarettes per day
C&D	cystoscopy and dilatation
CD_{50}	median curative dose
CDC	calculated day of confinement
	chenodeoxycholate
	Communicable Disease Center
CDD	certificate of disability for discharge
CDE	canine distemper encephalitis
	chlordiazepoxide
	common duct exploration
CDH	ceramide dihexoside
	congenital dislocation of the hip
CDL	chlorodeoxylincomycin
CDP	coronary drug project
CDSS	clinical decision support system
CE	California encephalitis
	cardiac enlargement
	chick embryo
	cholesterol esters
	contractile element
CEA	carcino-embryonic antigen

CEA *(continued)* . . crystalline egg albumin
CEEV . . . . .Central European encephalitis virus
CEF . . . . chick embryo fibroblast
Cel. . . . . Celsius
Cent. . . . . Centigrade
cent . . . . centimeter
centi- . . . . hundred
Ceph floc. . . . . cephalin flocculation
Cert. . . . . certified
CES . . . . central excitatory state
CF . . . . carbolfuchsin
                           cardiac failure
                           carrier-free
                           chemotactic factor
                           chest and left leg
                           Chiari-Frommel syndrome
                           Christmas factor
                           citrovorum factor
                           compare
                           complement fixation
                           complement-fixing
                           contractile force
                           count fingers
                           counting finger
                           cystic fibrosis
CFA . . . . complement-fixing antibody
                           complete Freund adjuvant
CFF . . . . critical flicker fusion test
                           critical fusion frequency
CFP . . . . chronic false-positive
                           cystic fibrosis of the pancreas
CFT . . . . clinical full-time
                           complement fixation test
CFU . . . . colony-forming units
                           color-forming units
CFWM . . . . cancer-free white mouse
CG . . . . cardio-green
                           chorionic gonadotropin

CG *(continued)* . . . chronic glomerulonephritis
colloidal gold
phosgene
cg. . . . . centigram
CGD . . . . chronic granulomatous disease
CGI . . . . clinical global impression
CGL . . . . chronic granulocytic leukemia
cgm . . . . centigram
CGN . . . . chronic glomerulonephritis
CG/OQ . . . . cerebral glucose oxygen quotient
CGP . . . . choline glycerophosphatide
chorionic growth hormone prolactin
circulating granulocyte pool
CGS . . . . centimeter-gram-second
CGT . . . . chorionic gonadotropin
CGTT . . . . cortisone glucose tolerance test
CH . . . . cholesterol
crown-heel (length of fetus)
wheelchair
CHA . . . . congenital hypoplastic anemia
cyclohexylamine
Chart . . . . paper (charta)
CHB . . . . complete heart block
CHD . . . . congestive heart disease
CHE . . . . cholinesterase
CHF . . . . congestive heart failure
CHH . . . . cartilage-hair hypoplasia
CHL . . . . chloramphenicol
CHO . . . . carbohydrate
Chol. . . . . cholesterol
Chol. est. . . . . cholesterol esters
CHP . . . . child psychiatry
comprehensive health planning
Chr. . . . . Chromobacterium
chronic
CHS . . . . Chediak-Higashi syndrome
CI . . . . cardiac index
cardiac insufficiency

CI *(continued)* . . . . cerebral infarction
chemotherapeutic index
clinical investigator
colloidal iron
color index
coronary insufficiency
crystalline insulin
Cib. . . . . food (cibus)
CICU . . . . cardiology intensive care unit
coronary intensive care unit
CID . . . . cytomegalic inclusion disease
CIDS . . . . cellular immunity deficiency syndrome
CIN . . . . cervical intra-epithelial neoplasia
Circ. . . . . circulation
CIS . . . . carcinoma in situ
central inhibitory state
CIXA . . . . constant infusion excretory urogram
CK . . . . check
creatine kinase
CL . . . . chest and left arm
Clostridium
Cl. . . . . chloride
cl . . . . centiliter
CLAS . . . . congenital localized absence of skin
CLBBB . . . . complete left bundle branch block
CLD . . . . chronic liver disease
chronic lung disease
cldy. . . . . cloudy
Clin . . . . clinic
clinical
CLL . . . . chronic lymphatic leukemia
chronic lymphocytic leukemia
CLO . . . . cod liver oil
CLSL . . . . chronic lymphosarcoma (cell) leukemia
CLT . . . . clot-lysis time
CM . . . . capreomycin
chloroquine-mepacrine
cochlear microphonic

CM *(continued)* . . . complications
costal margin
cow's milk
tomorrow morning (cras mane)
cm . . . . centimeter
cm³ . . . . cubic centimeter
CMB . . . . carbolic methylene blue
CMC . . . . carboxymethyl cellulose
critical micellar concentration
CMF . . . . chondromyxoid fibroma
CMGN . . . . chronic membranous glomerulonephritis
CMI . . . . carbohydrate metabolism index
cellular-mediated immune (response)
CMID . . . . cytomegalic inclusion disease
C/min . . . . cycles per minute
CML . . . . chronic myelocytic leukemia
chronic myelogenous leukemia
CMM . . . . cutaneous malignant melanoma
cmm . . . . cubic millimeter
CMN . . . . cystic medial necrosis
CMN-AA . . . . cystic medial necrosis of the
ascending aorta
CMO . . . . cardiac minute output
card made out
CMP . . . . cytidine monophosphate
CMR . . . . cerebral metabolic rate
crude mortality ratio
CMRG . . . . cerebral metabolic rate of glucose
CMRO . . . . cerebral metabolic rate of oxygen
CMS . . . . Clyde Mood Scale
to be taken tomorrow morning (cras
mane sumendus)
CMU . . . . chlorophenyldimethylurea
CMV . . . . cytomegalovirus
CN . . . . clinical nursing
cyanogen
tomorrow night (cras nocte)
CNE . . . . chronic nervous exhaustion

CNH	community nursing home
CNHD	congenital nonspherocytic hemolytic disease
CNL	cardiolipin natural lecithin
CNS	central nervous system
	to be taken tomorrow night (cras nocte sumendus)
CNV	conative negative variation
	contingent negative variation
CO	carbon monoxide
	cardiac output
	castor oil
	cervicoaxial
	coenzyme
	corneal opacity
	compound
C/O	complains of
	complaints
COA	coenzyme A
Coag.	coagulation
COC	cathodal opening clonus
	coccygeal
	combination-type oral contraceptive
Cochl	spoonful (cochleare)
Cochl. amp	heaping spoonful (cochleare amplum)
Cochl. mag	tablespoonful (cochleare magnum)
Cochl. med.	dessertspoonful (cochleare medium)
Cochl. parv.	teaspoonful (cochleare parvum)
COCL	cathodal opening clonus
Coct.	boiling (coctio)
COD	cause of death
COGTT	cortisone-primed oral glucose tolerance test
COHB	carboxyhemoglobin
Col.	strain (cola)
Colat.	strained (colatus)
COLD	chronic obstructive lung disease
Coll.	eyewash (collyrium)

Collut. . . . . mouthwash (collutorium)
Collyr. . . . . eyewash (collyrium)
COMP. . . . . complaint
                       complication
                       compound
COMT . . . . catechol-O-methyl transferase
Conc. . . . . concentration
Concis . . . . cut (concisus)
cong . . . . gallon (congius)
Cont. . . . . continue
                       continuously
Cont. rem. . . . . let the medicine be continued
                       (continuetur remedium)
Conv. . . . . conventional (rat)
COP . . . . colloid osmotic pressure
COPD. . . . . chronic obstructive pulmonary disease
Coq. . . . . boil (coque)
Coq. in s.a. . . . . boil in sufficient water (coque in
                       sufficiente aqua)
Coq. s.a. . . . . boil properly (coque secundum artem)
Cor . . . . heart
CORA . . . . conditioned orientation reflex audiometry
Cort. . . . . bark (cortex)
                       cortex
COT . . . . critical off-time
CP . . . . candle power
                       cerebral palsy
                       chemically pure
                       chloropurine
                       chloroquine and primaquine
                       chronic pyelonephritis
                       closing pressure
                       cochlear potential
                       combination product
                       combining power
                       coproporphyrin
                       creatine phosphate
C/P. . . . . cholesterol-phospholipid ratio

C&P . . . . compensation and pension
CPA . . . . cerebellar pontine angle
               chlorophenylalanine
CPB . . . . cardiopulmonary bypass
CPC . . . . cetylpyridinium chloride
               chronic passive congestion
               clinicopathologic conference
CPD . . . . cephalopelvic disproportion
               citrate-phosphate-dextrose
               compound
CPE . . . . chronic pulmonary emphysema
               compensation, pension, and education
               cytopathic effect
CPI . . . . constitutional psychopathic inferiority
               coronary prognostic index
CPIB . . . . chlorophenoxyisobutyrate
CPK . . . . creatine phosphokinase
cpm . . . . counts per minute
CPN . . . . chronic pyelonephritis
CPP . . . . cyclopentenophenanthrene
CPPB . . . . continuous positive-pressure breathing
CPPD . . . . calcium pyrophosphate dihydrate
CPR . . . . cerebral-cortex perfusion rate
               cortisol production rate
CPS . . . . clinical performance score
               cumulative probability of success
cps . . . . cycles per second
CPT . . . . chest physiotherapy
CPZ . . . . chlorpromazine
CQ . . . . chloroquine-quinine
               circadian quotient
CR . . . . calculus removed
               chest and right arm
               clinical research
               colon resection
               complete remission
               conditioned reflex
               crown-rump (length of fetus)

Cr.	chromium
CRA	central retinal artery
Cran.	cranial
CRBBB	complete right bundle branch block
CRD	chronic renal disease
	complete reaction of degeneration
Creat.	creatinine
CRF	chronic renal failure
	corticotropin-releasing factor
CRI	concentrated rust-inhibitor
CRM	cross-reacting material
CROS	contralateral routing of signal
CRP	C-reactive protein
CRS	colon-rectal surgery
CRST	calcinosis cutis, Raynaud's phenomenon, sclerodactyly, and telangiectasis
CRT	cathode ray tube
CRU	clinical research unit
CRV	central retinal vein
CRYS	crystal
CS	Central Service
	Central Supply
	cesarean section
	chondroitin sulfate
	conditioned stimulus
	conscious
	coronary sinus
	corticosteroid
	current strength
	cycloserine
C&S	culture and sensitivity
CSA	canavaninosuccinic acid
	chondroitin sulfate-A
CSF	cerebrospinal fluid
	colony-stimulating factor
CSH	chronic subdural hematoma
	cortical stromal hyperplasia
CSL	cardiolipin synthetic lecithin

CSM . . . . cerebrospinal meningitis
                     corn-soy milk
CSN . . . . carotid sinus nerve
CSR . . . . Cheyne-Stokes respiration
                     corrected sedimentation rate
                     cortisol secretion rate
CSS . . . . carotid sinus stimulation
CST . . . . convulsive shock therapy
CT . . . . cardiothoracic (ratio)
                     carotid tracing
                     carpal tunnel
                     cerebral thrombosis
                     chlorothiazide
                     circulation time
                     classic technique
                     clotting time
                     coagulation time
                     collecting tubule
                     connective tissue
                     contraction time
                     Coombs' test
                     coronary thrombosis
                     corrected transposition
                     corrective therapy
                     crest time
                     cytotechnologist
CTAB . . . . cetyltrimethylammonium bromide
CTC . . . . chlortetracycline
CTD . . . . carpal tunnel decompression
                     congenital thymic dysplasia
CTFE . . . . chlorotrifluoroethylene
CTH . . . . ceramide trihexoside
CTR . . . . cardiothoracic ratio
CTZ . . . . chlorothiazide
CU . . . . color unit
                     convalescent unit
cu. cm. . . . . cubic centimeter
cu. mm. . . . . cubic millimeter

CUC . . . . chronic ulcerative colitis
CUG . . . . cystourethrogram
Cuj. . . . . of which (cujus)
Cuj. lib. . . . . of any you desire (cujus libet)
CV . . . . cardiovascular
                        cell volume
                        central venous
                        cerebrovascular
                        coefficient of variation
                        color vision
                        conjugate diameter of pelvic inlet
                        conversational voice
                        corpuscular volume
                        cresyl violet
                        tomorrow evening (cras vespere)
CVA . . . . cardiovascular accident
                        cerebrovascular accident
                        costovertebral angle
CVD . . . . cardiovascular disease
                        color vision deviant
                        color vision deviate
                        curved
CVH . . . . combined ventricular hypertrophy
CVO . . . . conjugate diameter of pelvic inlet
CVP . . . . cell volume profile
                        central venous pressure
CVR . . . . cardiovascular-renal
                        cerebrovascular resistance
CVRD . . . . cardiovascular renal disease
CVS . . . . cardiovascular surgery
                        cardiovascular system
                        clean-voided specimen
CW . . . . cardiac work
                        casework
                        chemical warfare
                        chest wall
                        children's ward
                        clockwise

CW *(continued)* . . . continuous wave
CWDF . . . . cell wall-deficient bacterial forms
CWI . . . . cardiac work index
CWP . . . . childbirth without pain
cwt. . . . . hundredweight
CX . . . . cervix
      chest x-ray
      convex
Cy. . . . . copy
      cyanogen
Cyclo. . . . . cyclophosphamide
      cyclopropane
Cyl. . . . . cylinder
D . . . . daughter
      day
      dead
      deciduous
      density
      dermatology
      deuterium
      deuteron
      dextro
      died
      diopter
      diplomate
      distal
      divorced
      dorsal
      dose
      duration
      give (da)
      right (dexter)
      vitamin D unit
D_{CO} . . . . diffusing capacity for carbon monoxide
D_L . . . . diffusing capacity of the lung
D in p. aeq. . . . . . . divide in equal parts (divide in
        partes aequales)
D time . . . . dream time

DA . . . . degenerative arthritis
                  dental assistant
                  direct agglutination
                  disaggregated
                  dopamine
                  ductus arteriosus
DAB . . . . dimethylaminoazobenzene
DAH . . . . disordered action of the heart
DALA . . . . delta-aminolevulinic acid
DAM . . . . degraded amyloid
                  diacetyl monoxime
DAO . . . . diamine oxidase
DAP . . . . dihydroxyacetone phosphate
                  direct agglutination pregnancy (test)
Dapt. . . . . Daptazole
DAPT. . . . . direct agglutination pregnancy test
DAT. . . . . differential agglutination titer
                  diphtheria antitoxin
DB . . . . date of birth
                  dextran blue
                  disability
                  distobuccal
db. . . . . decibel
DBA. . . . . dibenzanthracene
DBC . . . . dye binding capacity
DBCL. . . . . dilute blood clot lysis (method)
DBI . . . . development-at-birth index
DBM . . . . dibromomannitol
DBO. . . . . distobucco-occlusal
DBP . . . . diastolic blood pressure
                  distobuccopulpal
DC . . . . daily census
                  deoxycholate
                  diagnostic code
                  dilation and curettement
                  diphenylarsine cyanide
                  direct current
                  discontinue

DC *(continued)* . . . distocervical
D&C. . . . . dilation and curettement
DCA. . . . . deoxycholate-citrate agar
.... desoxycorticosterone acetate
DCC . . . . double concave
DCF . . . . direct centrifugal flotation
DCG. . . . . disodium cromoglycate
DCHFB . . . . dichlorohexafluorobutane
DCI . . . . dichloroisoproterenol
DCT . . . . direct Coombs' test
DCTMA . . . . desoxycorticosterone trimethylacetate
DCTPA . . . . desoxycorticosterone triphenylacetate
DCX. . . . . double convex
DD . . . . died of the disease
.... differential diagnosis
.... disk diameter
.... let it be given to (detur ad)
DDC. . . . . diethyldithiocarbamic acid
DDD. . . . . dichlorodiphenyldichloroethane
DDS . . . . diaminodiphenylsulfone
.... dystrophy-dystocia syndrome
DDT. . . . . dichlorodiphenyltrichloroethane
DE . . . . dream elements
.... duration of ejection
D&E. . . . . dilation and evacuation
De d. in d. . . . . from day to day (de die in diem)
DEA. . . . . dehydroepiandrosterone
DEAE . . . . diethylaminoethanol
.... diethylaminoethyl
DEAE-D. . . . . diethylaminoethyl dextran
DEBA . . . . diethylbarbituric acid
Dec. . . . . deceased
.... deciduous
.... decrease
.... pour off (decanta)
deca-. . . . . ten
deci-. . . . . a tenth
Decoct. . . . . decoction

Decr. . . . . decrease
Decub. . . . . lying down (decubitus)
Def. . . . . deficiency
Deg. . . . . degeneration
　　　　　　　　　　　　degree
Deglut. . . . . let it be swallowed (deglutiatur)
deka- . . . . ten
Del. . . . . delivery
Dem. . . . . Demerol (meperidine)
Dep. . . . . dependents
DER. . . . . reaction of degeneration
Derm . . . . dermatology
DEST . . . . distilled (destilla)
Det. . . . . diethyltryptamine
Det. . . . . give (detur)
DEV. . . . . duck embryo vaccine
DF . . . . decapacitation factor
　　　　　　　　　　　　degree of freedom
　　　　　　　　　　　　desferrioxamine
　　　　　　　　　　　　diabetic father
　　　　　　　　　　　　discriminant function
　　　　　　　　　　　　disseminated foci
DFDT . . . . difluorodiphenyltrichloroethane
DFO. . . . . deferoxamine
DFP . . . . diisopropylfluorophosphate
DFU. . . . . dead fetus in utero
　　　　　　　　　　　　dideoxyfluorouridine
DG . . . . deoxyglucose
　　　　　　　　　　　　diagnosis
　　　　　　　　　　　　diastolic gallop
　　　　　　　　　　　　diglyceride
　　　　　　　　　　　　distogingival
dg. . . . . decigram
dgm . . . . decigram
DH . . . . delayed hypersensitivity
DHA . . . . dehydroepiandrosterone
　　　　　　　　　　　　dihydroxyacetone
DHAP . . . . dihydroxyacetone phosphate

DHAS . . . . dehydroepiandrosterone sulfate
DHE. . . . . dihydroergotamine
DHEA . . . . dehydroepiandrosterone
DHEAS . . . . dehydroepiandrosterone sulfate
DHFR . . . . dihydrofolate reductase
DHIA . . . . dehydroisoandrosterone
DHT. . . . . dihydrotachysterol
DI . . . . diabetes insipidus
Diag. . . . . diagnosis
DIC . . . . diffuse intravascular coagulation
                        disseminated intravascular coagulation
DID . . . . dead of intercurrent disease
DIE . . . . died in Emergency Room
Dieb. alt. . . . . on alternate days (diebus alternis)
Dieb. tert. . . . . . . every third day (diebus tertiis)
Diff. . . . . differential
Dig. . . . . let it be digested (digeratur)
Dil. . . . . dilute
DILD . . . . diffuse infiltrative lung disease
Diluc . . . . at daybreak (diluculo)
Dilut. . . . . dilute
DIM . . . . divalent ion metabolism
Dim. . . . . one half (dimidius)
DIP. . . . . desquamative interstitial pneumonia
                        diisopropyl phosphate
                        distal interphalangeal
DIPJ. . . . . distal interphalangeal joint
Dir. prop. . . . . with a proper direction (directione propria)
Dis. . . . . disease
Disc. . . . . discontinue
disch. . . . . discharge
Disp. . . . . dispensatory
                        dispense
Dist. . . . . distill
DIT . . . . diiodotyrosine
Div. . . . . divide
DJD . . . . degenerative joint disease
DK . . . . decay

DK *(continued)* .. diseased kidney
                       dog kidney
DL . . . . danger list
                       difference limen
                       diffusing capacity of the lung
                       distolingual
                       Donath-Landsteiner (test)
dl . . . . deciliter
DLA. . . . . distolabial
DLAI . . . . distolabioincisal
DLCO . . . . diffusing capacity of the lung for
                       carbon monoxide
DLE . . . . discoid lupus erythematosus
                       disseminated lupus erythematosus
DLI . . . . distolinguoincisal
DLO. . . . . distolinguo-occlusal
DLP . . . . distolinguopulpal
DM . . . . diabetes mellitus
                       diabetic mother
                       diastolic murmur
                       dopamine
DMA . . . . dimethyladenosine
DMAB . . . . dimethylaminobenzaldehyde
DMBA . . . . dimethylbenzanthracene
DMCT . . . . demethylchlortetracycline
DMD . . . . Duchenne's muscular dystrophy
DME . . . . dimethyl ether (of d-tubocurarine)
DMF . . . . decayed, missing or filled (teeth)
DMM . . . . dimethylmyleran
DMN . . . . dimethylnitrosamine
DMO . . . . dimethyloxazolidinedione
DMPA . . . . depomedroxyprogesterone acetate
DMPE . . . . dimethoxyphenylethylamine
DMPEA . . . . dimethoxyphenylethylamine
DMPP . . . . dimethylphenylpiperazinium
DMS . . . . dimethylsulfoxide
DMSO . . . . dimethylsulfoxide
DMT . . . . dimethyltryptamine

DN .... dextrose-nitrogen (ratio)
DNA............. deoxyribonucleic acid
DNase........... deoxyribonuclease
DNB............. dinitrobenzene
DNC............. dinitrocarbanilide
DNCB .... dinitrochlorobenzene
DND............. died a natural death
DNFB .... dinitrofluorobenzene
DNP............. deoxyribonucleoprotein
                 dinitrophenol
DNPH .... dinitrophenylhydrazine
DNPM........... dinitrophenylmorphine
DNT............. did not test
DO .... diamine oxidase
                 disto-occlusal
DOA .... dead on arrival
DOB .... date of birth
DOC .... deoxycholate
                 deoxycorticosterone
                 died of other causes
Doc............. doctor
DOCA .... deoxycorticosterone acetate
DOCS........... deoxycorticoids
DOD............. date of death
                 dead of disease
DOE............. dyspnea on exercise
                 dyspnea on exertion
DOET .... dimethoxyethyl amphetamine
DOM .... deaminated-O-methyl metabolite
                 dimethoxymethyl amphetamine
DOMA .... dihydroxymandelic acid
DON .... diazo-oxonorleucine
Donec alv. sol.
    Fuerit........ until the bowels are open (donec alvus
                 soluta fuerit)
DOPA .... dihydroxyphenylalanine
DOPAC   dihydroxyphenylacetic acid
DP .... dementia praecox

DP *(continued)* . . . diastolic pressure
directional preponderance
disability pension
distopulpal
with proper direction
DPA . . . . dipropylacetate
DPC . . . . delayed primary closure
DPD . . . . diffuse pulmonary disease
DPG . . . . diphosphoglycerate
displacement placentogram
DPGM . . . . diphosphoglyceromutase
DPGP . . . . diphosphoglycerate phosphatase
DPH . . . . diphenylhydantoin
DPI . . . . disposable personal income
DPL . . . . distopulpolingual
dpm . . . . disintegrations per minute
DPN . . . . diphosphopyridine nucleotide
DPNH . . . . diphosphopyridine nucleotide
DPO . . . . dimethoxyphenyl penicillin
DPS . . . . dimethylpolysiloxane
DPT . . . . diphtheria, pertussis, and tetanus
dipropyltryptamine
DPTA . . . . diethylenetriamine pentaacetic acid
DQ . . . . developmental quotient
DR . . . . diabetic retinopathy
doctor
reaction of degeneration
dr . . . . drachm
dram
DRF . . . . dose-reduction factor
DRI . . . . Discharge Readiness Inventory
DS . . . . dead space
dehydroepiandrosterone sulfate
dextrose-saline
Down's syndrome
dry swallow
D&S . . . . dermatology and syphilology
DSAP . . . . disseminated superficial actinic porokeratosis

DSC . . . . disodium cromoglycate
DSCG. . . . . disodium cromoglycate
DSM. . . . . dextrose solution mixture
DST . . . . dexamethasone suppression test
DT . . . . delirium tremens
                    distance test
                    duration tetany
                    dye test
DTBC . . . . d-tubocurarine
DTBN . . . . di-t-butyl nitroxide
DTC. . . . . d-tubocurarine
D.T.D. No. vi. . . . . let six such doses be given
DTM. . . . . dermatophyte test medium
DTMP. . . . . deoxythymidine monophosphate
DTN. . . . . diphtheria toxin normal
DTNB . . . . dithiobisnitrobenzoic acid
DTP . . . . diphtheria, tetanus, and pertussis
                    distal tingling on percussion
DTPA . . . . diethylenetriaminepentacetic acid
DTR. . . . . deep tendon reflex
DTZ. . . . . diatrizoate
DU. . . . . deoxyuridine
                    diagnosis undetermined
                    dog unit
                    duodenal ulcer
DUMP . . . . deoxyuridine monophosphate
Duod. . . . . duodenum
Dur. dolor . . . . while the pain lasts (durante dolore)
DV . . . . double vibration
DVA. . . . . distance visual acuity
DW. . . . . distilled water
                    dry weight
D/W . . . . dextrose in water
D-5-W . . . . 5 per cent dextrose in water
D_5W. . . . . 5 per cent dextrose in water
DX . . . . dextran
                    diagnosis
DXD. . . . . discontinued

DXM . . . . dexamethasone
DXT. . . . . deep x-ray therapy
DZ . . . . dizygous
E . . . . cortisone (compound E)
                       electric charge
                       electromotive force
                       electron
                       emmetropia
                       energy
                       Entamoeba
                       epinephrine
                       Escherichia
                       experimenter
                       eye
                       from
EA . . . . each
                       ethacrynic acid
EAC. . . . . Ehrlich ascites carcinoma
                       external auditory canal
EACA . . . . epsilon aminocaproic acid
Ead. . . . . the same (eadem)
EAE. . . . . experimental allergic encephalomyelitis
EAHF . . . . eczema, asthma, hay fever
EAHLG . . . . equine antihuman lymphoblast globulin
EAHLS . . . . equine antihuman lymphoblast serum
EAM . . . . external auditory meatus
EAP . . . . epiallopregnanolone
EAR. . . . . reaction of degeneration
EB . . . . elementary body
                       epidermolysis bullosa
                       Epstein-Barr (virus)
                       estradiol benzoate
EBI . . . . emetine bismuth iodide
EBV. . . . . Epstein-Barr virus
EC . . . . electron capture
                       enteric-coated
                       entrance complaint
                       Escherichia coli

EC *(continued)*. . . . excitation–contraction
extracellular
eyes closed
ECA . . . . ethacrynic acid
ECBV. . . . . effective circulating blood volume
ECF . . . . effective capillary flow
extended care facility
extracellular fluid
ECFV. . . . . extracellular fluid volume
ECG . . . . electrocardiogram
ECHO . . . . enteric cytopathogenic human
orphan (virus)
ECI . . . . extracorporeal irradiation (of blood)
ECIB . . . . extracorporeal irradiation of blood
ECIL . . . . extracorporeal irradiation of lymph
Eclec . . . . eclectic
ECLT. . . . . euglobulin clot lysis time
ECM. . . . . extracellular material
ECS . . . . electroconvulsive shock
ECT . . . . electroconvulsive therapy
ECV . . . . extracellular volume
ECW. . . . . extracellular water
ED . . . . effective dose
Ehlers–Danlos syndrome
epileptiform discharge
erythema dose
ED_{50} . . . . median effective dose
EDC. . . . . estimated date of confinement
expected date of confinement
EDD. . . . . effective drug duration
expected date of delivery
EDP . . . . electronic data processing
end-diastolic pressure
EDS . . . . Ehlers–Danlos syndrome
EDTA . . . . edetic acid
ethylenediamine tetraacetic acid
EDV. . . . . end-diastolic volume
EE . . . . Eastern equine encephalitis

EE *(continued)*. . . . end to end
                           eye and ear
EEA . . . . electroencephalic audiometry
EEC . . . . enteropathogenic Escherichia coli
EEE . . . . Eastern equine encephalitis
EEG . . . . electroencephalogram
EEME . . . . ethinylestradiol methyl ether
EENT . . . . eyes, ears, nose and throat
EER . . . . electroencephalic response
EF . . . . ectopic focus
                           ejection fraction
                           encephalitogenic factor
EFA . . . . essential fatty acids
                           extrafamily adoptees
EFC . . . . endogenous fecal calcium
EFE . . . . endocardial fibroelastosis
EFV . . . . extracellular fluid volume
EFVC . . . . expiratory flow-volume curve
EG . . . . esophagogastrectomy
EGG . . . . electrogastrogram
EGL . . . . eosinophilic granuloma of the lung
EGM. . . . . electrogram
EGOT . . . . erythrocyte glutamic oxaloacetic
                             transaminase
EH . . . . essential hypertension
EHBF. . . . . estimated hepatic blood flow
                           exercise hyperemia blood flow
EHC . . . . enterohepatic circulation
                           essential hypercholesterolemia
EHDP. . . . . ethane hydroxydiphosphate
EHF. . . . . exophthalmos-hyperthyroid factor
EHL. . . . . endogenous hyperlipidemia
EHO. . . . . extrahepatic obstruction
EHP . . . . excessive heat production
EI . . . . enzyme inhibitor
E/I . . . . expiration-inspiration ratio
EID . . . . egg infective dose
                           electroimmunodiffusion

EIP.	extensor indicis proprius
EK	erythrokinase
EKC.	epidemic keratoconjunctivitis
EKG.	electrocardiogram
EKY.	electrokymogram
El.	elixir
Elb.	elbow
Elix.	elixir
ELT	euglobulin lysis time
EM	ejection murmur
	electron microscopy
	emmetropia
	erythrocyte mass
EMB.	embryology
	eosin methylene blue
	ethambutol
	ethambutol–myambutol
EMC.	electron microscopy
	encephalomyocarditis
EMF.	electromagnetic flowmeter
	electromotive force
	endomyocardial fibrosis
	erythrocyte maturation factor
EMG.	electromyogram
	exophthalmos, macroglossia, gigantism
Emp.	a plaster (emplastrum)
	as directed
Emul.	emulsion
EN	enema
	erythema nodosum
ENA.	extractable nuclear antigen
Enem.	enema
ENG.	electronystagmograph
ENL.	erythema nodosum leproticum
ENT.	ear, nose, and throat
EO	eosinophils
	ethylene oxide
	eyes open

EOD . . . . entry on duty
                          every other day
EOG . . . . electro–oculogram
EOM . . . . extraocular movement
Eos. . . . . eosinophils
EOT . . . . effective oxygen transport
EP . . . . ectopic pregnancy
                          erythrocyte protoporphyrin
EPC . . . . epilepsia partialis continua
EPEC . . . . enteropathogenic Escherichia coli
EPF . . . . exophthalmos-producing factor
Epi. . . . . epinephrine
epith. . . . . epithelium
EPP . . . . erythropoietic protoporphyria
EPR . . . . electron paramagnetic resonance
                          electrophrenic respiration
                          estradiol production rate
EPS . . . . exophthalmos-producing substance
EPTE . . . . existed prior to enlistment
EPTS . . . . existed prior to service
Eq. . . . . equivalent
ER . . . . ejection rate
                          emergency room
                          endoplasmic reticulum
                          external resistance
                          evoked response
ERA . . . . evoked response audiometry
ERBF . . . . effective renal blood flow
ERG . . . . electroretinogram
ERP . . . . effective refractory period
                          equine rhinopneumonitis
ERPF . . . . effective renal plasma flow
ERV . . . . expiratory reserve volume
ES . . . . end to side
                          Expectation Score
ESB . . . . electrical stimulation to the brain
ESC . . . . electromechanical slope computer
Esch. . . . . Escherichia

ESD . . . . electronic summation device
ESE . . . . electrostatic unit
ESF . . . . erythropoietic-stimulating factor
ESL . . . . end-systolic length
ESM . . . . ejection systolic murmur
Eso. . . . . esophagoscopy
                            esophagus
ESP . . . . end-systolic pressure
                            extrasensory perception
ESR . . . . erythrocyte sedimentation rate
ESS . . . . erythrocyte-sensitizing substance
                            essential
Ess. neg. . . . . essentially negative
EST . . . . electroshock therapy
Est. . . . . estimated
ESU . . . . electrostatic unit
ESV . . . . end-systolic volume
ET . . . . and
                            effective temperature
                            ejection time
                            endotracheal
                            etiology
                            eustachian tube
Et. . . . . and
                            ethyl
Et al . . . . and others (et alii)
ETA . . . . ethionamide
ETH . . . . elixir terpin hydrate
ETH/C . . . . elixir terpin hydrate with codeine
Etiol. . . . . etiology
ETKM . . . . every test known to man
ETM . . . . erythromycin
ETOH. . . . . ethyl alcohol
ETOX . . . . ethylene oxide
ETP . . . . entire treatment period
                            eustachian tube pressure
ETT . . . . extrathyroidal thyroxine
ETV . . . . educational television

EU . . . . Ehrlich units
                     enzyme units
EUA. . . . . examination under anesthesia
EV . . . . extravascular
ev . . . . electron volt
Eval. . . . . evaluation
EW . . . . elsewhere
                     Emergency Ward
EWB. . . . . estrogen withdrawal bleeding
EWL. . . . . egg-white lysozyme
Ex. . . . . excision
                     exophthalmos
                     from
Exam. . . . . examination
EXBF. . . . . exercise hyperemia blood flow
Exc. . . . . excision
Exhib. . . . . let it be given (exhibeatur)
Exp. . . . . expired
Expir. . . . . expiration
                     expiratory
Ext. . . . . exterior
                     external
                     extract
                     spread (extende)
F . . . . Fahrenheit
                     fat
                     father
                     fellow
                     female
                     field of vision
                     Filaria
                     foramen
                     formula
                     French (catheter size)
                     Fusiformis
                     gilbert (unit of magnetomotive force)
                     hydrocortisone (compound F)
                     make (fiat)

F_1 . . . . first filial generation
F_2 . . . . second filial generation
F. pil . . . . let pills be made (fiant pilulae)
F. vs. . . . . let the patient be bled (fiat venaesectio)
FA . . . . far advanced
                fatty acid
                femoral artery
                field ambulance
                first aid
                fluorescent antibody
                forearm
                free acid
FAD . . . . flavin adenine dinucleotide
FADF . . . . fluorescent antibody darkfield
Fahr . . . . Fahrenheit
Fam. doc. . . . . family doctor
FAN . . . . fuchsin, amido black, and naphthol yellow
FANA . . . . fluorescent antinuclear antibody
FAT . . . . fluorescent antibody test
FAV . . . . feline ataxia virus
FB . . . . fingerbreadth
                foreign body
FBE . . . . full blood examination
FBP . . . . femoral blood pressure
                fibrinogen breakdown products
FBS . . . . fasting blood sugar
                fetal bovine serum
FC . . . . finger clubbing
                finger counting
fc . . . . foot candles
FCA . . . . ferritin-conjugated antibodies
FD . . . . fatal dose
                focal distance
                foot drape
                forceps delivery
                freeze-dried
FD_{50} . . . . median fatal dose
FDA . . . . frontodextra anterior

FDE . . . . final drug evaluation
FDP . . . . fibrin degradation product
                 flexor digitorum profundus
                 frontodextra posterior
                 fructose 1, 6-diphosphate
FDS . . . . flexor digitorum superficialis
FDT . . . . frontodextra transversa
Feb. dur. . . . . while the fever lasts (febre durante)
FEC . . . . free erythrocyte coproporphyrin
FECG . . . . fetal electrocardiogram
FECP . . . . free erythrocyte coproporphyria
FECVC . . . . functional extracellular fluid volume
FEF . . . . forced expiratory flow
FEKG . . . . fetal electrocardiogram
Fem . . . . female
FEP . . . . free erythrocyte protoporphyrin
FEPP . . . . free erythrocyte protoporphyrin
FES . . . . forced expiratory spirogram
FET . . . . forced expiratory time
FETS . . . . forced expiratory time, in seconds
FEV . . . . forced expiratory volume
FF . . . . fat free
                 father factor
                 fecal frequency
                 filtration fraction
                 finger to finger
                 flat feet
                 force fluids
                 forearm flow
                 foster father
FFA . . . . free fatty acids
FFDW . . . . fat-free dry weight
FFM . . . . fat-free mass
FFP . . . . fresh frozen plasma
FFT . . . . flicker fusion threshold
FFWW . . . . fat-free wet weight
FG . . . . fibrinogen
FGD . . . . fatal granulomatous disease

FGF . . . . father's grandfather
fresh gas flow
FGM . . . . father's grandmother
FH . . . . family history
fetal head
fetal heart
let a draft be made (fiat haustus)
FHR. . . . . fetal heart rate
FHS . . . . fetal heart sound
FHT . . . . fetal heart
fetal heart tones
FI. . . . . fever caused by infection
fibrinogen
Fib. . . . . fibrillation
fibrinogen
FID . . . . flame ionization detector
FIF. . . . . forced inspiratory flow
Fig. . . . . figure
FIGLU. . . . . formiminoglutamic acid
Filt. . . . . filter
Fist. . . . . fistula
FJN . . . . familial juvenile nephrophthisis
Fl. . . . . fluid
fl. dr. . . . . fluid dram
fl. oz. . . . . fluid ounce
Fl. up. . . . . flare-up
follow-up
FLA . . . . according to rule (fiat lege artis)
frontolaeva anterior
Fld. . . . . fluid
Flor. . . . . flowers
FLP . . . . frontolaeva posterior
FLSA . . . . follicular lymphosarcoma
FLT . . . . frontolaeva transversa
FM . . . . flowmeter
make a mixture (fiat mistura)
FME. . . . . full-mouth extraction
FMF. . . . . familial Mediterranean fever

FMG.	foreign medical graduate
FMN	flavin mononucleotide
FMS	fat-mobilizing substance
	full-mouth series
FN	false-negative
	finger to nose
FO	foramen ovale
	fronto-occipital
FOAVF	failure of all vital forces
FOD.	free of disease
Fol..	leaves (folia)
FP.	false-positive
	family practice
	freezing point
	frontoparietal
	frozen plasma
	let a potion be made (fiat potio)
FPA	fluorophenylalanine
FPC	fish protein concentrate
FPM	filter paper microscopic (test)
fps	frames per second
FR	Fisher-Race (notation)
	flocculation reaction
	French (catheter gauge)
Fr. BB	fracture of both bones
F & R	force and rhythm
Fract.	fracture
Fract. dos.	in divided doses (fracta dosi)
Frag.	fragility
FRC.	frozen red cells
	functional reserve capacity
	functional residual capacity
Frict.	friction
FROM	full range of motion
FRP	functional refractory period
FRS	furosemide
FS	full scale (IQ)
	function study

FSA . . . . let it be made skillfully (fiat secundum artem)
FSD . . . . focus to skin distance
FSF . . . . fibrin-stabilizing factor
FSH . . . . follicle stimulating hormone
FSP . . . . fibrinogen-split products
                  fibrinolytic split products
FSW . . . . field service worker
FT . . . . false transmitter
                  family therapy
                  fibrous tissue
                  free thyroxine
                  full term
                  make (fiat)
ft . . . . foot
Ft mas div in pil . . . make a mass and divide into pills (fiat massa dividenda in pilulae)
Ft pulv . . . . make a powder (fiat pulvis)
FTA . . . . fluorescent treponemal antibody
FTA-AB . . . . fluorescent treponemal antibody absorption test
FTA-ABS . . . . fluorescent treponemal antibody absorption test
FTI . . . . free thyroxine index
FTLB . . . . full term living birth
FTND . . . . full term normal delivery
FTT . . . . failure to thrive
FU . . . . fecal urobilinogen
                  fluorouracil
                  follow-up
FUDR . . . . fluorodeoxyuridine
FUO . . . . fever of undetermined origin
                  fever of unknown origin
FUR . . . . fluorouracil riboside
FV . . . . fluid volume
FVC . . . . forced vital capacity
FVL . . . . femoral vein ligation
FW . . . . Felix-Weil (reaction)

FW *(continued)*. . . . Folin and Wu's (method)
                         fragment wound
FWR. . . . . Felix-Weil reaction
FX . . . . fracture
                         frozen section
FY . . . . fiscal year
FYI . . . . for your information
G . . . . an immunoglobulin
                         force (the pull of gravity)
                         gauge
                         gingival
                         gonidial colony
                         good
                         gravida
                         Greek
g. . . . . gram
GA . . . . Gamblers Anonymous
                         gastric analysis
                         general anesthesia
                         gestational age
                         gingivoaxial
                         glucuronic acid
                         gut-associated
GABA. . . . . gamma-aminobutyric acid
gal . . . . gallon
GALT. . . . . gut-associated lymphoid tissue
Galv . . . . galvanic
GAPD . . . . glyceraldehyde phosphate dehydrogenase
Garg . . . . gargle
GB . . . . gallbladder
                         Guillain-Barré syndrome
GBA. . . . . ganglionic-blocking agent
                         gingivobuccoaxial
GBH. . . . . graphite-benzalkonium-heparin
GBM. . . . . glomerular basement membrane
GBS . . . . gallbladder series
GC . . . . ganglion cells
                         gas chromatography

GC *(continued)*. . . . glucocorticoid
gonococcus
gonorrhea
granular casts
guanine cytosine
g-cal . . . . gram-calorie
g-cm . . . . gram-centimeter
GCS . . . . general clinical service
GDA. . . . . germine diacetate
GDH. . . . . glycerophosphate dehydrogenase
GDS . . . . Gradual Dosage Schedule
GE . . . . gastroemotional
gastroenterology
gastroenterostomy
G/E . . . . granulocyte-erythroid ratio
Gel. quav . . . . any kind of jelly (gelatina quavis)
GEMS . . . . good emergency mother substitute
Gen . . . . general
Ger . . . . geriatrics
GET . . . . gastric emptying time
GET½ . . . . gastric emptying half-time
GF . . . . germ-free
gluten-free
grandfather
GFD. . . . . gluten-free diet
GFR. . . . . glomerular filtration rate
GG . . . . gamma globulin
GG or S . . . . glands, goiter, or stiffness (the neck)
GGA . . . . general gonadotropic activity
GGG . . . . gamboge
GGTP. . . . . gamma-glutamyl transpeptidase
GH . . . . growth hormone
GHD. . . . . growth hormone deficiency
GHRF . . . . growth hormone-releasing factor
GI. . . . . gastrointestinal
globin insulin
giga- . . . . one-billion
GIK . . . . glucose, insulin, and potassium

GIM . . . . gonadotropin-inhibitory material
GIS . . . . gas in stomach
                         gastrointestinal system
GIT. . . . . gastrointestinal tract
GITT . . . . glucose-insulin tolerance test
GK . . . . glycerol kinase
Gl. . . . . gill
                         gland
GL . . . . greatest length
GLA. . . . . gingivolinguoaxial
GLC . . . . gas-liquid chromatography
Glob. . . . . globulin
GLP . . . . group-living program
Glu. . . . . glucose
Gluc. . . . . glucose
GM . . . . gastric mucosa
                         general medical
                         geometric mean
                         grandmother
                         grand multiparity
gm . . . . gram
GMA . . . . glyceryl methacrylate
GMC . . . . general medical council
GMK. . . . . green monkey kidney
gm-m . . . . gram-meter
GM & S . . . . general medical and surgical
GMT. . . . . geometric mean titer
GMW. . . . . gram-molecular weight
GN . . . . glomerulonephritis
                         glucose nitrogen (ratio)
                         gram-negative
GNID . . . . gram-negative intracellular diplococci
GOE. . . . . gas, oxygen and ether
GOK. . . . . God only knows
GOT. . . . . glutamic oxaloacetic transaminase
GP . . . . general paresis
                         general practice
                         general practitioner

GP *(continued)*. . . . glycoprotein
group (muscle)
guinea pig
gutta-percha
GPA . . . . grade-point averages
GPAIS . . . . guinea pig anti-insulin serum
GPD . . . . glucose phosphate dehydrogenase
G6PD . . . . glucose-6-phosphate dehydrogenase
GPI. . . . . general paralysis of the insane
glucose phosphate isomerase
GPIPID. . . . . guinea pig intraperitoneal infectious dose
GPK . . . . guinea pig kidney (antigen)
GPKA. . . . . guinea pig kidney absorption test
GPS . . . . guinea pig serum
GPT . . . . glutamic pyruvic transaminase
GPUT. . . . . galactose phosphate uridyl transferase
GR . . . . gastric resection
glutathione reductase
gr. . . . . grain
GRA . . . . gonadotropin-releasing agent
Grad. . . . . gradually, by degrees
GRAS . . . . generally recognized as safe
Grav. I. . . . . pregnancy one
primigravida
GRF. . . . . gonadotropin-releasing factor
GS . . . . general surgery
G/S . . . . glucose and saline
GSA . . . . Gross virus antigen
guanidinosuccinic acid
GSC . . . . gas-solid chromatography
gravity-settling culture
GSD . . . . genetically significant dose
glycogen storage disease
GSE . . . . gluten-sensitive enteropathy
GSH . . . . glomerular-stimulating hormone
reduced glutathione
GSR . . . . galvanic skin response
generalized Shwartzman reaction

GSSG . . . . oxidized glutathione
GSSR . . . . generalized Sanarelli-Shwartzman reaction
GSW . . . . gunshot wound
GT . . . . gingiva, treatment of
                     glucose tolerance
                     glutamyl transpeptidase
G & T . . . . gowns and towels
gt. . . . . drop
GTH . . . . gonadotropic hormone
GTN . . . . glyceryl trinitrate
GTP . . . . glutamyl transpeptidase
                     guanosine triphosphate
GTT . . . . glucose tolerance test
gtt. . . . . drops
GU . . . . gastric ulcer
                     genitourinary
                     gonococcal urethritis
GUS . . . . genitourinary system
GV . . . . gentian violet
GVH . . . . graft versus host
GVHR . . . . graft-versus-host reaction
GW . . . . group work
GXT . . . . graded exercise test
GYN . . . . gynecology
GZ . . . . Guilford-Zimmerman personality test
H . . . . Hauch (motile)
                     haustus (a draft)
                     height
                     Hemophilus
                     henry
                     high
                     Holzknecht unit
                     horizontal
                     hormone
                     hour
                     hypermetropia
                     hypo
H^+ . . . . hydrogen ion

HA . . . . headache
height age
hemagglutinating antibody
hemagglutination
hemolytic anemia
high anxiety
hospital admission
hydroxyapatite
HAA. . . . . hepatitis associated antigen
HABA . . . . hydroxybenzeneazobenzoic acid
HAD. . . . . hemadsorption
HAHTG . . . . horse antihuman thymus globulin
HAI . . . . hemagglutination inhibition
hemagglutinin inhibition
Hal. . . . . halothane
HAP . . . . heredopathia atactica polyneuritiformis
histamine phosphate acid
HAPA . . . . hemagglutinating antipenicillin antibody
HASHD . . . . hypertensive arteriosclerotic heart disease
Haust. . . . . a draft (haustus)
HB . . . . heart block
hemoglobin
housebound
HBABA . . . . hydroxybenzeneazobenzoic acid
HBB . . . . hydroxybenzyl benzimidazole
HBD. . . . . hydroxybutyrate dehydrogenase
HBDH . . . . hydroxybutyrate dehydrogenase
HBF . . . . hepatic blood flow
HBI. . . . . high serum-bound iron
HBO. . . . . hyperbaric oxygen
HBP . . . . high blood pressure
HBW. . . . . high birth weight
HC . . . . hair cell
head compression
hepatic catalase
house call
Huntington's chorea
hyaline casts

HC	hydroxycorticoid
HCC.	hydroxycholecalciferol
HCG.	human chorionic gonadotropin
HCH.	hexachlorocyclohexane
HCP	hepatocatalase peroxidase
	hereditary coproporphyria
HCS	human chorionic somatomammotropin
HCSM	human chorionic somatomammotropin
HCT	hematocrit
	homocytotrophic
	hydrochlorothiazide
HCU.	homocystinuria
HCVD	hypertensive cardiovascular disease
HD	at bedtime (hora decubitus)
	hearing distance
	heart disease
	high dosage
	Hodgkin's disease
	hydatid disease
HDBH	hydroxybutyric dehydrogenase
HDC.	histidine decarboxylase
HDH.	heart disease history
HDL.	high density lipoprotein
HDLP.	high density lipoprotein
HDLW	distance at which a watch is heard by the left ear
HDN.	hemolytic disease of the newborn
HDP	hydroxydimethylpyrimidine
HDRW	distance at which a watch is heard by the right ear
HDS	herniated disk syndrome
HE	human enteric
H & E	hematoxylin and eosin
HEAT	human erythrocyte agglutination test
Hebdom.	a week (hebdomada)
HEC.	hydroxyergocalciferol
HED.	unit of roentgen-ray dosage
HEENT	head, ears, eyes, nose and throat

HEK . . . . human embryo kidney
                       human embryonic kidney
Hematol . . . . hematology
HEPA . . . . high-efficiency particulate air (filter)
HES . . . . hydroxyethyl starch
HET . . . . helium equilibration time
HETP . . . . hexaethyltetraphosphate
HF . . . . Hageman factor
                       hay fever
                       heart failure
                       hemorrhagic fever
                       high flow
                       high frequency
HFI . . . . hereditary fructose intolerance
HFP . . . . hexafluoropropylene
HG . . . . hemoglobin
HGB . . . . hemoglobin
HGF . . . . hyperglycemic-glycogenolytic factor
HGG . . . . human gamma globulin
HGH . . . . human growth hormone
HGPRT . . . . hypoxanthine guanine phosphoribosyl
                               transferase
HH . . . . hydroxyhexamide
HHA . . . . hereditary hemolytic anemia
HHB . . . . un-ionized hemoglobin
HHD . . . . hypertensive heart disease
H & Hm . . . . compound hypermetropic astigmatism
HHT . . . . hereditary hemorrhagic telangiectasia
HI . . . . hemagglutination inhibition
                       high impulsiveness
                       hydroxyindole
HIA . . . . hemagglutination-inhibition antibody
HIAA . . . . hydroxyindoleacetic acid
HIHA . . . . high impulsiveness, high anxiety
HILA . . . . high impulsiveness, low anxiety
HIOMT . . . . hydroxyindole-O-methyl transferase
HIT . . . . hemagglutination-inhibition test
                       hypertrophic infiltrative tendinitis

HJ . . . . Howell-Jolly (bodies)
HK . . . . heat-killed
                 heel to knee
                 hexokinase
HKLM . . . . heat-killed Listeria monocytogenes
HL . . . . hearing level
                 hearing loss
                 histocompatibility locus
                 hypermetropia, latent
H & L . . . . heart and lungs
HLH . . . . human luteinizing hormone
H-L-K . . . . heart, liver, kidney
HLR . . . . heart-lung resuscitator
HLT . . . . human lymphocyte transformation
Hlth.. . . . . health
HLV . . . . herpes-like virus
HM . . . . hand movement(s)
                 human milk
                 hydatidiform mole
                 manifest hypermetropia
HMD. . . . . hyaline membrane disease
HME. . . . . heat and moisture exchanger
HMF. . . . . hydroxymethylfurfural
HMG . . . . human menopausal gonadotropin
                 hydroxymethylglutaryl
HML . . . . human milk lysozyme
HMM . . . . hexamethylolmelamine
HMP. . . . . hexose monophosphate
                 hexose monophosphate pathway
                 hot moist packs
HMPG . . . . hydroxymethoxyphenylglycol
HMPS . . . . hexose monophosphate shunt
HMSAS . . . . hypertrophic muscular subaortic stenosis
Hmt. . . . . hematocrit
HN . . . . hereditary nephritis
                 hilar node
                 tonight (hac nocte)
HN_2 . . . . nitrogen mustard, mechlorethamine

HNP . . . . herniated nucleus pulposus
HNSHA . . . . hereditary nonspherocytic
                       hemolytic anemia
HO . . . . high oxygen
                       hyperbaric oxygen
H/O . . . . history of
H_2O . . . . water
HOC . . . . hydroxycorticoid
HOCM . . . . hypertrophic obstructive cardiomyopathy
HOOD . . . . hereditary osteo-onycho dysplasia
HOP . . . . high oxygen pressure
Hor. decub. . . . . . . at bedtime (hora decubitus)
Hor. interm. . . . . . . at intermediate hours (horis intermediis)
Hor. som. . . . . at bedtime (hora somni)
Hor. un spatio . . . . at the end of an hour (horae unius spatio)
Hosp. . . . . hospital
HP . . . . high protein
                       human pituitary
H & P . . . . history and physical
Hp . . . . haptoglobin
HPA . . . . hypothalamic-pituitary-adrenal
HPAA . . . . hydroxyphenylacetic acid
HPB . . . . high blood pressure
HPE . . . . history and physical examination
HPF . . . . heparin-precipitable fraction
                       high power field
HPFSH. . . . . human pituitary follicle-stimulating
                       hormone
HPG . . . . human pituitary gonadotropin
HPI . . . . history of present illness
HPL . . . . human placental lactogen
HPLA . . . . hydroxyphenyllactic acid
HPO . . . . high pressure oxygen
HPP. . . . . hydroxypyrazolopyrimidine
HPPA . . . . hydroxyphenylpyruvic acid
HPPH . . . . hydroxyphenyl-phenylhydantoin
HPS . . . . hematoxylin-phloxine-saffron
                       hypertrophic pyloric stenosis

HPT . . . . hyperparathyroidism
HPV . . . . Hemophilus pertussis vaccine
HPVD . . . . hypertensive pulmonary vascular disease
HPVG . . . . hepatic portal venous gas
HR . . . . heart rate
                         hospital record
                         hospital report
Hr. . . . . blood type factor
                         hour
H & R . . . . hysterectomy and radiation
HRBC . . . . horse red blood cells
HRIG . . . . human rabies immune globulin
HRS . . . . Hamilton Rating Scale
HRT . . . . heart rate
HS . . . . heat stable
                         heme synthetase
                         hereditary spherocytosis
                         herpes simplex
                         horse serum
                         Hurler's syndrome
                         on retiring (hora somni)
HSA . . . . human serum albumin
HSG . . . . hysterosalpingogram
HSV . . . . herpes simplex virus
HT . . . . heart
                         height
                         hemagglutination titer
                         Histologic technician
                         hydroxytryptamine
                         hypermetropia, total
                         hypertension
                         hypodermic tablet
HTA . . . . hydroxytryptamine
HTHD . . . . hypertensive heart disease
HTOH . . . . hydroxytryptophol
HTP . . . . hydroxytryptophan
HTV . . . . herpes-type virus
HU . . . . hemagglutinating unit

HU *(continued).* . . . hydroxyurea
                hyperemia unit
HUS . . . . hemolytic-uremic syndrome
                hyaluronidase unit for semen
HUTHAS . . . . human thymus antiserum
HV . . . . hepatic vein
                herpes virus
                hospital visit
H & V . . . . hemigastrectomy and vagotomy
HVA . . . . homovanillic acid
HVD . . . . hypertensive vascular disease
HVE . . . . high-voltage electrophoresis
HVH . . . . herpes virus hominis
HVL . . . . half-value layer
HVM . . . . high velocity missile
HVSD . . . . hydrogen-detected ventricular septal defect
HX . . . . history
Hy . . . . hypermetropia
                hysteria
Hypo . . . . injection
                under
Hys . . . . hysteria
Hz . . . . Hertz
I . . . . intensity of magnetism
                permanent incisor
^{131}I . . . . radioactive iodine
i . . . . optically inactive
IA . . . . impedance angle
                internal auditory
                intra-aortic
                intra-arterial
IABP . . . . intra-aortic balloon pumping
IAC . . . . internal auditory canal
IADH . . . . inappropriate antidiuretic hormone
IADHS . . . . inappropriate antidiuretic hormone
                syndrome
IAM . . . . internal auditory meatus
IAS . . . . interatrial septum

IAS . . . . intra-amniotic saline infusion
IASD . . . . interatrial septal defect
IAT . . . . invasive activity test
                       iodine-azide test
IB. . . . . inclusion body
IBB . . . . intestinal brush border
IBC . . . . iron-binding capacity
IBR . . . . infectious bovine rhinotracheitis
IBU . . . . international benzoate unit
IC. . . . . inspiratory capacity
                       intensive care
                       intercostal
                       intermediate care
                       intermittent claudication
                       intracavitary
                       intracellular
                       intracerebral
                       intracranial
                       intracutaneous
                       irritable colon
                       isovolumic contraction
ICA . . . . intracranial aneurysm
ICC . . . . immunocompetent cells
                       Indian childhood cirrhosis
                       intensive coronary care
ICCU . . . . intensive coronary care unit
ICD . . . . isocitric dehydrogenase
ICDH . . . . isocitric dehydrogenase
ICF. . . . . intensive care facility
                       intracellular fluid
ICG . . . . indocyanine green
ICM . . . . intercostal margin
ICS. . . . . intercostal space
ICSH . . . . interstitial cell-stimulating hormone
ICT. . . . . indirect Coombs' test
                       inflammation of connective tissue
                       insulin coma therapy
                       isovolumic contraction time

Ict ind . . . . icterus index
ICU . . . . intensive care unit
ICW. . . . . intracellular water
ID. . . . . identification
　　　　　　　　　　　infant deaths
　　　　　　　　　　　infective dose
　　　　　　　　　　　inside diameter
　　　　　　　　　　　internal diameter
　　　　　　　　　　　intradermal
　　　　　　　　　　　the same (idem)
I & D . . . . incision and drainage
ID_{50} . . . . median infective dose
IDA . . . . image display and analysis
　　　　　　　　　　　iron deficiency anemia
IDI . . . . induction-delivery interval
IDM . . . . infant of diabetic mother
IDP . . . . initial dose period
IDR . . . . intradermal reaction
IDS . . . . immunity deficiency state
IDU. . . . . idoxuridine
　　　　　　　　　　　iododeoxyuridine
IDVC . . . . indwelling venous catheter
IE. . . . . immunizing unit
　　　　　　　　　　　(Immunitäts Einheit)
I/E . . . . inspiratory-expiratory ratio
IEMG . . . . integrated electromyogram
IEOP . . . . immunoelectro-osmophoresis
IEP. . . . . immunoelectrophoresis
IF. . . . . immunofluorescence
　　　　　　　　　　　interstitial fluid
　　　　　　　　　　　intrinsic factor
IFA . . . . indirect fluorescent antibody
IFC . . . . intrinsic factor concentrate
IFR . . . . inspiratory flow rate
IFRA . . . . indirect fluorescent rabies antibody (test)
IFV . . . . intracellular fluid volume
IG. . . . . immune globulin
　　　　　　　　　　　intragastric

Ig . . . . immunoglobulin
IgA. . . . . gamma A immunoglobulin
IgD. . . . . gamma D immunoglobulin
IgE. . . . . gamma E immunoglobulin
IgG. . . . . gamma G immunoglobulin
IgM . . . . gamma M immunoglobulin
IGDM . . . . infant of gestational diabetic mother
IGV . . . . intrathoracic gas volume
IH. . . . . infectious hepatitis
               inner half
IHA . . . . indirect hemagglutination
IHBTD . . . . incompatible hemolytic blood transfusion
               disease
IHC . . . . idiopathic hypercalciuria
               inner hair cell
IHD . . . . ischemic heart disease
IHO . . . . idiopathic hypertrophic osteoarthropathy
IHR . . . . intrinsic heart rate
IHSA . . . . iodinated human serum albumin
IHSS . . . . idiopathic hypertrophic subaortic stenosis
IIF . . . . indirect immunofluorescent
IJP . . . . internal jugular pressure
ILA . . . . insulin-like activity
ILB . . . . infant, low birth weight
ILBW . . . . infant, low birth weight
ILD . . . . ischemic leg disease
               ischemic limb disease
IM . . . . infectious mononucleosis
               internal medicine
               intramedullary
               intramuscular
im . . . . (indicates presence of) NH group
IMA . . . . internal mammary artery
IMAA . . . . iodinated macroaggregated albumin
IMB . . . . intermenstrual bleeding
IMBC . . . . indirect maximum breathing capacity
IMH . . . . idiopathic myocardial hypertrophy
IMI. . . . . intramuscular injection

Imp. . . . . impression
improved
IMR . . . . infant mortality rate
IMRAD . . . . introduction, methods, results, and
discussion
IMS . . . . incurred in military service
IN. . . . . intranasal
in . . . . inch
INAD . . . . infantile neuroaxonal dystrophy
INAH . . . . isonicotinic acid hydrazide
Inc . . . . increase
incurred
Incr . . . . increase
Ind . . . . independents
In d . . . . daily (in die)
INDM . . . . infant of nondiabetic mother
INE . . . . infantile necrotizing encephalomyelopathy
Inf . . . . inferior
infusion
pour in (infunde)
Info . . . . information
INH . . . . isoniazid
(isonicotinic acid hydrazide)
Inj . . . . inject
Inj enem . . . . let an enema be injected (injiciatur enema)
Inl . . . . inlay
Inoc . . . . inoculate
INPV . . . . intermittent negative-pressure assisted
ventilation
INS . . . . idiopathic nephrotic syndrome
Inspir . . . . inspiration
Int . . . . intermediates
intermittent
internal
Int med . . . . internal medicine
IO . . . . internal os
intestinal obstruction
intraocular

I & O . . . . in and out
                     intake and output
IOFB . . . . intraocular foreign body
IOP . . . . intraocular pressure
IOU . . . . intensive therapy observation unit
IP . . . . incisoproximal
                     incubation period
                     instantaneous pressure
                     interphalangeal
                     intraperitoneal
                     isoelectric point
I-para . . . . primipara
IPC . . . . isopropyl chlorophenyl
IPD . . . . inflammatory pelvic disease
IPG . . . . impedance plethysmography
IPH . . . . idiopathic pulmonary hemosiderosis
IPL . . . . intrapleural
IPP . . . . intermittent positive pressure
IPPB . . . . intermittent positive pressure breathing
IPPI . . . . interruption of pregnancy for psychiatric
                     indication
IPPO . . . . intermittent positive-pressure inflation
                     with oxygen
IPPR . . . . intermittent positive-pressure respiration
IPPV . . . . intermittent positive-pressure ventilation
IPRT . . . . interpersonal reaction test
IPS . . . . initial prognostic score
IPU . . . . inpatient unit
IPV . . . . inactivated poliovaccine
IQ . . . . intelligence quotient
IR . . . . immunoreactive
                     index of response
                     internal resistance
IRBBB . . . . incomplete right bundle branch block
IRDS . . . . idiopathic respiratory distress syndrome
IRG . . . . immunoreactive glucagon
IRHCS . . . . immunoradioassayable human chorionic
                     somatomammotropin

IRHGH . . . . immunoreactive human growth hormone
IRI . . . . immunoreactive insulin
Irr. . . . . irradiation
IRS . . . . infrared spectrophotometry
IRV . . . . inspiratory rerserve volume
IS . . . . in situ
                      intercostal space
                      interspace
ISC . . . . irreversibly sickled cells
ISD . . . . isosorbide dinitrate
ISDN . . . . isosorbide dinitrate
ISF . . . . interstitial fluid
ISG . . . . immune serum globulin
ISH . . . . icteric serum hepatitis
Iso . . . . isoproterenol
ISP . . . . interspace
IST . . . . insulin sensitivity test
                      insulin shock therapy
ISW . . . . interstitial water
IT . . . . implantation test
                      inhalation test
                      inhalation therapy
                      intradermal test
                      intrathecal
                      intratracheal
                      intratracheal tube
                      intratumoral
                      isomeric transition
ITC . . . . Imidazolyl-thio-guanine chemotherapy
ITLC . . . . instant thin-layer chromatography
ITP . . . . idiopathic thrombocytopenic purpura
ITPA . . . . Illinois Test of Psycholinguistic Abilities
ITT . . . . insulin tolerance test
ITU . . . . intensive therapy unit
IU . . . . immunizing unit
                      international unit
                      intrauterine
IUCD . . . . intrauterine contraceptive device

IUD . . . . intrauterine death
intrauterine device
IUDR . . . . iododeoxyuridine
IUFB . . . . intrauterine foreign body
IUGR . . . . intrauterine growth rate
IUM . . . . intrauterine fetally malnourished
IUT. . . . . intrauterine transfusion
IV. . . . . interventricular
intervertebral
intravascular
intravenous
intraventricular
invasive
in vitro
in vivo
IVAP. . . . . in vivo adhesive platelet
IVC . . . . inferior vena cava
IVCC . . . . intravascular consumption coagulopathy
IVCD . . . . intraventricular conduction defect
IVCP . . . . inferior vena cava pressure
IVCV . . . . inferior venacavography
IVD. . . . . intervertebral disk
IVF. . . . . intravascular fluid
IVGTT . . . . intravenous glucose tolerance test
IVH . . . . intraventricular hemorrhage
IVM . . . . intravascular mass
IVP . . . . intravenous pyelogram
IVS . . . . interventricular septum
IVSD . . . . interventricular septal defect
IVT . . . . intravenous transfusion
IVTTT . . . . intravenous tolbutamide tolerance test
IVU . . . . intravenous urography
IWL . . . . insensible water loss
IWMI . . . . inferior wall myocardial infraction
J. . . . . Joule's equivalent
journal
JBE . . . . Japanese B encephalitis
Jej . . . . jejunum

JG. . . . . juxtaglomerular
JGC . . . . juxtaglomerular cell
JGI. . . . . juxtaglomerular granulation index
JND . . . . just noticeable difference
JPS. . . . . joint position sense
Jt . . . . joint
JV. . . . . jugular vein
. . . . jugular venous
JVP . . . . jugular venous pulse
K . . . . absolute zero
. . . . electrostatic capacity
. . . . kathode (cathode)
. . . . Kell blood system
. . . . Kelvin
. . . . potassium
KA . . . . kathode
. . . . ketoacidosis
. . . . King-Armstrong (units)
KAP . . . . knowledge, attitudes, and practice
KAU. . . . . King-Armstrong units
KB . . . . ketone bodies
KC . . . . kathodal closing
kc . . . . kilocycle
kcal . . . . kilocalorie
KCC . . . . kathodal closing contraction
KCG . . . . kinetocardiogram
KC1 . . . . potassium chloride
kcps . . . . kilocycles per second
KCT . . . . kathodal closing tetanus
KD . . . . kathodal duration
KDT . . . . kathodal duration tetanus
KE . . . . kinetic energy
KFAB . . . . kidney-fixing antibody
KFS . . . . Klippel-Feil syndrome
kg . . . . kilogram
kg-cal . . . . kilogram-calorie
KGS . . . . ketogenic steroid
KHZ . . . . kilohertz

KIA . . . . Kliger iron agar
KIU . . . . kallikrein-inhibiting unit
KJ . . . . knee jerk
KK . . . . knee kick
KLH . . . . keyhole-limpet hemocyanin
KLS . . . . kidney, liver, spleen
KM . . . . kanamycin
km . . . . kilometer
KMnO . . . . potassium permanganate
KMV . . . . killed measles-virus vaccine
Kn . . . . knee
KOC . . . . kathodal opening contraction
KP . . . . keratitic precipitates
KPTT . . . . kaolin partial thromboplastin time
KRB . . . . Krebs-Ringer bicarbonate buffer
KRP . . . . Kolmer's test with Reiter protein
                     Krebs-Ringer phosphate
KS . . . . ketosteroid
                     Klinefelter's syndrome
                     Kveim-Siltzbach (test)
KSC . . . . kathodal closing contraction
KST . . . . kathodal closing tetanus
KU . . . . Karmen units
KUB . . . . kidney, ureter and bladder
KV . . . . killed vaccine
kv . . . . kilovolt
kvp . . . . kilovolt peak
KW . . . . Keith-Wagener
kw . . . . kilowatt
KWB . . . . Keith, Wagener, Barker (classification)
kw-hr . . . . kilowatt-hour
L . . . . coefficient of induction
                     Lactobacillus
                     Latin
                     left
                     Leishmania
                     length
                     lethal

L *(continued)* . . . . . levo
ligament
light sense
liter
low
lower
lumbar
pound (libra)
LA . . . . lactic acid
left arm
left atrial
left atrium
leucine aminopeptidase
linguoaxial
local anesthesia
low anxiety
L & A . . . . light and accommodation
LAA . . . . leukocyte ascorbic acid
Lab. . . . . laboratory
LAD . . . . left anterior descending
left axis deviation
LAE . . . . left atrial enlargement
LAF . . . . laminar air flow
LAG . . . . labiogingival
lymphangiogram
LAH . . . . lactalbumin hydrolysate
left atrial hypertrophy
LAI . . . . labioincisal
LAIT . . . . latex agglutination-inhibition test
LAO . . . . left anterior oblique
LAP . . . . left atrial pressure
leucine aminopeptidase
leukocyte alkaline phosphatase
lyophilized anterior pituitary
LAR . . . . left arm recumbent
LAS . . . . linear alkylate sulfonate
LASER . . . . light amplification by stimulated emission
of radiation

LAT . . . . lateral
LATS . . . . long-acting thyroid stimulator
LB . . . . laboratory data
                lipid body
                live births
                loose body
lb . . . . pound (libra)
LBB . . . . left bundle branch
LBBB . . . . left bundle branch block
LBCD . . . . left border of cardiac dullness
LBF . . . . Lactobacillus bulgaricus factor
LBI . . . . low serum-bound iron
LBM . . . . lean body mass
LBNP . . . . lower-body negative pressure
LBW . . . . low birth weight
LBWI . . . . low birth weight infant
LBWR . . . . lung-body weight ratio
LC . . . . late clamped
                lethal concentration
                lipid cytosomes
                living children
LCA . . . . left coronary artery
LCD . . . . Liquor Carbonis Detergens
LCFA . . . . long-chain fatty acid
LCL . . . . Levinthal-Coles-Lillie (bodies)
                lymphocytic lymphosarcoma
LCM . . . . left costal margin
                lymphatic choriomeningitis
                lymphocytic choriomeningitis
LCT . . . . long-chain triglyceride
LD . . . . labyrinthine defect
                lactic dehydrogenase
                left deltoid
                lethal dose
                light difference
                linguodistal
                living donor
                low dosage

```
L-D. . . . . . . . . . . . Leishman-Donovan (bodies)
L/D. . . . . . . . . . . . light-dark ratio
LD₅₀ . . . . . . . . . . median lethal dose
LDA . . . . . . . . . . . left dorsoanterior
                         linear displacement analysis
LDD. . . . . . . . . . . light-dark discrimination
LDDS. . . . . . . . . . local dentist
LDH. . . . . . . . . . . lactic dehydrogenase
LDL . . . . . . . . . . . loudness discomfort level
                         low density lipoprotein
LDLP. . . . . . . . . . low density lipoprotein
LDP . . . . . . . . . . . left dorsoposterior
LDV. . . . . . . . . . . lactic dehydrogenase virus
LE . . . . . . . . . . . . left eye
                         leukoerythrogenetic
                         lower extremity
                         lupus erythematosus
LED . . . . . . . . . . . lupus erythematosus disseminatus
LES . . . . . . . . . . . local excitatory state
LET . . . . . . . . . . . linear energy transfer
LF . . . . . . . . . . . . larynogofissure
                         limit flocculation
                         low forceps
LFA . . . . . . . . . . . left femoral artery
                         left frontoanterior
LFD . . . . . . . . . . . lactose-free diet
                         least fatal dose
                         low forceps delivery
LFN . . . . . . . . . . . lactoferrin
LFP . . . . . . . . . . . left frontoposterior
LFT . . . . . . . . . . . latex flocculation test
                         left frontotransverse
                         liver function test
LG . . . . . . . . . . . . laryngectomy
                         left gluteal
                         linguogingival
Lg . . . . . . . . . . . . large
LGB . . . . . . . . . . . Landry-Guillain-Barré (syndrome)
```

LGN. . . . . lateral geniculate nucleus
LGV. . . . . lymphogranuloma venereum
LH . . . . lower half
                    luteinizing hormone
LHL. . . . . left hepatic lobe
LHRF. . . . . luteinizing hormone-releasing factor
LI. . . . . linguoincisal
                    low impulsiveness
LIAFI . . . . late infantile amaurotic familial idiocy
Lib. . . . . pound (libra)
LIBC . . . . latent iron-binding capacity
LIF. . . . . left iliac fossa
Lig . . . . ligament
LIHA . . . . low impulsiveness, high anxiety
LILA . . . . low impulsiveness, low anxiety
Liq. . . . . liquid
                    liquor
LIQ . . . . lower inner quadrant
LIS. . . . . lobular in situ
LK . . . . left kidney
LL . . . . left leg
                    left lower
                    left lung
                    lower lobe
                    lysolecithin
LLC . . . . lymphocytic leukemia
LLF . . . . Laki-Lorand factor
LLL . . . . left lower lobe
LLM. . . . . localized leukocyte mobilization
LLQ . . . . left lower quadrant
LM . . . . light microscopy
                    linguomesial
LMA . . . . left mentoanterior
LMD . . . . local medical doctor
                    low molecular weight dextran
LMDX . . . . low molecular weight dextran
LMP. . . . . last menstrual period
                    left mentoposterior

LMT. . . . . left mentotransverse
LMW . . . . low molecular weight
LMWD . . . . low molecular weight dextran
LN . . . . lipoid nephrosis
               lupus nephritis
               lymph node
L/N . . . . letter-numerical (system)
LNMP. . . . . last normal menstrual period
LNPF . . . . lymph node permeability factor
LO . . . . linguo-occlusal
               low
LOA . . . . leave of absence
               left occipitoanterior
Loc dol . . . . to the painful spot (loco dolenti)
LOD. . . . . line of duty
LOM. . . . . limitation of motion
               loss of motion
LOP . . . . left occipitoposterior
LOQ. . . . . lower outer quadrant
LOT . . . . left occipitotransverse
LOWBI . . . . low birth weight infant
LP . . . . latency period
               leukocyte-poor
               light perception
               linguopulpal
               lipoprotein
               low protein
               lumbar puncture
               lymphoid plasma
L/P . . . . lactate-pyruvate ratio
LPA . . . . left pulmonary artery
LPC . . . . late positive component
LPE . . . . lipoprotein electrophoresis
LPF . . . . leukocytosis-promoting factor
               localized plaque formation
               low power field
LPL . . . . lipoprotein lipase
lpm . . . . liters per minute

LPO	light perception only
LPS	lipopolysaccharide
LPV	left pulmonary veins
LR	laboratory references
	lactated Ringer's solution
	light reaction
L/R	left to right ratio
L & R	left and right
L→R	left to right
LRF	luteinizing hormone-releasing factor
LRH	luteinizing hormone-releasing hormone
LRQ	lower right quadrant
LRS	lactated Ringer's solution
LRT	lower respiratory tract
LS	left side
	legally separated
	liver and spleen
	lumbosacral
	lymphosarcoma
LSA	left sacroanterior
	lymphosarcoma
LSA/RCS	lymphosarcoma-reticulum cell sarcoma
LSB	left sternal border
LSCA	left scapuloanterior
LSCP	left scapuloposterior
LSCS	lower segment cesarean section
LSD	lysergic acid diethylamide
LSM	late systolic murmur
LSP	left sacroposterior
LST	left sacrotransverse
LSV	left subclavian vein
LT	left
	left thigh
	levothyroxine
	longterm
	lymphotoxin
LTB	laryngotracheobronchitis
LTH	lactogenic hormone

LTH . . . . luteotropic hormone
Lt lat . . . . left lateral
LTPP . . . . lipothiamide pyrophosphate
LU . . . . left upper
L & U . . . . lower and upper
LUL . . . . left upper lobe
LUQ . . . . left upper quadrant
LV . . . . left ventricle
　　　　　　　　　　leukemia virus
　　　　　　　　　　live virus
LVDP . . . . left ventricular diastolic pressure
LVE . . . . left ventricular enlargement
LVEDP . . . . left ventricular end-diastolic pressure
LVEDV . . . . left ventricular end-diastolic volume
LVET . . . . left ventricular ejection time
LVF . . . . left ventricular failure
　　　　　　　　　　low-voltage fast
　　　　　　　　　　low-voltage foci
LVH . . . . left ventricular hypertrophy
LVP . . . . left ventricular pressure
　　　　　　　　　　lysine-vasopressin
LVS . . . . left ventricular strain
LVSP . . . . left ventricular systolic pressure
LVSV . . . . left ventricular-stroke volume
LVSW . . . . left ventricular stroke work
LVW . . . . left ventricular work
LVWI . . . . left ventricular work index
LW . . . . lacerating wound
　　　　　　　　　　Lee-White (method)
L & W . . . . living and well
L/W . . . . living and well
LX . . . . local irradiation
Lymphs . . . . lymphocytes
Lzm . . . . lysozyme
M . . . . handful (manipulus)
　　　　　　　　　　macerate
　　　　　　　　　　male
　　　　　　　　　　married

M *(continued)* . . . . Micrococcus
Microsporum
minute
mix
molar
month
mother
multipara
murmur
muscle
Mycobacterium
Mycoplasma
myopia
strength of pole
thousand

m . . . . meter
minim

M_1 . . . . mitral first

M dict . . . . as directed (moro dicto)

M et sig . . . . mix and label (misce et signa)

M ft . . . . make a mixture (mistura fiat)

MA . . . . mandelic acid
mean arterial (blood pressure)
medical audit
mental age
Miller-Abbott (tube)
moderately advanced

ma . . . . meter-angle
milliampere

MAA . . . . macroaggregated albumin

MABP . . . . mean arterial blood pressure

Mac . . . . macerate

MAC . . . . maximum allowable concentration
minimum alveolar concentration

MAFH . . . . macroaggregated ferrous hydroxide

Magn . . . . large (magnus)

MAM . . . . methylazomethanol

M+AM . . . . myopic astigmatism

mam. . . . . milliampere minute
Man . . . . handful (manipulus)
　　　　　　　　　　 manipulate
Manip. . . . . manipulation
MANOVA . . . . multivariate analysis of variance
Man pr . . . . early in the morning (mane primo)
MAO . . . . maximal acid output
　　　　　　　　　　 monoamine oxidase
MAOI. . . . . monoamine oxidase inhibitor
MAP. . . . . mean aortic pressure
　　　　　　　　　　 mean arterial pressure
　　　　　　　　　　 megaloblastic anemia of pregnancy
　　　　　　　　　　 methylacetoxyprogesterone
　　　　　　　　　　 methylaminopurine
　　　　　　　　　　 muscle-action potential
MAPF. . . . . microatomized protein food
mas . . . . milliampere second
MASER . . . . microwave amplification by stimulated
　　　　　　　　　　　　 emission of radiation
　　　　　　　　　　 molecular application by stimulated
　　　　　　　　　　　　 emission of radiation
Matut. . . . . in the morning
Max . . . . maximum
MB. . . . . mesiobuccal
　　　　　　　　　　 methylene blue
　　　　　　　　　　 mix well
MBA . . . . methylbovine albumin
MBAS . . . . methylene blue active substance
MBC. . . . . maximal breathing capacity
　　　　　　　　　　 minimal bactericidal concentration
MBD. . . . . methylene blue dye
　　　　　　　　　　 minimal brain dysfunction
　　　　　　　　　　 Morquio-Brailsford disease
MBF. . . . . myocardial blood flow
MBFLB . . . . monaural bifrequency loudness balance
MBL. . . . . minimal bactericidal level
MBO. . . . . mesiobucco-occlusal
MBP. . . . . antigen prepared from melitensis

MBP *(continued)* . . mean blood pressure
                  mesiobuccopulpal
MBSA . . . . methylated bovine serum albumin
MC . . . . mast cell
                  maximum concentration
                  megacurie
                  megacycle
                  metacarpal
                  mineralocorticoid
                  myocarditis
                  mytomycin-C
mc . . . . millicurie
MCA. . . . . methylcholanthrene
MCB. . . . . membranous cytoplasmic body
MCBR . . . . minimum concentration of bilirubin
MCC. . . . . mean corpuscular-hemoglobin
                     concentration
                  minimum complete-killing concentration
MCCU . . . . mobile coronary care unit
MCD. . . . . mean cell diameter
                  mean corpuscular diameter
                  medullary cystic disease
MCFA . . . . medium-chain fatty acid
mcg . . . . microgram
MCH . . . . mean corpuscular hemoglobin
mch . . . . millicurie hour
MCHC . . . . mean corpuscular hemoglobin
                     concentration
MCI . . . . mean cardiac index
MCL. . . . . midclavicular line
                  midcostal line
                  most comfortable loudness level
MCP . . . . metacarpophalangeal
                  mitotic-control protein
MC P S . . . . megacycles per second
MCQ. . . . . multiple choice question
MCR. . . . . message competition ratio
                  metabolic clearance rate

MCT. . . . . mean circulation time
mean corpuscular thickness
medium-chain triglyceride
MCV. . . . . mean clinical value
mean corpuscular volume
MD. . . . . malic dehydrogenase
manic depressive
Mantoux diameter
Marek's disease
maternal deprivation
medium dosage
movement disorder
muscular dystrophy
myocardial damage
myocardial disease
MDA . . . . mentodextra anterior
methylenedioxyamphetamine
motor discriminative acuity
MDC. . . . . minimum detectable concentration
MDD . . . . mean daily dose
MDF. . . . . mean dominant frequency
myocardial depressant factor
MDH. . . . . malic dehydrogenase
MDHV . . . . Marek's disease herpesvirus
MDM . . . . minor determinant mixture
MDP. . . . . mentodextra posterior
MDT. . . . . median detection threshold
mentodextra transversa
MDTR . . . . mean diameter-thickness ratio
MDUO . . . . myocardial disease of unknown origin
MDY . . . . month, date, year
ME . . . . medical education
mercaptoethanol
middle ear
M/E . . . . myeloid-erythroid ratio
Me . . . . methyl
MEA . . . . mercaptoethylamine
multiple endocrine adenomatosis

Med . . . . median
                        medical
                        medicine
MED . . . . minimal effective dose
                        minimal erythema dose
Meds . . . . medications
                        medicines
MEF. . . . . maximal expiratory flow
MEFR . . . . maximum expiratory flow rate
MEG. . . . . mercaptoethylguanidine
mega- . . . . one-million
megalo- . . . . great size
MEM. . . . . minimum essential medium
Mep . . . . meperidine
MEPP. . . . . miniature end-plate potential
mEq. . . . . milliequivalents
MER . . . . mean ejection rate
                        methanol-extruded residue
MER-29 . . . . for elevated serum cholesterol
mev. . . . . million electron volts
MF . . . . medium frequency
                        mycosis fungoides
                        myelin figures
M/F . . . . male-female ratio
M & F . . . . mother and father
Mf . . . . microfilaria
MFB . . . . metallic foreign body
MFD . . . . midforceps delivery
                        minimal fatal dose
mfd. . . . . microfarad
MFP. . . . . monofluorophosphate
MFR . . . . mucus flow rate
MFW . . . . multiple fragment wounds
MG . . . . mesiogingival
                        methyl glucoside
                        muscle group
Mg. . . . . magnesium
mg. . . . . milligram

MGF. . . . . mother's grandfather
MGGH . . . . methylglyoxal guanylhydrazone
Mgh . . . . milligram/hour
MGM . . . . mother's grandmother
mgm . . . . milligram
MGN . . . . membranous glomerulonephritis
MGP . . . . marginal granulocyte pool
mg% . . . . milligrams per 100 milliliters
MGR . . . . modified gain ratio
Mgtis . . . . meningitis
MH. . . . . mammotropic hormone
　　　　　　　　　　marital history
　　　　　　　　　　medical history
　　　　　　　　　　mental health
MHA . . . . methemalbumin
　　　　　　　　　　microangiopathic hemolytic anemia
　　　　　　　　　　mixed hemadsorption
MHB . . . . maximum hospital benefit
MHb . . . . methemoglobin
MHD . . . . mean hemolytic dose
　　　　　　　　　　minimum hemolytic dose
mHg. . . . . millimeters of mercury
MHN . . . . massive hepatic necrosis
MHP. . . . . mercurihydroxypropane
MHPG . . . . methoxyhydroxyphenylglycol
MHR . . . . maximal heart rate
MI . . . . mercaptoimidazole
　　　　　　　　　　mitral incompetence
　　　　　　　　　　mitral insufficiency
　　　　　　　　　　myocardial infarction
MIC . . . . Maternity and Infant Care
　　　　　　　　　　minimum inhibitory concentration
Mic pan . . . . bread crumb (mica panis)
micro- . . . . one-millionth
MICU . . . . mobile intensive care unit
MID . . . . maximum inhibiting dilution
　　　　　　　　　　mesioincisodistal
　　　　　　　　　　minimum infective dose

Midnoc . . . . midnight
MIF . . . . macrophage-inhibiting factor
                      migration-inhibition factor
                      mixed immunofluorescence
MIFR . . . . maximal inspiratory flow rate
milli- . . . . one-thousandth
Min . . . . minim
                      minimal
                      minute
min . . . . drops of water
                      minim
                      minute
MIO . . . . minimum identifiable odor
MIP . . . . maximum inspiratory pressure
MIRD . . . . medical internal radiation dose
MIRU . . . . myocardial infarction research unit
Mist . . . . mixture (mistura)
MIT . . . . monoiodotyrosine
                      send (mitte)
Mixt . . . . mixture
MK . . . . monkey kidney
MKS . . . . meter-kilogram-second
MKV . . . . killed measles vaccine
ML . . . . mesiolingual
                      middle lobe
                      midline
M:L . . . . monocyte-lymphocyte ratio
ml. . . . . milliliter
MLA . . . . mentolaeva anterior
                      monocytic leukemia, acute
MLa . . . . mesiolabial
MLaI . . . . mesiolabioincisal
MLAP . . . . mean left atrial pressure
MLC . . . . mixed leukocyte culture
                      mixed lymphocyte culture
                      multilamellar cytosome
                      myelomonocytic leukemia, chronic
MLD . . . . metachromatic leukodystrophy

MLD. . . . . minimum lethal dose
MLI . . . . mesiolinguoincisal
MLO. . . . . mesiolinguo-occlusal
MLP . . . . mentolaeva posterior
       mesiolinguopulpal
MLS . . . . mean lifespan
       myelomonocytic leukemia, subacute
MLT. . . . . mentolaeva transversa
MLV. . . . . Moloney's leukemogenic virus
       mouse leukemia virus
MM. . . . . malignant melanoma
       Marshall-Marchetti
       medial malleolus
       mucous membrane
       multiple myeloma
       muscles
       muscularis mucosa
       myeloid metaplasia
M & M . . . . milk and molasses
mm . . . . millimeter
mM . . . . millimol
       millimolar
MMA . . . . methylmalonic acid
MMC . . . . minimal medullary concentration
MMD . . . . minimum morbidostatic dose
MMEF . . . . maximal midexpiratory flow rate
MMEFR . . . . maximal midexpiratory flow rate
MMF. . . . . maximal midexpiratory flow
MMFR . . . . maximal midexpiratory flow rate
       maximal midflow rate
mM/L. . . . . millimols per liter
MMM . . . . myeloid metaplasia with myelofibrosis
       myelosclerosis with myeloid metaplasia
mmm . . . . micromillimeter
       millimicron
MMPI . . . . Minnesota Multiphasic Personality
        Inventory
mmpp . . . . millimeters partial pressure

MMPR . . . . methylmercaptopurine riboside
MMR . . . . mass miniature radiography
mobile mass x-ray
myocardial metabolic rate
MN . . . . midnight
multinodular
myoneural
M/N . . . . midnight
M & N . . . . morning and night
Mn . . . . manganese
mN . . . . millinormal
MNA . . . . maximum noise area
MNCV . . . . motor nerve conduction velocity
MNU . . . . methylnitrosourea
MO . . . . mesio-occlusal
mineral oil
month
MOD . . . . mesio-occlusodistal
moderate
Mod praesc . . . . . . in the way directed (modo praescripto)
Mol wt . . . . molecular weight
Moll . . . . soft (mollis)
MOM . . . . milk of magnesia
MOMA . . . . methoxyhydroxymandelic acid
Mono . . . . monocyte
MOPV . . . . monovalent oral poliovirus vaccine
Mor dict . . . . in the manner directed (more dicto)
Mor sol . . . . in the usual way (more solito)
mOs . . . . milliosmolal
mOsm . . . . milliosmol
MP . . . . as directed (modo prescripto)
mean pressure
melting point
menstrual period
mercaptopurine
mesiopulpal
metacarpophalangeal
monophosphate

MP *(continued)* ... mucopolysaccharide
multiparous
MPA............ main pulmonary artery
medroxyprogesterone acetate
methylprednisolone acetate
MPAP.......... mean pulmonary arterial pressure
MPC............ marine protein concentrate
maximum permissible concentration
meperidine, promethazine, chlorpromazine
minimum mycoplasmacidal concentration
MPD............ maximum permissible dose
MPEH .... methylphenylethylhydantoin
MPJ .... metacarpophalangeal joint
MPL............ mesiopulpolingual
MPLa .... mesiopulpolabial
MPN .... most probable number
MPO .... myeloperoxidase
MPP............ mercaptopyrazidopyrimidine
MPS .... mucopolysaccharide
MR............. mental retardation
metabolic rate
methyl red
mitral reflux
mitral regurgitation
mortality rate
mortality ratio
muscle relaxant
mr .... milliroentgen
MRAP .... mean right atrial pressure
MRD .... minimum reacting dose
MRF............ mesencephalic reticular formation
mitral regurgitant flow
MRT............ median recognition threshold
milk-ring test
MRVP .... mean right ventricular pressure
MS .... manuscript
mental status
mitral stenosis

MS *(continued)*. . . . morphine sulfate
　　　　　　　　　　 mucosubstance
　　　　　　　　　　 multiple sclerosis
　　　　　　　　　　 musculoskeletal
msec. . . . . milliseconds
MSER . . . . mean systolic ejection rate
MSG. . . . . monosodium glutamate
MSH. . . . . medical self-help
　　　　　　　　　　 melanocyte-stimulating hormone
　　　　　　　　　　 melanophore-stimulating hormone
MSK. . . . . medullary sponge kidney
MSL. . . . . midsternal line
MSLA . . . . mouse-specific lymphocyte antigen
MSN. . . . . mildly subnormal
MSRPP . . . . multidimensional scale for rating
　　　　　　　　　　　 psychiatric patients
MSS . . . . mental status schedule
MSU . . . . monosodium urate
MSUD . . . . maple syrup urine disease
MSV. . . . . Moloney sarcoma virus
　　　　　　　　　　 murine sarcoma virus
MT . . . . empty
　　　　　　　　　　 malignant teratoma
　　　　　　　　　　 maximal therapy
　　　　　　　　　　 medical technologist
　　　　　　　　　　 membrana tympani
　　　　　　　　　　 metatarsal
　　　　　　　　　　 methyltyrosine
　　　　　　　　　　 more than
　　　　　　　　　　 music therapy
MTD. . . . . maximum tolerated dose
MTDT . . . . modified tone decay test
MTF. . . . . maximum terminal flow
　　　　　　　　　　 modulation transfer function
MTHF. . . . . methyltetrahydrofolic acid
MTI . . . . malignant teratoma intermediate
　　　　　　　　　　 minimum time interval
MTP　　　　　　　　 metatarsophalangeal

MTR	Meinicke turbidity reaction
MTT	malignant teratoma trophoblastic
	monotetrazolium
MTU	methylthiouracil
MTV	mammary tumor virus
MTX	methotrexate
MU	Mache unit
	Montevideo unit
	mouse unit
mU	milliunit
mu	micron
MUC	mucilage
Multip	pregnant woman who has borne two or more children
MUST	medical unit, self-contained, transportable
MUU	mouse uterine units
MV	minute volume
	mitral valve
	mixed venous
mv	millivolt
MVM	microvillose membrane
MVR	massive vitreous retraction
MVV	maximum voluntary ventilation
MW	molecular weight
mw	microwave
My	myopia
my	mayer (unit of heat capacity)
MyG	myasthenia gravis
MZ	monozygotic
N	nasal
	Neisseria
	nerve
	neurology
	Nocardia
	normal
	unit for fast neutrons
n	index of refraction
	size of sample

n_D . . . . refractive index
NA . . . . neutralizing antibody
                     Nomina Anatomica
                     noradrenaline
                     not admitted
                     not applicable
                     not available
                     numeric aperture
Na . . . . sodium
NAA . . . . no apparent abnormalities
NAD . . . . nicotinamide adenine dinucleotide
                     no appreciable disease
                     normal axis deviation
NADH . . . . nicotinamide adenine dinucleotide
                     (reduced form)
NADP . . . . nicotinamide adenine dinucleotide
                     phosphate
NADPH . . . . nicotinamide adenine dinucleotide
                     phosphate (reduced form)
NANA . . . . N-acetylneuraminic acid
nano- . . . . one-billionth
NAPA . . . . N-acetyl-p-aminophenol
NB . . . . newborn
                     nitrous oxide-barbiturate
                     note well (nota bene)
NBM . . . . nothing by mouth
NBO . . . . nonbed occupancy
NBS . . . . normal burro serum
NBT . . . . nitroblue tetrazolium
NBTE . . . . nonbacterial thrombotic endocarditis
NBW . . . . normal birth weight
NC . . . . no casualty
                     no change
                     noise criterion
                     noncontributory
                     not cultured
N/C . . . . no complaints
nc . . . . nanocurie

NCA. . . . . neurocirculatory asthenia
NCD. . . . . not considered disabling
ND . . . . neonatal death
                      neurotic depression
                      Newcastle disease
                      New Drugs
                      no data
                      no disease
                      nondisabling
                      normal delivery
                      not detectable
                      not detected
                      not determined
                      not done
NDA. . . . . no data available
                      no demonstrable antibodies
NDF. . . . . new dosage form
NDGA . . . . nordihydroguaiaretic acid
NDI . . . . nephrogenic diabetes insipidus
NDMA . . . . nitrosodimethylaniline
NDP. . . . . net dietary protein
NDV. . . . . Newcastle disease virus
NE . . . . nerve ending
                      neurologic examination
                      no effect
                      nonelastic
                      norepinephrine
                      not evaluated
                      not examined
NEC. . . . . not elsewhere classifiable
                      not elsewhere classified
NED. . . . . no evidence of disease
NEFA . . . . nonesterified fatty acid
NEG. . . . . negative
NEM. . . . . N-ethylmaleimide
Ne tr s num . . . . . . do not deliver unless paid (ne tradas
                      sine nummo)
Neur. . . . . neurology

Neuro	neurologic
Neurol	neurologic
NF	none found
	normal flow
	not found
NFTD	normal full-term delivery
NG	nasogastric
ng	nanogram
NGF	nerve growth factor
NGU	nongonococcal urethritis
NH	nonhuman
	nursing home
NHA	nonspecific hepatocellular abnormality
NHS	normal horse serum
	normal human serum
NI	no information
	not identified
	not isolated
NIA	no information available
NIH	National Institutes of Health
NK	not known
NKH	nonketotic hyperosmotic
Nl	normal
NLA	neuroleptanalgesia
NLP	no light perception
NLT	normal lymphocyte transfer test
NM	neuromuscular
	not measurable
	not measured
	not mentioned
	nuclear medicine
Nm	nutmeg
nm	nanometer
NMA	neurogenic muscular atrophy
NMP	normal menstrual period
N:N	(indicates presence of) the azo group
nn	nerves
NND	neonatal death

NND. . . . . New and Nonofficial Drugs
NNI . . . . noise and number index
NNN . . . . Nicolle-Novy-MacNeal (medium)
NO . . . . none obtained
No. . . . . number
Noc . . . . night
Noct . . . . at night (nocte)
Noct maneq . . . . . . at night and in the morning (nocte
                      maneque)
Non-REM . . . . nonrapid eye movement
Non rep . . . . do not repeat (non repetatur)
Non repetat . . . . . . do not repeat (non repetatur)
NOS . . . . not otherwise specified
NP . . . . nasopharyngeal
                      nasopharynx
                      neuropathology
                      neuropsychiatric
                      normal plasma
                      not performed
                      nucleoplasmic index
                      nucleoprotein
                      nursing procedure
NPB . . . . nodal premature beat
NPC . . . . near point of convergence
NPD . . . . Niemann-Pick disease
NPH . . . . neutral protamine Hagedorn (Insulin)
NPN . . . . nonprotein nitrogen
NPO . . . . nothing by mouth (nulla per os)
NPO/HS . . . . nothing by mouth at bedtime (nulla per os
                      hora somni)
NPT . . . . neoprecipitin test
NPU . . . . net protein utilization
NR . . . . do not repeat (non repetatur)
                      no radiation
                      no response
                      nonreactive
                      normal
                      not readable

NR *(continued)*. . . . not recorded
       not resolved
NRBC. . . . . nucleated red blood cell
NRC. . . . . normal retinal correspondence
NRD. . . . . nonrenal death
NREM . . . . nonrapid eye movement
NRS . . . . normal rabbit serum
       normal reference serum
NS . . . . nephrotic syndrome
       nervous system
       neurologic survey
       neurosurgery
       no sample
       no specimen
       nonspecific
       nonsymptomatic
       normal saline
       not significant
       not sufficient
N/S . . . . normal saline
NSA . . . . no serious abnormality
       no significant abnormality
NSC . . . . no significant change
       not service-connected
NSCD. . . . . nonservice-connected disability
NSD . . . . no significant defect
       no significant deviation
       no significant difference
       no significant disease
       normal spontaneous delivery
NSG . . . . nursing
NSM. . . . . neurosecretory material
NSND. . . . . nonsymptomatic, nondisabling
NSQ . . . . not sufficient quantity
NSR . . . . normal sinus rhythm
NSS . . . . normal saline solution
       not statistically significant
NSU . . . . nonspecific urethritis

NT . . . . nasotracheal
neutralization test
neutralizing
nontypable
not tested
NTAB. . . . . nephrotoxic antibody
NTG. . . . . nontoxic goiter
NTN. . . . . nephrotoxic nephritis
NTP . . . . normal temperature and pressure
NV . . . . negative variation
N & V. . . . . nausea and vomiting
Nv. . . . . naked vision
NVA. . . . . near visual acuity
NVD. . . . . nausea, vomiting and diarrhea
Newcastle virus disease
NWB. . . . . no weight bearing
NYD. . . . . not yet diagnosed
O . . . . eye (oculus)
none
nonmotile
obstetrics
opening
oral
orderly
pint (octarius)
respirations (anesthesia chart)
suture size
O_2 . . . . both eyes
oxygen
O_2Cap . . . . oxygen capacity
O_2saturation . . . . . oxygen saturation
O-. . . . . ortho
OA . . . . osteoarthritis
oxalic acid
OAAD . . . . ovarian ascorbic acid depletion
OAD. . . . . obstructive airway disease
OAP. . . . . osteoarthropathy
OAR . . . . other administrative reasons

OB . . . . objective benefit
                         obstetrics
O & B . . . . opium and belladonna
OBG . . . . obstetrics and gynecology
Ob-Gyn . . . . obstetrics and gynecology
Obl . . . . oblique
OBS . . . . obstetrical service
                         organic brain syndrome
Obs . . . . obstetrics
Obst . . . . obstetrics
OC . . . . occlusocervical
                         office call
                         on call
                         oral contraceptive
                         original claim
Occ. . . . . occasional
OCR . . . . optical character recognition
OCT . . . . ornithine carbamyl transferase
OCV . . . . ordinary conversational voice
OD . . . . once a day
                         optical density
                         outside diameter
                         overdose
od . . . . right eye (oculus dexter)
ODA . . . . occipitodextra anterior
ODM . . . . ophthalmodynamometry
ODP . . . . occipitodextra posterior
ODT . . . . occipitodextra transversa
O & E . . . . observation and examination
OEF . . . . oil emersion field
OER . . . . oxygen enhancement ratio
OF . . . . Ovenstone factor
Of . . . . official
OFC . . . . occipitofrontal circumference
OFD . . . . oral-facial-digital
OG . . . . obstetrics and gynecology
O & G . . . . obstetrics and gynecology
OGS . . . . oxogenic steroid

OGTT. . . . . oral glucose tolerance test
OH . . . . occupational history
OHC. . . . . outer hair cell
OHCS. . . . . hydroxycorticosteroid
OHP . . . . oxygen under high pressure
OIH . . . . orthoiodohippurate
OJ . . . . orange juice
OKN . . . . optokinetic nystagmus
OL . . . . left eye
Ol. . . . . oil
Ol res . . . . oleoresin
OLA . . . . occipitolaeva anterior
OLH . . . . ovine lactogenic hormone
OLP . . . . occipitolaeva posterior
OL & T . . . . owners, landlords, and tenants
OM . . . . otitis media
O M . . . . every morning (omni mane)
OMD. . . . . ocular muscle dystrophy
OMI . . . . old myocardial infarction
Omn bih. . . . . every two hours (omni bihora)
Omn hor. . . . . every hour (omni hora)
Omn noct. . . . . . . every night (omni nocte)
OMPA . . . . octamethylpyrophosphoramide
                       otitis media, purulent, acute
Om quar hor . . . . . every quarter of an hour (omni quarta
                       hora)
O N . . . . every night (omni nocte)
OOB . . . . out of bed
OP . . . . opening pressure
                       operation
                       osmotic pressure
                       outpatient
O & P . . . . ova and parasites
OPC . . . . Outpatient Clinic
OPD . . . . outpatient department
OPG . . . . oxypolygelatin
Oph . . . . ophthalmology
Ophth . . . . ophthalmology

OPK	optokinetic
OPS	Outpatient Service
OPT	outpatient
	outpatient treatment
OPV	oral poliovaccine
	oral poliovirus vaccine
OR	operating room
ORS	orthopedic surgery
Orth	orthopedics
Ortho	orthopedics
OS	mouth
	opening snap
	oral surgery
os	left eye (oculus sinister)
OSM	oxygen saturation meter
OST	object sorting test
OT	occlusion time
	occupational therapy
	old term
	old terminology
	old tuberculin
	orotracheal
	otolaryngology
OTC	ornithine transcarbamylase
	over the counter
	oxytetracycline
OTD	organ tolerance dose
Oto	otolaryngology
	otology
Otol	otology
Otolar	otolaryngology
OTR	Ovarian Tumor Registry
ou	both eyes (oculi unitas)
OURQ	outer upper right quadrant
OV	office visit
Ov	egg (ovum)
OW	out of wedlock
O/W	oil in water

O/W . . . . oil-water ratio
Ox . . . . oxymel
oz. . . . . ounce
P. . . . . after (post)
                            handful (pugillus)
                            near point
                            Para
                            partial pressure
                            Pasteurella
                            pharmacopeia
                            phosphorus
                            Plasmodium
                            position
                            postpartum
                            premolar
                            presbyopia
                            pressure
                            primipara
                            protein
                            Proteus
                            psychiatry
                            pulse
                            pupil
                            weight (pondus)
P_{NA} . . . . plasma sodium
P_1 . . . . parental generation
P_2 . . . . pulmonic second sound
^{32}P . . . . radioactive phosphorus
P ae . . . . in equal parts (partes aequales)
P rat aetat . . . . in proportion to age (pro ratione aetatis)
p. . . . . probability
p- . . . . para
P_{CO_2} . . . . carbon dioxide pressure
PA . . . . paralysis agitans
                            pathology
                            per annum
                            pernicious anemia
                            phakic-aphakic

PA *(continued)*. . . . posteroanterior
primary amenorrhea
primary anemia
pulmonary artery
pulpoaxial
P & A . . . . percussion & auscultation
PAB . . . . para-aminobenzoic acid
PABA . . . . para-aminobenzoic acid
PAC . . . . premature auricular contraction
PAF . . . . pulmonary arteriovenous fistula
PAFIB . . . . paroxysmal atrial fibrillation
PAGMK . . . . primary African green monkey kidney
PAH . . . . para-aminohippurate
polycyclic aromatic hydrocarbon
pulmonary artery hypertension
PAHA . . . . para-aminohippuric acid
PAL . . . . posterior axillary line
PAM . . . . crystalline penicillin G in 2 per cent
aluminum monostearate
phenylalanine mustard
pralidoxime chloride
pulmonary alveolar microlithiasis
pyridine aldoxime methiodide
PAN . . . . periodic alternating nystagmus
peroxyacetyl nitrate
PANS . . . . puromycin aminonucleoside
PAOD . . . . peripheral arterial occlusive disease
peripheral arteriosclerotic occlusive
disease
PAP . . . . Papanicolaou (stain, smear, test)
primary atypical pneumonia
prostatic acid phosphatase
pulmonary alveolar proteinosis
pulmonary artery pressure
PAPP . . . . para-aminopropiophenone
PAPS . . . . phosphoadenosyl-phosphosulfate
PAPVC . . . . partial anomalous pulmonary venous
connection

PAR	postanesthesia room
	pulmonary arteriolar resistance
Par aff	the part affected (pars affecta)
Para	number of pregnancies
Part aeq	equal parts (partes aequales)
Part vic	in divided doses (partibus vicibus)
PAS	para-aminosalicylic acid
	periodic acid-Schiff (method, stain, technique, test)
	pulmonary artery stenosis
PASA	para-aminosalicylic acid
PAS-C	para-aminosalicylic acid crystallized with ascorbic acid
PASD	after diastase digestion
	periodic acid-Schiff technique
PASM	periodic acid-silver methenamine
Past	Pasteurella
PAT	paroxysmal atrial tachycardia
Path	pathology
PB	phenobarbital
	phonetically balanced
PBA	pulpobuccoaxial
PBC	prebed care
	primary biliary cirrhosis
PBF	pulmonary blood flow
PBG	porphobilinogen
PBI	protein bound iodine
PBN	paralytic brachial neuritis
PBO	penicillin in beeswax
	placebo
PBS	phosphate-buffered saline
PBSP	prognostically bad signs during pregnancy
PBT_4	protein-bound thyroxine
PBV	predicted blood volume
	pulmonary blood volume
PBZ	pyribenzamine
PC	after meals (post cibum)
	per cent

PC *(continued)*.... phosphate cycle
phosphocreatine
platelet count
platelet concentrate
portacaval
pubococcygeus
pulmonic closure
weight (pondus civile)
pc . . . . picocurie
PCA . . . . passive cutaneous anaphylaxis
PCB . . . . paracervical block
PcB . . . . near point of convergence
PCc . . . . periscopic concave
PCD . . . . phosphate-citrate-dextrose
polycystic disease
posterior corneal deposits
PCF . . . . posterior cranial fossa
PCG . . . . phonocardiogram
PCH . . . . paroxysmal cold hemoglobinuria
PCM . . . . protein-calorie malnutrition
PCN . . . . penicillin
pCO_2 . . . . carbon dioxide pressure
PCP . . . . parachlorophenate
PCPA . . . . parachlorophenylalanine
Pcpt . . . . perception
PCS . . . . portacaval shunt
Pcs . . . . preconscious
PCT . . . . plasmacrit
porphyria cutanea tarda
portacaval transposition
PCV . . . . packed cell volume
polycythemia vera
PCV-M . . . . myeloid metaplasia with polycythemia vera
PCx . . . . periscopic convex
PD . . . . papilla diameter
Parkinson's disease
patent ductus
pediatrics

PD *(continued)*. . . . phosphate dehydrogenase
plasma defect
poorly differentiated
potential difference
pressor dose
prism diopter
progression of disease
psychotic depression
pulmonary disease
pulpodistal
pupillary distance
PDA . . . . patent ductus arteriosus
pediatric allergy
PDAB . . . . para-dimethylaminobenzaldehyde
PDC . . . . pediatric cardiology
PDD . . . . pyridoxine-deficient diet
PDH . . . . packaged disaster hospital
phosphate dehydrogenase
Pdl . . . . pudendal
PDP . . . . piperidino-pyrimidine
PE . . . . pharyngoesophageal
phenylephrine
physical evaluation
physical examination
pleural effusion
polyethylene
probable error
pulmonary edema
pulmonary embolism
PEBG . . . . phenethylbiguanide
Ped. . . . . pediatrics
Peds . . . . pediatrics
PEF . . . . peak expiratory flow
PEFR . . . . peak expiratory flow rate
PEG . . . . pneumoencephalography
polyethylene glycol
PEI. . . . . phosphate excretion index
physical efficiency index

Pen. . . . . penicillin
Pent . . . . pentothal
PEO . . . . progressive external ophthalmoplegia
PEP . . . . pre-ejection period
PEPP . . . . positive expiratory pressure plateau
PER . . . . protein efficiency ratio
Per . . . . by
                     for each
                     through
Per os . . . . by mouth
Percuss. . . . . percussion
PERLA . . . . pupils equal, react to light and
                     accommodation
Perpad . . . . perineal pad
PERRLA . . . . pupils equal, round, regular, react to light
                     and accommodation
PET . . . . pre-eclamptic toxemia
PETN. . . . . pentaerythritol tetranitrate
PF . . . . personality factor
                     picture-frustration (study)
                     platelet factor
P/F. . . . . pass-fail system
PFC . . . . plaque-forming cell
PFIB . . . . perfluoroisobutylene
PFK . . . . phosphofructokinase
PFO . . . . patent foramen ovale
PFQ . . . . personality factor questionnaire
PFR . . . . peak flow rate
PFT . . . . posterior fossa tumor
                     pulmonary function test
PFU . . . . plaque-forming units
PG . . . . plasma triglyceride
                     postgraduate
                     pregnant
                     prostaglandin
                     pyoderma gangrenosum
pg. . . . . picogram
PGA. . . . . pteroylglutamic acid

PGD . . . . phosphogluconate dehydrogenase
　　　　　　　　　　　 phosphoglyceraldehyde dehydrogenase
PGDH . . . . phosphogluconate dehydrogenase
PGDR . . . . plasma-glucose disappearance rate
PGH . . . . pituitary growth hormone
PGI . . . . phosphoglucoisomerase
　　　　　　　　　　　 potassium, glucose, and insulin
PGK . . . . phosphoglycerate kinase
PGM . . . . phosphoglucomutase
PGP . . . . postgamma proteinuria
PGTR . . . . plasma glucose tolerance rate
PH . . . . past history
　　　　　　　　　　　 personal history
　　　　　　　　　　　 pharmacopeia
　　　　　　　　　　　 phenyl
　　　　　　　　　　　 prostatic hypertrophy
　　　　　　　　　　　 public health
　　　　　　　　　　　 pulmonary hypertension
pH . . . . hydrogen ion concentration
PHA . . . . phytohemagglutinin
Phar . . . . pharmacy
Pharm . . . . pharmacy
PHBB . . . . propylhydroxybenzyl benzimidazole
PHC . . . . posthospital care
PHI . . . . phosphohexoisomerase
PHK . . . . platelet phosphohexokinase
PHLA . . . . postheparin lipolytic activity
PHP . . . . primary hyperparathyroidism
　　　　　　　　　　　 pseudohypoparathyroidism
Phys . . . . physiology
PI . . . . pacing impulse
　　　　　　　　　　　 performance intensity
　　　　　　　　　　　 pre-induction (examination)
　　　　　　　　　　　 present illness
　　　　　　　　　　　 protamine insulin
　　　　　　　　　　　 pulmonary incompetence
　　　　　　　　　　　 pulmonary infarction
PIA . . . . plasma insulin activity

pico-	one-trillionth
PICU	pulmonary intensive care unit
PID	pelvic inflammatory disease
	plasma-iron disappearance
PIDT	plasma-iron disappearance time
PIE	pulmonary infiltration and eosinophilia
	pulmonary interstitial emphysema
PIF	peak inspiratory flow
	prolactin-inhibiting factor
PIFR	peak inspiratory flow rate
PII	plasma inorganic iodine
Pil.	pill
PIP	proximal interphalangeal (joint)
PIPJ	proximal interphalangeal joint
PIT	plasma iron turnover
PITR	plasma iron turnover rate
PK	Prausnitz-Küstner (reaction)
	psychokinesis
	pyruvate kinase
PKU	phenylketonuria
PKV	killed poliomyelitis vaccine
PL	light perception
	phospholipid
	placebo
	placental lactogen
	pulpolingual
PLA	pulpolinguoaxial
PLa	pulpolabial
PLD	platelet defect
Pls	please
	prostaglandin-like substance
PLV	live poliomyelitis vaccine
	panleukopenia virus
	phenylalanine-lysine-vasopressin
PM	night
	physical medicine
	polymorphs
	postmortem

PM . . . . pulpomesial
PMA . . . . prevalence of gingivitis (papillary, marginal, attached)
progressive muscular atrophy
PMB . . . . para-hydroxymercuribenzoate
polymorphonuclear basophil
PMD . . . . primary myocardial disease
progressive muscular dystrophy
PME . . . . polymorphonuclear eosinophil
PMH . . . . past medical history
PMI . . . . point of maximal impulse
point of maximum intensity
PML . . . . progressive multifocal leukoencephalop-athy
PMN . . . . polymorphonuclear neutrophil
PMP . . . . past menstrual period
previous menstrual period
PMR . . . . perinatal mortality rate
physical medicine and rehabilitation
proportionate morbidity ratio
PMS . . . . phenazine methosulfate
postmitochondrial supernatant
pregnant mare serum
PMSG . . . . pregnant mare serum gonadotropin
PMT . . . . Porteus maze test
PN . . . . perceived noise
percussion note
periarteritis nodosa
peripheral neuropathy
pneumonia
positional nystagmus
pyelonephritis
PND . . . . paroxysmal nocturnal dyspnea
postnasal drainage
postnasal drip
pound
PNH . . . . paroxysmal nocturnal hemoglobinuria
PNP   para-nitrophenol

PNPP . . . . para-nitrophenylphosphate
PNU . . . . protein nitrogen unit
PO . . . . by mouth (per os)
                            parieto-occipital
                            period of onset
                            phone order
                            posterior
                            postoperative
pO_2 . . . . partial pressure of oxygen
POA . . . . point of application
POB . . . . phenoxybenzamine
                            place of birth
POC . . . . postoperative care
Pocul . . . . cup (poculum)
Pod. . . . . place of death
                            postoperative day
PODx . . . . preoperative diagnosis
pOH . . . . hydroxyl concentration
Poik . . . . poikilocyte
Polio . . . . poliomyelitis
Poly . . . . polymorphonuclear leukocyte
POP . . . . plasma oncotic pressure
Pos . . . . positive
Pos pr . . . . positive pressure
Poss . . . . possible
Post . . . . posterior
                            postmortem
Postop . . . . postoperative
Pot . . . . potassa
                            potion
PP. . . . . after shaking (phiala prius agitata)
                            near point (punctum proximum)
                            partial pressure
                            pauperismus
                            pellagra preventive
                            permanent partial
                            pink puffers (emphysema)
                            pinpoint

PP *(continued)* . . . . postpartum
postprandial
private practice
prothrombin-proconvertin
protoporphyrin
proximal phalanx
pulse pressure
pyrophosphate
PPA . . . . phenylpyruvic acid
shake well (phiala prius agitata)
PPB . . . . parts per billion
platelet-poor blood
positive-pressure breathing
PPBS . . . . postprandial blood sugar
PPC . . . . progressive patient care
PPD . . . . paraphenylenediamine
purified protein derivative
PPD-S . . . . Purified Protein Derivative-Standard
ppg. . . . . picopicogram
PPH . . . . primary pulmonary hypertension
protocollagen proline hydroxylase
postpartum hemorrhage
PPHP . . . . pseudopseudohypoparathyroidism
PPLO . . . . pleuropneumonia-like organism
PPM . . . . parts per million
PPP. . . . . pentose phosphate pathway
PPPI . . . . primary private practice income
PPR . . . . Price precipitation reaction
PPS. . . . . postpump syndrome
PPT. . . . . plant protease test
precipitate
prepared
PPV . . . . positive-pressure ventilation
PQ . . . . permeability quotient
pyrimethamine-quinine
PR . . . . far point (punctum remotum)
partial remission
peer review

PR *(continued)*. . . . peripheral resistance
pregnancy rate
presbyopia
production rate
professional relations
public relations
pulse rate
through the rectum (per rectum)
Pr . . . . prism
protein
PRA . . . . plasma renin activity
PRBV . . . . placental residual blood volume
PRC . . . . packed red cells
PRCA . . . . pure red cell agenesis
PRD . . . . partial reaction of degeneration
postradiation dysplasia
Pre . . . . preliminary
Preg . . . . pregnant
Preop . . . . preoperative
Prep . . . . prepare
PRFM . . . . prolonged rupture of fetal membranes
PRI . . . . phosphoribose isomerase
Primip . . . . woman bearing first child
PRM . . . . phosphoribomutase
preventive medicine
PRN . . . . as the occasion arises (pro re nata)
Pro . . . . prothrombin
Proct . . . . proctology
Prog . . . . prognosis
PROM . . . . premature rupture of membranes
prolonged rupture of membranes
Pro time . . . . prothrombin time
Prot . . . . protein
Prox . . . . proximal
PRP . . . . pityriasis rubra pilaris
platelet-rich plasma
Psychotic Reaction Profile
PRPP . . . . phosphoribosylpyrophosphate

PRT . . . . phosphoribosyltransferase
PRU . . . . peripheral resistance unit
PS . . . . chloropicrin
                      per second
                      performing scale (IQ)
                      periodic syndrome
                      physical status
                      plastic surgery
                      population sample
                      Porter-Silber (chromogen)
                      prescription
                      Pseudomonas
                      psychiatric
                      pulmonary stenosis
                      pyloric stenosis
P/S . . . . polyunsaturated to saturated fatty acids
                      ratio
PSA . . . . apply to the affected region
                      polyethylene sulfonic acid
PSC . . . . Porter-Silber chromogen
                      posterior subcapsular cataract
PSE . . . . portal-systemic encephalopathy
PSG . . . . peak systolic gradient
                      presystolic gallop
PSGN . . . . poststreptococcal glomerulonephritis
psi . . . . pounds per square inch
PSP . . . . periodic short pulse
                      phenolsulfonphthalein
                      positive spike pattern
                      progressive supranuclear palsy
PSS. . . . . physiological saline solution
                      progressive systemic sclerosis
PST . . . . penicillin, streptomycin, and tetracycline
Psy . . . . psychiatry
                      psychology
Psych . . . . psychiatry
                      psychology
PT . . . . parathyroid

PT *(continued)*. . . . paroxysmal tachycardia
permanent and total
pharmacy and therapeutics
physical therapy
physical training
pneumothorax
prothrombin time
Pt . . . . patient
pint
PTA . . . . persistent truncus arteriosus
phosphotungstic acid
plasma thromboplastin antecedent
post-traumatic amnesia
prior to admission
prior to arrival
PTAH. . . . . phosphotungstic acid hematoxylin
PTB . . . . patellar tendon bearing
prior to birth
PTC . . . . phenylthiocarbamide
plasma thromboplastin component
PTD . . . . permanent and total disability
PTE . . . . parathyroid extract
pulmonary thromboembolism
PTED . . . . pulmonary thromboembolic disease
PTH . . . . parathormone
parathyroid hormone
post transfusion hepatitis
PTHS . . . . parathyroid hormone secretion (rate)
PTI. . . . . persistent tolerant infection
PTM . . . . post-transfusion mononucleosis
PTMA. . . . . phenyltrimethylammonium
PTP . . . . post-tetanic potentiation
prior to program
PTR . . . . peripheral total resistance
PTS . . . . para-toluenesulfonic acid
PTT . . . . partial thromboplastin time
particle transport time
PTU . . . . propylthiouracil

PTX . . . . parathyroidectomy
PU . . . . peptic ulcer
                  pregnancy urine
PUD . . . . pulmonary disease
PUE . . . . pyrexia of unknown etiology
PUFA. . . . . polyunsaturated fatty acid
Pul . . . . pulmonary
Pulm . . . . gruel (pulmentum)
                  pulmonary
Pulv . . . . powder (pulvis)
PUO . . . . pyrexia of unknown origin
PV . . . . peripheral vascular
                  peripheral vein
                  peripheral vessels
                  plasma volume
                  polycythemia vera
                  portal vein
                  postvoiding
                  through the vagina (per vaginam)
P & V . . . . pyloroplasty and vagotomy
PVA . . . . polyvinyl alcohol
PVC . . . . polyvinyl chloride
                  premature ventricular contraction
                  pulmonary venous congestion
PVD . . . . peripheral vascular disease
PVF . . . . portal venous flow
PVM. . . . . pneumonia virus of mice
PVP . . . . penicillin V potassium
                  peripheral vein plasma
                  polyvinylpyrrolidone
                  portal venous pressure
PVR . . . . peripheral vascular resistance
                  pulmonary vascular resistance
PVS . . . . premature ventricular systole
PVT . . . . paroxysmal ventricular tachycardia
                  portal vein thrombosis
Pvt . . . . private
PW . . . . posterior wall

PWB . . . . partial weight-bearing
PWC . . . . physical work capacity
PWI . . . . posterior wall infarct
PX . . . . physical examination
　　　　　　　　　　　 pneumothorax
　　　　　　　　　　　 prognosis
PXE . . . . pseudoxanthoma elasticum
PZ . . . . pancreozymin
PZA . . . . pyrazinamide
PZ-CCK . . . . pancreozymin-cholecystokinin
PZI . . . . protamine zinc insulin
Q . . . . coulomb (electric quantity)
　　　　　　　　　　　 every (quaque)
　　　　　　　　　　　 quart
QAM . . . . every morning
QC . . . . quinine-colchicine
QD . . . . every day (quaque die)
QH . . . . every hour (quaque hora)
Q2H . . . . every two hours
Q3H . . . . every three hours
Q4H . . . . every four hours
QHS . . . . every hour of sleep
QID . . . . four times a day (quater in die)
QL . . . . as much as desired (quantum libet)
QM . . . . every morning (quaque mane)
QN . . . . every night
QNS . . . . quantity not sufficient
QOD . . . . every other day
qO_2 . . . . oxygen quotient
QP . . . . at will (quantum placeat)
　　　　　　　　　　　 quanti-Pirquet reaction
QPM . . . . every night
QQ . . . . each
QQH . . . . every four hours (quaque quarta hora)
QQHOR . . . . every hour (quaque hora)
QRZ . . . . wheal reaction time
QS . . . . enough (quantum satis)
QSAD . . . . to a sufficient quantity

QSuff . . . . as much as suffices (quantum sufficit)
Qt. . . . . quiet
qt . . . . quart
Quant . . . . quantity
Quat . . . . four
QUICHA . . . . quantitative inhalation challenge apparatus
Quint . . . . fifth
Quotid . . . . daily (quotidie)
QV . . . . as much as you like (quantum vis)
q. v. . . . . which see (quod vide)
R . . . . Behnken's unit
                organic radical
                radiology
                Rankine (scale)
                Réaumur (scale)
                rectal
                regression coefficient
                remote
                resistance
                respiration
                Rickettsia
                right
                Rinne test
                roentgen
                rough (colony)
                take (recipe)
R_A . . . . airway resistance
R_P . . . . pulmonary resistance
RA . . . . renal artery
                rheumatoid arthritis
                right arm
                right atrial
                right atrium
RAD . . . . radial
                radiation absorbed dose
                right axis deviation
                root
RADTS . . . . rabbit antidog-thymus serum

RAE............ right atrial enlargement
RAF............ rheumatoid arthritis factor
RAH............ right atrial hypertrophy
RAI .... radioactive iodine
RAIU........... radioactive iodine uptake
RAMT .... rabbit antimouse thymocyte
RAO............ right anterior oblique
RAP............ right atrial pressure
RAR............ right arm recumbent
RARLS .... rabbit antirat lymphocyte serum
RAS............ renal artery stenosis
               scrapings (rasurae)
Ras............ scrapings (rasurae)
RAST........... radioallergosorbent test
RATHAS .... rat thymus antiserum
RB .... rating board
RBA........... rose bengal antigen
RBB........... right bundle branch
RBBB.......... right bundle branch block
RBC........... red blood cell
               red blood count
RBCM .... red blood cell mass
RBCV .... red blood cell volume
RBE........... relative biological effectiveness
RBF........... renal blood flow
RC .... red cell
               red cell casts
               retrograde cystogram
RCA........... right coronary artery
RCBV.......... regional cerebral blood volume
RCC........... red cell count
RCD........... relative cardiac dullness
RCF........... red cell folate
               relative centrifugal force
RCM........... red cell mass
               right costal margin
RCR........... respiratory control ratio
RCS .... reticulum cell sarcoma

RCU. . . . . respiratory care unit
RCV. . . . . red cell volume
RD . . . . Raynaud's disease
                         reaction of (to) degeneration
                         resistance determinant
                         respiratory disease
                         right deltoid
rd . . . . rutherford
RDA. . . . . recommended daily allowance
                         recommended dietary allowance
                         right dorsoanterior
RDDA . . . . recommended daily dietary allowance
RDE. . . . . receptor destroying enzyme
RDI . . . . rupture-delivery interval
RDP. . . . . right dorsoposterior
RDS. . . . . respiratory distress syndrome
RE . . . . radium emanation
                         regional enteritis
                         resting energy
                         reticuloendothelial
                         right eye
R & E . . . . Research and Education
Rec . . . . fresh (recens)
Rect . . . . rectified
Red in pulv . . . . . . reduced to powder (reductus in pulverem)
REF. . . . . renal erythropoietic factor
Ref doc . . . . referring doctor
REFRAD . . . . released from active duty
REG. . . . . radioencephalogram
Reg umb. . . . . umbilical region
Rehab . . . . rehabilitation
REM. . . . . rapid eye movement
                         roentgen-equivalent – man
Rem . . . . removal
REMP. . . . . roentgen-equivalent – man period
REP . . . . roentgen equivalent – physical
Rep. . . . . let it be repeated (repetatur)
Rept . . . . let it be repeated

RER . . . . rough endoplasmic reticulum
Res . . . . research
RES . . . . reticuloendothelial system
RESP . . . . respectively
         respiratory
Retic . . . . reticulocyte
RF . . . . Reitland-Franklin (unit)
         relative fluorescence
         releasing factor
         rheumatic fever
         rheumatoid factor
         root canal, filling of
RFA . . . . right femoral artery
         right frontoanterior
RFB . . . . retained foreign body
RFLA . . . . rheumatoid factor-like activity
RFP . . . . right frontoposterior
RFS . . . . renal function study
RFT . . . . right frontotransverse
         rod-and-frame test
RFW . . . . rapid filling wave
RG . . . . right gluteal
RH . . . . reactive hyperemia
         relative humidity
Rh . . . . Rhesus (factor)
         rheumatic
Rh neg . . . . Rhesus factor negative
Rh pos . . . . Rhesus factor positive
RHBF . . . . reactive hyperemia blood flow
RHD . . . . relative hepatic dullness
         rheumatic heart disease
Rheum . . . . rheumatic
RHL . . . . right hepatic lobe
RHLN . . . . right hilar lymph node
rhm . . . . roentgen (per) hour (at one) meter
RI . . . . refractive index
         regional ileitis
         respiratory illness

RIA . . . . radioimmunoassay
RIF . . . . right iliac fossa
RIFA . . . . radioiodinated fatty acid
RIHSA . . . . radioactive iodinated human serum
                       albumin
RISA . . . . radioiodine serum albumin
RITC . . . . rhodamine isothiocyanate
RIU . . . . radioactive iodine uptake
RK . . . . rabbit kidney
                       right kidney
RKY . . . . roentgen kymography
RL . . . . right leg
                       right lung
R-L . . . . right to left
R→L . . . . right to left
RLC . . . . residual lung capacity
RLD . . . . related living donor
RLF . . . . retrolental fibroplasia
RLL . . . . right lower lobe
RLN . . . . recurrent laryngeal nerve
RLP . . . . radiation-leukemia-protection
RLQ . . . . right lower quadrant
RLS . . . . Ringer's lactate solution
RM . . . . radical mastectomy
                       respiratory movement
RMA . . . . right mentoanterior
RMK . . . . rhesus monkey kidney
RML . . . . right middle lobe
RMP . . . . rapidly miscible pool
                       right mentoposterior
RMS . . . . root-mean-square
RMSF . . . . Rocky Mountain spotted fever
RMT . . . . retromolar trigone
                       right mentotransverse
RMV . . . . respiratory minute volume
RNA . . . . ribonucleic acid
RNase . . . . ribonuclease
RND . . . . radical neck dissection

RNP . . . . ribonucleoprotein
RO . . . . Ritter-Oleson (technique)
                         rule out
ROA . . . . right occipitoanterior
Roent . . . . roentgenology
ROH . . . . rat ovarian hyperemia (test)
ROM . . . . range of motion
                         rupture of membranes
ROP . . . . right occipitoposterior
ROS . . . . review of systems
ROT . . . . right occipitotransverse
                         rotating
RP . . . . reactive protein
                         refractory period
                         rest pain
                         resting pressure
RPA . . . . right pulmonary artery
RPCF . . . . Reiter protein complement fixation
RPCFT . . . . Reiter protein complement fixation test
RPE . . . . retinal pigment epithelium
RPF . . . . renal plasma flow
RPG . . . . retrograde pyelogram
RPGN . . . . rapidly progressive glomerulonephritis
rpm . . . . revolutions per minute
RPR . . . . rapid plasma reagin
RPS . . . . renal pressor substance
RPV . . . . right pulmonary veins
RQ . . . . respiratory quotient
RR . . . . radiation response
                         Recovery Room
                         renin release
                         respiratory rate
                         response rate
R & R . . . . rest and recuperation
RR & E . . . . round, regular, and equal
RR-HPO . . . . rapid recompression-high pressure oxygen
RRP . . . . relative refractory period
RRR . . . . renin-release rate

RS . . . . Rating Schedule
respiratory syncytial
right side
RSA . . . . relative specific activity
reticulum cell sarcoma
right sacroanterior
RSB . . . . right sternal border
RSC . . . . rested-state contraction
RScA . . . . right scapuloanterior
RScP . . . . right scapuloposterior
RSP . . . . right sacroposterior
RSR . . . . regular sinus rhythm
RST . . . . radiosensitivity test
right sacrotransverse
RSV . . . . respiratory syncytial virus
right subclavian vein
Rous sarcoma virus
RT . . . . radiation therapy
radiotherapy
radium therapy
reaction time
reading test
recreational therapy
right
right thigh
room temperature
Rt lat . . . . right lateral
RTA . . . . renal tubular acidosis
RTD . . . . routine test dilution
Rtd . . . . retarded
RTF . . . . replication and transfer
resistance transfer factor
respiratory tract fluid
Rtn . . . . return
RU . . . . rat unit
resistance unit
retrograde urogram
right upper

RU . . . . roentgen unit
Rub . . . . red (ruber)
RUL . . . . right upper lobe
RUQ . . . . right upper quadrant
RUR . . . . resin-uptake ratio
RURTI . . . . recurrent upper respiratory tract infection
RV . . . . rat virus
       residual volume
       respiratory volume
       right ventricle
       rubella virus
RVB . . . . red venous blood
RVD . . . . relative vertebral density
RVE . . . . right ventricular enlargement
RVEDP . . . . right ventricular end-diastolic pressure
RVH . . . . right ventricular hypertrophy
RVI . . . . relative value index
RVP . . . . red veterinary petrolatum
RVR . . . . renal vascular resistance
       resistance to venous return
RVRA . . . . renal vein renin activity
       renal venous renin assay
RVRC . . . . renal vein renin concentration
RVS . . . . Relative Value Study (Schedule)
RVT . . . . renal vein thrombosis
RW . . . . ragweed
Rx . . . . take (recipe)
       therapy
       treatment
S . . . . half (semis)
       label (signa)
       left (sinister)
       sacral
       Salmonella
       Schistosoma
       second
       single
       smooth

S *(continued)* . . . . . soluble
spherical lens
Spirillum
Staphylococcus
Streptococcus
subject
supravergence
surgery
Svedberg unit of sedimentation coefficient
without (sine)
write (signa)
S OP S . . . . if it is necessary (si opus sit)
S Romanum . . . . . . sigmoid colon
SA . . . . according to art (secundum artem)
salicylic acid
sarcoma
secondary amenorrhea
secondary anemia
sensation unit
serum albumin
sinoatrial
slightly active
specific activity
Stokes-Adams
surface area
sustained action
sympathetic activity
SAB . . . . significant asymptomatic bacteriuria
SACD . . . . subacute combined degeneration
SAD . . . . source to axis distance
SAG . . . . Swiss agammaglobulinemia
SAH . . . . subarachnoid hemorrhage
SAL . . . . according to the rules of art (secundum
artis leges)
saline
SAM . . . . sulfated acid mucopolysaccharide
SAP . . . . serum alkaline phosphatase
systemic arterial pressure

SAS . . . . supravalvular aortic stenosis
SAT . . . . Scholastic Aptitude Test
Sat . . . . saturated
SB . . . . serum bilirubin
                  single breath
                  Stanford-Binet (test)
                  sternal border
                  stillbirth
SBE . . . . subacute bacterial endocarditis
SBF . . . . splanchnic blood flow
SBP . . . . systemic blood pressure
                  systolic blood pressure
SBS . . . . social-breakdown syndrome
SBT . . . . single-breath test
SBTI . . . . soy-bean trypsin inhibitor
SC . . . . closure of the semilunar valves
                  sacrococcygeal
                  Self-Care
                  semicircular
                  semiclosed
                  service connected
                  sick call
                  sickle cell
                  single chemical
                  Special Care
                  sternoclavicular
                  subcutaneous
                  succinylcholine
                  sugar-coated
SCAT . . . . sheep cell agglutination test
Scat . . . . a box (scatula)
SCC . . . . squamous cell carcinoma
SCD . . . . service-connected disability
ScDA . . . . scapulodextra anterior
ScDP. . . . . scapulodextra posterior
SCH . . . . succinylcholine
Sched . . . . schedule
Schiz . . . . schizophrenia

SCI	structured clinical interview
SCK	serum creatine kinase
ScLA	scapulolaeva anterior
ScLP	scapulolaeva posterior
Scop	scopolamine
SCP	single-celled protein
SCPK	serum creatine phosphokinase
Scr	scruple
SCT	sex chromatin test
	staphylococcal clumping test
SCUBA	self-contained underwater breathing apparatus
SD	septal defect
	serum defect
	skin dose
	spontaneous delivery
	standard deviation
	streptodornase
	sudden death
S/D	systolic to diastolic
SDA	sacrodextra anterior
	specific dynamic action
SDCL	symptom distress check list
SDH	serine dehydrase
	sorbitol dehydrogenase
	succinate dehydrogenase
SDM	standard deviation of the mean
SDO	sudden-dosage onset
SDP	sacrodextra posterior
SDS	Self-Rating Depression Scale
	sensory deprivation syndrome
	sodium dodecyl sulfate
	sudden death syndrome
SDT	sacrodextra transversa
SE	himself
	standard error
	Starr-Edwards (prosthesis)
sec	second

SED . . . . skin erythema dose
                       spondyloepiphyseal dysplasia
Sed. . . . . stool (sedes)
Sed rate . . . . sedimentation rate
SEE . . . . standard error of the estimate
Seg. . . . . segmented (leukocyte)
                       sonoencephalogram
SEGS . . . . segmented neutrophils
SEM. . . . . scanning electron miscroscopy
                       standard error of the mean
Semi. . . . . half
Semid. . . . . half a drachm
Semih . . . . half an hour
SEP . . . . sensory evoked potential
                       systolic ejection period
Seq. . . . . sequela
                       sequestrum
Seq luce . . . . the next day (sequenti luce)
SER . . . . smooth endoplasmic reticulum
                       systolic ejection rate
Serv . . . . keep (serva)
                       preserve
SES . . . . socioeconomic status
SET . . . . systolic ejection time
Sev. . . . . severe
                       severed
SF . . . . scarlet fever
                       shell fragment
                       shrapnel fragment
                       spinal fluid
Sf. . . . . Svedberg flotation units
SFD . . . . short food drape
SFF . . . . specific-pathogen free
SFP . . . . screen filtration pressure
                       spinal fluid pressure
SFS . . . . split function study
SFT . . . . skinfold thickness
SFW. . . . . shell fragment wound

SFW . . . . shrapnel fragment wound
SG . . . . serum globulin
                signs
                skin graft
                specific gravity
S-G . . . . Sachs-Georgi (test)
SGA . . . . small for gestational age
SGOT . . . . serum glutamic oxalic transaminase
                serum glutamic oxaloacetic transaminase
SGP . . . . serine glycerophosphatide
SGPT . . . . serum glutamic pyruvic transaminase
SGV . . . . salivary gland virus
SH . . . . serum hepatitis
                sex hormone
                sinus histiocytosis
                social history
                sulfhydryl
                surgical history
Sh . . . . shoulder
SHB . . . . sulfhemoglobin
SHBD . . . . serum hydroxybutyrate dehydrogenase
SHG . . . . synthetic human gastrin
SHO . . . . secondary hypertrophic osteoarthropathy
SI . . . . sacro-iliac
                saturation index
                self-inflicted
                seriously ill
                serum iron
                soluble insulin
                stroke index
Si non val . . . . if it is not enough (si non valeat)
Si op sit . . . . if it is necessary (si opus sit)
Si vir perm . . . . if the strength will permit (si vires
                permittant)
SIADH . . . . syndrome of inappropriate antidiuretic
                hormone
SICD . . . . serum isocitric dehydrogenase
SID . . . . sudden infant death

SIDS . . . . sudden infant death syndrome
Sig . . . . let it be labeled (signetur)
        significant
Sig n pro . . . . label with the proper name (signa nomine
        proprio)
SIJ . . . . sacro-iliac joint
Simul . . . . at the same time
Sing . . . . of each
SISI . . . . short-increment sensitivity index
SIW . . . . self-inflicted wound
SJR . . . . Shinawora-Jones-Reinhart (units)
SK . . . . streptokinase
SKSD . . . . streptokinase-streptodornase
SL . . . . according to law (secundum legem)
        sensation level
        streptolysin
Sl . . . . slight
SLA . . . . sacrolaeva anterior
SLD . . . . serum lactic dehydrogenase
SLDH . . . . serum lactic dehydrogenase
SLE . . . . St. Louis encephalitis
        systemic lupus erythematosus
SLEV . . . . St. Louis encephalitis virus
SLI . . . . splenic localization index
SLKC . . . . superior limbic keratoconjunctivitis
SLN . . . . superior laryngeal nerve
SLO . . . . streptolysin-O
SLP . . . . sacrolaeva posterior
SLR . . . . straight leg raising
        Streptococcus lactis R
SLT . . . . sacrolaeva transversa
SM . . . . simple mastectomy
        skim milk
        small
        streptomycin
        submucous
        suction method
        symptoms

SM *(continued)*. . . . systolic mean
systolic murmur
SMA. . . . . superior mesenteric artery
SMC. . . . . special monthly compensation
SMO. . . . . slip made out
SMON . . . . subacute myelo-optical neuropathy
SMP . . . . slow-moving protease
special monthly pension
SMR. . . . . somnolent metabolic rate
standard mortality ratio
standardized mortality ratio
submucous resection
submucous resection and rhinoplasty
SN . . . . according to nature (secundum naturam)
serum-neutralizing
suprasternal notch
SNB . . . . scalene node biopsy
SO . . . . salpingo-oophorectomy
SOB . . . . short of breath
SOC . . . . sequential-type oral contraceptive
Sol . . . . solution
space-occupying lesion
SOL . . . . space-occupying lesion
Soln . . . . solution
Solv . . . . dissolve (solve)
SOM. . . . . secretory otitis media
serous otitis media
sulformethoxine
SOP . . . . standing operative procedure
SOS . . . . if it is necessary (si opus sit)
SOTT. . . . . synthetic medium old tuberculin
trichloracetic acid precipitated
SP . . . . shunt procedure
skin potential
steady potential
summating potential
suprapubic
symphysis pubis

SP . . . . systolic pressure
Sp . . . . species
                     spirit (spiritus)
Sp gr . . . . specific gravity
Sp gravity . . . . specific gravity
SPA . . . . suprapubic aspiration
SPAI . . . . steroid protein activity index
SPBI . . . . serum protein-bound iodine
SPCA . . . . serum prothrombin conversion accelerator
SPCK . . . . serum creatine phosphokinase
SPF . . . . specific-pathogen free
                     split products of fibrin
SPH . . . . secondary pulmonary hemosiderosis
Sph. . . . . spherical
                     spherical lens
SPI . . . . serum precipitable iodine
Spir . . . . spirit (spiritus)
SPL . . . . sound pressure level
                     spontaneous lesion
Spont . . . . spontaneous (delivery)
SPP. . . . . suprapubic prostatectomy
Spt . . . . spirit
SQ . . . . social quotient
                     square
                     subcutaneous
SR . . . . sarcoplasmic reticulum
                     secretion rate
                     sedimentation rate
                     sensitization response
                     service record
                     sigma reaction
                     sinus rhythm
                     skin resistance
                     superior rectus
                     system review
                     systemic resistance
                     systems research
SRBC . . . . sheep red blood cells

SRC . . . . sedimented red cells
                sheep red cells
SRF . . . . somatotropin-releasing factor
                split renal function
SRFS . . . . split renal function study
SRNA. . . . . soluble ribonucleic acid
SRR . . . . slow rotation room
SRS . . . . slow-reacting substance
SRSA. . . . . slow-reacting substance of anaphylaxis
SRT . . . . speech reception test
                speech reception threshold
SS . . . . saturated solution
                side to side
                signs and symptoms
                soapsuds
                statistically significant
                subaortic stenosis
                sum of squares
                supersaturated
ss . . . . one-half (semis)
SSA . . . . salicylsalicylic acid
                skin-sensitizing antibody
                sulfosalicylic acid (test)
SSD . . . . source to skin distance
                sum of square deviations
SSE . . . . soapsuds enema
SSKI . . . . saturated solution of potassium iodide
SSN . . . . severely subnormal
SSP. . . . . Sanarelli-Shwartzman phenomenon
                subacute sclerosing panencephalitis
SSPE . . . . subacute sclerosing panencephalitis
SSS . . . . layer upon layer (stratum super stratum)
                specific soluble substance
SSU . . . . sterile supply unit
SSV . . . . under a poison label (sub signo veneni)
ST . . . . esotropia
                sternothyroid
                subtalar

ST *(continued)*.... subtotal
                     surface tension
St.............. let it stand (stet)
                     straight
STA........... serum thrombotic accelerator
Stab........... stabnuclear neutrophil
Staph.......... staphylococcus
Stat .... immediately (statim)
stat .... German unit of radium emanation
STC........... soft tissue calcification
Std............ saturated
STD........... skin test dose
                     skin to tumor distance
Stet .... let it stand
STH........... somatotropic hormone
STK........... streptokinase
STM........... streptomycin
STP .... scientifically treated petroleum
                     standard temperature and pressure
STPD........... standard temperature and pressure, dry
                     ($0°C.$, 760 mm. Hg)
Str .... streptococcus
Strep .... streptococcus
STS .... serologic test for syphilis
                     standard test for syphilis
STSG .... split thickness skin graft
STT .... serial thrombin time
STU .... skin test unit
STVA.......... subtotal villose atrophy
Su .... let him take (sumat)
SUA........... serum uric acid
                     single umbilical artery
Subcu.......... subcutaneous
Subling......... under the tongue
Subq........... subcutaneous
SUD........... sudden unexpected death
                     sudden unexplained death
SUID .... sudden unexplained infant death

Sum . . . . let him take (sumat)
SUN . . . . serum urea nitrogen
SUP . . . . superficial
        superior
Surg . . . . surgery
SUS . . . . stained urinary sediment
SUUD . . . . sudden unexpected, unexplained death
SV . . . . alcoholic spirit (spiritus vini)
        severe
        simian virus
        snake venom
        stroke volume
        subclavian vein
        supravital
SVAS . . . . supravalvular aortic stenosis
SVC . . . . slow vital capacity
        superior vena cava
SVCG . . . . spatial vectorcardiogram
SVD . . . . spontaneous vaginal delivery
        spontaneous vertex delivery
SVI . . . . stroke volume index
SVM . . . . syncytiovascular membrane
SVR . . . . rectified spirit of wine (spiritus vini
         rectificatus)
        systemic vascular resistance
SVT . . . . proof spirit (spiritus vini tenuis)
SW . . . . spiral wound
        stroke work
SWI . . . . stroke work index
SX . . . . signs
        symptoms
Sym . . . . symmetrical
        symptoms
Symp . . . . symptoms
Syr . . . . syrup
SZ . . . . schizophrenia
T . . . . Taenia
        temperature

T *(continued)* . . . . . tension, intraocular
thoracic
time
Treponema
Trichophyton
Trypanosoma
tumor

t . . . . temporal
ter- (three times)
tertiary
test of significance

T+ . . . . increased tension
T− . . . . decreased tension
T½ . . . . half-life
T$_3$ . . . . triiodothyronine
T$_4$ . . . . thyroxine, levothyroxine, tetraiodo-
thyronine
TA . . . . alkaline tuberculin
therapeutic abortion
titratable acid
toxin-antitoxin
T & A . . . . tonsillectomy & adenoidectomy
Tab. . . . . tablet
TAB . . . . typhoid, paratyphoid A, and paratyphoid B
TACE . . . . tripara-anisylchloroethylene
TAD . . . . thoracic asphyxiant dystrophy
TAF . . . . albumose-free tuberculin
toxoid-antitoxin floccules
trypsin-aldehyde-fuchsin
TAH . . . . total abdominal hysterectomy
Tal . . . . of such (talis)
TAL . . . . tendo Achilles lengthening
thymic alymphoplasia
TAM . . . . toxoid-antitoxin mixture
TAME . . . . toluene-sulpho-trypsin arginine methyl
ester
TAO . . . . thromboangiitis obliterans
triacetyloleandomycin

TAPVD . . . . total anomalous pulmonary venous
        drainage
TAR . . . . thrombocytopenia with absence of the
        radius
TAT . . . . tetanus antitoxin
        thematic apperception test
        thromboplastin activation test
        total antitryptic activity
        toxin-antitoxin
        tyrosine aminotransferase
TB . . . . toluidine blue
        total base
        total body
        tracheobronchitis
        tubercle bacillus
        tuberculosis
TBA . . . . tertiary butylacetate
        testosterone-binding affinity
        thiobarbituric acid
TBC . . . . tuberculosis
TBD . . . . total body density
TBF . . . . total body fat
TBG . . . . thyroxine-binding globulin
TBGP . . . . total blood granulocyte pool
TBI . . . . thyroid-binding index
        total body irradiation
TBK . . . . total body potassium
TBM . . . . tuberculous meningitis
TBN . . . . bacillus emulsion
TBP . . . . thyroxine-binding protein
TBPA . . . . thyroxine-binding prealbumin
TB-RD . . . . tuberculosis-respiratory disease
TBS . . . . total body solute
        tribromosalicylanilide
        triethanolamine-buffered saline
tbsp . . . . tablespoonful
TBT . . . . tolbutamide test
        tracheobronchial toilet

TBV . . . . total blood volume
TBW . . . . total body water
total body weight
TBX . . . . whole body irradiation
TC . . . . taurocholate
temperature compensation
tetracycline
tissue culture
to contain
total capacity
total cholesterol
tubocurarine
TCA . . . . tricarboxylic acid
trichloroacetate
trichloroacetic acid
TCAP . . . . trimethylcetylammonium
pentachlorophenate
TCC . . . . trichlorocarbanilide
TCD . . . . tissue culture dose
TCD_{50} . . . . median tissue culture dose
TCE . . . . trichloroethylene
TCF . . . . total coronary flow
TCH . . . . total circulating hemoglobin
TCI . . . . to come in
transient cerebral ischemia
TCID . . . . tissue culture infective dose
$TCID_{50}$ . . . . median tissue culture infective dose
TCIE . . . . transient cerebral ischemic episode
TCM . . . . tissue culture medium
TCP . . . . therapeutic continuous penicillin
TCSA . . . . tetrachlorosalicylanilide
TCT . . . . thrombin clotting time
thyrocalcitonin
TD . . . . tetanus-diptheria
therapy discontinued
thoracic duct
three times a day
threshold of discomfort

TD *(continued)*. . . . thymus-dependent
time disintegration
to deliver
tone decay
torsion dystonia
total disability
transverse diameter
treatment discontinued
TDF . . . . thoracic duct fistula
thoracic duct flow
TDI . . . . toluene-diisocyanate
total-dose infusion
TDL . . . . thoracic duct lymph
TDP . . . . thoracic duct pressure
thymidine diphosphate
TDS . . . . three times a day (ter die sumendum)
TDT . . . . tone decay test
TE . . . . tetanus
threshold energy
tissue-equivalent
tooth extracted
total estrogen (excretion)
tracheo-esophageal
TEA . . . . tetraethylammonium
TEAC. . . . . tetraethylammonium chloride
TEE . . . . tyrosine ethyl ester
TEEP . . . . tetraethyl pyrophosphate
TEF . . . . tracheo-esophageal fistula
TEIB . . . . triethyleneiminobenzoquinone
TEL . . . . tetraethyl lead
TEM. . . . . transmission electron microscopy
triethylenemelamine
TEN . . . . toxic epidermal necrolysis
Tenac. . . . . tenaculum
TEP . . . . thromboendophlebectomy
TEPP . . . . tetraethyl pyrophosphate
TER . . . . three times
threefold

TES . . . . trismethylaminoethanesulfonic acid
Tet . . . . tetralogy of Fallot
TETD . . . . tetraethylthiuram-disulfide
TF . . . . tactile fremitus
                   tetralogy of Fallot
                   thymol flocculation
                   tissue-damaging factor
                   to follow
                   total flow
                   transfer factor
                   tuberculin filtrate
                   tubular fluid
TFA . . . . total fatty acids
TFE . . . . tetrafluoroethylene
TFS . . . . testicular feminization syndrome
TG . . . . thioguanine
                   thyroglobulin
                   toxic goiter
                   triglyceride
TGA . . . . transposition of the great arteries
TGAR . . . . total graft area rejected
TGFA . . . . triglyceride fatty acid
TGL . . . . triglyceride
                   triglyceride lipase
TGT . . . . thromboplastin generation test
                   thromboplastin generation time
TGV . . . . thoracic gas volume
                   transposition of the great vessels
TH . . . . thoracic
                   thyrohyoid
THA . . . . total hydroxyapatite
THAM . . . . trihydroxymethylaminomethane
THC . . . . tetrahydrocannabinol
THDOC . . . . tetrahydrodeoxycorticosterone
THE . . . . tetrahydrocortisone
er . . . . therapy
F . . . . humoral thymic factor
                   tetrahydrocortisol

THF . . . . tetrahydrofolic acid
THFA . . . . tetrahydrofolic acid
THO . . . . tritiated water
THP . . . . total hydroxyproline
TI . . . . thoracic index
                        time interval
                        tricuspid incompetence
                        tricuspid insufficiency
TIA . . . . transient ischemic attack
TIBC . . . . total iron-binding capacity
TIC . . . . trypsin-inhibitory capacity
TID . . . . three times a day (ter in die)
                        titrated initial dose
TIE . . . . transient ischemic episode
TIN . . . . three times a night (ter in nocte)
Tinct . . . . tincture
TIS . . . . tumor in situ
TIVC . . . . thoracic inferior vena cava
TKA . . . . transketolase activity
TKD . . . . tokodynamometer
TKG . . . . tokodynagraph
TL . . . . time lapse
                        time-limited
                        total lipids
                        tubal ligation
TLA . . . . translumbar aortogram
TLC . . . . tender loving care
                        thin-layer chromatography
                        total L-chain concentration
                        total lung capacity
                        total lung compliance
TLD . . . . thermoluminescent dosimeter
T/LD_{100} . . . . minimum dose causing death or
                        malformation of 100 per cent of
                        fetuses
TLE . . . . thin-layer electrophoresis
TLQ . . . . total living quotient
TLV . . . . threshold limit value

TM . . . . temporomandibular
trademark
transmetatarsal
tympanic membrane
Tm . . . . maximal tubular excretory capacity of the
kidneys
TMAS . . . . Taylor Manifest Anxiety Scale
TmG. . . . . maximal tubular reabsorption of glucose
TMJ . . . . temporomandibular joint
TML. . . . . tetramethyl lead
TMP . . . . thymidine monophosphate
trimethoprim
TMTD . . . . tetramethylthiuram disulfide
TMV. . . . . tobacco mosaic virus
TN . . . . total negatives
true-negative
Tn . . . . normal intraocular tension
TND. . . . . term normal delivery
TNI . . . . total nodal irradiation
TNM . . . . (primary) tumor, (regional lymph) nodes,
(remote) metastases (system)
TNT . . . . trinitrotoluene
TNTC. . . . . too numerous to count
TO . . . . original tuberculin
telephone order
tincture of opium
TOA. . . . . tubo-ovarian abscess
TOCP . . . . triorthocresyl phosphate
Tonoc. . . . . tonight
TOPS . . . . Take Off Pounds Sensibly
TOPV. . . . . trivalent oral poliovirus vaccine
Tot prot . . . . total protein
TP . . . . temperature and pressure
thrombocytopenic purpura
total positives
total protein
true-positive
tryptophan

TP *(continued)*.... tube precipitin
tuberculin precipitation
TPA .... Treponema pallidum agglutination
TPBF .... total pulmonary blood flow
TPCF .... Treponema pallidum complement fixation
TPG .... transplacental gradient
TPH .... transplacental hemorrhage
TPI .... Treponema pallidium immobilization
treponemal immobilization test
(cardiolipin)
triose phosphate isomerase
TPIA .... Treponema pallidum immobilization
(immune) adherence
TPM .... triphenylmethane
TPN .... triphosphopyridine nucleotide
TPNH........... reduced triphosphopyridine nucleotide
TPP .... thiamine pyrophosphate
TPR .... temperature, pulse, and respiration
testosterone production rate
total peripheral resistance
total pulmonary resistance
TPS .... tumor polysaccharide substance
TPT .... typhoid-paratyphoid (vaccine)
TPTZ .... tripyridyltriazine
TPVR .... total pulmonary vascular resistance
TQ .... tourniquet
TR .... tetrazolium reduction
therapeutic radiology
time released
tincture
total resistance
total response
trace
tuberculin R (new tuberculin)
TRA............ transaldolase
TRAM .... Treatment Rating Assessment Matrix
Treatment Response Assessment Method
TRBF........... total renal blood flow

TRC . . . . tanned red cell
　　　　　　　　　　 total ridge-count
TRF . . . . thyrotropin-releasing factor
TRH . . . . thyrotropin-releasing hormone
TRI . . . . tetrazolium-reduction inhibition
TRIC . . . . trachoma-inclusion conjunctivitis
Trit . . . . triturate
TRK . . . . transketolase
TRMC . . . . tetramethylrhodamino-isothiocyanate
Troch . . . . trochiscus
TRP . . . . tubular reabsorption of phosphate
TRPT . . . . theoretical renal phosphorus threshold
TRU . . . . turbidity-reducing unit
TS . . . . test solution
　　　　　　　　　　 thoracic surgery
　　　　　　　　　　 total solids
　　　　　　　　　　 triple strength
　　　　　　　　　　 tropical sprue
TSA . . . . technical surgical assistance
　　　　　　　　　　 trypticase soy agar
T_4SA . . . . thyroxine-specific activity
TSB . . . . trypticase soy broth
TSC . . . . thiosemicarbizide
TSD . . . . target skin distance
　　　　　　　　　　 Tay-Sachs disease
　　　　　　　　　　 theory of signal detectability
TSE . . . . trisodium edetate
TSF . . . . tissue coding factor
TSH . . . . thyroid stimulating hormone
TSI . . . . triple sugar iron (agar)
TSP . . . . total serum protein
tsp . . . . teaspoonful
TSPAP . . . . total serum prostatic acid phosphatase
TSR . . . . thyroid to serum ratio
TSS . . . . tropical splenomegaly syndrome
TST . . . . tumor skin test
TSTA . . . . tumor-specific transplantation antigen
TSY . . . . trypticase soy yeast

TT . . . . tetrazol
thrombin time
thymol turbidity
tooth, treatment of
total thyroxine
total time
transit time
transthoracic
TTC . . . . triphenyltetrazolium chloride
TTH . . . . thyrotropic hormone
tritiated thymidine
TTI . . . . time-tension index (tension time index)
TTP . . . . thrombotic thrombocytopenic purpura
thymidine triphosphate
TTS . . . . temporary threshold shift
TTT . . . . tolbutamide tolerance test
TU . . . . thiouracil
toxic unit
tuberculin unit
Tuberc . . . . tuberculosis
TUG . . . . total urinary gonadotropin
TUR . . . . transurethral resection
TURB . . . . transurethral resection of the bladder
TURP . . . . transurethral resection of the prostate
Tus . . . . cough (tussis)
TV . . . . tidal volume
trial visit
tuberculin volutin
TVC . . . . timed vital capacity
total volume capacity
transvaginal cone
TVH . . . . total vaginal hysterectomy
TW . . . . tap water
TWL . . . . transepidermal water loss
TX . . . . traction
treatment
Ty . . . . type
typhoid

TZ . . . . tuberculin zymoplastic
U . . . . unit
                            unknown
                            upper
                            urology
UA . . . . umbilical artery
                            unaggregated
                            uric acid
                            urine analysis
                            uterine aspiration
UB . . . . ultimobranchial body
UBBC . . . . unsaturated vitamin B_{12}-binding capacity
UBF . . . . uterine blood flow
UBI . . . . ultraviolet blood irradiation
UC . . . . ulcerative colitis
                            ultracentrifugal
                            unchanged
                            unclassifiable
                            unit clerk
                            urea clearance
                            urethral catheterization
U & C . . . . usual and customary
UCD . . . . usual childhood diseases
UCG . . . . urinary chorionic gonadotropin
UCHD . . . . usual childhood diseases
UCO . . . . urethral catheter out
UCP . . . . urinary coproporphyrin
UCS . . . . unconditioned stimulus
                            unconscious
UD . . . . urethral discharge
                            uroporphyrinogen decarboxylase
UDP . . . . uridine diphosphate
UDPG . . . . uridine diphosphoglucose
UDPGA . . . . uridine diphosphoglucuronic acid
UDPGT . . . . uridine diphosphoglycyronyl transferase
UE . . . . upper extremity
UFA . . . . unesterified fatty acid
UG . . . . urogenital

UGI . . . . upper gastrointestinal
UH . . . . upper half
UI . . . . uroporphyrin isomerase
UIBC . . . . unsaturated iron-binding capacity
UIF . . . . undergraded insulin factor
UIQ . . . . upper inner quadrant
UK . . . . unknown
                 urokinase
UL . . . . upper lobe
U & L . . . . upper and lower
ULQ . . . . upper left quadrant
UM . . . . uracil mustard
Umb . . . . umbilicus
UMP . . . . uridine monophosphate
UN . . . . urea nitrogen
Ung . . . . ointment (unguentum)
uni- . . . . one
Unk . . . . unknown
Unkn . . . . unknown
UOQ . . . . upper outer quadrant
UP . . . . upright posture
                 ureteropelvic
                 uroporphyrin
U/P . . . . urine-plasma ratio
UPG . . . . uroporphyrinogen
UPI . . . . uteroplacental insufficiency
UPJ . . . . ureteropelvic junction
UPOR . . . . upper place of residence
UR . . . . upper respiratory
                 urine
                 utilization review
URD . . . . upper respiratory disease
URI . . . . upper respiratory infection
Urol . . . . urology
URQ . . . . upper right quadrant
URTI . . . . upper respiratory tract infection
US . . . . ultrasonic
USN . . . . ultrasonic nebulizer

USO . . . . unilateral salpingo-oophorectomy
USR . . . . unheated serum reagin (test)
Ut dict . . . . as directed (ut dictum)
UTBG . . . . unbound thyroxine-binding globulin
Utend . . . . to be used (utendus)
UTI . . . . urinary tract infection
UTP . . . . uridine triphosphate
UU . . . . urine urobilinogen
UUN . . . . urine urea nitrogen
UV . . . . ultraviolet
                        umbilical vein
                        urinary volume
UVL . . . . ultraviolet light
V . . . . see (vide)
                        vein
                        Vibrio
                        vision
                        visual acuity
                        voice
                        volume
V_T . . . . tidal volume
v . . . . very
                        volt
VA . . . . vacuum aspiration
                        ventriculoatrial
                        vertebral artery
                        visual acuity
Va . . . . alveolar ventilation
                        visual acuity
Vag . . . . vagina
                        vaginal
Vag hyst . . . . vaginal hysterectomy
VALE . . . . visual acuity, left eye
VAMP . . . . vincristine, amethopterine,
                        6-mercaptopurine, and prednisone
Var . . . . variation
VARE . . . . visual acuity, right eye
Vasc . . . . vascular

VASC	Verbal Auditory Screen for Children
VB	viable birth
	vinblastine
VBL	vinblastine
VBS	veronal-buffered saline
VBS:FBS	veronal-buffered saline-fetal bovine serum
VC	acuity of color vision
	vena cava
	ventilatory capacity
	vincristine
	vital capacity
VCG	vectorcardiogram
VCR	vincristine
VD	vapor density
	venereal disease
VDA	visual discriminatory acuity
VDBR	volume of distribution of bilirubin
VDG	veneral disease – gonorrhea
Vdg	voiding
VDH	valvular disease of the heart
VDL	visual detection level
VDM	vasodepressor material
VDP	vincristine, daunorubicin, prednisone
VDRS	Verdun Depression Rating Scale
VDS	venereal disease – syphilis
VE	visual efficiency
	volumic ejection
V & E	Vinethene and ether
VEE	Venezuelan equine encephalomyelitis
VEM	vasoexcitor material
Vent	ventricular
VEP	visual evoked potential
VER	visual evoked response
Ves	bladder
	vesicular
Vesic	blister (vesicula)
VF	left leg (electrode)
	ventricular fibrillation

VF *(continued)*. . . . ventricular fluid
visual field
vocal fremitus
VFP . . . . ventricular fluid pressure
VG . . . . ventricular gallop
VH . . . . vaginal hysterectomy
venous hematocrit
viral hepatitis
VHD. . . . . viral hematodepressive disease
VHF. . . . . visual half-field
VI . . . . volume index
VIA . . . . virus-inactivating agent
Vib. . . . . vibration
VIG . . . . vaccinia-immune globulin
Vin. . . . . wine (vinum)
VIP . . . . very important patient
VIS . . . . vaginal irrigation smear
Vit . . . . vitamin
yolk (vitellus)
Vit cap . . . . vital capacity
VL . . . . left arm (electrode)
VLDL . . . . very low-density lipoprotein
VLDLP . . . . very low density lipoprotein
VM . . . . viomycin
voltmeter
VMA. . . . . vanillylmandelic acid
VN . . . . virus neutralizing
VO . . . . verbal order
VOD . . . . vision, right eye
Vol. . . . . volume
VOS . . . . dissolved in yolk of egg (vitello ovi
solutus)
vision, left eye
VP . . . . vasopressin
venipuncture
venous pressure
Voges-Proskauer (reaction)
volume-pressure

VP . . . . vulnerable period
V & P . . . . vagotomy and pyloroplasty
VPB . . . . ventricular premature beat
VPC . . . . ventricular premature contraction
                 volume per cent
VPRC . . . . volume of packed red cells
V/Q . . . . ventilation-perfusion
VR . . . . right arm (electrode)
                 valve replacement
                 vascular resistance
                 venous return
                 ventilation ratio
                 vocal resonance
                 vocational rehabilitation
VRBC . . . . red blood cell volume
VR & E . . . . vocational rehabilitation and education
VRI . . . . viral respiratory infection
VRP . . . . very reliable product (written on
                 prescription)
VS . . . . vaccination scar
                 venisection
                 verbal scale (IQ)
                 vital signs
                 volumetric solution
                 without glasses
Vs . . . . against
                 voids
vs . . . . vibration seconds
VsB . . . . bleeding in the arm (venaesectio brachii)
VSD . . . . ventricular septal defect
VSOK . . . . vital signs normal
VSS . . . . vital signs stable
VSULA . . . . vaccination scar upper left arm
VSV . . . . vesicular stomatitis virus
VSW . . . . ventricular stroke work
VT . . . . tidal volume
                 vacuum tuberculin
                 ventricular tachycardia

V & T. . . . . volume and tension
VTSRS. . . . . Verdun Target Symptom Rating Scale
VV. . . . . veins
                  viper venom
v/v . . . . volume for volume
V/VI. . . . . grade 5 on a 6 grade basis
VW. . . . . vessel wall
                  von Willebrand's disease
VZ . . . . varicella-zoster
W . . . . water
                  Weber (test)
                  week
                  wehnelt (unit of roentgen rays hardness)
                  weight
                  widowed
                  wife
                  with
W+ . . . . weakly positive
w . . . . watt
WAIS . . . . Wechsler's Adult Intelligence Scale
WB . . . . weight bearing
                  Willowbrook (virus)
                  whole blood
                  whole body
WBC . . . . white blood cell
                  white blood count
WBF. . . . . whole-blood folate
WBH. . . . . whole-blood hematocrit
WBR . . . . whole body radiation
WC. . . . . water closet
                  white cell
                  white cell casts
                  whooping cough
                  work capacity
WC'. . . . . whole complement
WCC . . . . white cell count
WD. . . . . wallerian degeneration
                  well-developed

WD *(continued)* . . . well-differentiated
with disease
WDWN . . . . well-developed, well-nourished
WE . . . . Western encephalitis
Western encephalomyelitis
WEE . . . . Western equine encephalomyelitis
WF . . . . Weil-Felix (reaction)
white female
WFR . . . . Weil-Felix reaction
WG . . . . water gauge
WH . . . . well-healed
WIA . . . . wounded in action
WISC . . . . Wechsler's Intelligence Scale for Children
Wk . . . . weak
week
WK . . . . Wernicke-Korsakoff (syndrome)
WL . . . . waiting list
wavelength
work load
WM . . . . white male
whole milk
WMF . . . . white middle-aged female
WMM . . . . white middle-aged male
WMR . . . . work metabolic rate
WN . . . . well-nourished
WNF . . . . well-nourished female
WNL . . . . within normal limits
WNM . . . . well-nourished male
WO . . . . without
W/O . . . . water in oil
WP . . . . weakly positive
working point
WPRS . . . . Wittenborn Psychiatric Rating Scale
WPW . . . . Wolff-Parkinson-White (syndrome)
WR . . . . Wassermann reaction
weakly reactive
Wr . . . . wrist
WRC . . . . washed red cells

WRE	whole ragweed extract
WS	water swallow
ws	watts second
Wt	weight
	white
WV	whispered voice
w/v	weight per volume
X	homeopathic symbol for the decimal scale of potencies
	Kienböck's unit of x-ray dosage
	magnification
	removal of
	respirations (anesthesia chart)
	start of anesthesia
	times
XDP	xeroderma pigmentosum
XM	crossmatch
XP	xeroderma pigmentosum
XR	x-ray
XS	excess
	xiphisternum
XT	exotropia
XU	excretory urogram
Y	year
yd	yard
YF	yellow fever
YO	year old
YOB	year of birth
yr	year
YS	yellow spot (of the retina)
	yolk sac
Z	zero
	Zuckung (contraction)
z	atomic number
Z/D	zero defects
ZE	Zollinger-Ellison (syndrome)
Z/G	zoster immune globulin
ZIG	zoster immune globulin

Zz . . . . ginger
Z, Z', Z″. . . . . increasing degrees of contraction

SYMBOLS

$\mathrm{\textcircled{L}}$	left	$\bar{c}$	with
$\mathrm{\textcircled{M}}$	murmur	$\bar{s}$	without
$\mathrm{\textcircled{R}}$	right trademark	?	question of questionable possible
$\odot$	start of operation	~	approximate
$\mathrm{\textcircled{X}}$	end of operation	±	not definite
□	male	↓	decreased depression
○	female	↑	elevation increased
♂	male	⇧	up
♀	female	→	causes transfer to
*	birth	←	is due to
†	death	⊖	normal
τ	life (time)	$\sqrt{\bar{c}}$	check with
$\tau^{\frac{1}{2}}$	half-life (time)	φ	none
$\bar{p}$	after		
$\bar{a}$	before		

$\vee$	systolic blood pressure	$1\times$	once
		$^{\circ}$	degree
$\wedge$	diastolic blood pressure	$'$	foot
#	gauge number weight	$''$	inch
		$\ddot{\text{ii}}$	two
24°	24 hours	$/$	of per
Δt	time interval	$:$	ratio (is to)
$3 = D$	delayed double diffusion (test)	$+$	positive present
606	arsphenamine	$-$	absent negative
914	neoarsphenamine		
		$\overline{X}$	average of all X's
℞	take		
		α	alpha particle is proportional to
6-MP	6-mercaptopurine		
^{3}HT	H_3T, triated thymidine	$\neq$	does not equal
		$>$	greater than
2d	second		
		$<$	less than
2°	secondary		
		χ^2	chi square (test)
2ndry	secondary		
		σ	1/100 of a second standard deviation
$2\times$	twice		
$\times2$	twice	℈	scruple

Symbol	Meaning	Symbol	Meaning
ℨ	ounce	μu	microunit
f ℨ	fluid ounce	μv	microvolt
μ	micron	μw	microwatt
μμ	micromicron	μV	milligamma (micromicrogram, picogram)
μc	microcurie		
μEq	microequivalent	mμc	millimicrocurie (nanocurie)
μf	microfarad	mμg	millimicrogram (nanogram)
μg	microgram		
μl	microliter	mμ	millimicron
μμc	micromicrocurie (picocurie)	ʒ	drachm dram
μμg	micromicrogram (picogram)	f ʒ	fluidrachm fluidram
μM	micromolar	△	prism diopter
μr	microroentgen	∞	infinity
μsec	microsecond	⌣	combined with